T0342123

Chest Imaging Case Atlas
Second Edition

Mark S. Parker, MD
Professor, Diagnostic Radiology and Internal Medicine
Department of Radiology
VCU Medical Center
Richmond, Virginia

Melissa L. Rosado-de-Christenson, MD, FACR
Section Chief
Department of Thoracic Imaging
Saint Luke's Hospital of Kansas City
Professor of Radiology
University of Missouri–Kansas City
Kansas City, Missouri

Gerald F. Abbott, MD
Associate Professor of Radiology
Harvard University
Associate Radiologist
Massachusetts General Hospital
Boston, Massachusetts

Thieme
New York · Stuttgart

Thieme Medical Publishers, Inc.
333 Seventh Ave.
New York, NY 10001

Executive Editor: Timothy Hiscock
Managing Editor: J. Owen Zurhellen IV
Editorial Assistant: Michael Rowley
Production Editor: Kenneth L. Chumbley
International Production Director: Andreas Schabert
Senior Vice President, International Marketing and Sales: Cornelia Schulze
Vice President, Finance and Accounts: Sarah Vanderbilt
President: Brian D. Scanlan
Compositor: Prairie Papers Inc.
Printer: Sheridan Books, Inc.

Library of Congress Cataloging-in-Publication Data

Parker, Mark S.
 Chest imaging case atlas / Mark S. Parker, Melissa L. Rosado-de-Christenson, Gerald F. Abbott. — 2nd ed.
   p. ; cm.
 Rev. ed. of: Teaching atlas of chest imaging. c2006.
 Includes bibliographical references and index.
 ISBN 978-1-60406-590-9 (alk. paper)
 I. Rosado de Christenson, Melissa L. II. Abbott, Gerald F. III. Parker, Mark S. Teaching atlas of chest imaging.
 IV. Title.
 [DNLM: 1. Diagnostic Imaging—Atlases. 2. Diagnostic Imaging—Case Reports. 3. Thoracic Diseases—
diagnosis—Atlases. 4. Thoracic Diseases—diagnosis—Case Reports. 5. Radiography, Thoracic—Atlases.
6. Radiography, Thoracic—Case Reports. WF 17]
 617.5'407572—dc23

                                                                                    2011052038

Copyright © 2012 by Thieme Medical Publishers, Inc. This book, including all parts thereof, is legally protected by copyright. Any use, exploitation, or commercialization outside the narrow limits set by copyright legislation without the publisher's consent is illegal and liable to prosecution. This applies in particular to photostat reproduction, copying, mimeographing or duplication of any kind, translating, preparation of microfilms, and electronic data processing and storage.

Important note: Medical knowledge is ever-changing. As new research and clinical experience broaden our knowledge, changes in treatment and drug therapy may be required. The authors and editors of the material herein have consulted sources believed to be reliable in their efforts to provide information that is complete and in accord with the standards accepted at the time of publication. However, in view of the possibility of human error by the authors, editors, or publisher of the work herein or changes in medical knowledge, neither the authors, editors, nor publisher, nor any other party who has been involved in the preparation of this work, warrants that the information contained herein is in every respect accurate or complete, and they are not responsible for any errors or omissions or for the results obtained from use of such information. Readers are encouraged to confirm the information contained herein with other sources. For example, readers are advised to check the product information sheet included in the package of each drug they plan to administer to be certain that the information contained in this publication is accurate and that changes have not been made in the recommended dose or in the contraindications for administration. This recommendation is of particular importance in connection with new or infrequently used drugs.

Some of the product names, patents, and registered designs referred to in this book are in fact registered trademarks or proprietary names even though specific reference to this fact is not always made in the text. Therefore, the appearance of a name without designation as proprietary is not to be construed as a representation by the publisher that it is in the public domain.

Printed in the United States of America

5 4 3 2 1

ISBN 978-1-60406-590-9
eISBN 978-1-60406-591-6

To my heavenly Father, for the innumerable blessings He has afforded me in life. To my grandparents, for their love and encouragement from the beginning of my journey. To my parents, for the opportunities they provided and encouragement they offered. To my wife Cindy, for whom nothing in my personal or professional life would be possible without her unwavering love, support, and patience. To my son, Steven, and my daughter, Casey, for their love, support, and countless sacrificed hours of family time. To my colleagues and friends, Melissa and Gerry, for their friendship, dedication, and conscientious work on this project.

Mark S. Parker, MD

To my husband, Paul J. Christenson, MD, my daughters, Jennifer and Heather, for their love, support, and encouragement. And to the countless radiology residents it has been my privilege to teach over the course of my career and to my colleagues at the Saint Luke's Hospital of Kansas City, Missouri, whose curiosity, enthusiasm, and thirst for knowledge greatly enrich my academic life.

Melissa L. Rosado-de-Christenson, MD, FACR

To the many radiology residents I have had the pleasure and honor of teaching at Massachusetts General Hospital, Rhode Island Hospital, and the Armed Forces Institute of Pathology. Your spirit and enthusiasm make it all enjoyable.

Gerald F. Abbott, MD

CONTENTS

SECTION VIII
Diffuse Lung Disease **505**

SECTION XIII

FOREWORD

Cardiothoracic radiology is at the "heart" of radiology, with no single examination being performed more often in private or academic practice environments than the chest radiograph. A survey of X-ray use in the early 1960s by the National Center for Health Statistics reported that medical radiation accounted for half of human radiation exposure, and that of the 85 million visits for X-rays, 51 million (60%) were for chest X-rays (Health Statistics, US National Health Survey, Volume of X-ray Visits, U.S. Department of Health, Education and Welfare, October 1962). Today, estimates are that over 100 million chest X-rays are performed annually in the United States. While seemingly simple and straightforward, it can be argued that there is no exam more complex and nuanced in the entire field of radiology. I remember attending an American College of Radiology Intersociety Conference in 1998 on the topic of "Are today's residents ready for tomorrow's practice?," the summary of which concluded that residents not only needed to be prepared to read large numbers of "films" accurately and efficiently, but that they be able to recognize normal, with all of its variations, in order to minimize recommendations for more complex and expensive testing, only to discover there was nothing of clinical significance.

Today, more attention is paid to the judicious use of computed tomography (CT) as the largest source of medical radiation exposure, with significant advances in the last few years to minimize radiation exposure, while maintaining diagnostic accuracy. Rapid advances in CT technology have taken chest CT from a basic examination to one that is commonly tailored to the specific clinical question, and uses advanced three-dimensional viewing methods and quantitative tools to render diagnosis and report their clinical significance. Together, the chest x-ray and chest CT are the mainstays of cardiothoracic imaging, and their judicious and appropriate use is an important aspect of safe radiology practice.

Just as technology has advanced, so also have educational techniques. One such educational advance is the use of a case-based approach to convey practical, clinically relevant knowledge, using an initial case supplemented by image-rich companion cases. This is a technique that the talented authors of *Chest Imaging Case Atlas, Second Edition,* have made famous through their teachings at educational courses far and wide. Dr. Melissa Rosado-de-Christenson is an internationally renowned, passionate, articulate, organized, and tireless educator, sought the world over for her precise approach to delivering educational content. I remember when she proposed a case-based approach to teaching for the annual meeting of the American Roentgen Ray Society. Not surprisingly, Dr. Rosado-de-Christenson selected another outstanding and focused educator, Dr. Gerald Abbott, as her partner in developing the inaugural course in 2006, entitled "Approach to Diagnosis: A Case-Based Imaging Review." Together and in record time, with attention to detail, while assembling an outstanding cadre of both seasoned and talented younger educators, the Case-Based Review Course was born and is now an essential educational element to the annual meeting, accompanied by an enduring syllabus. Brought together by Dr. Mark S. Parker, himself a renowned and decorated educator who has received awards such as "The Teacher's Teacher Award for Extraordinary Educator in Thoracic Medicine," these three professors and veteran educators collaborated on the *Teaching Atlas of Chest Imaging*, the earlier edition of this book.

The authors' experience, honing their skills with the case-based teaching format, forms the foundation of *Chest Imaging Case Atlas, Second Edition*. The readers of this book, novice and experienced radiologist alike, as well as non-radiologists interested in a practical, clinically relevant approach and format, will enjoy learning through this image-rich format that replicates how we practice radiology every day: through the comparison to databanks of images either accumulated in memory over time or available in an instant through the Internet, contrasting different diagnoses in the clinical context of each patient, and synthesizing the information to provide a clinically relevant interpretation and radiology report.

Each section begins with brief fundamentals, followed by the relevant cases presented in a standardized format. Each case begins with clinical presentation, akin to the history provided on radiology requisitions with images, allowing the reader to make an assessment before the radiologic findings are described and the diagnosis is revealed. Differential diagnosis and discussion follow, including background, etiology, clinical findings, scope of imaging findings for the diagnosis presented, management, and prognosis. Pearls for each case represent the synthesized and salient take-home messages. The section on developmental anomalies and the new section on postprocedure findings should be committed to memory, as they aid readers in not mistaking normal variants and postoperative findings for significant disease. New to this edition are updates related to advances in medicine, such as revised classifications of malignancies such as lung cancer and thymoma, and illustrations of entities unknown to us at the time of the first publication, such as H1N1 infection. Also new are improved illustrations of both normal anatomy and disease processes using multiplanar (MPR) and three-dimensional CT-reformatted images. The coronal and sagittal MPRS are particularly useful as the CT equivalent of the posteroanterior and lateral chest radiographs, aiding the reader in understanding how the gray and white shadows are formed on this enduring, fundamental radiology examination.

I want to personally congratulate Drs. Parker, Rosado-de-Christenson, and Abbott for preparing and illustrating this wonderful case-based approach to cardiothoracic radiology. Sit back and enjoy as you learn!

Ella A. Kazerooni, MD, MS
Professor and Associate Chair for Clinical Affairs
Director, Cardiothoracic Radiology Division
University of Michigan Medical School/Health System
Ann Arbor, Michigan

PREFACE

Chest imaging remains one of the most challenging subspecialties of diagnostic radiology. It has become further complicated by the rapid evolution and clinical demand for advanced cardiothoracic imaging, and multiplanar, three-dimensional, and volume-rendered as well as CT-angiographic techniques. Advances in the use of diagnostic imaging for the evaluation of airways disease, infectious disease, diffuse lung disease, thoracic trauma, and critical care, and the recently released data on the positive impact lung cancer screening may have on the mortality of current and past heavy tobacco smokers, introduce additional complexity to the study and understanding of these disease processes. The successful delivery of thoracic imaging services is also restricted by the marked shortage of thoracic radiologists and residents pursuing advanced cardiothoracic imaging fellowships. Diagnostic radiology residents must be exposed to a large volume of thoracic imaging cases in order to hone their diagnostic interpretative skills; generate appropriate, differential diagnoses; and positively impact patient care by being a valuable clinical consultant and colleague rather than simply a film reader. As the shortage in thoracic radiologists continues, general radiologists and body imagers continue to find themselves in the uncomfortable position of covering the "chest service" and interpretating complex studies often without adequate resources. Our earlier book, *Teaching Atlas of Chest Imaging*, was conceived and developed with those needs in mind. This new book, *Chest Imaging Case Atlas*, Second Edition, has been further tailored based on insightful comments and observations from our readers, radiology residents, and radiologists across the country, and input from many clinical colleagues in pulmonary medicine, thoracic surgery, cardiothoracic surgery, and critical care, to address the ever growing demand placed on diagnosticians. We appreciate your guidance in the development of this new edition. We are also indebted to thirty-four academic colleagues for their contribution of figures to this book.

In accordance with requests from candidates preparing for their diagnostic radiology boards and their preference to view *Atlas* cases as "unknowns," the specific case diagnosis is no longer listed immediately after the case number, and we have limited but not eliminated the use of extensive annotations. We have also added more tables for quick and concise reference. In keeping with our rapidly changing diagnostic imaging technology, most of our CT images were acquired from 64-MDCT scanners, and we have incorporated more multiplanar, CT angiographic (CTA) and 3D imaging. The growing need for donor hearts with limited availability for patients awaiting transplantation has prompted novel approaches to the management of patients with univentricular and biventricular or end-stage heart failure, including various ventricular assist devices and the Total Artificial Heart. Thus, we expanded the "Adult Cardiovascular Disease Section" to include a discussion on these devices, their imaging features, and complications associated with their use. Requests from radiology residents, cardiothoracic imaging, and pulmonary medicine fellows prompted the inclusion of more CT in the "Pulmonary Infections Section." We also added a discussion on the Novel Swine-Origin Influenza A (H1N1) Virus and on parasitic diseases. We likewise expanded the "Diffuse Lung Disease Section" and also added an approach to HRCT interpretation as requested. The "Neoplastic Diseases Section" has been revised to include the most recent TNM staging system (seventh edition) for lung cancer, recently adopted by the International Association for the Study of Lung Cancer (IASLC), International Union against Cancer (UICC), and American Joint Committee on Cancer (AJCC). The "Neoplastic Diseases Section" also includes a discussion on the new classification system of mediastinal lymph nodes; the new, soon to be released, classification system for adenocarcinoma and bronchioloalveolar cell carcinoma, and the recent classification of thymoma by the World Health Organization. Post-operative chest examinations can be very difficult to interpret. The nature and complexity of thoracic interventional procedures is never ending, and the complications associated with these procedures can be devastating. As such, we have added a new section on the "Post-Thoracotomy Chest."

The overall format of our book has not changed. We continue to believe a strong foundation in normal anatomy is essential to the understanding of chest diseases and their various imaging manifestations. Thus, once again, the atlas begins with an overview of normal chest radiography, CT, and MRI. The remainder of the atlas is formulated as a case-based-review of numerous congenital, traumatic, and acquired thoracic conditions. Most sections begin with an overview of disease entities and processes that will be discussed in further detail in the section itself. Each case is supported by a brief discussion of the etiology, imaging features, management, and prognosis of the disease process illustrated in a concise, bulleted format. Case discussions are based on up-to-date reviews of the current literature, as well as classic landmark articles. Additional supplementary images illustrate other manifestations of a given entity or similar entities in the differential diagnosis. Major teaching points ("PEARLS") are provided for most cases to emphasize those features that may strongly support a specific diagnosis. Suggested readings are provided for the interested reader desiring additional in-depth information on the subject matter. It is our sincere hope that our book will prove to be an invaluable teaching tool for you whether you are still in residency, in fellowship training, or practicing in an academic university hospital or in private practice.

Mark S. Parker, MD
Richmond, Virginia

Melissa L. Rosado-de-Christenson, MD, FACR
Kansas City, Missouri

Gerald F. Abbott, MD
Boston, Massachusetts

Acknowledgments

The authors wish to thank Rob Walker of Walker Illustration, for his exceptional efforts in creating the graphic illustrations for this project, and Betty Arkwright, chief administrative assistant, for her immense assistance in the final preparation of the manuscript of this book.

WITH SUPPLEMENTAL FIGURES KINDLY PROVIDED BY

Michael Atalay, MD, PhD
Department of Diagnostic Imaging
Brown Medical School, Rhode Island Hospital
Providence, Rhode Island

Susan J. Back, MD
Department of Diagnostic Radiology
VCU Medical Center
Richmond, Virginia

Susan W. Bennett, MD
Department of Diagnostic Radiology, Thoracic Imaging
VCU Medical Center
Richmond, Virginia

Sonya Bhole, BS
VCU Medical Center
Richmond, Virginia

Phillip Boiselle, MD
Harvard Medical School and Beth Israel Deaconess
    Medical Center
Department of Diagnostic Radiology, Thoracic Imaging
Boston, Massachusetts

Anthony D. Cassano, MD
Department of Thoracic Surgery
VCU Medical Center
Richmond, Virginia

Alpha A. Fowler III, MD
Division of Pulmonary Medicine and Critical Care
    Medicine
VCU Medical Center
Richmond, Virginia

Judson Frye, MD
Department of Diagnostic Radiology
VCU Medical Center
Richmond, Virginia

John D. Grizzard, MD
Department of Diagnostic Radiology, Non-Invasive
    Cardiovascular Imaging
VCU Medical Center
Richmond, Virginia

Jud W. Gurney MD [deceased]
Department of Diagnostic Radiology
University of Nebraska Hospital
Omaha, Nebraska

Daniel A. Henry, MD
Department of Diagnostic Radiology, Thoracic Imaging
VCU Medical Center
Richmond, Virginia

Laura E. Heyneman, MD
Department of Radiology
University of North Carolina
Wilmington, North Carolina

Jennifer Hubert, MD
Department of Diagnostic Radiology, Thoracic Imaging
VCU Medical Center
Richmond, Virginia

Janae Johnson, MD
Department of Diagnostic Radiology
VCU Medical Center
Richmond, Virginia

Nicole M. Kelleher-Linkonis, MD
Department of Diagnostic Radiology
VCU Medical Center
Richmond, Virginia

Wanda M. Kirejczyk, MD
Department of Diagnostic Radiology
New Britain General Hospital
New Britain, Connecticut

Maysiang Lesar, MD
National Naval Medical Center
Bethesda, Maryland

Gael J. Lonergan, MD
Austin Radiological Association
Austin, Texas

Santiago Martínez-Jiménez, MD
Duke University Medical Center
Durham, North Carolina

H. Page McAdams, MD
Duke University Medical Center
Durham, North Carolina

James Messmer, MD
Department of Diagnostic Radiology
VCU Medical Center
Richmond, Virginia

Kristin Miller, MD
Department of Pulmonary and Critical Care
    Medicine
VCU Medical Center
Richmond, Virginia

Lakshmana Das Narla, MD
Department of Diagnostic Radiology; Pediatric
    Imaging
VCU Medical Center
Richmond, Virginia

Janet Pinson, NP
Division of Pulmonary Medicine and Critical Care
    Medicine
VCU Medical Center
Richmond, Virginia

Santiago Rossi, MD
Buenos Aires, Argentina

Jeffery D. Settles II, MD
Department of Diagnostic Radiology
VCU Medical Center
Richmond, Virginia

Rosita M. Shah, MD
University of Pennsylvania Abramson Cancer Center
Philadelphia, Pennsylvania

Stephanie E. Spottswood, MD, MSPH
Department of Pediatric Radiology
Vanderbilt Children's Hospital
Nashville, Tennessee

Diane C. Strollo, MD
University of Pittsburgh Medical Center
Department of Diagnostic Radiology; Thoracic
    Imaging
Pittsburgh, Pennsylvania

Malcolm K. Sydnor Jr., MD
Department of Diagnostic Radiology; Interventional
    Radiology
VCU Medical Center
Richmond, Virginia

Jaime Tisnado, MD
Department of Diagnostic Radiology; Interventional
    Radiology
VCU Medical Center
Richmond, Virginia

Roger Tutton, MD
Department of Diagnostic Radiology; Thoracic Imaging
VCU Medical Center
Richmond, Virginia

Helen T. Winer-Muram, MD
Indiana University Medical Center
Indianapolis, Indiana

Jill D. Wruble, DO
Danbury Radiology Associates
Danbury, Connecticut

Section I

Normal Thoracic Anatomy

OVERVIEW

■ Airways

Trachea and Main Bronchi (Fig. I.1)

The trachea is a midline structure 6 to 9 cm in length. On posteroanterior (PA) chest radiography, the tracheal walls are parallel except on the *left side* just above the bifurcation, where the thoracic aorta smoothly indents the airway (**Fig. I.1A**). Slight deviation of the trachea to the right at the aortic arch is normal and should not be misinterpreted as pathology. This deviation becomes more exaggerated with advancing age. On lateral radiography, the airways line up in a vertically oriented plane (**Fig. I.1B**). This relationship may become altered with volume loss or mediastinal pathology. The *anterior* and *lateral* tracheal walls are composed of regularly spaced, horseshoe-shaped cartilaginous rings, whereas the *posterior* wall is membranous. These regularly spaced cartilaginous rings give the trachea and main bronchi a smoothly serrated contour on radiography. Tracheal diameter varies with both age and sex and is usually larger in men. Coronal and sagittal diameters of the trachea as measured 2.0 cm above the aortic arch on chest radiography and chest CT are provided in **Table I.1**.

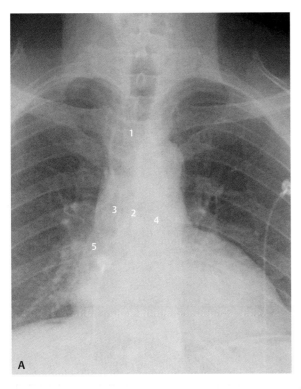
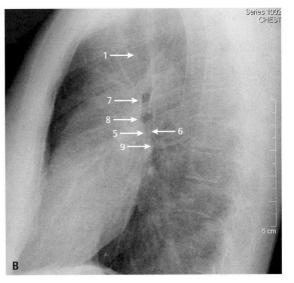

Fig. I.1 **(A)** Trachea and main bronchi, coned-down PA and **(B)** lateral chest radiographs. **(A)** Note the normal smooth indentation on the left side of the trachea by the transverse aorta on the frontal exam. **(B)** Observe the relationship between the right and left upper lobe bronchi on the lateral exam. *1*, trachea; *2*, carina; *3*, right main bronchus; *4*, left main bronchus; *5*, bronchus intermedius; *6*, posterior wall bronchus intermedius; *7*, right upper lobe bronchus; *8*, left upper lobe bronchus; *9*, lower lobe bronchi.

Table I.1 Normal Tracheal Air Column Dimensions on Chest Imaging

Individual Sex	Coronal Diameter (mm)	Sagittal Diameter (mm)
Men	13–25	13–27
Women	10–21	10–23

3

The trachea divides into right and left main bronchi at the carina (**Fig. I.1A**). Before 15 years of age, the right and left main bronchi follow a relatively vertical course. This explains the relatively equal incidence of right- and left-sided foreign body aspirations in younger children. In adolescence and adulthood, the right main bronchus assumes a more vertical course than the left, which is more horizontal, predisposing these individuals to an increased incidence of right-sided aspiration. The *subcarinal angle* (angle of divergence of right and left main bronchi measured along their inferior borders) is in the range of 41–71° in *men* and 41–74° in *women* (**Fig. I.2**). The right main bronchus is shorter but wider than the left. The *right main bronchus* averages 2.2 cm in length and 15.3 mm in diameter. The *left main bronchus* averages 5 cm in length and 13.0 mm in diameter.

Lobar and Segmental Bronchi (Fig. I.3)

There is considerable anatomic variation in the pattern of bronchial branching, especially with respect to the subsegmental airways. Variations also involve the lobar and segmental airways to a lesser degree. In most cases, such variations are of little clinical significance. Despite these anatomic variations, the anatomic location of the bronchopulmonary segments is relatively consistent.

Right Upper Lobe (Fig. I.3)

The right upper lobe bronchus arises from the lateral wall of the right main bronchus 2.0 cm below the carina. Approximately 1.0 cm from its origin, it divides into three segmental branches, the *anterior, posterior,* and *apical* divisions. Rarely, the upper lobe bronchus or one of its segmental divisions (e.g., apical) arises directly off the lateral wall of the trachea, forming an anatomic variant, the "tracheal bronchus" (**Fig. I.4**) (also see Section II).

Right Middle Lobe (Fig. I.3)

The *bronchus intermedius* extends 3–4 cm distally from the right upper lobe bronchus takeoff and then bifurcates to supply both the middle and right lower lobes. The middle lobe bronchus arises from the anterolateral wall of the bronchus intermedius, directly opposite the superior segmental bronchus origin to the lower lobe. The middle lobe bronchus extends 1–2 cm before bifurcating into *lateral* and *medial* segmental divisions.

Right Lower Lobe (Fig. I.3)

The right lower lobe has five segmental branches. The *superior segment* is the first branch, and arises from the posterior wall of the lower lobe bronchus just beyond its origin. The four basal branches sequentially arise, lateral to medial, from the lower lobe bronchus in the following order: *anterior, lateral, posterior,* and *medial.*

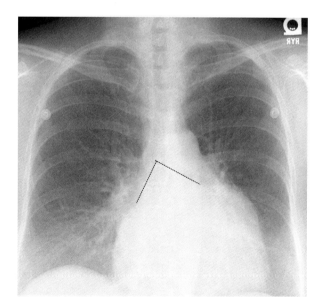

Fig. I.2 Subcarinal angle. Coned-down PA chest radiograph demonstrates an accentuated subcarinal angle (*line annotations*) in this 53 year old woman with underlying mitral stenosis and left atrial enlargement.

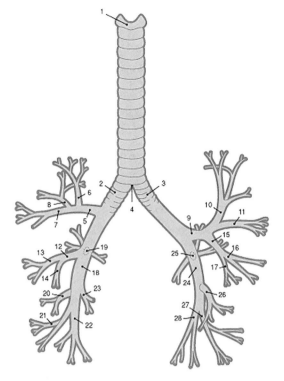

Fig. I.3 Lobar and segmental bronchial anatomy (*artist's illustration*). *1*, trachea; *2*, right main bronchus; *3*, left main bronchus; *4*, carina; *5*, right upper lobe bronchus; *6*, apical segmental bronchus, right upper lobe; *7*, anterior segmental bronchus, right upper lobe; *8*, posterior segmental bronchus, right upper lobe; *9*, left upper lobe bronchus; *10*, apical-posterior segmental bronchus, left upper lobe; *11*, anterior segmental bronchus, left upper lobe; *12*, right middle lobe bronchus; *13*, lateral segmental bronchus, right middle lobe; *14*, medial segmental bronchus, right middle lobe; *15*, lingular bronchus; *16,* superior lingular segmental bronchus; *17*, inferior lingular segmental bronchus; *18*, right lower lobe bronchus; *19*, superior segmental bronchus, right lower lobe; *20*, anterior basal segmental bronchus, right lower lobe; *21*, lateral basal segmental bronchus, right lower lobe; *22*, posterior basal segmental bronchus, right lower lobe; *23*, medial basal segmental bronchus, right lower lobe; *24*, left lower lobe bronchus; *25*, superior segmental bronchus, left lower lobe; *26*, anteromedial basal segmental bronchus, left lower lobe; *27*, lateral basal segmental bronchus, left lower lobe; *28*, posterior basal segmental bronchus, left lower lobe.

Left Upper Lobe (Fig. I.3)

The left upper lobe bronchus arises from the anterolateral wall of the left main bronchus and then either bifurcates or, less frequently, trifurcates into branches to supply the upper lobe and lingula. In the *bifurcation pattern*, the *upper division* immediately divides into *anterior* and *apical posterior* segments. The *lower division* is the *lingular bronchus* (right middle lobe bronchus analogue). The *lingular bronchus* extends anteroinferiorly 2–3 cm before bifurcating into *superior* and *inferior* segmental branches. When the *trifurcation pattern* exists, the *apical posterior*, *anterior*, and *lingular* bronchi originate simultaneously off the upper lobe bronchus to supply their respective segments.

Left Lower Lobe (Fig. I.3)

The left lower lobe has four segmental divisions. These divisions are similar in name and anatomic distribution to those of the right lower lobe. The major difference is the absence of a separate *medial basal bronchus.* In the left lower lobe, the anterior and medial portions of the lower lobe are supplied by a single, combined *anteromedial basal segmental* bronchus. The *superior segment* and the remaining two basal segments, the *lateral basal* and *posterior basal*, arise sequentially in a manner similar to the basal divisions of the right lower lobe.

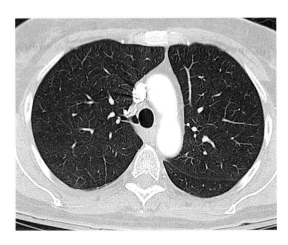

Fig. I.4 Tracheal bronchus. Axial chest CT (lung windows) of an asymptomatic 71-year-old woman demonstrates an incidental tracheal bronchus emanating off the lateral wall of the trachea.

Bronchial Anatomy on CT (Figs. I.5, I.6, I.7)

Visualization of bronchi on CT is affected by slice collimation, and by the size and orientation of the bronchus relative to the CT plane of section. The thinner the slice collimation, the more bronchi visualized. Bronchi coursing *horizontal* to the CT plane are seen in their *long axes* (**Fig. I.5**). These include the right and left upper lobe bronchi, the anterior segmental bronchi of both upper lobes, the middle lobe bronchus, and both lower lobe superior segmental bronchi (**Fig. I.5**). Bronchi coursing *vertically* are cut in cross-section and appear as variable-size circular lucencies. These include the right upper lobe apical segmental bronchus, the left upper lobe apical posterior segmental bronchus, the bronchus intermedius, both lower lobe bronchi, and the basal segmental bronchi of the lower lobes (**Fig. I.6**). Those bronchi coursing *obliquely* appear as stretched oval lucencies and are less well visualized. These include the lingular bronchus, along with its superior and inferior segmental branches, and the medial and lateral right middle lobe segmental branches (**Fig. I.7**). High-resolution CT (HRCT) more clearly depicts the segmental and subsegmental bronchial anatomy.

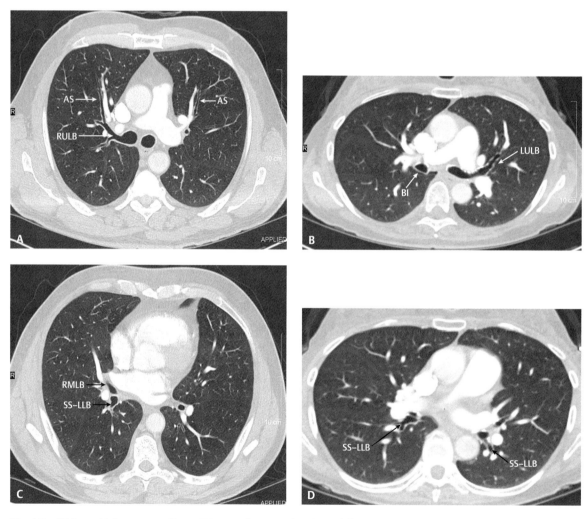

Fig. I.5 CT bronchial anatomy. Chest CT scans (lung windows) on different patients illustrate bronchi and segmental branches at various anatomic levels. **(A)** Immediately below the carinal bifurcation, the horizontal orientation of the anterior segmental bronchi of both upper lobes (*AS*) and that of the right upper lobe bronchus (*RULB*) are seen. **(B)** The horizontal lie of the left upper lobe bronchus (*LULB*) is demonstrated more inferiorly at the bronchus intermedius (*BI*). **(C)** More caudad, the origins of both the right middle lobe bronchus (*RMLB*) and the superior segment of the right lower lobe (*SS-LLB*) are identified. **(D)** Still more caudad, the horizontal orientation of the superior segmental bronchi of both lower lobes (*SS-LLB*) is seen.

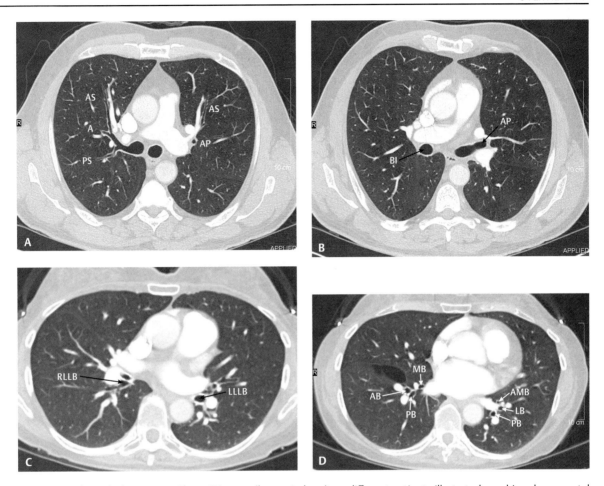

Fig. I.6 CT bronchial anatomy. Chest CT scans (lung windows) on different patients illustrate bronchi and segmental branches at various anatomic levels. **(A)** Immediately below the carinal bifurcation, the apical posterior segmental bronchus of the left upper lobe (*AP*) is seen as a spherical lucency. The horizontal orientation of the anterior segmental bronchi of both upper lobes (*AS*) and the posterior segment of the right upper lobe (*PS*) is also seen. **(B)** More caudad, one can identify the apical posterior segmental bronchus (*AP*) joining the left upper lobe bronchus. The bronchus intermedius (*BI*) is seen as a spherical lucency. **(C)** More inferiorly, the origins of both the right (*RLLB*) and left (*LLLB*) lower lobe bronchi are seen on end. **(D)** Still more inferiorly, several of the basilar segmental bronchi of both lower lobes can be identified. (*MB*, medial basal; *AB*, anterobasal; *PB*, posterobasal; *AMB*, anteromedial basal; *LB*, lateral basal.)

Lung Parenchyma Subdivisions

Primary Lobule

This lung unit consists of all alveolar ducts, alveolar sacs, and alveoli, along with their respective nerves, blood vessels, and connective tissue distal to the last respiratory bronchiole. There are approximately 20–25 million primary lobules in the lung. However, they are all below the limits of conventional radiographic and radiologic resolution.

Secondary Lobule (Fig. I.8)

The secondary pulmonary lobule (SPL) represents the *fundamental unit* of lung structure from a radiologic perspective. It is the *smallest* discrete anatomic lung unit surrounded by connective tissue that can be identified on HRCT. An analysis of abnormalities within the secondary lobule is useful in the diagnosis of many diseases (see Section VIII). The SPL is polyhedral in shape, averages 1.0–2.5 cm in size, and is supplied by three to five terminal bronchioles. The central or *core structures* include the centrilobular bronchus and its

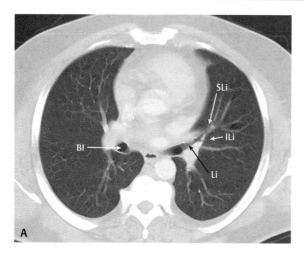

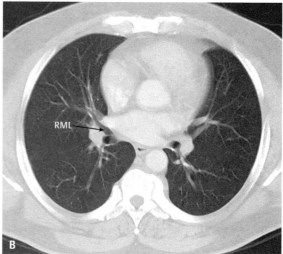

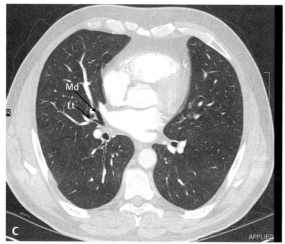

Fig. I.7 CT bronchial anatomy. Chest CT scans (lung windows) on different patients illustrate bronchi and segmental branches at various anatomic levels. **(A)** At the bronchus intermedius (*BI*) level one can see the lingular bronchus (*Li*), along with its superior (*SLi*) and inferior (*ILi*) segmental branches. **(B)** The horizontal orientation of the right middle lobe (*RML*) bronchus is clearly seen. **(C)** More inferiorly, the medial (*Md*) and lateral (*Lt*) segmental branches of the right middle lobe are identified.

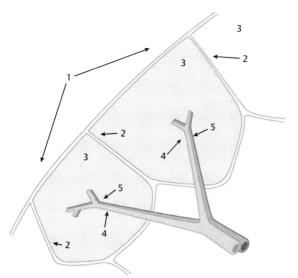

Fig. I.8 Secondary pulmonary lobule (*artist's illustration*). *1*, visceral pleura; *2*, interlobular septa; *3*, individual secondary pulmonary lobules; *4*, centrilobular bronchus; *5*, centrilobular artery.

accompanying centrilobular artery, and lymphatics. The *peripheral structures* include the interlobular septa, which are continuous with the visceral pleura, pulmonary veins, and lymphatics. The interlobular septa are most numerous in the apical, anterior, and lateral regions of the upper lobes, and in the lateral and anterior regions of the right middle lobe, lingula, and the lower lobes.

Although the normal SPL is inconspicuous on conventional imaging, it is readily identified on HRCT (**Fig. I.9**). Interlobular septa are most commonly identified in the lateral aspect of the lung as straight lines 1.0–2.5 cm in length (**Fig. I.9**).

The SPL may also be seen on HRCT when it becomes opacified by an inflammatory exudate or blood (**Fig. I.10**). Disease processes affecting the core and peripheral structures of the SPL are discussed in further detail in Section VIII.

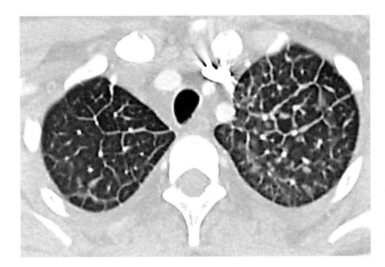

Fig. I.9 Interlobular septal thickening. HRCT (1 mm collimation) scan through the upper lung zones in a patient with hydrostatic edema shows interlobular septal thickening. Individual pulmonary lobules are variable in size and have an irregular polyhedral shape.

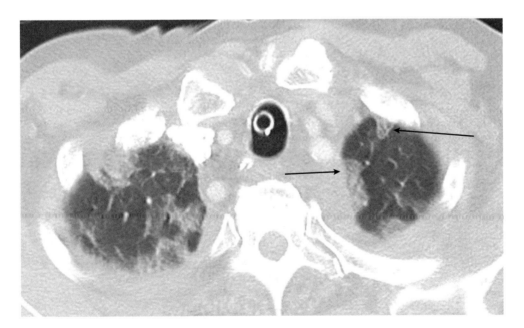

Fig. I.10 Opacified secondary pulmonary lobules. HRCT (1 mm collimation) through the upper lung zones in an elderly intubated man diagnosed with acute interstitial pneumonia (AIP) demonstrates multi-focal ground glass opacities, the distribution and morphology of which correspond to individual secondary pulmonary lobules (*arrows*).

Acinus (Fig. I.11)

The acinus represents that portion of the lung located *distal* to the terminal bronchiole (i.e., last conducting airway) and is comprised of the respiratory bronchioles, alveolar ducts, alveolar sacs, alveoli, and their accompanying blood vessels and connective tissue. A given acinus ranges between 6 and 10 mm in diameter and contains 7,100 to 20,000 alveoli. Normal acini are not conspicuous on conventional chest radiography or even on HRCT.

■ Hilar Anatomy

The hilum (root) represents the junction of the lung and the mediastinum. The normal hilum contains bronchi, pulmonary and systemic arteries, pulmonary and systemic veins, lymphatics, lymph nodes, and autonomic nerves. The hila are divided into upper and lower zones. The *upper zone* of the right hilum contains the superior pulmonary vein, the truncus anterior, a short portion of the right upper lobe bronchus, and the anterior segmental artery and bronchus (visualized *en face*). The *upper zone* of the left hilum contains the distal left pulmonary artery and the superior pulmonary vein. The *lower zone* of the right hilum contains the right interlobar (descending) pulmonary artery, which lies medial to the bronchus intermedius. The inferior pulmonary vein is horizontally oriented and lies posterior and inferior to the hilum. The *lower zone* of the left hilum contains the distal interlobar (descending) pulmonary artery, the inferior pulmonary vein, and lingular and lower lobe bronchi.

Normal Hilar Relationships

Frontal Radiography (Fig. I.12)

On frontal chest radiography, the right and left pulmonary arteries form most of the normal hilar opacity. The superior pulmonary veins, lobar bronchi, bronchopulmonary lymph nodes, and associated fat contribute little to the overall opacity. In 97% of individuals, the proximal left pulmonary artery is higher than the right interlobar pulmonary artery. This is because the left pulmonary artery, which creates most of the left hilar opacity, ascends *over* the left main and upper lobe bronchus (*hyparterial*), whereas the right pulmonary artery lies *inferior* to the right upper lobe bronchus (*eparterial*). In 3% of individuals, the proximal left pulmonary artery and the right interlobar pulmonary artery lie at approximately the same horizontal level on frontal chest radiographs. The right pulmonary artery never normally lies higher than the left. Such a relationship suggests either right upper or left lower lobe volume loss (see Section IV).

The normal *right hilar* opacity on frontal chest radiography has a sideways V-shaped morphology (**Figs. I.12.A, I.12.B**). The upper portion of this "V" is created by the truncus anterior and posterior division of the right superior pulmonary vein. The superior pulmonary vein forms the lateral margin of the upper right hilum. The apical segmental bronchus of the upper lobe may be seen interposed between these two vessels

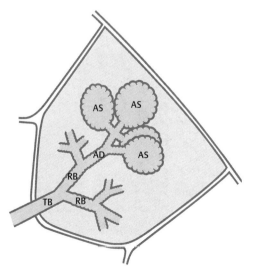

Fig. I.11 Pulmonary acinus (*artist's illustration*). *TB*, terminal bronchiole; *RB*, respiratory bronchiole; *AD*, alveolar duct; *AS*, alveolar sac.

(**Figs. I.12A, I.12B**). The right descending pulmonary artery forms the lower portion of the V-shaped hilar opacity as it descends lateral to the bronchus intermedius (**Figs. I.12A, I.12B**). Although the right inferior pulmonary vein crosses the lower portion of the right hilum, it does not contribute to its overall opacity.

The normal *left hilar* opacity on frontal chest radiography is created by the distal left pulmonary artery centrally and one or more of its upper lobe arterial divisions and the posterior division of the superior pulmonary vein more peripherally (**Figs. I.12A, I.12B**). The lateral margin of the upper hilar shadow is formed by either the superior pulmonary vein or the apical posterior segmental artery (**Figs. I.12A, I.12B**). The upper lobe bronchus can be identified centrally where it is encircled by the left pulmonary artery. The anterior segmental bronchus and its accompanying artery may be seen *en face* at the lateral margin of the upper left hilar opacity (**Fig. I.12C**). The descending pulmonary artery forms the lower portion of the left hilar opacity as it descends behind the cardiac silhouette (**Figs. I.12A, I.12B**). The adjacent left lower lobe bronchus lies anterior and medial to this artery and therefore may not always be conspicuous.

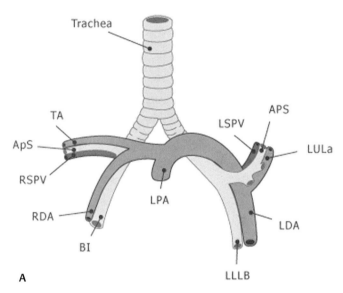

Fig. I.12 Normal hilar anatomy—frontal chest radiography. **(A)** Artist's illustration of the anatomic structures typically visualized: *ApS*, apical segmental bronchus; *APS*, posterior segmental bronchus; *BI*, bronchus intermedius; *LDA*, left descending pulmonary artery; *LLLB*, left lower lobe bronchus; *LPA*, left pulmonary artery; *LULa*, left upper lobe pulmonary artery; *LSPV*, left superior pulmonary vein; *RDA*, right descending pulmonary artery; *RSPV*, right superior pulmonary vein; *TA*, truncus anterior. **(B)** Coned-down frontal chest radiograph over the hila. Correlate the anatomy with that depicted in the artist's illustration **(A)**. **(C)** Coned-down frontal chest radiograph over the left hilum demonstrates the left upper lobe anterior segmental artery (*ASa*) and bronchus (*ASb*) in the lateral margin of the left hilar opacity. Correlate the anatomy with that depicted in the artist's illustration **(A)**.

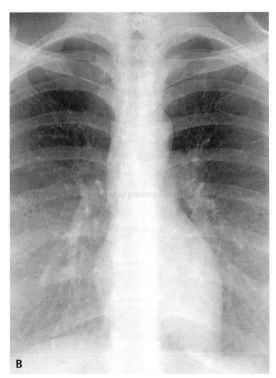

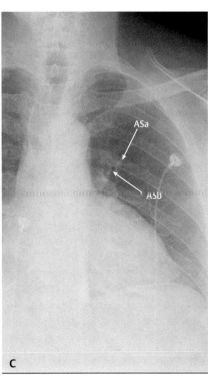

Normal Hilar Relationships

Lateral Radiography (Fig. I.13)

On lateral chest radiographs, the normal right and left hilar opacities are created by the superimposed opacities of the right and left pulmonary arteries and the accompanying superior pulmonary veins (**Fig. I.13A**). The anterior aspect of the *right hilar opacity* is formed by the transverse portion of the right pulmonary artery, and appears as an *oval-shaped opacity* anterior to the bronchus intermedius. The confluence of the right superior pulmonary veins overlapping the lower portion of the right pulmonary artery also contributes to this opacity (**Figs. I.13A, I.13B**). The *left hilar opacity* projects more superiorly and posteriorly, appearing as a *comma-shaped opacity* above and behind the oval lucency representing the left upper lobe bronchus. The left pulmonary artery then descends behind the left lower lobe bronchus. The confluence of the left superior pulmonary veins overlapping the left pulmonary artery posteriorly and inferiorly also contributes to this opacity (**Figs. I.13A, I.13B**). A lucent triangle *inferior* to the right pulmonary artery and veins and *anterior* to the descending left pulmonary artery and left superior pulmonary vein represents the *inferior hilar window*. The *apex* of the inferior hilar window is located at the confluence of the left upper lobe and left lower lobe bronchi. The *base* is located more anteriorly and inferiorly (**Figs. I.13A, I.13B**). Obscuration of the lucent inferior hilar window is an important radiographic clue to underlying subcarinal pathology.

The tracheal air column ends in two rounded lucencies. The uppermost lucency is the *right upper lobe bronchus*, and the lowermost lucency the *left upper bronchus*, both projected *en face* (**Figs. I.13A, I.13B**). The orifice of the *right upper lobe bronchus* is visualized on 50% of well-centered lateral radiographs, whereas that of the *left upper lobe bronchus* is seen more than 75% of the time. The *left upper lobe bronchus* appears better circumscribed and is seen more frequently because of its relationship to the surrounding vasculature. As a caveat, if the *right upper lobe bronchus* is circumferentially sharply marginated or becomes more conspicuous than on previous lateral exams, the radiologist should be suspicious of a possible central hilar tumor or evolving right hilar lymphadenopathy. The normal upper lobe bronchial orifices range between 7 and 12 mm in diameter. Aerated lung in the azygoesophageal recess outlines the posterior wall of the bronchus interme-

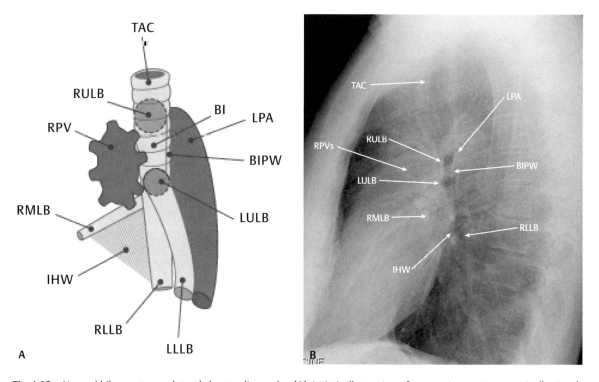

Fig. I.13   Normal hilar anatomy—lateral chest radiography. **(A)** Artist's illustration of anatomic structures typically visualized. *BI*, bronchus intermedius; *BIPW*, bronchus intermedius posterior wall; *IHW*, inferior hilar window; *LPA*, left pulmonary artery; *LULB*, left upper lobe bronchus; *RMLB*, middle lobe bronchus; *RLLB*, right lower lobe bronchus; *RPV*, summation right pulmonary vessels; *RULB*, right upper lobe bronchus; *TAC*, tracheal air column. **(B)** Coned down lateral chest radiograph over the hila. Correlate the anatomy with that depicted in the artist's illustration in **(A)**.

dius, which is seen in up to 95% of lateral chest exams and should not exceed 3 mm in diameter (**Figs. I.13A, I.13B**). Increased thickness of the posterior wall may be seen with various inflammatory and neoplastic diseases. The right lower lobe bronchus is seen on only 8% of lateral exams. Its posterior wall should have the same orientation as the posterior wall of the bronchus intermedius.

Hilum Overlay

The *hilum overlay sign* can be used to differentiate an anterior mediastinal mass from an enlarged heart or pericardial sac. The proximal segment of the left or right pulmonary artery lies lateral to the cardiac silhouette (or just within its edge) on normal frontal chest radiography (**Figs. I.1A, I.2, I.12B**). As the myocardium enlarges (e.g., cardiomyopathy, cardiomegaly) or as the pericardial sac distends with fluid (e.g., pericardial effusion), the pulmonary artery segments are displaced outward but maintain this same relationship to the cardiac silhouette. Alternatively, if either the left or right pulmonary artery is seen 1.0 cm or more within the lateral edge of an opacity that appears to represent the cardiac silhouette, that opacity represents an anterior mediastinal mass (**Fig. I.14**).

Hilum Convergence

The *hilum convergence sign* is useful in distinguishing an enlarged pulmonary artery from a true hilar mass. Because the pulmonary artery branches arise from the pulmonary artery, an enlarged pulmonary artery will have branches that arise from its outer margin and its vessels will converge toward the pulmonary artery. Alternatively, a true hilar mass may simulate an enlarged pulmonary artery; however, the vessels will not arise from its outer margin but rather seem to pass through the margin converging on the true pulmonary artery.

CT Imaging

The hila are optimally imaged with thin collimated and contrast-enhanced CT. Although intravenous contrast is not necessary in all cases, it simplifies interpretation, improves diagnostic accuracy and confidence, and provides insight into the potential nature of various structures. Magnetic resonance imaging (MRI) is com-

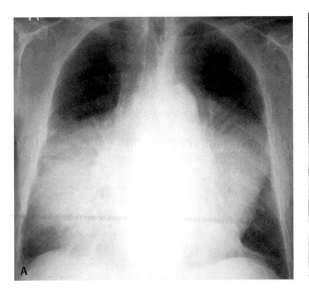 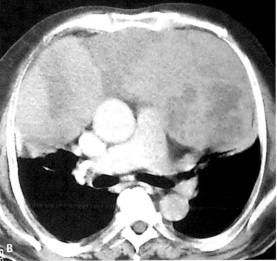

Fig. I.14 **(A)** PA chest radiograph demonstrates a massively enlarged cardiomediastinal silhouette. Lateral chest radiography (not illustrated) demonstrated complete obliteration of the retrosternal clear space. The right and left pulmonary arteries and their respective interlobar divisions are seen well within what appears to be the peripheral margin of the cardiomediastinal silhouette. **(B)** Contrast-enhanced CT (mediastinal windows) through the main pulmonary artery level shows a large, aggressive anterior mediastinal mass intimately related to the ascending aorta and main pulmonary artery. Diagnosis: Malignant peripheral nerve sheath tumor of the vagus nerve with mediastinal invasion. (Reprinted with permission from ARJII.)

parable to CT and may be used in patients in whom iodinated contrast media are contraindicated or ionizing radiation is a concern (e.g., children, pregnant women, serial exams).

■ Pulmonary Vessels

Pulmonary Arteries (Fig. I.15)

The *main pulmonary artery* or *trunk* (MPA) originates within the mediastinum at the pulmonary valve. It measures 5 cm in length and initially courses superiorly and to the left. Before exiting the pericardium, the MPA bifurcates into long (right) and short (left) pulmonary arteries.

The *right pulmonary artery* courses behind the ascending aorta. Behind the superior vena cava, and in front of the right main bronchus (*eparterial*), it divides into *ascending* (truncus anterior) and *descending* (interlobar) rami. Although anatomic variations exist, most commonly the *ascending artery* subdivides into three segments (e.g., apical, anterior, posterior) supplying the three bronchopulmonary segments of

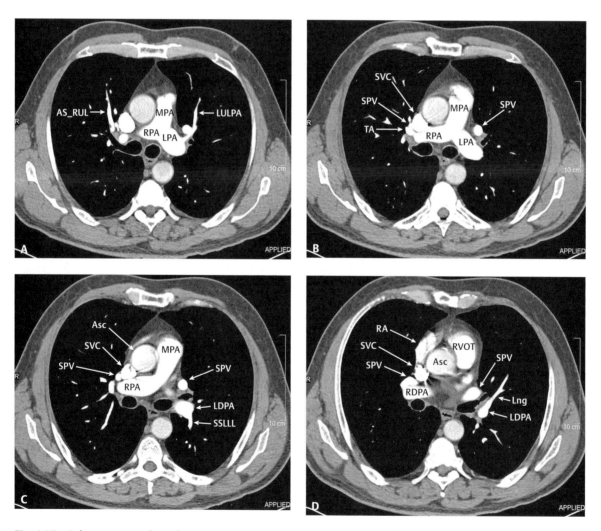

Fig. I.15 Pulmonary vessels—pulmonary artery anatomy. Contrast-enhanced chest CT (mediastinal windows) illustrating the main pulmonary artery, its lobar and segmental branches, and their relationship to various mediastinal structures. *AB*, right lower lobe anterobasal segmental artery; *AMB*, left lower lobe anteromedial basal segmental artery; *AR*, aortic root; *Asc*, ascending aorta; *AS–RUL*, right upper lobe anterior segmental artery; *IPV*, inferior pulmonary vein; *LA*, left atrium; *LB*, right lower lobe lateral basal segmental artery; *LDPA*, left descending pulmonary artery; *LRML*, right middle lobe lateral segmental artery; *Lng*, lingular artery; *LPA*, left main pulmonary artery; *LULPA*, left upper lobe

the right upper lobe. The *descending artery* supplies the segmental arteries to the right middle and lower lobes. In 90% of individuals, a portion of the posterior segment of the right upper lobe is also supplied by a separate branch arising from the *descending artery*. The first portion of the right *descending artery* is horizontal and interposed between the superior vena cava and bronchus intermedius. It then abruptly courses downward and backward, assuming a vertical orientation in the oblique fissure, where it gives off one or two segmental divisions to the middle lobe (e.g., medial and lateral) and usually five single branches, one to each of the five lower lobe bronchopulmonary segments (e.g., superior, medial basal, anterobasal, lateral basal, and posterior basal).

The *left pulmonary artery* courses over the left main bronchus (*hyparterial*). It sometimes gives off a short *ascending branch* that divides into segmental branches supplying the left upper lobe (e.g., anterior, apicoposterior). More often, however, the left pulmonary artery continues directly into the vertically oriented *descending* (interlobar) *artery*, from which segmental arteries to both the upper and lower lobes arise. Posterolateral to the lower lobe bronchus, the *descending artery* supplies branches to the lingula (e.g., superior, inferior) and the lower lobe bronchopulmonary segments (e.g., superior, anteromedial, lateral basal, posterobasal).

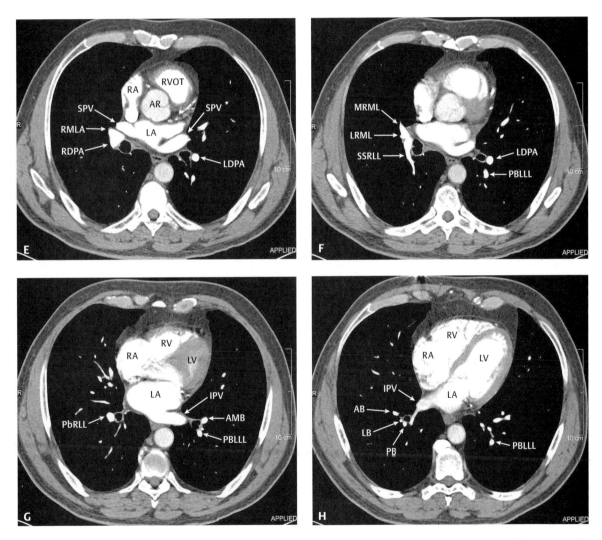

Fig. I.15 *(Continued)*   pulmonary artery; *LV*, left ventricle; *MPA*, main pulmonary artery; *MRML*, right middle lobe medial segmental artery; *PB*, right lower lobe posterior basal segmental artery; *PBLLL*, left lower lobe posterobasal segmental artery; *PbRLL*, proximal basilar arterial divisions right lower lobe; *RA*, right atrium; *RMLA*, right middle lobe artery; *RDPA*, right descending pulmonary artery; *RPA*, right main pulmonary artery; *RV*, right ventricle; *RVOT*, right ventricular outflow tract; *SPV*, superior pulmonary vein; *SSLLL*, left lower lobe superior segmental artery; *SSRLL*, right lower lobe superior segmental artery; *SVC*, superior vena cava; *TA*, truncus anterior.

The recognition of dimensional changes in the MPA and its descending lobar divisions, as well as alterations in the normal pulmonary artery to bronchus ratio, is useful in diagnosing pulmonary artery hypertension or pulmonary edema, respectively, and is discussed later (see Section X). The normal transverse diameter of the *right descending pulmonary artery* measured from its lateral aspect tangential to the bronchus intermedius on frontal chest radiography is 16 mm in males and 15 mm in females (**Fig. I.16**).

The normal diameters of the pulmonary arteries have also been determined on CT. The *MPA* should be measured perpendicular to its long axis at the bifurcation into the right and left main lobar arteries (**Fig. I.17A**). The normal maximal diameter (mean ± 2 SD) is 28.6 mm. The *descending pulmonary artery* should be measured at the right middle lobe bronchus origin (**Fig. I.17B**) and should not exceed 16.8 mm. There is no statistical difference in measurements between men and women.

The *pulmonary artery-to-bronchus ratio* can be calculated on frontal chest radiography (**Fig. I.18**). In otherwise healthy *erect* individuals, the ratio is 0.85 ± 0.15 (mean ± SD) (i.e., slightly less than 1:1) *above* the right hilar angle and 1.34 ± 0.25 (i.e., slightly greater than 1:1) *below* the right hilar angle. When the individual is *supine*, the ratios change to 1.01 ± 0.13 *above* and 1.05 ± 0.13 *below* the right hilar angle, or roughly 1:1 in both anatomic locations. Changes in these ratios are helpful when assessing patients for vascular engorgement from volume overloading (e.g., aggressive volume resuscitation) or cardiac decompensation (see Section X).

Bronchial Arteries (Fig. I.19)

The bronchial arteries are the primary nutrient vessels of the lung. Not only do the bronchial arteries supply blood to the terminal bronchioles, but they also partially supply the trachea, thymus, middle one-third of the esophagus, mediastinal lymph nodes, visceral pleura, pericardium, and the vagus nerve. Their site of origin is somewhat variable. These arteries arise from the proximal descending thoracic aorta usually between the T3 and T8 vertebral body levels. Most often, one *right-sided* and two *left-sided* bronchial arteries are present. The

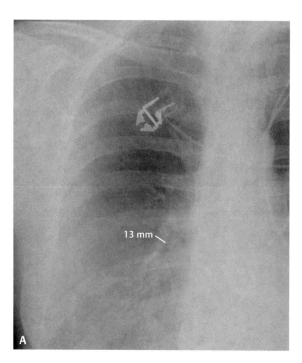
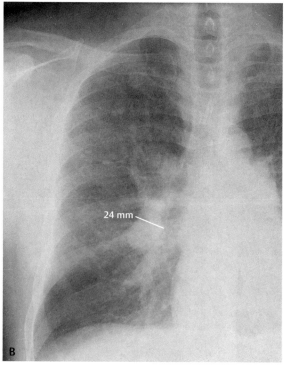

Fig. I.16   Descending pulmonary artery at the bronchus intermedius (CXR). **(A)** Coned-down PA chest radiograph of a healthy young woman demonstrates a descending pulmonary artery diameter of 13 mm. **(B)** Contrast the former with this coned-down PA chest radiograph of a 40-year-old man with long-standing pulmonary artery hypertension and chronic pulmonary thromboembolic disease in which the descending pulmonary artery measures 24 mm.

right bronchial artery typically originates as a common intercostobronchial artery trunk (**Fig. I.19**). The left bronchial arteries usually arise individually from the anterolateral wall of the aorta at about the same anatomic level. Less often, the left bronchial arteries arise from an intercostal artery. Two-thirds of the bronchial arterial system blood returns to the pulmonary venous system via the bronchial veins. The remainder drains into the azygos and hemiazygos systems.

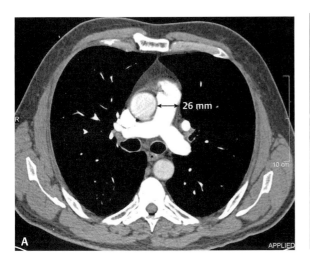
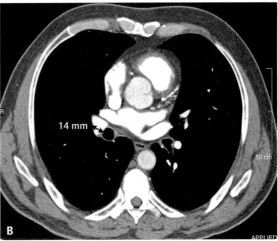

Fig. I.17 Measuring the pulmonary artery (CT). **(A)** The MPA is measured along its long axis at the bifurcation and 90° to the ascending aorta and measures 26 mm in this otherwise healthy man. **(B)** The descending pulmonary artery measures 14 mm at the right middle lobe bronchus origin.

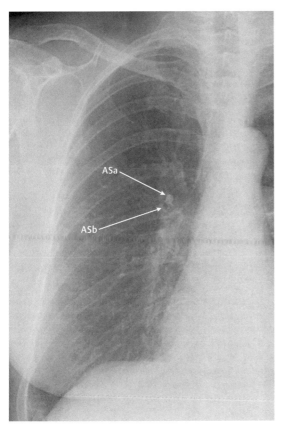

Fig. I.18 Assessing pulmonary artery-to-bronchus ratio. Coned-down frontal chest radiograph over the right hemithorax of this young woman shows the anterior segmental artery (*ASa*) and anterior segmental bronchus (*ASb*) projected en face. Note: the normal ratio is roughly 1:1.

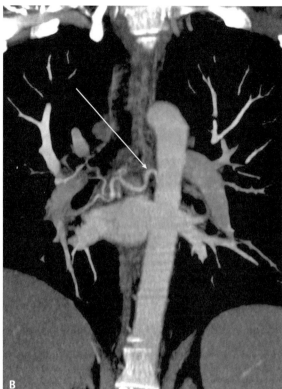

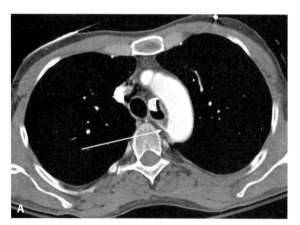

Fig. I.19 Right bronchial artery (CT). **(A)** Contrast-enhanced axial CT shows the normal common intercostobronchial artery trunk emanating off the posterolateral thoracic aorta (*arrow*). **(B)** Contrast-enhanced coronal MIP CT at the pericarinal level of a 40-year-old man with chronic pulmonary thromboembolic disease, pulmonary artery hypertension, and acute hemoptysis reveals a hypertrophied right bronchial artery originating off the posterolateral thoracic aorta (*arrow*).

Pulmonary Veins (Fig. I.20)

During early embryogenesis, the primitive lungs are initially drained by a *vascular plexus*, which has numerous connections with the *cardinal veins*. Later, a *common pulmonary vein* develops in the *sinoatrial region* that connects with this vascular plexus, and the cardinal vein connections involute. If the *vascular plexus–cardinal vein* connections fail to involute and persist, drainage from that portion of the lung may continue to flow into derivatives of the cardinal veins (e.g., left brachiocephalic vein, superior vena cava, azygos vein) rather than draining into the left atrium, resulting in either *complete* or *partial* forms of *anomalous pulmonary venous return* (see Section II).

Most of the left atrium develops from this *common pulmonary vein*. Initially, a single *common pulmonary vein* drains into the primitive left atrium. Later, as the left atrium expands, the proximal branches of the *common pulmonary vein* become incorporated into its wall, leaving four pulmonary veins with separate openings into the left atrium. *Accessory pulmonary veins* may develop and can induce regression of portions of the common pulmonary vein. This results in additional anomalous connections between the accessory pulmonary veins and the left atrium itself.

Conventional pulmonary venous anatomy is defined as a *single right* and *left superior* and *inferior pulmonary vein* that drain into the left atrium without any accessory veins (**Fig. I.20A**). Normally, the *right superior pulmonary vein* drains the right upper lobe and the right middle lobe, and descends medially into the superior aspect of the left atrium. The *left superior pulmonary vein* drains the left upper lobe and lingula, descends medially into the mediastinum, and drains into the superior portion of the left atrium. Both the *right* and *left inferior pulmonary veins* drain their respective lower lobes and follow a medial and oblique course into the posterolateral left atrial wall. The *ostia* of the *inferior pulmonary veins* are more posterior and medial relative to the *superior pulmonary veins*. The *superior pulmonary veins* tend to have a longer trunk and are larger in diameter (mean 21.6 mm ± 7.5 [SD] mm) than the *inferior pulmonary veins* (mean 14.0 mm ± 6.2 [SD] mm). There is no significant difference between the average diameters of the *right* and *left inferior pulmonary vein ostia* (mean 18.0 ± 3.7 [SD] mm).

A *common* or *conjoined pulmonary vein* occurs when the *superior* and *inferior pulmonary veins* combine *proximal* to the left atrium, resulting in a single broad *atriopulmonary venous junction* on the affected side (**Figs. I.20B, I.20C**). Such *conjoined pulmonary veins* occur more frequently on the left. A *common left pulmonary vein trunk* is one of the more common variants encountered. It is characterized by an ostial diameter greater than that of the other pulmonary veins (mean 32.5 mm ± [SD] 0.5 mm).

Supernumerary or *accessory pulmonary veins* represent "extra veins" with *independent atriopulmonary venous junctions* separate from the *superior* and *inferior pulmonary veins* (**Fig. I.20D**). *Accessory veins* are designated for the bronchopulmonary lobe or segment they drain. *Accessory drainage* can be complex but occurs more frequently on the right side. *Accessory veins* typically have a narrower *atriopulmonary venous junction* than do the *superior* and *inferior pulmonary veins*. An *accessory right middle lobe pulmonary vein* is the most common anatomic variant and may be identified in up to 16% of CT pulmonary vein examinations. In such cases, the *middle lobe pulmonary vein* passes underneath the middle lobe bronchus and drains into the left atrium at the base of the superior pulmonary venous confluence. The *middle lobe pulmonary vein* has an ostial diameter smaller than that of the other pulmonary veins (mean 9.9 mm ± 1.9 [SD] mm).

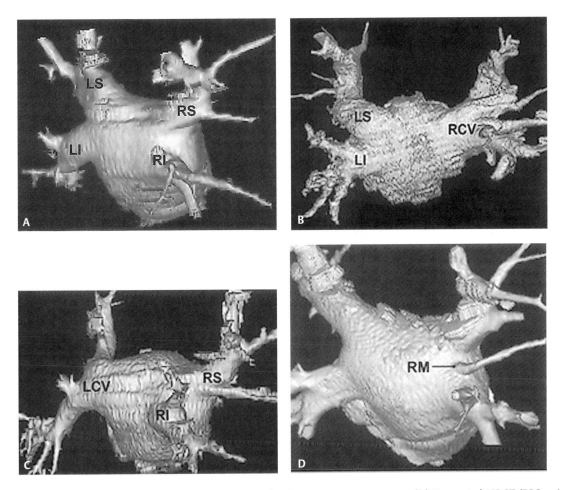

Fig. I.20 Pulmonary venous anatomy—conventional pulmonary venous anatomy. **(A)** Non-gated MDCT (RPO epicardial view) shows single right and left superior and inferior pulmonary veins draining into the left atrium without accessory veins. *LI*, left inferior pulmonary vein; *LS*, left superior pulmonary vein; *RI*, right inferior pulmonary vein; *RS*, right superior pulmonary vein. **(B)** Common (conjoined) veins. Volume rendered CT (PA epicardial view) from a non-gated MDCT shows a right common pulmonary vein (*RCV*). *LI*, left inferior pulmonary vein; *LS*, left superior pulmonary vein. **(C)** Common (conjoined) veins. Volume rendered CT (RPO epicardial view) from a non-gated MDCT performed in a different patient illustrates a left common pulmonary vein (*LCV*). *RI*, right inferior pulmonary vein; *RS*, right superior pulmonary vein. **(D)** Supernumerary or accessory pulmonary vein. Volume rendered CT image (epicardial view) from a non-gated MDCT shows an accessory right middle lobe pulmonary vein (*RM*). (*Images courtesy of John D. Grizzard, MD, VCU Medical Center, Richmond, Virginia.*)

■ Pleura

Anatomy

The pleura consist of two layers. The *parietal pleura* covers the non-pulmonary surfaces (e.g., ribs, mediastinum, and diaphragm). It has a systemic blood supply (via branches of the subclavian artery, internal mammary artery, and intercostal arteries) and venous drainage (via branches of the azygos and hemiazygos systems, and the internal mammary veins). The parietal pleura contains pain fibers, the irritation and inflammation of which cause pleuritic chest pain. The parietal pleura lymphatics communicate with the pleural space. The *visceral pleura* covers the surface of the lung. It has a dual blood supply. Branches of the bronchial circulation supply the apical, hilar, mediastinal, and interlobar visceral pleura, whereas branches from the pulmonary arteries supply the costal and diaphragmatic pleura. The visceral pleura also has a dual venous drainage (e.g., pulmonary and bronchial veins). Branches of the vagus nerve and sympathetic trunk innervate the visceral pleura. However, it does not contain pain fibers. Visceral pleura lymphatics do not communicate with the pleural space. Contiguous layers of visceral pleura form interlobar fissures that may be complete or incomplete.

Standard Fissures

The standard fissures divide the lung into lobes and include the minor (horizontal) and the major (oblique) fissures (**Fig. I.21**).

Minor Fissure (Figs. I.22.A, I.22B, I.22C, I.22D, I.22E, I.22F, I.22G)

This fissure separates the anterior segment of the right upper lobe from the middle lobe. It is seen in 44–88% of normal chest radiographs (**Figs. I.22A, I.22B**). In two-thirds of studies it lies at the fourth anterior intercostal space. On MDCT, it is most often recognized as an oval lucent area devoid of vasculature (**Fig. I.22C**). On 8% of studies, the fissure is seen as an oval area of ground glass attenuation. Coronal and sagittal MIP reconstructions clearly delineate the course and orientation of the horizontal fissure relative to the other standard fissures (**Figs. I.22D, I.22E**). On HRCT, the minor fissure often appears as a curvilinear line or C-shaped band of increased attenuation (**Fig. I.22F**). Incomplete minor fissure with resulting parenchymal fusion between the upper lobe anterior segment and the middle lobe (**Fig. I.22G**) is present in 60–90% of scans.

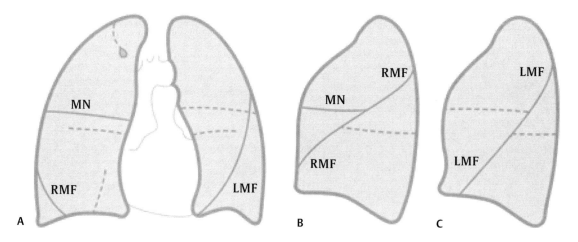

Fig. I.21 Standard fissures (*artist's illustration*). The standard fissures depicted in the coronal plane of **(A)** both lungs and the individual **(B)** right and **(C)** left lung in sagittal planes are illustrated by solid lines. *MN*, minor fissure; *LMF*, left major fissure; *RMF*, right major fissure.

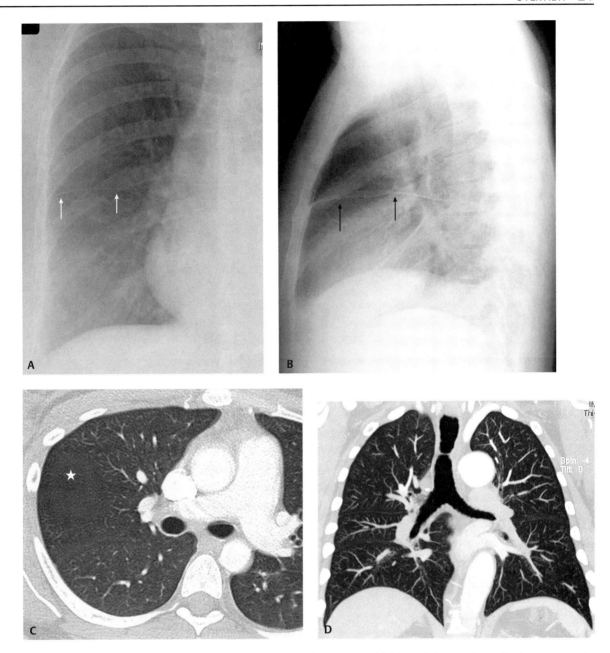

Fig. I.22 Radiologic features of the minor fissure. **(A)** Coned-down PA and **(B)** lateral chest radiographs demonstrate the normal course and position of the minor fissure (*arrows*). **(C)** Chest CT (lung windows) shows the minor fissure as a triangular area devoid of vasculature (*asterisk*). **(D)** Coronal MIP CT image (PA and lateral radiograph equivalents) depicting the course and orientation of the minor fissure and its relationship to the major fissure. *(Continued on page 22)*

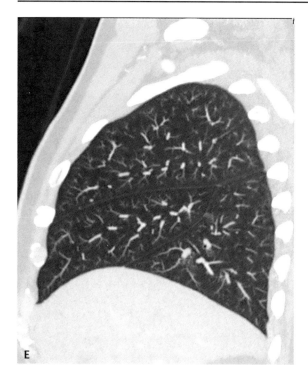

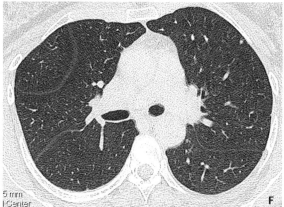

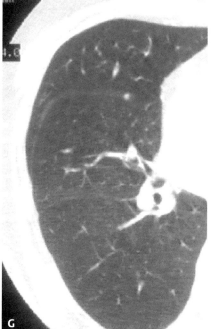

Fig. I.22 *(Continued)* Radiologic features of the minor fissure. **(E)** Sagittal MIP CT image (lateral radiograph equivalents) depicting the course and orientation of the minor fissure and its relationship to the major fissure. **(F)** HRCT shows the minor fissure as a reverse C-shaped band of increased attenuation. **(G)** Unenhanced axial CT reveals an incomplete minor fissure and parenchymal fusion between the right upper and middle lobes.

Major Fissures (Figs. I.23, I.24, I.25, I.26, I.27)

The *right major fissure* separates the combined upper and middle lobes from the lower lobe. The *left major fissure* separates the combined upper and lingular lobes from the lower lobe (**Fig. I.23**). The major fissures are best seen on lateral chest exams (**Fig. I.24**). The right major fissure originates at the level of T5, and the left at approximately T6. The major fissures parallel the sixth rib as they course obliquely and inferiorly. The right fissure follows a more oblique, anterior, and inferior course than its counterpart. Major fissures are seen on 80–90% of MDCT studies. Like the minor fissure, the major fissures most often appear as a lucent band devoid of vasculature. However, the major fissure may also appear as a well-defined line (**Fig. I.25A**), or as an ill-defined dense or somewhat fuzzy band (**Fig. I.25A**). On HRCT they are virtually always conspicuous, and most often appear as a single line (**Fig. I.25B**). Major fissures are incomplete on 12–75% of studies (**Fig. I.26**). *Incomplete fissures* are more frequently seen on the right, especially between the upper and lower lobes, and are least common between the left upper and lower lobes. The major fissures undulate through the lung and their morphology has been likened to that of a propeller blade or "figure 8" (**Figs. I.27A, I.27B**), an appearance better appreciated on CT. In the upper thorax, the fissure is anteriorly concave (*lateral facing orientation*) (**Fig. I.27C**). In the inferior thorax, the fissure is anteriorly convex (*medial facing orientation*) (**Fig. I.27D**). Alterations in this orientation serve as clues to underlying volume loss or lung disease.

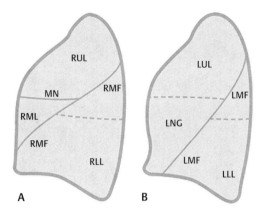

Fig. I.23 Standard fissures (*artist's illustration*). The standard fissures depicted in the individual **(A)** right and **(B)** left lung illustrated by solid lines. *LNG*, lingula; *LLL*, left lower lobe; *LUL*, left upper lobe; *MN*, minor fissure; *LMF*, left major fissure; *RMF*, right major fissure; *RLL*, right lower lobe; *RML*, right middle lobe; *RUL*, right upper lobe.

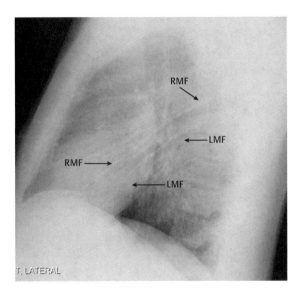

Fig. I.24 Coned-down lateral chest radiograph demonstrating the normal course and position of the right (RMF) and left (LMF) major fissures.

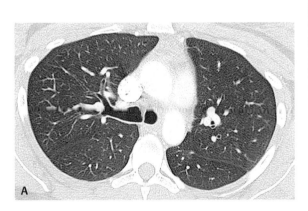
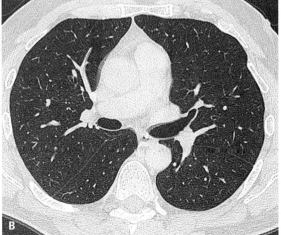

Fig. I.25 Variable appearances of major fissures on MDCT. **(A)** The right major fissure is somewhat fuzzy and ill-defined, whereas the left major fissure appears more linear. **(B)** On HRCT of another patient, both fissures are sharply defined and curvilinear.

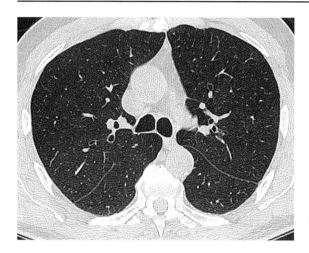

Fig. I.26 HRCT illustrating an incomplete right major fissure. Note this fissure fails to reach the ipsilateral hilum, resulting in a parenchymal bridge of communication between the upper and lower lobe. The left fissure is complete.

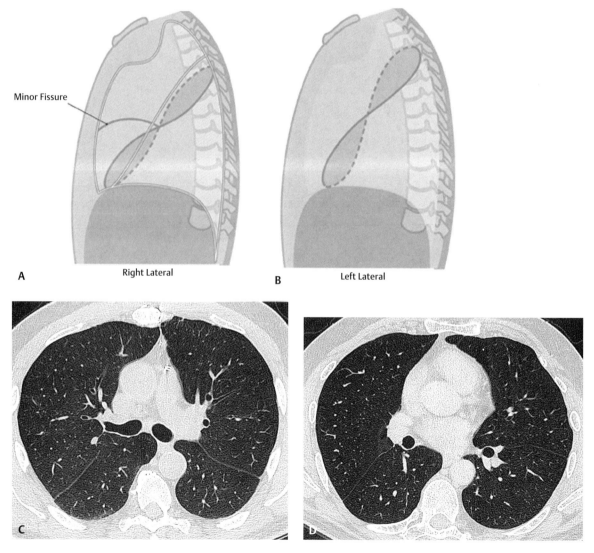

Fig. I.27 Propeller-like morphology of the major fissure. Artist's illustration depicts the undulating morphology of the major fissures through both the **(A)** right and the **(B)** left thorax. **(C)** HRCT through the upper thorax demonstrates the anterior concave (lateral facing orientation) of the major fissures. **(D)** HRCT through the lower thorax demonstrates the anterior convex (medial facing orientation) of the major fissures.

Accessory Fissures (Fig. I.28)

Accessory fissures occur within a given lobe itself, and may be seen on 10% of chest radiographs and 20% of CTs.

Accessory Azygos Fissure (Fig. I.29)

Embryologically, the *azygos fissure* results from abnormal migration of the right posterior cardinal vein (**Fig. I.29A**) directly into the lung apex, drawing in the layers of visceral and parietal pleura. The displaced azygos vein ultimately resides in a sling of four pleural layers (mesoazygos). This normal variant occurs in 1% of the population. It is seen on 1% of imaging studies and appears as a curvilinear opacity extending obliquely from the upper portion of the right lung, and terminates in a teardrop-shaped opacity 2–4 cm above the hilum (**Figs. I.29B, I.29E**), representing the displaced azygos vein. The lung residing medial to this fissure is referred to as the azygos lobe.

Inferior Accessory Fissure (Fig. I.30)

The *inferior accessory fissure* separates the medial basal segment of the lower lobe from the remaining basilar segments. It is the most common of the accessory fissures, seen in 30–45% of anatomic specimens, 5–10% of frontal radiographs (**Fig. I.30A**), and 15% of CT examinations (**Figs. I.30B, I.30C, I.30D**). Although it occurs with equal frequency in the two lungs, it is more conspicuous in the right hemithorax, extending superiorly and slightly medially from the hemidiaphragm toward the ipsilateral hilum (**Fig. I.30A**). The lung medial to this fissure is called the cardiac lobe (**Figs. I.30B, I.30C, I.30D**).

Superior Accessory Fissure (Fig. I.31)

The superior accessory fissure separates the superior segment of the lower lobe from the remainder of the lower lobe segments and is seen in 6% of anatomic specimens. On imaging, it lies in a horizontal plane and may mimic the minor fissure, but is typically lower, at the level of the lower lobe segmental bronchus (**Fig. I.31**). On lateral chest radiography, it extends further posteriorly than the minor fissure, often overlying the spine. The portion of lung isolated by this fissure is called the dorsal lobe of Nelson.

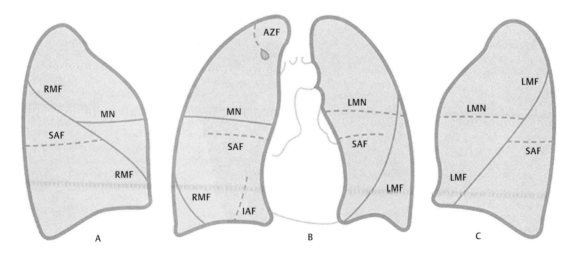

Fig. I.28 Accessory fissures (*artist's illustration*). The more commonly encountered accessory fissures are illustrated by the interrupted lines. Solid lines illustrate the standard fissures. *AZF*, azygos fissure; *IAF*, inferior accessory fissure; *LMF*, left major fissure; *LMN*, left minor fissure; *MN*, right minor fissure; *SAF*, superior accessory fissure; *RMF*, right major fissure.

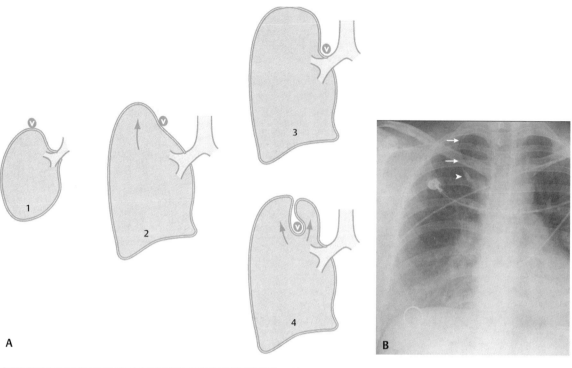

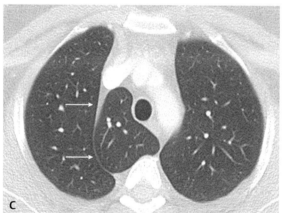

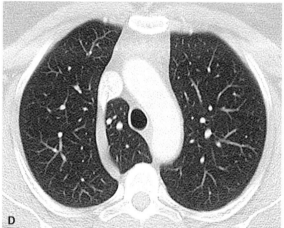

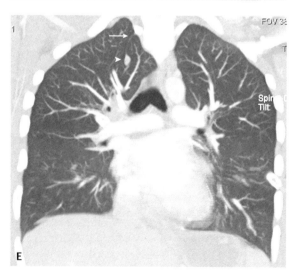

Fig. I.29 Azygos fissure. Abnormal right posterior cardinal vein (RPCV) migration results in formation of the azygos fissure and lobe. **(A)** Artist's illustration: (*1*) depicts the embryologic origin of the RPCV before its migration into the mediastinum. (*2*) Illustrates the normal migration of the RPCV along the mediastinal pleural reflection. (*3*) The RPCV subsequently comes to reside at the tracheobronchial angle; the normal anatomic location of the azygos vein. (*4*) Illustrates abnormal migration of the RPCV into the lung apex drawing in four layers of visceral and parietal pleura forming the mesoazygos. **(B)** Coned-down PA chest radiograph shows an azygos fissure (*arrows*). The tear-dropped opacity (*arrowhead*) represents the displaced azygos vein. **(C)** Axial chest CT (lung window) reveals the appearance, course and position of an azygos fissure (*arrows*) and **(D)** displaced azygos vein cradled in 4 layers of pleura more inferiorly. **(E)** Coronal MIP CT delineates an azygos fissure (*arrow*) and displaced azygos vein (*arrowhead*). Isolated lung tissue medial to this fissure is the azygos lobe.

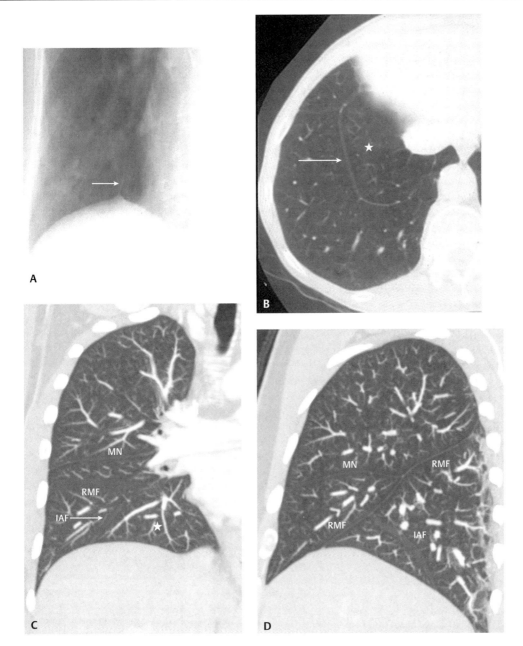

Fig. I.30 Inferior accessory fissure. **(A)** Coned-down PA chest radiograph shows the typical location and course of this fissure (*arrow*). **(B)** Axial chest CT (lung window) demonstrates the normal course and orientation of this accessory fissure (arrow) and the isolated cardiac lobe (*asterisk*). **(C)** Coronal and **(D)** sagittal MIP CT reveals an inferior fissure and its relationship to the standard fissures. *IAF*, inferior accessory fissure; *MN*, minor fissure; *RMF*, right major fissure; (*asterisk*) cardiac lobe.

Left Minor Fissure (Fig. I.32)

The left minor fissure is analogous to the right minor fissure. That is, it separates the lingula from the anterior segment of the left upper lobe. Although present in 8–18% of anatomic specimens, it is seen in only 1.5% of chest radiographs (**Fig. I.32A**). It usually lies more cephalad than its counterpart, and has a more medial sloping or oblique course. On MDCT and HRCT the left minor fissure appears similar to the right minor fissure (**Figs. I.32B, I.32C**). Additional unnamed, left upper lobe, accessory fissures or lung clefts are seen in up to 9% of studies (**Fig. I.32D**). Such fissures often separate the superior and inferior lingular segments or apical posterior and anterior segments of the upper lobe.

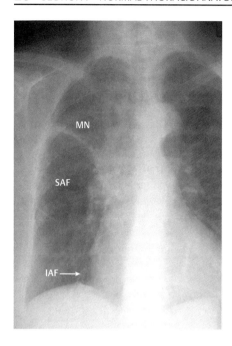

Fig. I.31 Superior accessory fissure. Coned-down PA chest radiograph shows the typical location and course of this fissure. Note its relationship to the displaced minor fissure in this patient with right upper lobe volume loss. *IAF*, inferior accessory fissure; *MN*, minor fissure; *SAF*, superior accessory fissure.

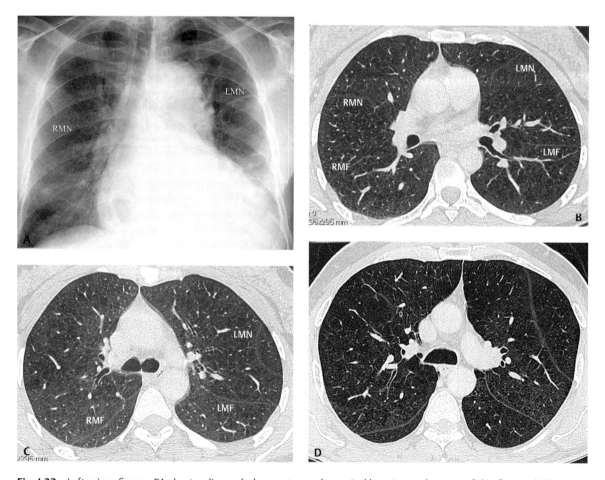

Fig. I.32 Left minor fissure. PA chest radiograph demonstrates the typical location and course of this fissure. **(A)** Note its relationship to the right minor fissure. HRCT shows a left minor fissure as an anteromedial straight line extending obliquely and medially from the **(B)** anterior chest wall and in another patient **(C)** as a C-shaped curvilinear opacity. **(D)** HRCT of an unnamed left upper lobe accessory fissure seen as a convex medial linear opacity. LMF, left major fissure; *LMN*, left minor fissure; *RMF*, right major fissure; *RMN*, right minor fissure.

Pulmonary Ligament (Fig. I.33)

This double layer of pleura tethers the medial aspect of the lower lobe to the mediastinum and diaphragm. It is formed by the union of parietal and visceral pleural at the hilum and extends from its inferior margin toward the ipsilateral hemidiaphragm. Although not conspicuous on radiography, the ligament is often seen on CT at or just above the hemidiaphragm. It appears as a small pyramidal opacity on the mediastinal surface (ligament) and as a thin, linear opacity that extends from the pyramid's apex to the lung (intersegmental septum). The *right pulmonary ligament* lies adjacent to the azygos vein and inferior vena cava and is seen on 40–60% of CTs. The *left pulmonary ligament* lies adjacent to the esophagus and descending thoracic aorta and is seen on 60–70% of CT exams. The septum created by these pleural reflections contains bronchial veins, lymphatics, and lymph nodes. The pulmonary ligament may serve as an anchor for the lower lobe, preventing torsion.

■ Lymphatic System

The pleuropulmonary lymphatics are not normally visible on radiography. However, their intrathoracic repository, the hilar and mediastinal lymph nodes, are frequently seen. Nodal enlargement is common and often serves as a diagnostic clue to underlying thoracic disease. On chest radiography, grossly enlarged mediastinal nodes manifest by increased opacity or alteration in normal mediastinal borders or contours. On CT, lymph nodes appear as oval or kidney bean–shaped soft tissue attenuation structures, with or without central or eccentric radiolucent fat. On MRI, lymph nodes often show soft tissue signal intensity and are easily distinguished from adjacent mediastinal vessels. Intrathoracic lymph nodes are broadly grouped as either parietal or visceral.

Parietal Lymph Nodes

Parietal nodes reside outside the parietal pleura in extramediastinal tissue and drain the thoracic wall and other extrathoracic structures. These nodes are divided into three subcategories (**Table I.2**).

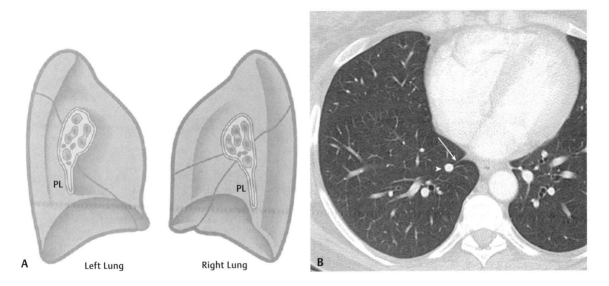

Fig. I.33 Pulmonary ligament. **(A)** Artist's illustration depicting the union of visceral and parietal pleural layers at the hilum forming the pulmonary ligament. Chest CT (lung window) caudad to the inferior pulmonary vein shows a thin white line extending from the mediastinum (*arrow*). **(B)** This represents the intersegmental septum of the lower lobe, bound at the mediastinum by the base of the pulmonary ligament and laterally by a vertically oriented vein (*arrowhead*). *PL*, pulmonary ligament.

Table I.2 Parietal Lymph Node Groups

Nodal Group	Location	Afferent Channels	Efferent Channels
Anterior (internal mammary)	Upper thorax, behind anterior intercostal spaces; parallels internal mammary vessels	Upper anterior abdominal wall Anterior thoracic wall Anterior diaphragm Medial breasts	Right lymphatic or thoracic duct Communicates with visceral nodes of anterior mediastinum and cervical nodes
Posterior	*Intercostal*—adjacent to rib heads posterior intercostal space *Juxtavertebral*—parallel thoracic spine	Intercostal spaces Parietal pleura Vertebral column	Thoracic duct—upper thorax Cisterna chyli—lower thorax Communicates with other posterior mediastinal nodes
Diaphragmatic	*Anterior (prepericardiac)*—immediately behind xyphoid; parallel anterior pericardium *Middle (juxtaphrenic)*—near phrenic nerves at diaphragm *Posterior (retrocrural)*—behind diaphragm crura	Diaphragm Anterior superior liver	Cisterna chyli

Visceral Lymph Nodes

Visceral lymph nodes are located in the mediastinum between the pleural membranes and primarily drain the intrathoracic structures. These nodes are also divided into three subcategories (**Table I.3**).

Table I.3 Visceral Lymph Node Groups

Nodal Group	Location	Afferent Channels	Efferent Channels
Anterosuperior mediastinal (prevascular)	Anterior to superior vena cava; innominate veins; ascending aorta; thymus; behind manubrium/sternum	Most anterior mediastinal structures; pericardium; thymus; diaphragmatic and mediastinal pleura; part of the heart; anterior hila	Right lymphatic or thoracic duct
Posterior mediastinal	*Periesophageal*—around esophagus	Posterior diaphragm; pericardium; esophagus; lower lobes of lungs via pulmonary ligament	Right lymphatic or thoracic duct
	Periaortic—anterior/lateral aspects descending thoracic aorta		Communicates with subcarinal tracheobronchial nodes
Tracheobronchial	*Paratracheal*—parallel trachea	Bronchopulmonary; tracheal bifurcation nodes; trachea; esophagus; right/left lung	Right lymphatic or thoracic duct
			Communicates with anterior/posterior visceral nodes
	Tracheal bifurcation (carinal)—precarinal/subcarinal fat; right/left main bronchi	Bronchopulmonary nodes; anterior/posterior mediastinal nodes; heart; pericardium; esophagus; esophagus; lungs	Primarily right paratracheal lymph nodes
	Aortopulmonary—Mediastinal fat between left pulmonary artery and aortic arch		
	Bronchopulmonary or hilar—main bronchi and vessels	All lung lobes	Carinal/paratracheal nodes

Lymph Node Stations

As opposed to the anatomic grouping of lymph nodes into parietal and visceral groups, radiologists and surgeons classify thoracic lymph nodes into stations relevant to the staging, management, and prognosis of neoplastic diseases associated with lymph node involvement. The recently revised 7th edition of the TNM classification for non–small cell lung cancer has placed thoracic lymph nodes into seven specific zones (**Table I.4**). Although the nomenclature has changed, the general concept has not. *N1* (hilar or peribronchial) nodes include lymph nodes distal to the mediastinal pleural reflection and within the visceral pleura (stations 10–14). *N2* (mediastinal) nodes include nodes within the mediastinal pleural reflection (stations 1–9) (see Section VI). Pathologic staging often requires lymph node tissue sampling. The radiologist can be instrumental in directing the most appropriate means of lymph node biopsy by understanding this nodal classification scheme and those stations most accessible to various sampling techniques (**Table I.5**).

■ Mediastinum

The mediastinum is the space between the lungs and pleural surfaces bound by the sternum anteriorly and the vertebral column posteriorly (**Fig. I.34A**). It extends from the thoracic inlet to the diaphragm and contains the thymus, lymph nodes, heart, great vessels, trachea, esophagus, and other soft tissues. The division of the mediastinum into compartments is arbitrary, as no anatomic boundaries divide the space. The method of mediastinal compartmentalization varies among the medical disciplines, and several radiologic classifications have been proposed.

Table I.4 International Association for Study of Lung Cancer Nodal Zones—Revised Staging System for Lung Cancer

Nodal Zones	Nodal Anatomic Locations	Nodal Stations
Supraclavicular	Supraclavicular	1
	Low cervical	1
	Sternal notch	1
Upper	Upper paratracheal (left)	2L
	Upper paratracheal (right)	2R
	Pre-vascular	3A
	Retrotracheal	3P
	Lower paratracheal (right)	4R
	Lower paratracheal (left)	4L
Aorticopulmonary	Subaortic (aorticopulmonary window)	5
	Para-aortic (ascending aorta/phrenic)	6
Lower	Para-esophageal (below carina)	8
	Pulmonary ligament	9
Subcarinal	Subcarinal	7
Hilar/interlobar	Hilar	10
	Interlobar	11
Peripheral	Lobar	12
	Segmental	13
	Subsegmental	14

Table I.5 Accessible Lymph Node Stations by Various Biopsy Techniques

Sampling Technique	Accessible Lymph Nodes via Station
Cervical mediastinoscopy	Upper right/left paratracheal[a] Lower right/left paratracheal[a] Anterior subcarinal Some anterosuperior mediastinal and pre-vascular
Anterior/parasternal mediastinoscopy (extended mediastinoscopy)	Subaortic Para-aortic
Parasternal mini-thoracotomy (Chamberlain procedure)	Subaortic Para-aortic
Endobronchial ultrasound biopsy (EBUS)	Some anterosuperior mediastinal Upper right/left paratracheal Lower right/left paratracheal Pre-vascular Retrotracheal Subcarinal Hilar Some interlobar
Esophageal endoscopic ultrasound biopsy (EUS)	Upper left paratracheal[c] Lower left paratracheal[c] Subcarinal[a] Para-esophageal[a] Left pulmonary ligament[a] Subaortic[b] Para-aortic[b] Left adrenal gland Left hepatic lobe Celiac axis nodes
Transbronchial biopsy	Lower paratracheal Subcarinal
Thoracoscopy and video assisted thoracoscopic surgery (VATS):	
Right hemithorax	Upper right paratracheal Lower right paratracheal Subcarinal Pulmonary ligament Hilar Interlobar
Left hemithorax	Subaortic Para-aortic Subcarinal Pulmonary ligament Hilar Interlobar
Mediastinal transthoracic FNA/core biopsy: CT or ultrasound guidance	Most all nodal stations; Subaortic can be difficult
Supranavigational electromagnetic biopsy	Some anterosuperior mediastinal Upper paratracheal Lower paratracheal Pre-vascular Subcarinal Hilar Interlobar Peripheral lung nodule(s)

[a] optimal nodes to biopsy
[b] difficult but possible in select cases
[c] requires punctures through pulmonary artery

Mediastinal Compartments

Anatomic Compartments

Anatomists recognize four mediastinal compartments: superior, anterior, middle, and posterior (**Fig. I.34B**). This classification excludes the paravertebral regions and locates the anterior, middle, and posterior compartments below the superior mediastinum. The *superior mediastinum* is located between the manubrium sternum and the first four thoracic vertebrae, from an oblique plane through the first rib superiorly to a horizontal plane through the sternal angle inferiorly. It contains thymus, portions of the great vessels, portions of the trachea and esophagus, portions of the vagus and phrenic nerves, and the recurrent laryngeal nerve. The *anterior mediastinum* is located between the sternum and the pericardium, and contains areolar tissue, lymphatics, and lymph nodes. The *middle mediastinum* is located between the anterior and posterior compartments, and contains the pericardium (in fact, the fibrous pericardium forms the borders of the anatomic middle mediastinum), heart, great vessel origins, tracheal bifurcation, lymph nodes, portions of the phrenic nerves, and azygos arch. The *posterior mediastinum* is located between the posterior aspect of the pericardium and the spine, and contains the descending aorta, a portion of the esophagus, thoracic duct, azygos and hemiazygos veins, portions of the vagus nerves, splanchnic nerves, and lymph nodes.

Surgical Compartments

Like anatomists, surgeons use four mediastinal compartments—superior, anterior, middle, and posterior (**Fig. I.34C**)—but the division of the mediastinum is based on areas of operability and includes the paravertebral regions. The surgical *superior mediastinum* is situated above the aortic arch. The anterior, middle, and posterior mediastinal compartments are located below the superior mediastinum. The *anterior mediastinum* is located between the sternum and pericardium. The *middle mediastinum* is located between the anterior mediastinum and the thoracic spine and includes structures in the anatomic middle mediastinum as well as the descending aorta, esophagus, azygos and hemiazygos veins, and thoracic duct. The *posterior mediastinum* consists of the paravertebral soft tissues, including proximal intercostal neurovascular structures, lymph nodes, and the sympathetic chain and its branches.

Radiographic Compartments

Felson

Benjamin Felson divided the mediastinum based on the lateral chest radiograph (**Fig. I.34D**). Because anterior mediastinal masses frequently projected over the heart on lateral radiography, the heart was included in the radiographic anterior mediastinum. The paravertebral region (not anatomically in the mediastinum) was included in the posterior mediastinum. The *anterior mediastinum* includes structures located anterior to a line drawn along the anterior tracheal wall and continued along the posterior heart border (**Fig. I.34D**). The posterior mediastinum includes structures located posterior to a line connecting points on each thoracic vertebral body approximately one centimeter behind their anterior margins. The *middle mediastinum* contains structures located between the above-mentioned lines.

Fraser, Müller, Colman, Paré

This mediastinal division recognizes that the distinction between compartments is difficult to establish on radiography and that mediastinal masses may occupy more than one compartment. It combines the middle and posterior compartments and describes a separate paravertebral region. Masses are described as occurring predominantly in one of the compartments (**Fig. I.34E**). The *anterior mediastinum* contains structures anterior to a line that extends along the anterior wall of the trachea and continues along the posterior heart border (as in the Felson mediastinal division). The *middle-posterior mediastinum* contains structures located between the above-mentioned line and a line drawn along the anterior aspects of the thoracic vertebral bodies. The *paravertebral region* overlaps the vertebral bodies on the lateral radiograph (**Fig. I.34E**).

Cross-Sectional Imaging Divisions

Cross-sectional imaging with CT and MR imaging allows visualization of the normal mediastinal structures, accurate localization of mediastinal abnormalities, and description of their relationship to normal structures within the mediastinum. The *anterior mediastinum* is located between the chest wall anteriorly and the an-

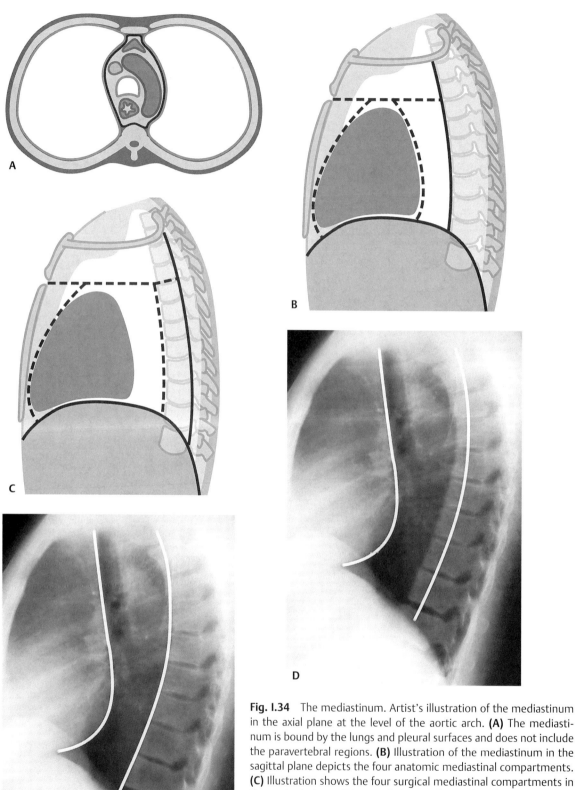

Fig. I.34 The mediastinum. Artist's illustration of the mediastinum in the axial plane at the level of the aortic arch. **(A)** The mediastinum is bound by the lungs and pleural surfaces and does not include the paravertebral regions. **(B)** Illustration of the mediastinum in the sagittal plane depicts the four anatomic mediastinal compartments. **(C)** Illustration shows the four surgical mediastinal compartments in the sagittal plane. **(D)** Lateral chest radiograph with superimposed lines illustrates the three radiographic mediastinal compartments (anterior, middle, posterior) according to Felson. **(E)** Lateral chest radiograph with superimposed lines illustrates the three radiographic mediastinal compartments (anterior, middle-posterior, paravertebral region) according to Fraser, Müller, Colman, and Paré.

terior aspects of the mediastinal great vessels and pericardium posteriorly. The *middle mediastinum* is bound anteriorly by the pericardium and posteriorly by the dorsal tracheal wall and pericardium. The *posterior mediastinum* is bound anteriorly by the plane between the trachea and esophagus and the pericardium, and posteriorly by the spine or the paravertebral regions.

The Cervicothoracic Sign

Understanding this radiographic sign is useful in the analysis of paravertebral masses located in the superior aspect of the mediastinum. Because the thoracic inlet is obliquely oriented, the paravertebral regions extend cephalad to the superior aspect of the anterior mediastinum. Thus, a mediastinal or paravertebral opacity that projects above the clavicles on a frontal chest radiograph must be posteriorly located (**Fig. I.35**), whereas an opacity that is effaced superiorly and appears to terminate at the clavicles must be located anteriorly. The location of such lesions can be confirmed on lateral radiography, but when such lesions are small or when only frontal radiography is available, this sign can be useful in localizing a lesion within the mediastinum or paravertebral region.

Mediastinal Borders and Interfaces

Contact of the air density lung with the water density mediastinum produces a series of radiographic interfaces. On the frontal radiograph these include the superior vena cava interface and the right atrium on the right, and the aortic arch, the pulmonary trunk, and the left ventricle on the left (**Fig. I.36A**). Normal interfaces on the lateral radiograph include the pulmonary trunk and the right ventricle anteriorly and the left atrium, left ventricle, and inferior vena cava posteriorly (**Fig. I.36B**).

Mediastinal Lines, Stripes, and Interfaces

The points of contact between the bilateral lungs (and pleural surfaces) anterior and posterior to the mediastinum and the contact between the air density lungs and the water density mediastinal structures result in a series of normal radiographic landmarks manifesting as lines, stripes, and interfaces. *Lines* characteristi-

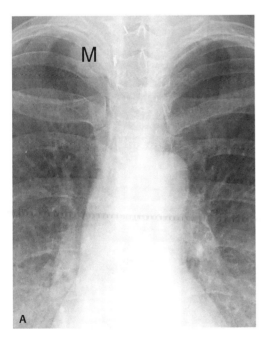
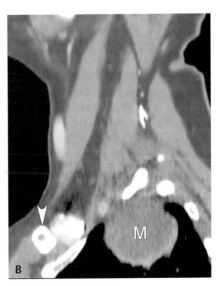

Fig. I.35 Cervicothoracic sign. **(A)** Coned-down view of a frontal chest radiograph shows a right paramediastinal mass (*M*) projecting above the level of the ipsilateral clavicle. **(B)** Sagittal chest CT (mediastinal window) demonstrates the lesion (*M*) is located within the posterior aspect of the mediastinum (paravertebral region) and located above the ipsilateral clavicle (*arrowhead*).

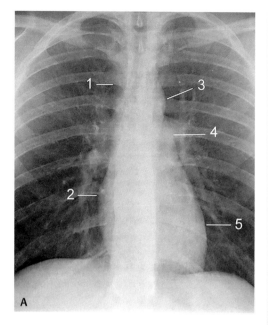

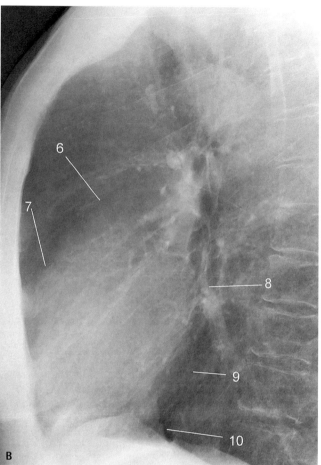

Fig. I.36 Normal mediastinal borders and interfaces. **(A)** Frontal chest radiograph labeled to show normal radiographic interfaces, including the (*1*) superior vena cava interface, (*2*) right atrium, (*3*) aortic arch, (*4*) pulmonary trunk, and (*5*) left ventricle. **(B)** Lateral chest radiograph labeled to show normal radiographic interfaces, including the (*6*) pulmonary trunk, (*7*) right ventricle, (*8*) left atrium, (*9*) left ventricle, and (*10*) inferior vena cava.

cally represent contact of the bilateral lungs and pleural surfaces, *stripes* generally represent contact of the lung and surrounding pleura with mediastinal mesenchymal tissues, and *interfaces* usually represent contact between the lung/pleura and specific mediastinal organs.

The Junction Lines

Anterior (**Fig. I.37**) and *posterior* (**Fig. I.38**) *junction lines* are formed by contact of the bilateral lungs anteriorly (posterior to the sternum and anterior to the mediastinum) or posteriorly (posterior to the mediastinum and anterior to the thoracic vertebrae), respectively. They comprise four layers of pleura (the visceral and parietal pleural surfaces around each lung) and are more frequently visualized in the setting of emphysema due to increased lung volumes. When mediastinal fat intervenes between the apposed lungs, anterior or posterior junction stripes may be visualized.

The *anterior junction line* (**Fig. I.37**) follows an oblique course from the caudal aspect of the manubrium sternum and extends inferiorly toward the left on frontal chest radiography (**Fig. I.37A**). It is visible in approximately 20% of subjects. In cases of upper lobe atelectasis, the junction line may manifest as an interface between normal aerated lung and the water density atelectatic lung.

The *posterior junction line* (**Fig. I.38**) is located in the superior aspect of the thorax, includes four layers of pleura and intervening mediastinal fat, and is visible in 40% of cases. It manifests as a vertical line or stripe usually visible through the tracheal air column and terminates at the level of the aortic arch (**Fig. I.38**). When the air-filled esophagus is contained within the posterior junction stripe, it is referred to as the right and/or left pleuroesophageal stripe.

The Paratracheal Stripes

Right and left paratracheal stripes (**Fig. I.39**) are formed by contact between the lung and the lateral trachea walls and their surrounding mediastinal soft tissues. The *right paratracheal stripe* courses between the

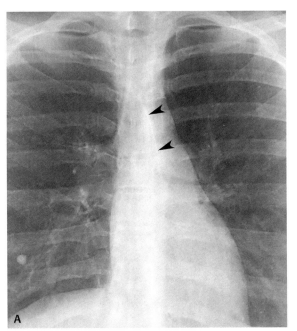

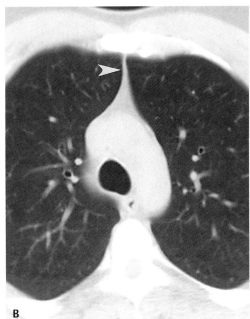

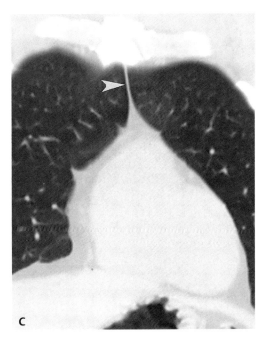

Fig. I.37 Radiologic depiction of the anterior junction line. **(A)** Anterior junction line (*black arrowheads*) formed by contact between the bilateral upper lobes anterior to the mediastinum on PA chest radiography. **(B)** Axial and **(C)** coronal chest CT (lung window) shows the anatomic basis for the anterior junction line (*white arrowheads*).

thoracic inlet and the azygos arch (**Figs. I.39A, I.39B, I.39C**) and is visible in approximately 95% of normal subjects and measures up to 4 mm in thickness. The *left paratracheal stripe* (**Figs. I.39A, I.39D, I.39E**) extends from the thoracic inlet to the aortic arch and is typically thicker than the right due to intervening fat and vascular structures (**Figs. I.39D, I.39E**), particularly the left subclavian artery.

The Aortopulmonary Window

The aortopulmonary (AP) window (**Fig. I.40**) is the interface formed by the contact between the left upper lobe and the mediastinal reflection between the aortic arch superiorly and the left pulmonary artery inferiorly (**Fig. I.40B**). It is characteristically either straight or concave laterally. On cross-sectional imaging, the aortopulmonary window refers to the mediastinal space bound laterally by the left parietal pleura and medially by the ligamentum arteriosum.

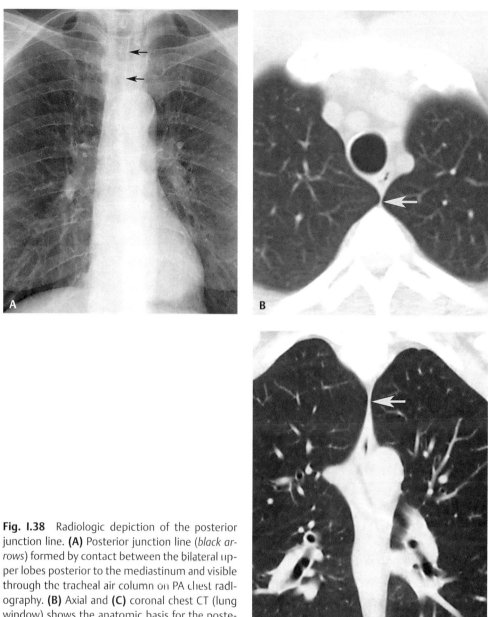

Fig. I.38 Radiologic depiction of the posterior junction line. **(A)** Posterior junction line (*black arrows*) formed by contact between the bilateral upper lobes posterior to the mediastinum and visible through the tracheal air column on PA chest radiography. **(B)** Axial and **(C)** coronal chest CT (lung window) shows the anatomic basis for the posterior junction line (*white arrows*).

The Paravertebral Stripes

The paravertebral stripes (**Fig. I.41**) are formed by contact between the lower lobes and the paravertebral soft tissues. The *right paravertebral stripe* is visualized more frequently and is often longer than the left. The right paravertebral stripe is typically visible adjacent to the inferior thoracic spine (**Figs. I.41A, I.41B**). The thickness of the right paravertebral stripe may be accentuated by osteophytes (**Fig. I.41C, I.41D**) whereas that of the left may be accentuated by aortic tortuosity.

The Posterior Tracheal Stripe

The posterior tracheal stripe (**Fig. I.42**), also known as the tracheoesophageal stripe, is formed by contact between the right upper lobe and the posterior wall of the trachea (**Figs. I.42A, I.42B, I.42C**) and occasionally the intervening esophagus, and has a variable length and thickness.

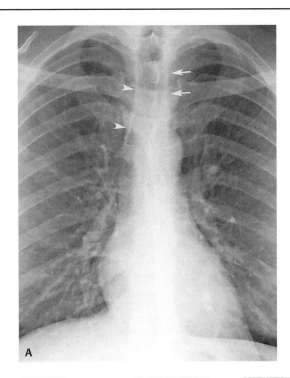

Fig. I.39 Radiologic depiction of the paratracheal stripes. **(A)** Normal PA chest radiograph showing the right (*arrowheads*) and left (*arrows*) paratracheal stripes. **(B)** Axial and **(C)** coronal chest CT (lung window) show the normal thin right paratracheal stripe. **(D)** Axial and **(E)** coronal chest CT (lung window) show the thicker left paratracheal stripe with intervening fat and vascular structures between the left tracheal wall and adjacent ipsilateral lung.

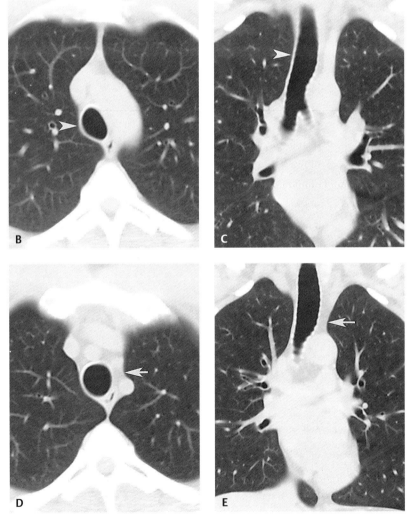

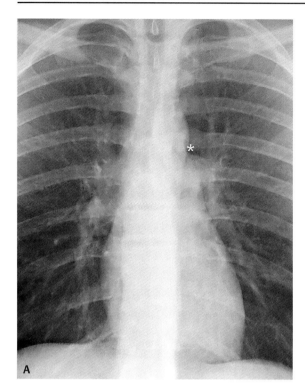
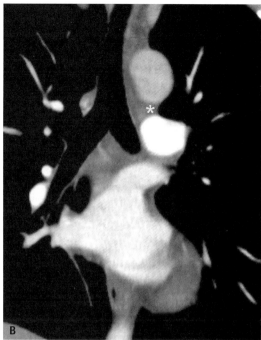

Fig. I.40 Radiologic depiction of the aortopulmonary window. **(A)** Normal PA chest radiograph and **(B)** coronal contrast-enhanced chest CT (mediastinal window) show the AP window (*asterisk*) between the aortic arch superiorly and the left pulmonary artery inferiorly.

The Retrotracheal Triangle

The retrotracheal triangle (also known as Raider's triangle) (**Fig. I.43**) is a lucent triangular area with a superiorly oriented apex located between the posterior tracheal stripe anteriorly and the thoracic vertebrae posteriorly (**Fig. I.43B**).

The Azygoesophageal Recess

The azygoesophageal recess (**Fig. I.44**) is the interface produced by contact between the right lower lobe and the adjacent mediastinum near the azygos vein and esophagus. This interface extends from the azygos arch to the diaphragm and normally exhibits a gentle laterally concave or S-shaped contour. When the adjacent esophagus contains air, it becomes the right inferior pleuroesophageal stripe.

The Pericardium

The pericardium is formed by an *outer fibrous pericardium* (**Fig. I.45**), which defines the boundaries of the anatomic middle mediastinum, and an *inner serous pericardium*. Like the pleura, the *serous pericardium* (**Fig. I.45**) is a continuous thin membrane composed of *parietal* (lining the fibrous pericardium) and *visceral* (lining the heart) components. The *visceral pericardium* is synonymous with the epicardium. Subjacent fat is referred to as subepicardial fat. The fat that surrounds the outer aspect of the pericardium is simply the mediastinal fat.

The *fibrous pericardium* is contiguous with the vascular adventitia of the ascending aorta (**Fig. I.45**) and the pulmonary artery. The *serous pericardium* forms reflections around the ascending aorta, pulmonary trunk and the pulmonary veins, and two sinuses, the oblique sinus and the transverse sinus (**Fig. I.46**). The transverse sinus and the pericardial space give rise to a series of *pericardial recesses*. These recesses have variable appearances based on the amount of pericardial fluid they contain and should not be mistaken for pathologic processes.

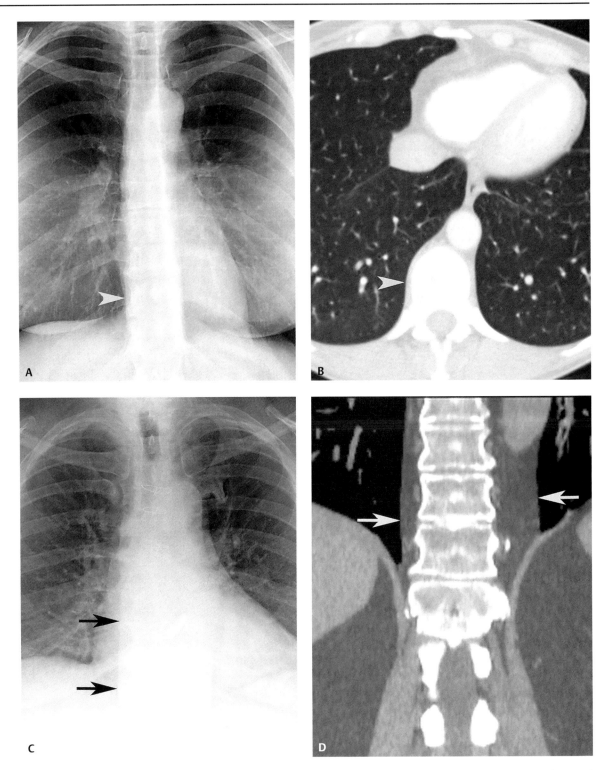

Fig. I.41 Radiologic depiction of the paravertebral stripes. **(A)** Normal PA chest radiograph and **(B)** corresponding axial chest CT (lung window) demonstrate the right paravertebral stripe (*arrowheads*). **(C)** PA chest radiograph of an elderly patient with large vertebral osteophytes shows thick bilateral paravertebral stripes (*arrows*) demonstrated on **(D)** coronal thoracoabdominal CT (soft-tissue window).

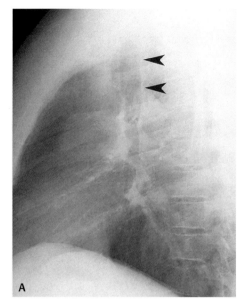

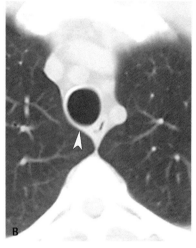

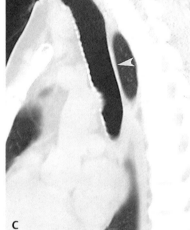

Fig. I.42   Radiologic depiction of the posterior tracheal stripe. **(A)** Normal lateral chest radiograph shows the posterior tracheal stripe (*black arrowheads*). **(B)** Axial and **(C)** sagittal chest CT (lung window) show the right upper lobe contact with the posterior tracheal wall to form the posterior tracheal stripe (*white arrowheads*).

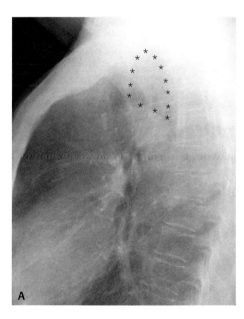

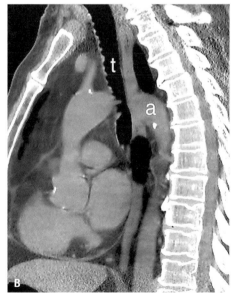

Fig. I.43   Radiologic depiction of the retrotracheal triangle. **(A)** Normal lateral chest radiograph and **(B)** unenhanced chest CT (mediastinal window) demonstrate the retrotracheal triangle (outlined by *asterisks*) situated posterior to the trachea (*t*) and superior to the dorsal aspect of the aortic arch (*a*).

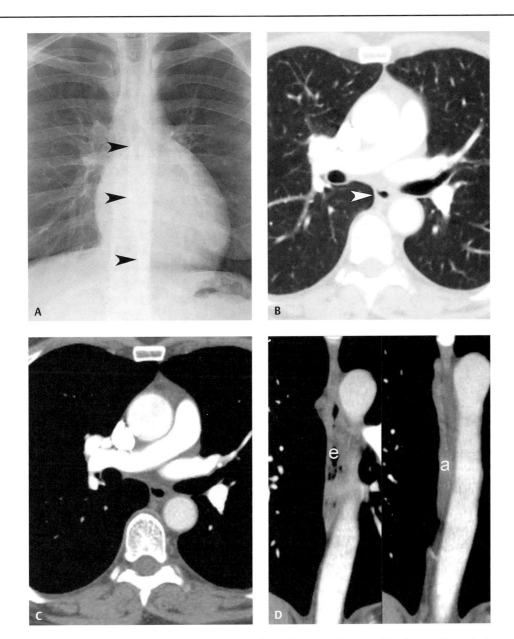

Fig. I.44 Radiologic depiction of the azygoesophageal recess. **(A)** Normal PA chest radiograph demonstrates the normal course and contour of the azygoesophageal recess (*black arrowheads*). **(B)** Axial contrast-enhanced chest CT (lung window and **(C)** mediastinal window) demonstrates the anatomic basis of the azygoesophageal recess (*white arrowhead*) formed by contact of the right lower lobe with the adjacent mediastinum near the esophagus anteriorly and the azygos vein posteriorly **(C)**. **(D)** Coronal chest CT demonstrates the course of the esophagus (*e*) and the azygos vein (*a*).

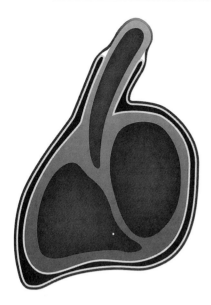

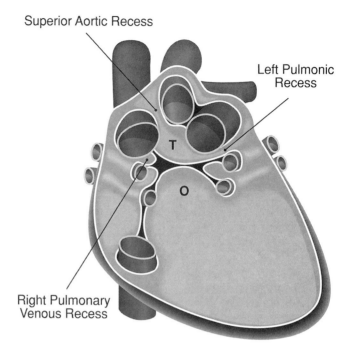

Fig. I.45 Pericardial layers. Artist's illustration of the pericardial layers shows the fibrous pericardium (outer pericardial layer), which defines the anatomic middle mediastinum and is contiguous with the aortic and pulmonary artery adventitia. The serous pericardium is a continuous membrane that lines the fibrous pericardium (serous parietal pericardium) and the heart (serous visceral pericardium).

Fig. I.46 Pericardial sinuses and recesses. Artist's illustration of the serous pericardium, its sinuses and recesses, formed by the pericardial reflections surrounding various vascular structures. Note the oblique sinus (*o*), the transverse sinus (*t*) and three of the pericardial recesses.

The *oblique sinus* is located immediately superior to the left atrium and anterior to the esophagus. It does not give rise to recesses (**Fig. I.47**). The *transverse sinus* is located anterior to the oblique sinus and does not communicate with it (**Fig. I.47**). It gives rise to the superior and inferior aortic recesses, the right and left pulmonic recesses, and the post-caval recess. The *superior aortic recess* (**Figs. I.48, I.49**) is frequently identified and has anterior (**Fig. I.49**), lateral (**Fig. I.49A**), and posterior portions (**Figs. I.48, I.49**). The anterior portion of the superior aortic recess insinuates between the pulmonary trunk and the ascending aorta (**Fig. I.49**). The posterior portion of the superior aortic recess has a semilunar shape and is intimately related to the posterior wall of the ascending aorta (**Figs. I.48, I.49**). The *right* and *left pulmonic recesses* (**Fig. I.50**) are located immediately below the respective pulmonary arteries. The *post-caval recess* is located posterior to the superior vena cava.

The pericardial space proper gives rise to the *right* and *left pulmonary venous recesses* (**Fig. I.51**). These are in close proximity to the bilateral pulmonary veins and may mimic lymph node enlargement.

■ Chest Wall

Various soft-tissue structures of the chest wall may be seen on chest radiography. Those most frequently observed include sternocleidomastoid muscles, breast tissue, and pectoralis muscles (anterior axillary fold) (**Fig. I.52**). *Companion shadows* are smooth, homogeneous opacities with a well-defined margin paralleling bony structures and should not be confused with chest wall or pleural pathology. The three most common companion shadows are the *clavicular companion shadow*, a thin soft-tissue stripe along the upper edge of the clavicle (**Fig. I.53A**); *rib companion shadows*, comprised of fat and muscles, which parallel ribs in the intercostal space and measure 1–5 mm in thickness, and are best seen adjacent to the inferior and inferolateral margins of the first and second ribs (**Fig. I.53B**) and axillary portions of the lower ribs; and the *scapular companion shadow*, which parallels the medial scapular border and can be mistaken for a pleural-based lesion.

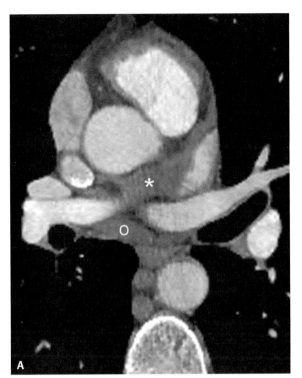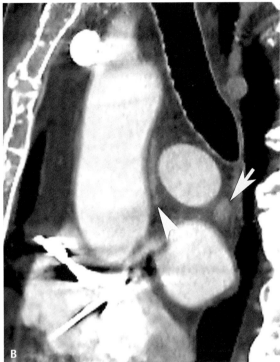

Fig. I.47 CT depiction of the oblique and transverse sinus. Axial contrast-enhanced chest CT (mediastinal window) demonstrates the oblique sinus (*o*) and the transverse sinus (*asterisk*). **(A)** These pericardial sinuses do not communicate with each other and are separated by a tissue plane. **(B)** Sagittal contrast-enhanced chest CT (mediastinal window) shows the oblique sinus (*arrow*) located above the left atrium and the transverse sinus (*arrowhead*).

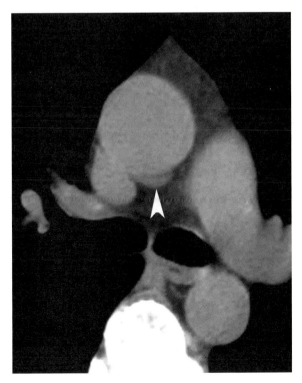

Fig. I.48 Superior aortic recess of the transverse sinus. Axial unenhanced chest CT (mediastinal window) shows the posterior portion of the superior aortic recess of the transverse sinus (*arrowhead*), manifesting as a water attenuation semilunar fluid collection located immediately posterior to the ascending aorta.

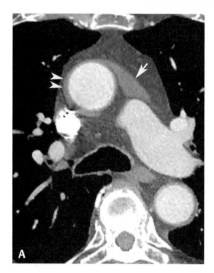
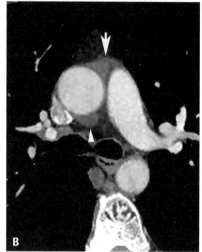

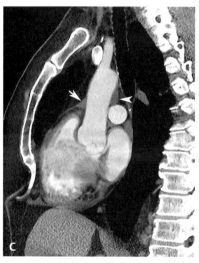

Fig. I.49 Components of the superior aortic recess on CT. **(A,B)** Axial and **(C)** sagittal contrast-enhanced chest CT (mediastinal window) demonstrate the components of the superior aortic recess: the posterior (*arrowheads*), anterior (*arrows*) and lateral (*double arrowheads*) portions.

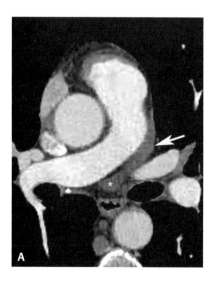
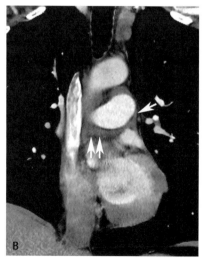

Fig. I.50 The pulmonic recesses on CT. **(A)** Axial and **(B)** coronal contrast-enhanced chest CT (mediastinal window) demonstrate the right (*arrow*) and left (*double arrows*) pulmonic recesses located below the corresponding pulmonary arteries and arising from the transverse sinus (*asterisk*).

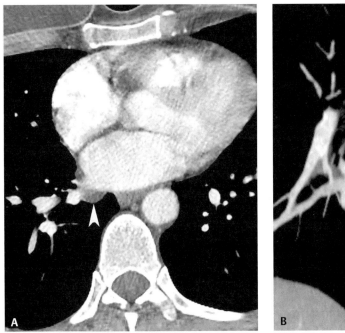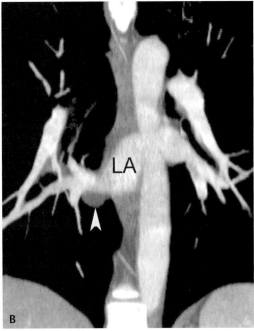

Fig. I.51 Right pulmonary venous recesses on CT. **(A)** Axial and **(B)** coronal contrast-enhanced chest CT (mediastinal window) demonstrate the right pulmonary venous recess (*arrowheads*). It is located adjacent to the right inferior pulmonary vein seen anastomosing with the adjacent left atrium (*LA*). Its characteristic location, attenuation and shape allows distinction from lymphadenopathy.

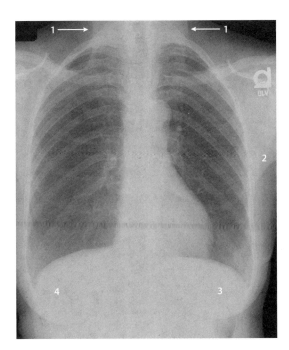

Fig. I.52 PA chest radiograph shows normal soft tissues of the chest wall. *1*, sternocleidomastoid muscles; *2*, axillary fold; *3*, left breast shadow; *4*, right breast shadow.

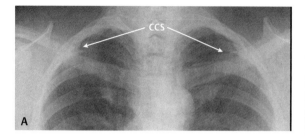

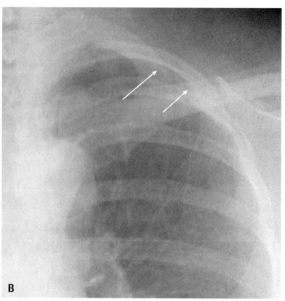

Fig. I.53 Normal companion shadows. **(A)** Coned-down PA chest radiograph over the upper thorax reveals a thin soft-tissue stripe paralleling the upper edge of each clavicle. *CCS*, clavicular companion shadows. **(B)** Coned-down PA chest X-ray over the upper left thorax reveals a radio-opaque stripe along the inferolateral margins of the first and second ribs representing the rib companion shadow (*arrows*).

Costochondral calcification is a common finding that increases in frequency with age. The pattern of calcification varies with the patient's sex. In men, the superior and inferior borders of the cartilage tend to calcify, whereas in women, the central cartilage calcifies.

The normal chest wall musculature is clearly demonstrated on both MDCT and MRI studies. Those muscles the radiologist should be most familiar with and able to recognize are highlighted in **Fig. I.54** and **Fig. I.55**. Congenital and pathologic processes affecting the chest wall are discussed further in Section XII.

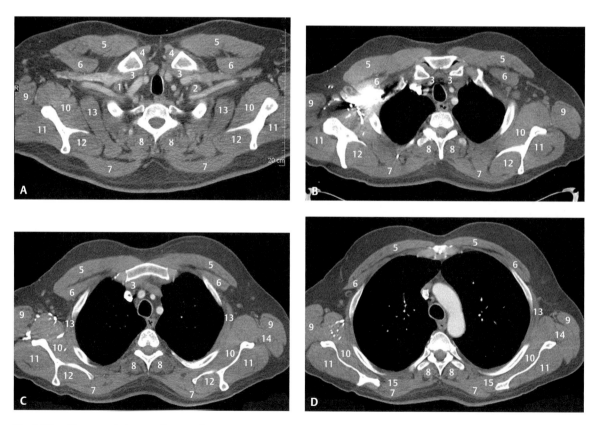

Fig. I.54 CT—normal chest wall musculature.

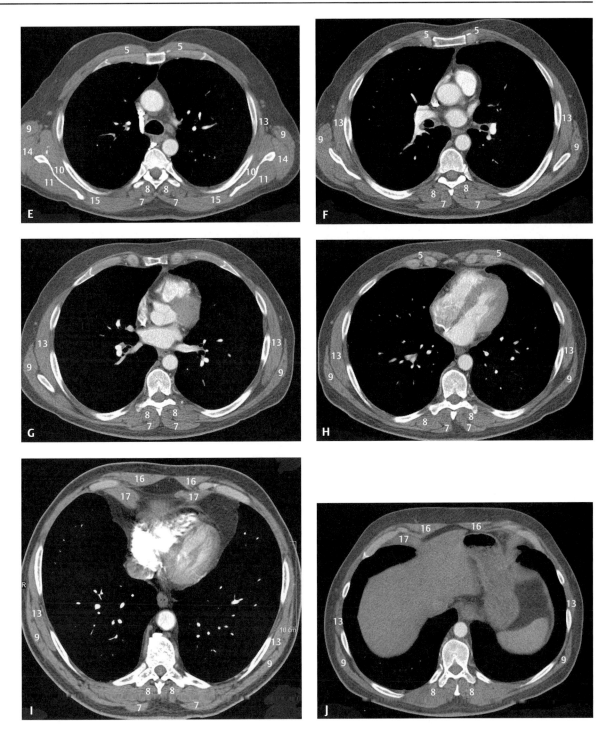

Fig. I.54 *(Continued)* CT—normal chest wall musculature. *1*, right anterior scalene muscle; *2*, left anterior scalene muscle; *3*, sternothyroid-sternohyoid muscles; *4*, sternocleidomastoid muscles; *5*, pectoralis major muscle; *6*, pectoralis minor muscle; *7*, trapezius muscle; *8*, erector spinae muscle; *9*, latissimus dorsi muscle; *10*, subscapularis muscle; *11*, infraspinatus muscle; *12*, supraspinatus muscle; *13*, serratus anterior muscle; *14*, teres major muscle; *15*, rhomboid major muscle; *16*, rectus abdominis muscle; *17*, diaphragm.

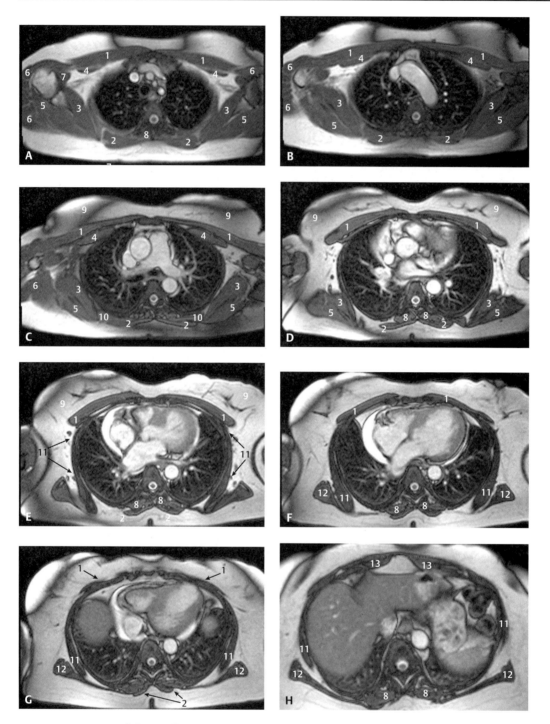

Fig. I.55 MRI—normal chest wall musculature (SSFP pulse sequence). *1*, pectoralis major muscle; *2*, trapezius muscle; *3*, subscapularis muscle; *4*, pectoralis minor muscle; *5*, infraspinatus muscle; *6*, deltoid muscle; *7*, coracobrachialis muscle; *8*, erector spinae muscle; *9*, breast tissue; *10*, rhomboid major muscle; *11*, serratus anterior muscle; *12*, latissimus dorsi muscle; *13*, rectus abdominis muscle.

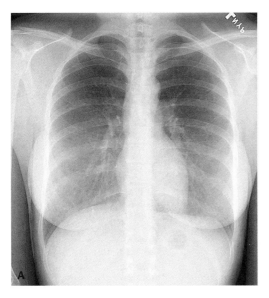 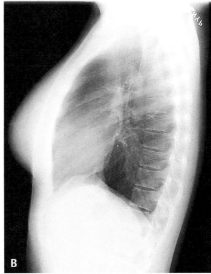

Fig. I.56 **(A)** PA and **(B)** lateral chest radiographs demonstrate the normal relationships of the right and left hemidiaphragms.

■ Diaphragm (Fig. I.56)

The diaphragm is a muscular tendinous sheath that separates the thorax from the abdomen. It is supplied by the phrenic and intercostal arteries, and branches of the internal mammary artery, and is innervated by the phrenic nerve. The right hemidiaphragm is usually one-half an interspace higher than the left, and the heart usually obscures the anterior and medial portion of the left hemidiaphragm. The diaphragm is usually smooth and uniform in contour, but arcuate elevations or scalloping may be seen in 5% of normal individuals. Diaphragmatic abnormalities are discussed further in Section XII.

Suggested Reading

1. Aquino SL, Duncan G, Taber KH, Sharma A, Hayman LA. Reconciliation of the anatomic, surgical, and radiographic classifications of the mediastinum. J Comput Assist Tomogr 2001;25(3):489–492

2. Berkmen T, Berkmen YM, Austin JH. Accessory fissures of the upper lobe of the left lung: CT and plain film appearance. AJR Am J Roentgenol 1994;162(6):1287–1293

3. Brant WE, Helms CA. Methods of examination and normal anatomy. In: Fundamentals of Diagnostic Radiology, 2nd ed. Philadelphia: Lippincott, William & Wilkins; 1999:295–318

4. Felson BF. Localization of intrathoracic lesions. In: Chest Roentgenology. Philadelphia: WB Saunders; 1973:39–41

5. Felson BF. The hila and pulmonary vessels. In: Chest Roentgenology. Philadelphia: WB Saunders; 1973:185–250

6. Felson B. The mediastinum. In: Chest Roentgenology. Philadelphia: WB Saunders; 1973:380–420

7. Franquet T, Erasmus JJ, Giménez A, Rossi S, Prats R. The retrotracheal space: normal anatomic and pathologic appearances. Radiographics 2002;22(Spec No):S231–S246

8. Fraser RS, Müller NL, Colman N, et al. The normal chest. In: Fraser RS, Müller NL, Colman N, Paré PD, eds. Fraser and Paré's Diagnosis of Diseases of the Chest, 4th ed. Philadelphia: Saunders; 1999:1–280

9. Fraser RS, Müller NL, Colman N, et al. Masses situated predominantly in the anterior compartment. In: Fraser RS, Müller NL, Colman N, Paré PD, eds. Fraser and Paré's Diagnosis of Diseases of the Chest, 4th ed. Philadelphia: Saunders; 1999: 2875–2937

10. Gibbs JM, Chandrasekhar CA, Ferguson EC, Oldham SA. Lines and stripes: where did they go?—From conventional radiography to CT. Radiographics 2007;27(1):33–48

11. Goldstraw P, Crowley JJ, Chansky K, et al; International Association for the Study of Lung Cancer International Staging Committee; Participating Institutions. The IASLC Lung Cancer Staging Project: proposals for the revision of the TNM stage groupings in the forthcoming (seventh) edition of the TNM Classification of Malignant Tumours. J Thorac Oncol 2007;2(8):706–714

12. Kligerman S, Abbott G. A radiologic review of the new TNM classification for lung cancer. AJR Am J Roentgenol 2010;194(3):562–573

13. Lacomis JM, Wigginton W, Fuhrman CR, Schwartzman D, Armfield DR, Pealer KM. Multi-detector row CT of the left atrium and pulmonary veins before radio-frequency catheter ablation for atrial fibrillation. Radiographics 2003;23(Spec No):S35–S48, discussion S48–S50

14. Moore KL, Dalley AF. Thorax. In: Moore KL, Dalley AF, eds. Clinically Oriented Anatomy, 5th ed. Philadelphia: Lippincott, Williams and Wilkins; 2006:75–191

15. Mountain CF, Dresler CM. Regional lymph node classification for lung cancer staging. Chest 1997;111(6): 1718–1723

16. Proto AV, Speckman JM. The left lateral radiograph of the chest. I. Med Radiogr Photogr 1979;55:30–42

17. Proto AV, Speckman JM. The left lateral radiograph of the chest. Med Radiogr Photogr 1980;56(3):38–64

18. Truong MT, Erasmus JJ, Gladish GW, et al. Anatomy of pericardial recesses on multidetector CT: implications for oncologic imaging. AJR Am J Roentgenol 2003;181(4):1109–1113

19. Whitten CR, Khan S, Munneke GJ, Grubnic S. A diagnostic approach to mediastinal abnormalities. Radiographics 2007;27(3):657–671

20. Woodburne RT, Burkel WE. Essentials of Human Anatomy, 9th ed. New York: Oxford University Press; 1994:370–371

Section II

Developmental Anomalies

OVERVIEW OF DEVELOPMENTAL ANOMALIES

Congenital lesions of the *thorax* include a variety of malformations that occur during various stages of embryologic development. Many of these lesions manifest in neonates, infants, and children, but in some cases, the first clinical manifestations may not occur until adulthood. This section discusses common congenital lesions that characteristically affect adults. These include abnormalities of the airways, heart, and thoracic vascular structures (**Table II.1**).

Many congenital lesions of the *airways* and *lungs* occur early in embryologic development and involve anomalous development of the primitive foregut. These lesions include variant tracheobronchial branching, tracheoesophageal abnormalities, congenital foregut cysts, and pulmonary sequestrations. Congenital tracheoesophageal abnormalities are typically diagnosed in infancy. Congenital foregut cysts are characteristically located in the mediastinum and are discussed in Section XI. Although intralobar sequestration is thought to represent an acquired condition in most instances, it will be discussed in this section to compare and contrast it with congenital extralobar sequestration, which typically affects neonates and young infants (**Table II.2**). Some congenital lesions of the airways (e.g., bronchial atresia) occur later in embryologic life with relatively normal distal bronchopulmonary development.

Vascular lesions comprise many of the congenital lesions characteristically diagnosed in adults. These include lesions related to abnormal development of the aorta and its branches as well as variant development of the pulmonary venous system, including both the systemic and pulmonary veins. While congenital heart disease is often diagnosed in infancy, some congenital anomalies may produce few symptoms and may remain clinically silent until adulthood. Various abnormalities of situs may be associated with non-cyanotic asymptomatic or minimally symptomatic congenital heart disease and may be incidentally diagnosed in asymptomatic adults.

Congenital lesions characteristically diagnosed in utero or in infancy and early childhood are beyond the scope of this book and belong in the discussion of pediatric conditions affecting the chest. It should be noted that some lesions (such as intralobar sequestration and pulmonary varix) may have both developmental and acquired etiologies, which complicates their classification.

Table II.1 Congenital Lesions in Adults

Airway/lung	Tracheal bronchus
	Bronchial atresia
	Pulmonary sequestration
Vascular	**Systemic arteries**
	Right aortic arch
	Aortic coarctation
	Marfan syndrome
	Aberrant right subclavian artery
	Systemic veins
	Persistent left superior vena cava
	Interruption of the IVC with azygos continuation
	Pulmonary arteries/veins
	Arteriovenous malformation
	Pulmonary veins
	Partial anomalous pulmonary venous return
	Scimitar syndrome
	Pulmonary varix
	Heart
	Heterotaxy
	Atrial septal defect
	Heart valves
	Pulmonic stenosis

Table II.2   Pulmonary Sequestrations

	Intralobar	Extralobar
Age	Children/adults	Neonate/infant
Gender	M = F	4M:1F
Clinical	Infection	Mass effect
Location	Lower lobe (L > R)	Extrapulmonary
Associated anomalies	Rare	Common
Blood supply	Systemic	Systemic
Venous drainage	Systemic	Pulmonary
Borders	Irregular	Well defined
Lesion	Heterogeneous: air, air-fluid levels	Homogeneous or fluid-filled cysts

CASE 1

■ Clinical Presentation

74-year-old man evaluated for exacerbation of chronic obstructive pulmonary disease

■ Radiologic Findings

Axial and coronal chest CT (lung window) (**Figs. 1.1, 1.2**) demonstrates a right tracheal bronchus. A normal right upper lobe apical segmental bronchus was not present. Volume-rendered surface display (**Fig. 1.3**) demonstrates an anomalous bronchus arising from the right lateral tracheal wall (*arrow*). Artist's illustration (**Fig. 1.4**) depicts variations of right-sided anomalous bronchial branching. The tracheal bronchus (TB) arises from the lateral tracheal wall. The pre-eparterial bronchus (Pre-EAB) arises from the right mainstem bronchus proximal to the origin of the right upper lobe bronchus. The post-eparterial bronchus (Post-EAB) arises distal to the origin of the right upper lobe bronchus. The accessory cardiac bronchus (ACB) arises from the medial wall of the right mainstem bronchus or the bronchus intermedius and is usually blind-ending.

■ Diagnosis

Tracheal Bronchus

■ Differential Diagnosis

- Tracheal Diverticulum
- Tracheal Air Cyst

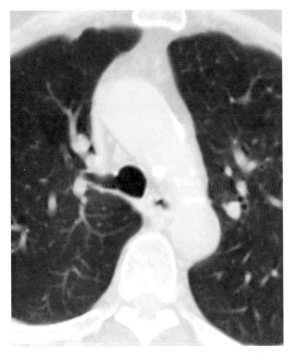

Fig. 1.1

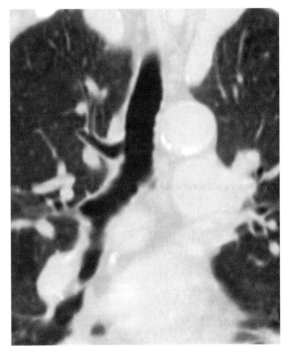

Fig. 1.2

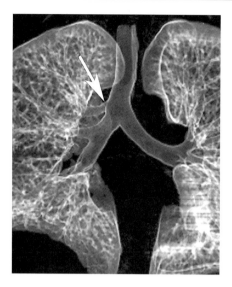

Fig. 1.3

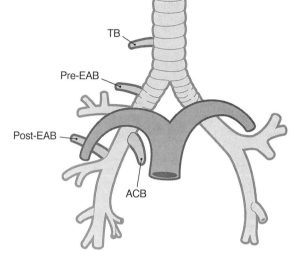

Fig. 1.4

■ Discussion

Background

Variations of bronchial branching are common, may affect all portions of the tracheobronchial tree, and are usually discovered incidentally. Tracheal bronchus is characterized by its anomalous origin from the lateral tracheal wall (usually within 2.0 cm from the carina) and typically supplies the right upper lobe. It is also known as "pig bronchus" or "bronchus suis" (the usual anatomic bronchial morphology in pigs and certain other mammals). Other right-sided anomalous bronchi are classified as *pre-eparterial* or *post-eparterial* if they arise proximal or distal to the origin of the right upper lobe bronchus respectively (and distal to the carina). The terms *pre-hyparterial* and *post-hyparterial* are used for left-sided anomalous bronchi that arise proximal or distal to the left upper lobe bronchus respectively. Upper lobe anomalous bronchi are seven times more common on the right than on the left. *Displaced* (absent equivalent lobar, segmental or subsegmental bronchus) and *supernumerary* (coexistent normal upper lobe bronchial anatomy) anomalous bronchi occur; the former are more frequent. A displaced pre-eparterial bronchus arising from the right mainstem bronchus to supply the apical segment of the right upper lobe is the most common variant (**Fig. 1.2**). Tracheobronchial diverticula are blind ending airway outpouchings not surrounded by lung parenchyma.

Etiology

Tracheobronchial development occurs during the early embryonic period (26 days to six weeks). The normal five lobar bronchi appear by 32 days of gestation. While the precise etiology of tracheal (and other anomalous) bronchi is not known, regression of anomalous bronchial buds, migration of primitive bronchi to anomalous positions, and induction of anomalous bronchial branches by surrounding primitive mesenchyme have all been suggested as possible mechanisms. Associated conditions include vascular abnormalities (e.g., anomalous venous drainage), accessory lobes and fissures, rib anomalies, tracheoesophageal fistula, tracheobronchial stenosis, and trisomy 21.

Clinical Findings

Most adults with anomalous bronchi are asymptomatic and are diagnosed incidentally on chest CT. The reported prevalence of tracheal bronchus in adults is 0.1%. However, affected patients may present in infancy or childhood with recurrent pulmonary infection, cough, stridor, hemoptysis, or respiratory distress. Recurrent upper lobe consolidation, bronchiectasis, atelectasis, and emphysema are reported in affected symptomatic children.

Imaging Findings

Radiography

- Normal chest radiograph
- Rare visualization of anomalous bronchi
- Segmental or lobar right upper lobe atelectasis/consolidation

MDCT

- Visualization of anomalous bronchus originating from lateral tracheal wall (**Figs. 1.1, 1.2, 1.3**) or proximal mainstem bronchus
- Multiplanar reformations, shaded surface displays (**Fig. 1.3**), volume rendering, and virtual bronchoscopy techniques useful in anatomic characterization and classification

Management

- None for asymptomatic individuals
- Excision of anomalous bronchus and associated lung tissue in patients with recurrent infection

Prognosis

- Good (particularly without associated anomalies)

PEARLS

- Recognition of asymptomatic tracheal bronchi is important in patients undergoing endotracheal intubation as an appropriately positioned endotracheal tube may occlude the anomalous bronchus with resultant obstruction and potential pulmonary infection.
- *Accessory cardiac bronchus* is an anomalous bronchus that arises from the medial aspect of the right mainstem or intermediate bronchus and courses caudally toward the heart and mediastinum (hence the "cardiac" designation) (**Fig. 1.5**). It is typically blind-ending but may be surrounded by normal or vestigial lung parenchyma. Affected patients are often asymptomatic, but hemoptysis and recurrent infection have been reported.
- Tracheobronchial diverticula are blind-ending airways that often arise from the mainstem bronchi (**Fig. 1.6**).
- Tracheal air cysts (**Fig. 1.7**) are tracheal diverticula manifesting as air-filled thin-walled blind-ending structures at the thoracic inlet. These exhibit a normal mucosal lining and cartilage within their walls.

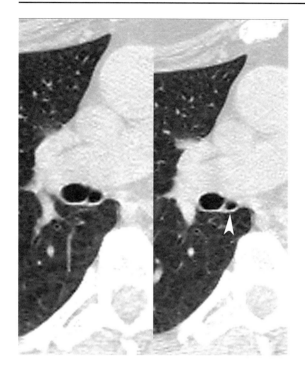

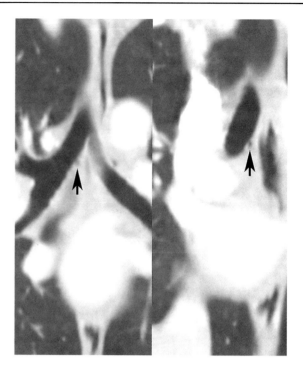

Fig. 1.5 Composite image from a chest CT (lung window) shows an incidental accessory cardiac bronchus found in a 52-year-old woman evaluated for chronic dyspnea. The accessory cardiac bronchus manifests as an air-filled tubular structure arising from the medial wall of the bronchus intermedius and coursing inferomedially (*arrowhead*).

Fig. 1.6 Composite image from a chest CT (lung window) with coronal and oblique reformatted images demonstrates a tiny tracheal diverticulum (*black arrows*) arising from the medial wall of the right mainstem bronchus.

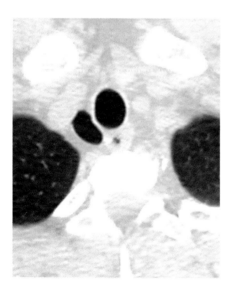

Fig. 1.7 Coned-down chest CT (lung window) shows a right tracheal air cyst manifesting as an ovoid air-filled structure located to the right of the trachea near the thoracic inlet.

Suggested Reading

1. Berrocal T, Madrid C, Novo S, Gutiérrez J, Arjonilla A, Gómez-León N. Congenital anomalies of the tracheobronchial tree, lung, and mediastinum: embryology, radiology, and pathology. Radiographics 2004;24(1):e17

2. Ghaye B, Szapiro D, Fanchamps J-M, Dondelinger RF. Congenital bronchial abnormalities revisited. Radiographics 2001;21(1):105–119

3. Yedururi S, Guillerman RP, Chung T, et al. Multimodality imaging of tracheobronchial disorders in children. Radiographics 2008;28(3):e29

4. Zylak CJ, Eyler WR, Spizarny DL, Stone CH. Developmental lung anomalies in the adult: radiologic-pathologic correlation. Radiographics 2002;22(Spec No):S25–S43

CASE 2

■ Clinical Presentation

Asymptomatic 42-year-old woman

■ Radiologic Findings

PA (**Fig. 2.1**) chest radiograph demonstrates a left lower lobe branching tubular opacity (*arrow*). Chest CT (lung window) (**Figs. 2.2, 2.3**) shows the branching tubular lesion (**Fig. 2.3**) surrounded by hyperlucent lung. Artist's illustration (**Fig. 2.4**) shows the proposed etiology of bronchial atresia: an interruption of the bronchial lumen produces a mucocele distal to the atresia formed by accumulation of secretions (carried centrally by the mucociliary escalator).

■ Diagnosis

Bronchial Atresia

■ Differential Diagnosis

*   Mucoid Impaction Distal to Bronchial Obstruction (e.g., endobronchial neoplasm)
*   Focal Bronchiectasis with Mucoid Impaction
*   Allergic Bronchopulmonary Fungal Disease
*   Vascular Malformation
*   Intralobar Sequestration

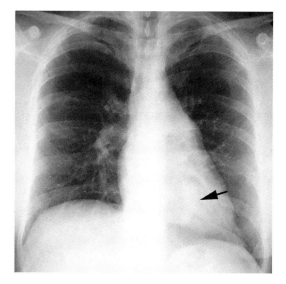

Fig. 2.1

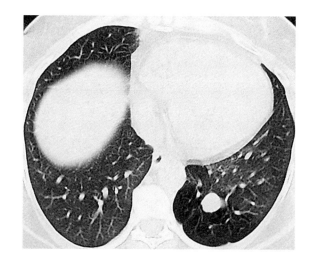

Fig. 2.2

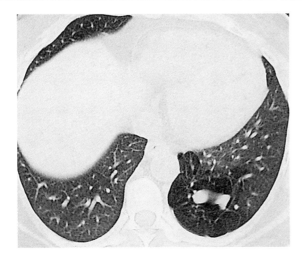

Fig. 2.3

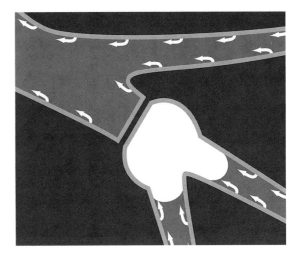

Fig. 2.4

■ Discussion

Background

Bronchial atresia is a rare congenital anomaly that typically affects segmental bronchi, although lobar and sub-segmental bronchi may also be involved. The left upper lobe bronchus (apical-posterior segment) is affected in approximately 64% of cases, followed by involvement of segmental right upper, middle, and lower lobe bronchi. Most cases of bronchial atresia are isolated, but associated congenital anomalies have been reported.

Etiology

Bronchial atresia is thought to result from an in-utero vascular insult that affects the blood supply to a small segment of the tracheobronchial tree, with resultant complete interruption (atresia/stenosis) of the airway lumen with development of the distal airways. The surrounding alveoli may fail to develop normally and may overinflate because of collateral air drift through pores of Kohn, canals of Lambert, or other communications. Endoluminal debris accumulating distal to the atresia may form a mucocele (**Fig. 2.4**). Another theory postulates multiplying bronchial bud cells that lose connection with the proximal tracheobronchial tree.

Clinical Findings

Patients with bronchial atresia exhibit a wide age range but are often asymptomatic adults diagnosed incidentally on chest radiography. Up to 40% present with cough, dyspnea, bronchospasm, or symptoms of pulmonary infection. Men are more frequently affected than women.

Imaging Findings

Radiography

- Focal pulmonary overinflation
- Rounded, tubular, or branching opacity (mucocele) (**Fig. 2.1**)
- Focal overinflation surrounding mucocele
- Expiratory air trapping surrounding mucocele
- Air-fluid level within mucocele (with superimposed infection)

MDCT

- Rounded (**Fig. 2.2**), branching (**Figs. 2.3, 2.5**), or tubular (**Fig. 2.6**) typically central opacity; low attenuation (–5 to 25 HU) (**Figs. 2.5, 2.6**)
- Absence of contrast enhancement within bronchus or mucocele (**Figs. 2.5, 2.6**)
- Overinflated lung surrounding mucocele (**Figs. 2.2, 2.3, 2.5, 2.6**)

MRI

- Visualization of mucocele with high signal intensity on T1- and T2-weighted images

Management

- Observation of asymptomatic patients (clinical/radiographic follow-up)
- Lobectomy/segmentectomy in chronically symptomatic patients

Prognosis

- Excellent

PEARLS

- Bronchial atresia is a radiologic diagnosis based on the demonstration of a central mucocele surrounded by pulmonary overinflation (**Figs. 2.2, 2.3, 2.5, 2.6**). The tubular morphology of the mucocele may suggest a vascular etiology, which is excluded by absence of contrast enhancement (**Figs. 2.5, 2.6**) and absence of communication with pulmonary vessels.
- Mucoid impaction may result from a slow-growing central obstructing endobronchial neoplasm. Thus, contrast-enhanced chest CT and/or endoscopic examination may be required.

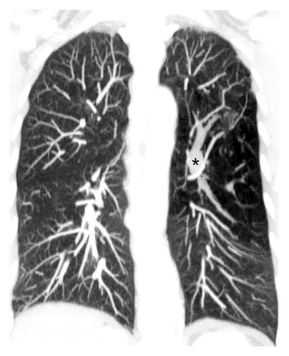

Fig. 2.5 Coronal MIP image from a contrast-enhanced chest CT (lung window) of an asymptomatic 52-year-old woman with left lower lobe bronchial atresia demonstrates a soft tissue branching opacity (*asterisk*) surrounded by hyperlucent lung.

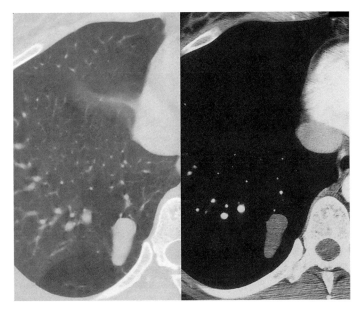

Fig. 2.6 Composite contrast-enhanced chest CT (lung and mediastinal window) of an asymptomatic young woman with bronchial atresia demonstrates a non-enhancing low-attenuation tubular opacity in the right lower lobe with surrounding pulmonary hyperlucency characteristic of bronchial atresia. Absence of enhancement or communication with pulmonary vessels excludes a vascular lesion. (*Images courtesy of Jill D. Wruble, DO, Danbury Radiology Associates, Danbury, CT.*)

Suggested Reading

1. Berrocal T, Madrid C, Novo S, Gutiérrez J, Arjonilla A, Gómez-León N. Congenital anomalies of the tracheobronchial tree, lung, and mediastinum: embryology, radiology, and pathology. Radiographics 2004;24(1):e17

2. Gipson MG, Cummings KW, Hurth KM. Bronchial atresia. Radiographics 2009;29(5):1531–1535

3. Yedururi S, Guillerman RP, Chung T, et al. Multimodality imaging of tracheobronchial disorders in children. Radiographics 2008;28(3):e29

4. Zylak CJ, Eyler WR, Spizarny DL, Stone CH. Developmental lung anomalies in the adult: radiologic-pathologic correlation. Radiographics 2002;22(Spec No):S25–S43

CASE 3

■ Clinical Presentation

37-year-old woman with recurrent pneumonia and productive cough

■ Radiologic Findings

PA (**Fig. 3.1**) and lateral (**Fig. 3.2**) chest radiographs demonstrate a left lower lobe thin-walled multilocular cystic lesion with a large air-fluid level. Contrast-enhanced chest CT (mediastinal window) (**Fig. 3.3**) through the inferior chest demonstrates a heterogeneously enhancing left lower lobe lesion with soft tissue, air, and fluid attenuation components, supplied by a branch of the descending thoracic aorta (*arrowhead*). Coronal gradient-echo MRA (**Fig. 3.4**) demonstrates the aortic arterial branch (*arrow*) that supplies the lesion.

■ Diagnosis

Intralobar Sequestration

■ Differential Diagnosis

- Pneumonia (including post-obstructive pneumonia from central obstruction)
- Lung Abscess
- Bronchiectasis (with secondary infection)
- Infected Bullae

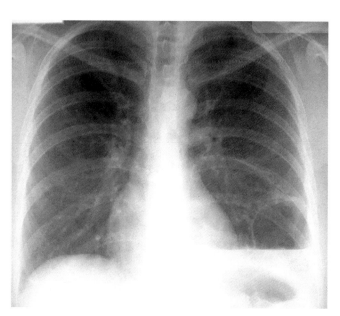

Fig. 3.1

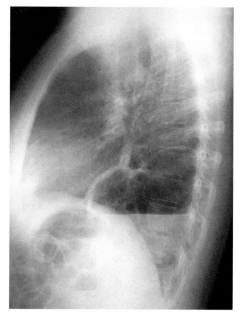

Fig. 3.2

66

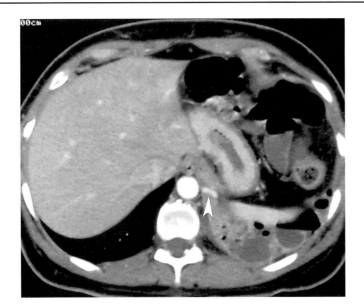

Fig. 3.3

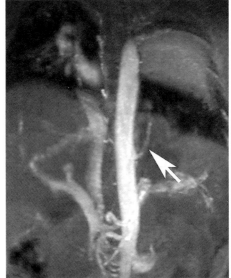

Fig. 3.4

■ Discussion

Background

The term *pulmonary sequestration* refers to lung parenchyma that does not communicate normally with the tracheobronchial tree and has a systemic blood supply. *Intralobar sequestrations* are four times more frequent than *extralobar sequestrations* and occur almost exclusively in the lower lobes, slightly more frequently on the left. The systemic arterial supply to the lesion often courses within the pulmonary ligament and typically originates from the descending aorta, although other systemic arteries (abdominal aorta, inferior phrenic, coronary) may participate. The venous drainage is typically (95%) normal into the pulmonary veins. The lesion is often heterogeneous due to acute and chronic inflammation and bronchopneumonia with resultant bronchiectasis, fibrosis, and cystic change. The lesion typically abuts adjacent normal (non-sequestered) lung.

Extralobar sequestrations represent accessory pulmonary lobes that result from abnormal foregut budding and are located outside the confines of normal lung. They may occur in the thorax, diaphragm, or abdomen; are characteristically supplied and drained by the systemic circulation; and represent true congenital anomalies. Affected patients are typically diagnosed within the first 6 months of life, but a small number of lesions (10%) are diagnosed in asymptomatic adults.

Etiology

The majority of intralobar sequestrations are thought to represent acquired lesions, which result from lower lobe bronchial obstruction and subsequent distal infection. It is postulated that the normal pulmonary arterial supply to the infected lung is obliterated by the inflammatory process, and that normal systemic pulmonary ligament arteries (which arise from the thoracic aorta) are parasitized to supply the affected lung. A small number of intralobar sequestrations represent true congenital anomalies.

Clinical Findings

Patients with intralobar sequestration are often older children and young adults, but approximately 50% are over the age of 20 years. Men and women are equally affected. Presenting symptoms include chronic cough, sputum production, recurrent pneumonia, chest pain, bronchospasm, and hemoptysis. Some patients present with acute, chronic, or recurrent lower lobe infection. A small percentage of patients (15%) are asymptomatic and are diagnosed because of an incidentally discovered radiographic abnormality.

Imaging Findings

Radiography

- Typical location: posterior basal segment of a lower lobe (98%), more frequently the left (**Figs. 3.1, 3.2**)
- Consolidation or mass; may contain air, fluid, and/or air-fluid levels (**Figs. 3.1, 3.2**), and multilocular cystic areas (**Figs. 3.1, 3.2**); irregular margins typical, but may exhibit well-defined borders
- Predominantly cystic lesions; exhibit a single cyst or multiple cysts of variable sizes
- Rarely, branching tubular opacities representing mucoid impacted bronchi
- Surrounding lung may be hyperlucent
- May produce mass effect on adjacent structures

MDCT

- Posteromedial lower lobe location (**Figs. 3.3, 3.5, 3.6**)
- Homogeneous or heterogeneous mass (**Fig. 3.5**)
- Homogeneous or heterogeneous consolidation
- Smooth, lobular, or irregular (**Fig. 3.5**) borders against adjacent lung
- Typically heterogeneous attenuation with air-filled and fluid-filled components, and/or air-fluid levels (**Figs. 3.3, 3.5**)
- Heterogeneous enhancement (**Figs. 3.3, 3.5**)
- Hyperlucent (**Fig. 3.6**) or predominantly cystic lesion with single or multiple thin-walled cysts; may contain air and/or fluid
- Demonstration of anomalous systemic arterial supply (usually from descending aorta) in up to 80% of cases (**Figs. 3.3, 3.6**); CT angiography with multiplanar reformatted images may enhance visualization of anomalous vessel

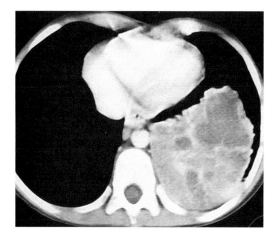

Fig. 3.5 Contrast-enhanced chest CT (mediastinal window) of a 6-year-old with a left lower lobe intralobar sequestration demonstrates a heterogeneously enhancing multicystic mass with irregular borders.

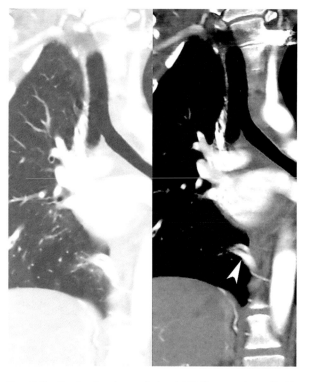

Fig. 3.6 Contrast-enhanced chest CT (lung and mediastinal window) of a 25-year-old woman with right lower lobe intralobar sequestration manifesting as hyperlucent lung parenchyma supplied by aberrant systemic vessels (*arrowhead*) arising from the celiac axis.

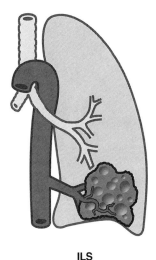

ILS

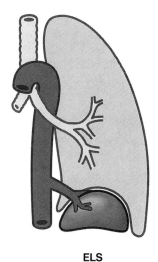

ELS

Fig. 3.7 Artist's illustration (*left*) depicts the heterogeneous morphology and typical lower lobe location of intralobar sequestration and the homogeneous morphology of extralobar sequestration (*right*) and its location outside the confines of the normal lung. Both lesions are supplied by systemic arteries. Intralobar sequestration has a normal (pulmonary) venous drainage and extralobar sequestration has a systemic venous drainage.

MRI

- Heterogeneous intrapulmonary lower lobe lesion; may exhibit cystic areas
- Gradient-echo sequences may demonstrate systemic blood supply (**Fig. 3.4**) and pulmonary venous drainage

Angiography

- Aortography for demonstration of anomalous systemic arterial supply (single or multiple vessels) arising from descending aorta in up to 73% of cases, or other systemic abdominal arteries
- Selective angiography of anomalous systemic artery may allow demonstration of pulmonary venous drainage

Management

- Surgical excision of affected lobe and ligation of anomalous feeding vessels

Prognosis

- Excellent

PEARLS

- Intralobar sequestration must be considered in the differential diagnosis of any patient who presents with recurrent infection or a chronic radiologic abnormality in a lower lobe. The diagnosis is based on identification of systemic arterial supply to the lesion (**Figs. 3.3, 3.4, 3.6**).
- Differentiation from extralobar sequestration is not always necessary but can usually be made based on clinical and morphologic features.
  - *Intralobar sequestration* typically manifests in children and adults with signs and symptoms of infection, while *extralobar sequestration* usually affects neonates and infants who present with respiratory distress.
  - As its name implies, *intralobar sequestration* is always located within lung, typically in a lower lobe (**Fig. 3.7,** left). As a result, it often exhibits irregular margins against the adjacent (non-sequestered) lung and may contain air. *Extralobar sequestration* occurs outside normal lung and typically demonstrates a well-defined border (**Fig. 3.7,** right) and does not contain air.

- ◦ Both lesions are supplied by the systemic circulation (**Fig. 3.7**), although the pulmonary arteries may partially supply both lesions.
- Preoperative imaging allows delineation of the number and location of systemic feeding arteries and may be helpful in surgical planning for ligation and control of these vessels.

Suggested Reading

1. Abbey P, Das CJ, Pangtey GS, Seith A, Dutta R, Kumar A. Imaging in bronchopulmonary sequestration. J Med Imaging Radiat Oncol 2009;53(1):22–31

2. Frazier AA, Rosado de Christenson ML, Stocker JT, Templeton PA. Intralobar sequestration: radiologic-pathologic correlation. Radiographics 1997;17(3):725–745

3. Lee EY, Boiselle PM, Cleveland RH. Multidetector CT evaluation of congenital lung anomalies. Radiology 2008;247(3): 632–648

4. Zylak CJ, Eyler WR, Spizarny DL, Stone CH. Developmental lung anomalies in the adult: radiologic-pathologic correlation. Radiographics 2002;22(Spec No):S25–S43

CASE 4

■ Clinical Presentation

43-year-old man evaluated prior to neck surgery

■ Radiologic Findings

PA (**Fig. 4.1**) chest radiograph demonstrates a right-sided aortic arch with a right descending aorta. Contrast-enhanced chest CT (mediastinal window) (**Figs. 4.2, 4.3**) demonstrates the right aortic arch (*asterisk*) and an aortic diverticulum (*arrowhead*) (**Fig. 4.2**) giving rise to an aberrant left subclavian artery (*arrow*) (**Fig. 4.3**).

■ Diagnosis

Right Aortic Arch with Aberrant Left Subclavian Artery

■ Differential Diagnosis

None

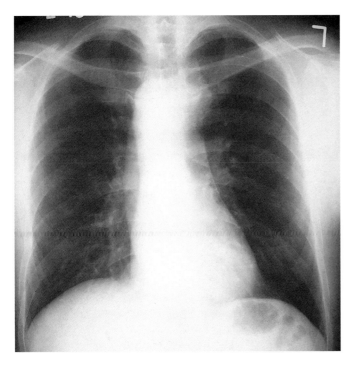

Fig. 4.1

71

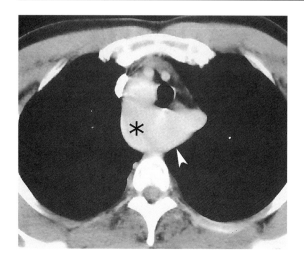

Fig. 4.2

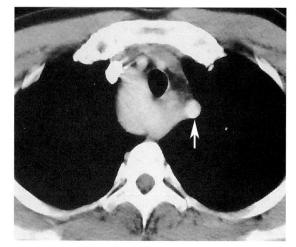

Fig. 4.3

■ Discussion

Background

The aorta and great vessels develop from primitive paired dorsal aortas, which sequentially give rise to six paired primitive arches (**Fig. 4.4**), portions of which sequentially regress. The normal left aortic arch results from persistence of the left fourth primitive arch (**Fig. 4.4**), regression of the right fourth arch beyond the right subclavian artery, and persistence of the left dorsal aorta and the left ductus arteriosus (the latter forms from the left sixth primitive arch). The brachiocephalic, left common carotid, and left subclavian arteries arise in succession from the normal left aortic arch (**Fig. 4.4**). Right aortic arch affects approximately 0.1% of the population. A right aortic arch may exhibit mirror image or non–mirror image branching of the great vessels. In right aortic arch with *mirror image branching*, the left brachiocephalic, right common carotid, and right subclavian arteries arise in succession. The most common type of right aortic arch exhibits *non–mirror image branching*, and the left common carotid, right common carotid, right subclavian, and aberrant left subclavian arteries arise in succession. The aberrant left subclavian artery may be associated with dilatation of its origin (diverticulum of Kommerell). A coexistent left ligamentum arteriosus results in a complete vascular ring.

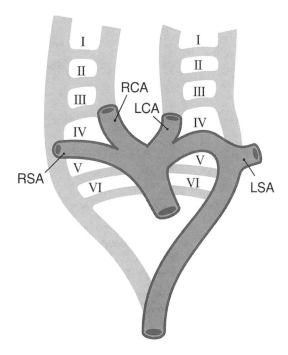

Fig. 4.4 Artist's illustration depicts the normal embryologic development of the aortic arch; several components of the system regress (*broken lines*). Paired dorsal aortas sequentially give rise to six paired arches (*roman numerals*). The normal left aortic arch results from persistence of the left fourth primitive arch and involution of part of the right fourth primitive arch. A portion of the right fourth primitive arch gives rise to the right subclavian artery. Precursors of the right subclavian artery (*RSA*), right carotid artery (*RCA*), left carotid artery (*LCA*), and left subclavian artery (*LSA*) are illustrated.

Etiology

The most common type of right aortic arch (non–mirror image branching) is thought to result from involution of the left fourth primitive arch and persistence of the right fourth arch, which is interrupted between the left common carotid and left subclavian arteries (**Fig. 4.4**), the latter arising from the dorsal aorta as its fourth branch. The diverticulum of Kommerell may be congenital, a remnant of the left fourth aortic arch, or acquired due to atherosclerotic dilatation.

Clinical Presentation

Right aortic arch with aberrant left subclavian artery (retroesophageal segment) and left ductus arteriosus results in a true vascular ring but is not usually associated with congenital heart disease. Affected patients may be asymptomatic or may present with cough, stridor, or dysphagia. Right aortic arch without a retroesophageal arterial segment (mirror image branching) is associated with congenital heart disease (seen in 1.4% of patients with congenital cardiac anomalies), particularly tetralogy of Fallot, persistent truncus arteriosus, transposition of the great vessels with pulmonic stenosis, and ventricular septal defect with infundibular pulmonic stenosis. Associated tracheomalacia may contribute to respiratory symptoms.

Imaging Findings

Radiography

- Right paratracheal soft-tissue mass (**Fig. 4.1**)
  - Vascular impression on the right side of the trachea
  - Rightward azygos vein displacement
- Right or left para-aortic interface depending on location of descending aorta
- Retrotracheal soft-tissue mass from Kommerell diverticulum (at origin of aberrant left subclavian artery) (**Fig. 4.5**)
- Visualization of oblique tubular opacity projecting over the trachea on frontal radiography and coursing toward the left (aberrant left subclavian artery)

MDCT/MRI

- Direct visualization of right aortic arch (**Figs. 4.2, 4.3**)
- Direct visualization of aortic diverticulum (**Fig. 4.3**)
- Direct visualization of aberrant left subclavian artery origin (**Fig. 4.3**)
- Evaluation of mass effect on adjacent mediastinal structures (trachea, esophagus) (**Figs. 4.2, 4.3**)
- Cardiac evaluation to exclude associated congenital heart disease

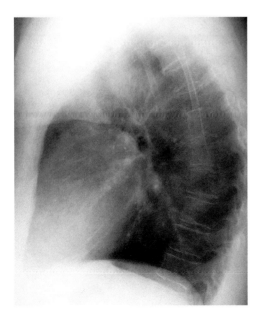

Fig. 4.5 Lateral chest radiograph of a patient with a right aortic arch and an aberrant left subclavian artery who presented with cough and dysphagia demonstrates mass effect on the posterior trachea produced by a diverticulum of Kommerell at the origin of the aberrant left subclavian artery.

Management

- Observation of asymptomatic patients
- Surgical reconstruction in symptomatic patients including arteriopexy, aortopexy, and tracheopexy

Prognosis

- Good for adults without associated congenital anomalies

PEARLS

- Patients with right aortic arch with non–mirror image branching may have a large aortic diverticulum, which may manifest as a left paratracheal soft-tissue mass and may mimic a left aortic arch.
- Double aortic arch results from persistence of both embryonic fourth aortic arches. The arches encircle the trachea and join posteriorly as a left or right descending aorta. The right arch is usually larger and situated more cephalad than the left in 75% of cases (**Fig. 4.6**), and each arch gives rise to ipsilateral common carotid and subclavian arteries. This is the most common cause of a symptomatic vascular ring in infants and young children. Radiographic findings may be similar to those of right aortic arch, but CT (**Fig. 4.7**) and MR demonstrate the patent left and right aortic arches and allow assessment of the origins of the great vessels.

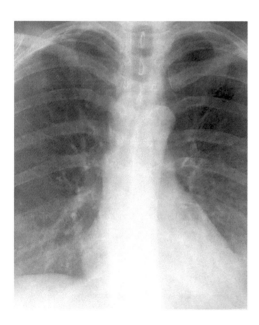

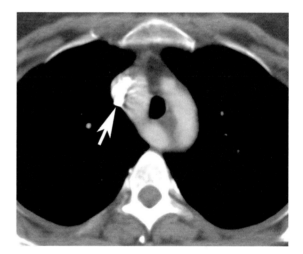

Fig. 4.6 PA chest radiograph of a woman with vague chest pain and a double aortic arch demonstrates bilateral indentations on the trachea produced by the two components of the double arch. Note the right arch is located slightly cephalad to the left. The resultant vascular ring (**Fig. 4.7**) produces mild mass effect on the trachea. Note the lateral displacement of the superior vena cava (*arrow*) by the right aortic arch (**Fig. 4.7**).

Fig. 4.7 Contrast-enhanced chest CT (mediastinal window) of the same woman in **Fig. 4.6** with vague chest pain and a double aortic arch. (*Images courtesy of Diane C. Strollo, MD, University of Pittsburgh Medical Center, Pittsburgh, Pennsylvania.*)

Suggested Reading

1. Kimura-Hayama ET, Meléndez G, Mendizábal AL, Meave-González A, Zambrana GF, Corona-Villalobos CP. Uncommon congenital and acquired aortic diseases: role of multidetector CT angiography. Radiographics 2010;30(1): 79–98

2. Russo V, Renzulli M, La Palombara C, Fattori R. Congenital diseases of the thoracic aorta. Role of MRI and MRA. Eur Radiol 2006;16(3):676–684

3. Salanitri J. MR angiography of aberrant left subclavian artery arising from right-sided thoracic aortic arch. Br J Radiol 2005;78(934):961–966

CASE 5

■ Clinical Presentation

18-year-old woman with differential upper and lower extremity blood pressures and stronger radial than femoral pulses

■ Radiologic Findings

PA (**Fig. 5.1**) chest radiograph demonstrates rib notching (*arrowhead*) and an inconspicuous aortic arch. The heart size and pulmonary vascularity are normal. The straight left superior mediastinal contour (*arrow*) is formed by an enlarged left subclavian artery. Artist's illustration (**Fig. 5.2**) depicts the collateral pathways that produce dilatation and tortuosity of the intercostal arteries and the radiographic finding of rib notching, which results from benign pressure erosion by the pulsatile collateral vessels on the adjacent ribs.

■ Diagnosis

Coarctation of the Aorta

■ Differential Diagnosis

- Pseudocoarctation
- Neurofibromatosis
- Pulmonary Atresia with Harvested Systemic Vessels Communicating with Pulmonary Vessels

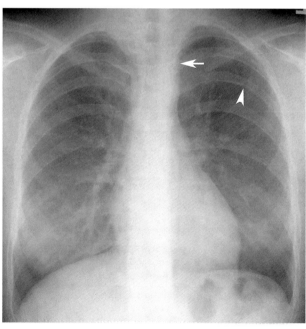

Fig. 5.1

Fig. 5.2

■ Discussion

Background

Coarctation of the aorta is a focal luminal narrowing distal to the left subclavian artery near the ligamentum arteriosum. Such luminal narrowing can be focal (coarctation), diffuse (hypoplastic isthmus), or complete (aortic interruption). It accounts for approximately 6% of congenital cardiac anomalies. While there is blood flow across the coarctation, it is supplemented by collateral blood flow that bypasses the obstruction through the spinal artery, intercostal arteries (**Fig. 5.2**), epigastric arteries, lateral thoracic artery, and periscapular arteries. These collateral vessels are not usually present at birth and develop over time.

Etiology

Coarctation of the aorta is a congenital anomaly of unknown etiology. Diffuse coarctation is thought to result from marked reduction of blood flow through the fetal aortic isthmus from associated congenital cardiac anomalies.

Clinical Findings

Aortic coarctation occurs slightly more commonly in males than in females (1.5:1 ratio), but coarctation associated with congenital cardiac anomalies affects males and females equally. Associated conditions include Turner syndrome, bicuspid aortic valve, intracranial aneurysm, atrial and ventricular septal defects, and various degrees of aortic hypoplasia. Patients with aortic coarctation and associated anomalies typically become symptomatic at birth. Patients with isolated coarctation may be asymptomatic or may become symptomatic in childhood or young adulthood. Symptoms include headache, claudication, and fatigue. Patients may also present with a murmur, systemic hypertension, or aortic dissection. Aortic coarctation in association with bicuspid aortic valve typically does not manifest with symptoms related to valvular stenosis but may manifest with bacterial endocarditis. On physical examination there are differential blood pressures between the upper and lower extremities (difference of at least 20 mm Hg) and radial pulses that are stronger than femoral pulses.

Imaging Findings

Radiography

- Infants
  - Cardiomegaly related to heart failure
    - Left ventricular dilatation
    - Right ventricular dilatation
    - Left atrial enlargement
  - Accentuated pulmonary vasculature from pulmonary venous hypertension
  - Pulmonary edema
- Older children and adults
  - Normal heart size, normal pulmonary vasculature (**Fig. 5.1**)
  - Left ventricular configuration from left ventricular hypertrophy
  - Cardiomegaly from left ventricular failure
  - Narrow cardiac waist and inconspicuous pulmonary trunk (**Fig. 5.1**)
  - Inconspicuous aortic arch (**Fig. 5.1**) obscured by enlarged left subclavian artery that forms a straight left superior mediastinal contour (**Fig. 5.1**)
  - "Figure-of-3" sign of the left lateral arch
  - Aortic valve calcification, wide ascending aorta from associated stenotic bicuspid aortic valve
  - Inferior rib notching (usually ribs 3 to 9) (**Fig. 5.1**)

MDCT

- Visualization of length and location of coarctation and evaluation of aortic size proximal and distal to the obstruction
- Visualization of aortic branches and their relationship to the coarctation
- Visualization of collateral vessels

MRI

- Oblique sagittal MRI (**Fig. 5.3**) and gadolinium-enhanced magnetic resonance angiography (**Fig. 5.4**) for visualization and measurement of length and location of coarctation and degree of luminal narrowing
- Visualization of aortic branches and their relationship to coarctation (**Figs. 5.3, 5.4**)
- Velocity-encoded cine MRI, flow mapping, and three-dimensional MRA for estimation of flow gradient across coarctation and estimation of collateral blood flow

Angiography

- Demonstration of location and length of coarctation
- Visualization of aortic branches and their relationship to the coarctation

Management

- Surgical treatment with resection or aortoplasty
- Balloon angioplasty of discrete luminal stenosis
- Endovascular stent placement

Prognosis

- Good with surgical treatment
- Early post-surgical complications: systemic hypertension and mesenteric arteritis
- Late post-surgical complications: aneurysm, pseudoaneurysm, re-coarctation, and infective endocarditis
- Poor prognosis without treatment, with over 90% of patients dying by 60 years of age

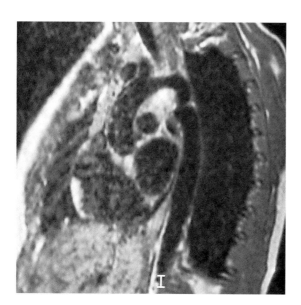

Fig. 5.3 Sagittal T1-weighted MRI of an 11-year-old boy with aortic coarctation demonstrates the location and degree of aortic stenosis and mild post-stenotic aortic dilatation.

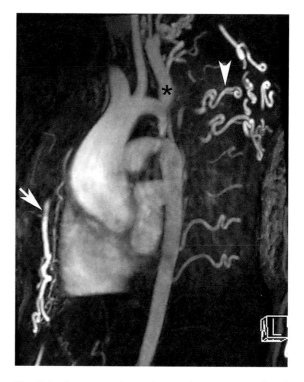

Fig. 5.4 Contrast-enhanced sagittal MR angiography of a patient with aortic coarctation demonstrates the location of the coarct (distal to the origin of the left subclavian artery [*asterisk*]), the major aortic branches, and numerous collateral vessels, including internal mammary (*arrow*) and intercostal (*arrowhead*) arteries.

PEARLS

- Rib notching is produced by pulsation of dilated intercostal arteries (**Figs. 5.1, 5.2, 5.4**), which provide collateral flow. It is rare before age 10 and most prominent along the posterior ribs and most visible in the upper ribs. The upper ribs (1 to 3) are usually free of notching because of communication between the intercostal arteries and the aorta above the coarctation (without a drop in systolic pressure). The lower ribs (10 to12) are free of notching because of communication between intercostal arteries and superior epigastric arteries without additional collateral flow. Unilateral rib notching results when one of the subclavian arteries arises distal to the coarctation.
- Aortic *pseudocoarctation* (**Fig. 5.5**) is elongation of the aortic arch and proximal descending aorta with a "kink" in the descending thoracic aorta at the ligamentum arteriosum without obstruction, pressure gradient, or collateral blood flow. Chest radiographs may demonstrate mediastinal abnormalities similar to those seen in coarctation, but there is no obstruction and no symptoms or signs related to aortic obstruction or collateral blood flow. With increasing age, flow turbulence may result in progressive aortic dilatation with reported cases of dissection.

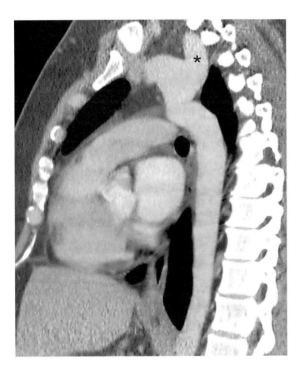

Fig. 5.5 Sagittal contrast-enhanced chest CT (mediastinal window) of an asymptomatic 25-year-old woman evaluated because an abnormal chest radiograph shows a pseudocoarctation of the aorta manifesting as a "kink" of the aorta just distal to the left subclavian artery (*asterisk*).

Suggested Reading

1. Ferguson EC, Krishnamurthy R, Oldham SAA. Classic imaging signs of congenital cardiovascular abnormalities. Radiographics 2007;27(5):1323–1334

2. Kimura-Hayama ET, Meléndez G, Mendizábal AL, Meave-González A, Zambrana GF, Corona-Villalobos CP. Uncommon congenital and acquired aortic diseases: role of multidetector CT angiography. Radiographics 2010;30(1): 79–98

3. Russo V, Renzulli M, La Palombara C, Fattori R. Congenital diseases of the thoracic aorta. Role of MRI and MRA. Eur Radiol 2006;16(3):676–684

4. Shih MC, Tholpady A, Kramer CM, Sydnor MK, Hagspiel KD. Surgical and endovascular repair of aortic coarctation: normal findings and appearance of complications on CT angiography and MR angiography. AJR Am J Roentgenol 2006;187(3):W302–W312

5. Steiner RM, Reddy GP, Flicker S. Congenital cardiovascular disease in the adult patient: imaging update. J Thorac Imaging 2002;17(1):1–17

CASE 6

■ Clinical Presentation

18-year-old man with recurrent pneumothorax

■ Radiologic Findings

PA (**Fig. 6.1**) and lateral (**Fig. 6.2**) chest radiographs demonstrate a right pneumothorax and thickening of the right apical pleura (**Fig. 6.1**). Note the abnormal cardiac contour, enlargement of the pulmonary trunk, and pectus excavatum deformity (**Figs. 6.1, 6.2**). Note left apical pleural thickening and metallic sutures (**Fig. 6.2**) (*arrow*) from previous lung resection for treatment of recurrent pneumothorax. Oblique sagittal gradient-echo MRA (**Fig. 6.3**) shows dilatation of the proximal ascending aorta and sinuses of Valsalva.

■ Diagnosis

Marfan Syndrome

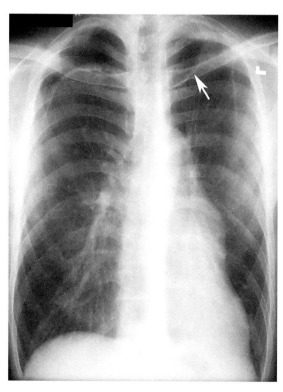

Fig. 6.1

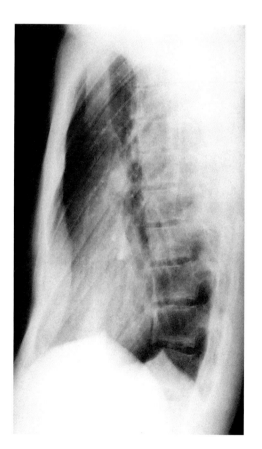

Fig. 6.2

80

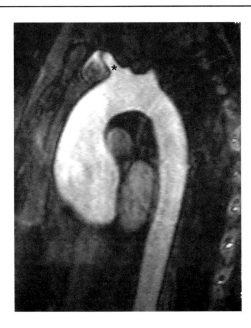

Fig. 6.3

■ Differential Diagnosis

- Primary Spontaneous Pneumothorax
- Annuloaortic Ectasia of Other Etiology (Ehlers-Danlos Syndrome, Turner Syndrome, Polycystic Kidney Disease, Osteogenesis Imperfecta)
- Aortic Stenosis with Post-Stenotic Dilatation
- Aortic Dissection

■ Discussion

Background

Marfan syndrome is a systemic connective tissue disorder involving primarily elastic tissues that affects the central nervous system, eye, skeleton, lung, and cardiovascular structures. Marfan syndrome is an autosomal dominant disorder, but may occur sporadically in up to 30% of cases.

Etiology

Marfan syndrome results from a genetic defect (linked to the fibrillin-1 [FBN1] gene on chromosome 15) in the production of glycoprotein fibrillin, which is important in the formation of elastic fibers found in normal connective tissue, and particularly affects the walls of major arteries. The resultant disruption of elastic fibers in the ascending aorta results in annuloaortic ectasia with dilatation of the ascending aorta, sinuses of Valsalva (formed by the aortic valve leaflets), and the aortic annulus. Myxomatous degeneration of the aortic and mitral valves is also described.

Clinical Findings

Marfan syndrome affects men and women equally, with an estimated prevalence of 2–3 persons per 10,000. Affected patients are typically tall, thin individuals and may exhibit arachnodactyly. Chest wall anomalies include scoliosis and pectus deformities. Ocular involvement manifests with subluxation of the optic lens in up to 80% of patients. Approximately 50% of patients have clinical evidence of cardiovascular disease by age 21 years. Children with Marfan syndrome typically exhibit auscultatory evidence of mitral insufficiency whereas aortic insufficiency is more commonly diagnosed in adults. Up to 15% of affected patients may have spontaneous pneumothorax resulting from bullous disease. The diagnosis is based on the presence of a combination of major and minor clinical features listed in the revised 1996 Ghent Nosology.

Imaging Findings

Radiography

- Narrow anteroposterior chest diameter, pectus (excavatum or carinatum) deformity, scoliosis, and long thin body habitus (**Figs. 6.1, 6.2**)
- Dilatation (aneurysm) of ascending thoracic aorta with normal caliber arch and descending aorta; may not be visible on radiography
- Cardiomegaly from aortic and less commonly mitral insufficiency and consequent left ventricular (**Fig. 6.1**) and left atrial enlargement
- Enlarged pulmonary trunk (**Fig. 6.1**)
- Spontaneous pneumothorax (may be recurrent) (**Fig. 6.1**)

MDCT

- Enlargement of ascending aorta from aortic valve to origin of brachiocephalic artery
- Normal aortic arch and descending aorta
- Left ventricular enlargement and hypertrophy
- Findings of aortic dissection (**Figs. 6.4A,B**): intimal flap, mural/mediastinal hemorrhage
- Pulmonary trunk dilatation

MRI

- Enlargement of ascending aorta from aortic valve to origin of brachiocephalic artery (**Fig. 6.3**)
- Left ventricular enlargement and hypertrophy
- Findings of aortic dissection: intimal flap, mural/mediastinal hemorrhage
- Valvular evaluation, demonstration of valvular insufficiency

Management

- Control of dysrhythmias and systemic hypertension to prevent further dilatation of ascending aorta and progression of aortic insufficiency
- Surgical graft placement within ascending aorta and aortic valve replacement

Prognosis

- Guarded; death from cardiovascular disease in over 90% of untreated patients
- Good results with early surgical aortic repair prior to onset of dissection

PEARLS

- Marfan syndrome is one of the most common causes of ascending aortic aneurysm in young adults. Aortic aneurysm in patients with Marfan syndrome is differentiated from atherosclerotic aneurysm by absence of involvement of the descending thoracic aorta in the former and universal involvement of the descending aorta in the latter.
- Aortic aneurysm is defined as permanent dilatation with resultant diameter of at least 50% greater than normal. Normal aortic measurements in young adults on CT are: 3.6 cm (aortic root), 3.5 cm (ascending aorta), 2.6 cm (proximal descending aorta), and 2.5 cm (distal descending aorta). There is progressive diameter enlargement with increasing age (approximately 0.1 cm per decade).

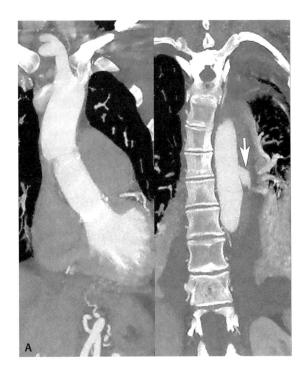
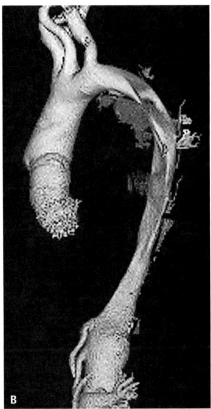

Figs. 6.4   Composite image (coronal reformations) of a contrast-enhanced chest CT (mediastinal window) **(A)** of a young woman with chest pain and known Marfan syndrome status post aortic valve replacement and ascending aorta repair (*left image*) for type A dissection **(A)** demonstrates an intimal tear of the descending aorta (*arrow*) communicating with the thrombosed false lumen of a descending aortic dissection. The ascending aortic repair and the morphology of the true lumen of the descending aorta are shown on the oblique sagittal volume-rendered CT aortogram **(B).** (*See color insert following page 108.*)

Suggested Reading

1. Fraser RS, Müller NL, Colman N, Paré PD. Hereditary anomalies of pulmonary connective tissue. In: Fraser RS, Müller NL, Colman N, Paré PD, eds. Fraser and Paré's Diagnosis of Diseases of the Chest, 4th ed. Philadelphia: WB Saunders; 1999;676–693

2. Ha HI, Seo JB, Lee SH, et al. Imaging of Marfan syndrome: multisystemic manifestations. Radiographics 2007;27(4): 989–1004

3. Kimura-Hayama ET, Meléndez G, Mendizábal AL, Meave-González A, Zambrana GF, Corona-Villalobos CP. Uncommon congenital and acquired aortic diseases: role of multidetector CT angiography. Radiographics 2010;30(1): 79–98

4. Loeys BL, Dietz HC, Braverman AC, et al. The revised Ghent nosology for the Marfan syndrome. J Med Genet 2010;47(7):476–485

5. Nguyen BT. Computed tomography diagnosis of thoracic aortic aneurysms. Semin Roentgenol 2001;36(4): 309–324

CASE 7

■ Clinical Presentation

Asymptomatic 42-year-old man

■ Radiologic Findings

Coned-down PA (**Fig. 7.1**) and lateral (**Fig. 7.2**) chest radiographs demonstrate a left aortic arch and a tubular opacity (*asterisk*) that arises from its superior aspect, projects over the tracheal lumen, and courses obliquely toward the right upper extremity (**Fig. 7.1**). Note the presence of an accessory azygos fissure. The lateral radiograph (**Fig. 7.2**) demonstrates a soft-tissue opacity (*double asterisk*) that produces mass effect on the dorsal trachea. Contrast-enhanced chest CT (mediastinal window) (**Figs. 7.3, 7.4**) demonstrates an aberrant right subclavian artery (*arrow*) (**Fig. 7.3**) that arises from a diverticulum of Kommerell (*arrowhead*) (**Fig. 7.4**).

■ Diagnosis

Aberrant Right Subclavian Artery

■ Differential Diagnosis

None

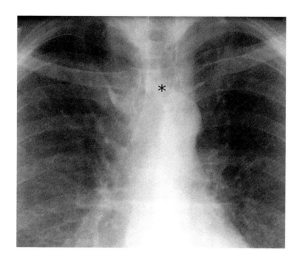

Fig. 7.1

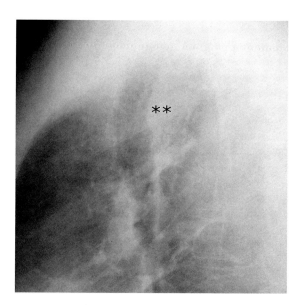

Fig. 7.2

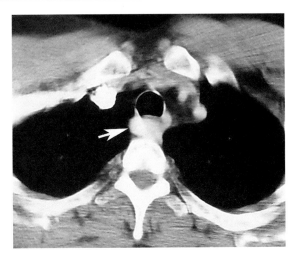

Fig. 7.3

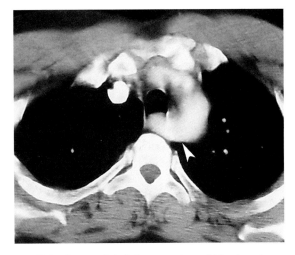

Fig. 7.4   (*Images 7.1–7.4 are courtesy of Maysiang Lesar, MD, National Naval Medical Center, Bethesda, Maryland.*)

■ Discussion

Background

An aberrant right subclavian artery arises as the last branch off a left-sided aortic arch and courses obliquely and superiorly behind the trachea and esophagus to resume its normal course. It is typically an isolated anomaly, represents one of the most common aortic arch branching anomalies, and affects up to 0.5% of the population, with a reported prevalence of 0.4–2%.

Etiology

An aberrant right subclavian artery results from involution of the entire right fourth embryonic arch with persistence of the right seventh intersegmental artery (which gives rise to the right subclavian artery); the latter maintains its attachment to the descending aorta. The aortic arch branches arise in the following order: right common carotid, left common carotid, left subclavian, and right subclavian arteries. The aberrant right subclavian artery may arise from an aortic diverticulum that may result from persistence of the dorsal portion of the embryonic arch.

Clinical Findings

Affected patients are typically asymptomatic adults. Patients with associated right ligamentum arteriosus have a complete vascular ring and may have symptoms. In addition, symptoms of tracheal compression have been described in affected children, particularly those with associated common origin of the carotid arteries. With aneurysmal dilatation of the aberrant vessel, esophageal compression may produce symptoms. In these cases, the aberrant vessel has been called "arteria lusoria" and the symptom "dysphagia lusoria" (from the Latin *lusus naturae*, meaning "game" or "freak of nature").

Imaging Findings

Radiography

- Tubular opacity arising from superior aspect of aortic arch and coursing obliquely toward the right over the tracheal air column on frontal radiography (**Fig. 7.1**)
- Soft-tissue opacity above the aortic arch; may produce mass effect on the dorsal aspect of the trachea on lateral radiography (**Fig. 7.2**)
- Lucent band coursing diagonally across the esophagus toward the right with focal mass effect on the dorsal esophagus on barium esophagography

MDCT/MRI

- Visualization of aberrant vessel arising from the distal posterior aortic arch and coursing superiorly and to the right behind the trachea and esophagus (**Figs. 7.3, 7.4, 7.5**)
- Visualization of aortic diverticulum when present (**Fig. 7.4**)

Angiography

- Demonstrates pattern of aortic branching—right carotid, left carotid, left subclavian, and right subclavian arteries, the latter coursing obliquely toward the right shoulder

Management

- None for asymptomatic patients
- Division of right-sided ligamentum arteriosum or resection of aortic diverticulum in symptomatic patients

Prognosis

- Excellent

PEARLS _____

- An aberrant right subclavian artery is a significant incidental finding in patients who undergo cardiac catheterization through the right arm as the catheter typically enters the descending aorta and cannot be maneuvered into the ascending aorta.

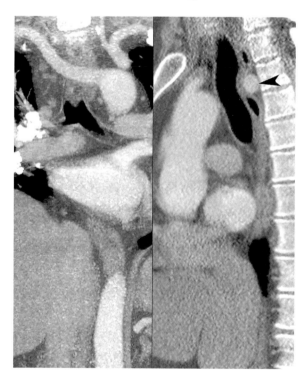

Fig. 7.5 Composite contrast-enhanced chest CT (mediastinal window) with coronal (*left*) and sagittal (*right*) reformatted images shows the oblique orientation of an aberrant right subclavian artery coursing behind the trachea and esophagus (*arrowhead*). (*Images courtesy of Michael Atalay, MD, PhD, Department of Diagnostic Imaging, Brown Medical School, Rhode Island Hospital, Providence, Rhode Island.*)

- The so-called diverticulum of Kommerell (**Fig. 7.4**) was first described on an esophagram of an asymptomatic patient with a left aortic arch and an aberrant right subclavian artery with a diverticulum at its origin, which produced mass effect on the esophagus. Interestingly, the aortic diverticulum occurs more frequently in patients with right aortic arch and aberrant left subclavian artery and is also referred to as diverticulum of Kommerell in these instances. It may be congenital or secondary to atherosclerotic dilatation.
- An aberrant right subclavian artery in a patient with aortic coarctation typically arises distal to the coarctation. A right vertebral subclavian steal may result in these cases from retrograde flow from the right subclavian artery into the descending thoracic aorta. Affected patients may exhibit unilateral left rib notching.
- Other minor anomalies of aortic arch branching occur relatively frequently. The most frequent are: common origin of the right brachiocephalic artery and the left common carotid artery (so-called bovine arch) (25% prevalence) (**Fig. 7.6**) and aberrant origin of the left vertebral artery proximal to origin of the left subclavian artery (**Fig. 7.7**) (2.4–5.8% prevalence).

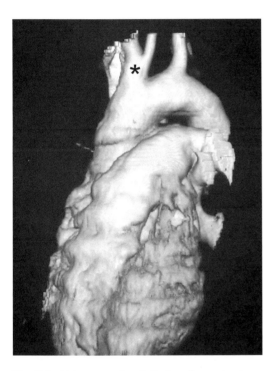

Fig. 7.6 Volume-rendered display of a contrast-enhanced chest CT of a patient with a so-called bovine arch demonstrates the common origin of the brachiocephalic and left carotid arteries (*asterisk*). Note: in a "true" bovine arch, all great vessels share a common origin.

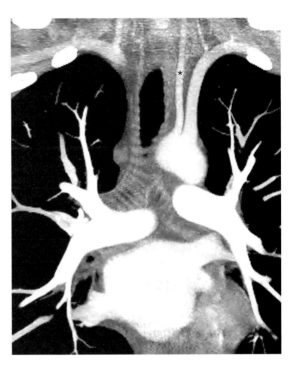

Fig. 7.7 Coronal MIP image of a contrast-enhanced chest CT (mediastinal window) shows an aberrant left vertebral artery (*asterisk*) arising directly from the aortic arch. (*Images courtesy of Michael Atalay, MD, PhD, Department of Diagnostic Imaging, Brown Medical School, Rhode Island Hospital, Providence, Rhode Island.*)

Suggested Reading

1. Amplatz K, Moller JH. Anomalies of the aortic arch system. In: Amplatz K, Moller JH, eds. Radiology of Congenital Heart Disease. St Louis: Mosby; 1993:995–1049

2. Gross GW, Steiner RM. Radiographic manifestations of congenital heart disease in the adult patient. Radiol Clin North Am 1991;29(2):293–317

3. Ka-Tak W, Lam WWM, Yu SCH. MDCT of an aberrant right subclavian artery and of bilateral vertebral arteries with anomalous origins. AJR Am J Roentgenol 2007;188(3):W274–W275

4. Russo V, Renzulli M, La Palombara C, Fattori R. Congenital diseases of the thoracic aorta. Role of MRI and MRA. Eur Radiol 2006;16(3):676–684

5. van Son JA, Konstantinov IE. Burckhard F. Kommerell and Kommerell's diverticulum. Tex Heart Inst J 2002;29(2): 109–112

CASE 8

■ Clinical Presentation

Asymptomatic 30-year-old man

■ Radiologic Findings

Coned-down PA chest radiograph (**Fig. 8.1**) demonstrates a subtle vertically oriented left paramediastinal interface lateral to the aortic arch (*arrow*). Contrast-enhanced chest CT (mediastinal window) (**Figs. 8.2, 8.3, 8.4**) demonstrates a persistent left superior vena cava (*arrow*) coursing vertically along the left superior mediastinum lateral to the aortic arch (**Fig. 8.2**). The vessel courses medial to the left superior pulmonary vein (*arrowhead*) (**Fig. 8.3**) and drains into a dilated coronary sinus (*S*) (**Fig. 8.4**). Note the coexistent small-caliber right superior vena cava (**Figs. 8.2, 8.3**)

■ Diagnosis

Persistent Left Superior Vena Cava

■ Differential Diagnosis

Left Upper Lobe Partial Anomalous Pulmonary Venous Return (PAPVR)

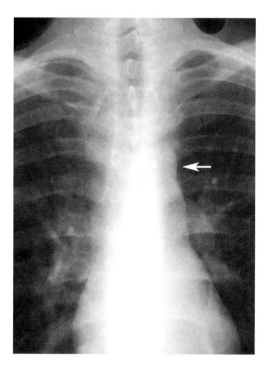

Fig. 8.1

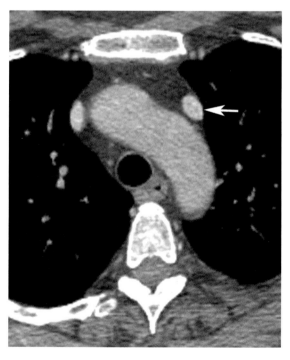

Fig. 8.2   (*Images courtesy of Maysiang Lesar, MD, National Naval Medical Center, Bethesda, Maryland.*)

88

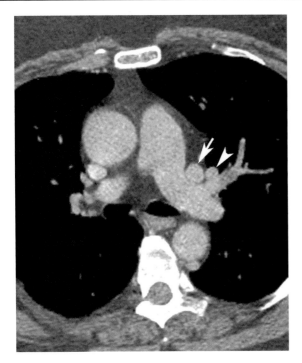

Fig. 8.3

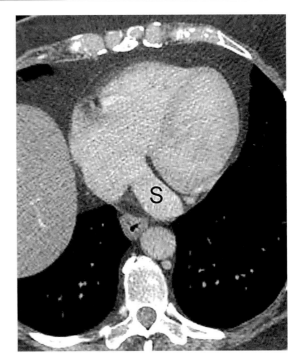

Fig. 8.4

■ Discussion

Background

A persistent left superior vena cava (PLSVC) is a relatively common anomaly and represents the most frequent form of anomalous venous return to the heart. It occurs in approximately 0.3–0.5% of the general population, with an increased prevalence (4.4%) in patients with congenital heart disease.

Etiology

The embryonic sinus venosus has right and left horns which receive blood from three major venous structures during the fourth week of embryonic development: the vitelline, umbilical, and common cardinal veins. The anterior cardinal veins are paired structures that drain the upper body while the posterior cardinal veins drain the lower body. The left anterior cardinal vein normally joins the right anterior cardinal vein to form the left brachiocephalic vein. The caudal portion of the right anterior cardinal vein forms the superior vena cava. The proximal left horn of the sinus venosus gives rise to the coronary sinus. The left anterior cardinal vein caudal to the brachiocephalic vein normally involutes, but its distal aspect persists as the ligament or oblique vein of Marshall. Failure of involution of the left anterior cardinal vein results in a PLSVC (**Fig. 8.5**). In many cases the left brachiocephalic vein is absent and the right superior vena cava is smaller than the left (**Fig. 8.5**). A bridging vein between the two superior vena cavae may be present. Obliteration of the right anterior cardinal vein results in absence or atresia of the right superior vena cava. PLSVC typically receives the accessory hemiazygos vein and continues vertically to drain into the coronary sinus.

Clinical Findings

Affected patients are typically asymptomatic adults. The diagnosis is often made incidentally in patients who undergo central venous catheterization (**Fig. 8.6**), pacemaker placement, or cardioverter defibrillator implantation when access to the heart is attempted via a jugular/subclavian venous approach. PLSVC is associated

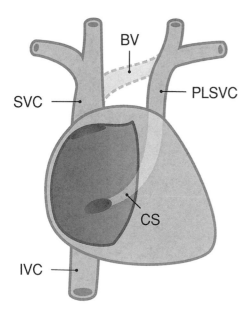

Fig. 8.5 Artist's illustration demonstrates the course of the persistent left superior vena cava (*PLSVC*), which arises at the anastomosis of the left jugular and subclavian veins. Note the PLSVC drains into the right atrium (*RA*) via the coronary sinus (*CS*). A normal right superior vena cava (*RSVC*) and a normal, small or atretic bridging vein (*BV*) are often found in association with a PLSVC.

with abnormal cardiac impulse formation/conduction related to abnormal development of the sinus node, the AV node, and the His bundle. Affected patients may be predisposed to dysrhythmias and sudden death. Patients with PLSVC may have associated congenital heart disease, including abnormal atrioventricular connections/situs ambiguous, anomalous pulmonary venous return, Ebstein anomaly, common atrioventricular valves, tetralogy of Fallot, subaortic stenosis, and ventricular/atrial septal defects.

Imaging Findings

Radiography

- Vertical left superior mediastinal interface lateral to aortic arch (**Fig. 8.1**)
- Abnormal course of venous catheters/leads introduced via jugular (**Fig. 8.6**) or subclavian vein approach; vertical left paramediastinal central catheter course (**Fig. 8.6**); catheter course into the coronary sinus to enter the right heart

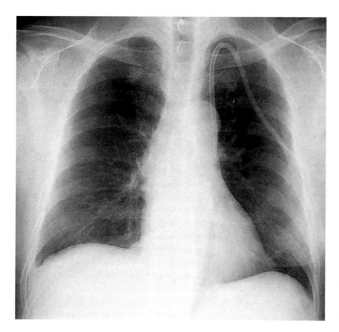

Fig. 8.6   PA chest radiograph of a 67-year-old man with chronic renal failure demonstrates a dialysis catheter placed via left internal jugular vein approach with its tip in a PLSVC.

MDCT/MRI

- Left superior vena cava; vertical course along left superior mediastinum lateral to aortic arch (**Fig. 8.2**)
- Vertical course posterior to left atrial appendage, anterior and medial to left superior pulmonary vein (**Fig. 8.3**)
- Drainage into coronary sinus, which may be enlarged and demonstrate dense contrast (**Fig. 8.4**)
- Identification and evaluation of coexistent right superior vena cava and bridging vein (**Figs. 8.2, 8.3, 8.7**); absence of right superior vena cava

Management

- Awareness of anatomic variant

Prognosis

- Excellent (in the absence of associated anomalies)

PEARLS

- Recognition of a PLSVC is important in patients undergoing placement of central venous catheters (**Fig. 8.6**), pacemaker electrodes, or cardioverter-defibrillator leads as special techniques may have to be employed. In affected patients undergoing open-heart surgery, special techniques must be used to avoid flooding of the cardiac chambers by systemic blood entering through the coronary sinus. Surgical ligation of the LSVC in cases in which there is no venous connection between the right and left superior vena cavae and/or absence of the right superior vena cava may result in venous engorgement of the head and upper extremities.
- PLSVC may be associated with atresia of the coronary sinus ostium without a left atrial connection, resulting in retrograde flow of cardiac blood into the PLSVC. In such cases, surgical ligation of the PLSVC may result in myocardial ischemia and infarction.
- PLSVC may be associated with coronary sinus–left atrium fenestration (unroofing) with resultant right-to-left shunt or an interatrial communication (coronary sinus atrial septal defect) at the mouth of the coronary sinus. In these cases the PLSVC drains into the left atrium and is associated with congenital heart disease.

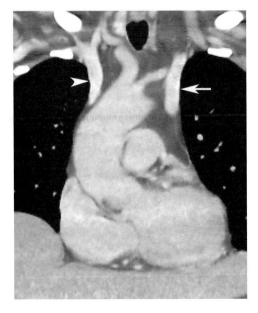

Fig. 8.7 Coronal contrast-enhanced chest CT (mediastinal window) of an asymptomatic 66-year-old woman with PLSVC (*arrow*) demonstrates a coexistent right superior vena cava (*arrowhead*). The vertical course of the PLSVC accounts for the left superior mediastinal interface seen on radiography

Suggested Reading

1. Biffi M, Boriani G, Frabetti L, Bronzetti G, Branzi A. Left superior vena cava persistence in patients undergoing pacemaker or cardioverter-defibrillator implantation: a 10-year experience. Chest 2001;120(1):139–144

2. Demos TC, Posniak HV, Pierce KL, Olson MC, Muscato M. Venous anomalies of the thorax. AJR Am J Roentgenol 2004;182(5):1139–1150

3. Dillman JR, Hernandez RJ. Role of CT in the evaluation of congenital cardiovascular disease in children. AJR Am J Roentgenol 2009;192(5):1219–1231

4. Jha NK, Gogna A, Tan TH, Wong KY, Shankar S. Atresia of coronary sinus ostium with retrograde drainage via persistent left superior vena cava. Ann Thorac Surg 2003;76(6):2091–2092

CASE 9

■ Clinical Presentation

22-year-old woman with postpartum dyspnea and hypoxemia

■ Radiologic Findings

Coned-down PA chest radiograph (**Fig. 9.1**) demonstrates a left lower lobe mass of lobular contours with tubular opacities (*arrowheads*) coursing between the mass and the left hilum. Left pulmonary arteriogram (**Figs. 9.2, 9.3**) demonstrates a pulmonary arteriovenous malformation supplied by two branches of the left interlobar pulmonary artery (**Fig. 9.2**) that drains into the left atrium (*LA*) via an enlarged pulmonary vein (**Fig. 9.3**).

■ Diagnosis

Pulmonary Arteriovenous Malformation

■ Differential Diagnosis

* Arteriovenous Fistula
* Pulmonary Artery Aneurysm

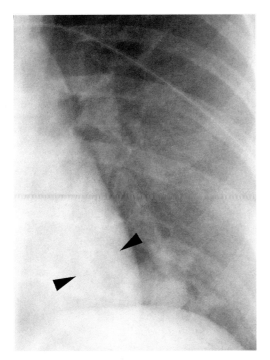

Fig. 9.1

93

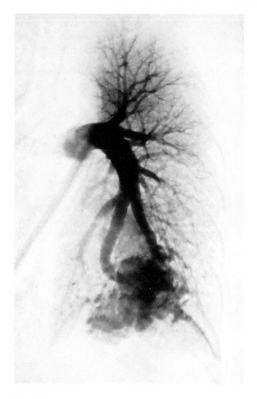

Fig. 9.2

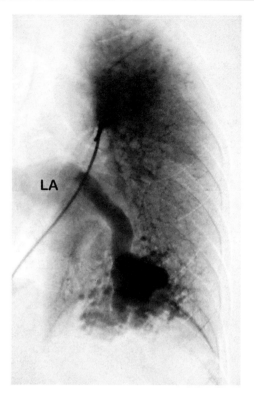

Fig. 9.3 *(Images 9.1–9.3 are courtesy of Wanda M. Kirejczyk, MD, New Britain General Hospital, New Britain, Connecticut.)*

■ Discussion

Background

A pulmonary arteriovenous malformation (PAVM) is an abnormal communication between a pulmonary artery and a pulmonary vein without an intervening capillary bed, and results in a right-to-left shunt. *Simple PAVMs* (90%) are defined as single or multiple feeding arteries originating from a single segmental pulmonary artery. *Complex PAVMs* (10%) are characterized by feeding arteries originating from two or more segmental pulmonary arteries. Approximately 33% are multiple; 20% are bilateral.

Etiology

PAVMs are thought to arise from congenital defects in the capillary bed, which result in a direct communication between the pulmonary arterial and venous circulations. Acquired arteriovenous communications also occur, usually follow trauma (non-iatrogenic or iatrogenic) or inflammation, and are designated arteriovenous fistulae. Rendu-Osler-Weber syndrome or hereditary hemorrhagic telangiectasia (HHT) is an autosomal dominant disorder characterized by recurrent epistaxis, mucocutaneous telangiectasias, and arteriovenous malformations, with an estimated prevalence of one in 5,000 to 10,000 persons. Approximately 60–90% of PAVMs occur in patients with HHT, up to 35% of patients with HHT have one or more PAVMs, and 60% of patients with HTT-related PAVMs have multiple lesions.

Clinical Findings

Over 50% of patients with PAVM are asymptomatic. Symptomatic patients are usually adults between the fourth and sixth decades of life. Symptoms include fatigue and exertional dyspnea (related to hypoxemia) and neurologic complaints and/or fever from paradoxical emboli. Affected patients may develop myocardial infarction and mesenteric, renal, or limb ischemia. Stroke occurs in up to 40% of patients with PAVM, brain abscess in 20%, and hemoptysis/hemothorax in 10%. Affected patients may have a family history of PAVM or HHT with associated clubbing, cyanosis, and mucosal telangiectasias. Approximately 40–60% of these patients have additional arteriovenous malformations in the skin and mucous membranes and may present with epistaxis, chronic gastrointestinal bleeding, and/or hematuria.

Imaging Findings

Radiography

- Lobular well-defined non-calcified nodule/mass (**Fig. 9.1**)
- Typically in peripheral lower lobe; often projects below dome of diaphragm (**Fig. 9.1**)
- Associated tortuous tubular opacities coursing to and from ipsilateral hilum representing feeding and draining vessels (**Fig. 9.1**)
- Rarely, multiple pulmonary nodules/masses

CT/MDCT

- Demonstration of PAVM manifesting as nodule with feeding and draining vessels (**Fig. 9.4**)
- Evaluation of origin, number, length, and diameter of feeding vessels and internal structure of vascular sac (**Figs. 9.4, 9.5**)
- Enhancing mass with vascular connections (**Fig. 9.4**)
- Rapid contrast enhancement and washout (**Fig. 9.4**)
- Unenhanced or enhanced multidetector CT imaging for screening (**Fig. 9.5**), characterization, and quantification of PAVM (**Fig. 9.8**)

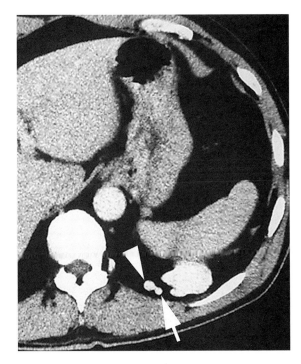

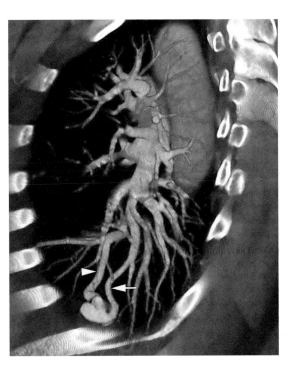

Fig. 9.4 Coned-down contrast-enhanced chest CT (soft-tissue window) of a man with an asymptomatic left lower lobe simple PAVM demonstrates intense lesion enhancement and allows identification of the feeding artery (*arrow*) and draining vein (*arrowhead*).

Fig. 9.5 Oblique sagittal volume-rendered CT image of a PAVM demonstrates its feeding artery (*arrow*) and draining vein (*arrowhead*).

MRI

- Low-signal flow void in PAVM; low to intermediate signal in PAVM with internal thrombus
- Three-dimensional contrast-enhanced MR angiography for non-invasive diagnosis of PAVM larger than 3 mm in size; high-signal-intensity nodule and associated vessels
- Evaluation of size and number of feeding vessels prior to embolotherapy

Angiography

- Opacification of feeding vessels and draining veins (**Figs. 9.2, 9.3, 9.6**)
- Confirmation of diagnosis, documentation of multiple lesions, and evaluation of origin, number, length, and diameter of the feeding vessels (**Figs. 9.2, 9.3**) for coil embolization therapy planning (**Figs. 9.6, 9.7**)

Other Modalities

- Contrast-enhanced two-dimensional echocardiography for screening (90% sensitivity for detection of intrapulmonary shunts)
- Lung perfusion scintigraphy for determination of shunt size

Management

- Embolotherapy with detachable coils or vascular plug for improvement of oxygenation and prevention of neurologic and systemic complications (**Fig. 9.7**)

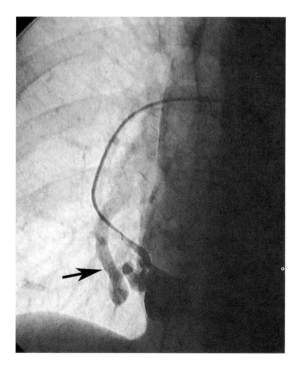 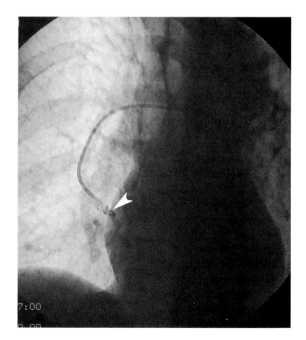

Figs. 9.6 Subtraction image from a pulmonary arteriogram of a 47-year-old man who developed a left temporoparietal brain abscess secondary to a right middle lobe PAVM demonstrates selective injection of the feeding pulmonary artery and the tortuous draining vein (*arrow*).

Fig. 9.7 Frontal coned-down subtraction radiograph demonstrates the pulmonary artery catheter within the feeding artery immediately after deployment of embolotherapy coils (*arrowhead*), which completely obliterated flow through the PAVM.

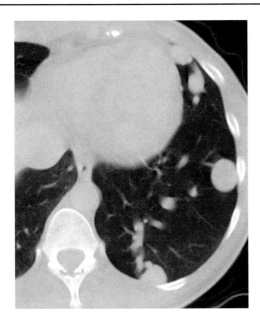

Fig. 9.8   Chest CT (lung window) of a 32-year-old woman with HHT demonstrates at least three PAVMs of various sizes affecting the left lung. The PAVMs manifest as peripheral sub-pleural pulmonary nodules with associated tubular opacities that represent the feeding pulmonary arteries and draining pulmonary veins.

Prognosis

- Guarded
- Significant morbidity and reported mortality rate of 10% for patients with HHT
- Complications of embolotherapy: paradoxical emboli, air emboli, transient ischemic attacks, angina, bradycardia, hypotension, and chest pain
- Complete obliteration of right-to-left shunt achieved in less than half of treated patients

PEARLS

- Patients with suspected HHT may undergo screening with arterial blood gas evaluation in room air and with 100% oxygen. Affected patients typically exhibit a 1–2% drop in O_2 saturation after standing and a further 8% drop in O_2 saturation after exercise. These findings are supplemented by imaging studies for definitive diagnosis.
- AVM in patients with HHT typically affects the lungs, brain, nose, and gastrointestinal system (including the liver).
- PAVM with feeding vessels ≥3 mm in diameter are traditionally treated with embolotherapy (**Figs. 9.6, 9.7**). However, patients with smaller lesions may suffer from clinically occult stroke. Thus, embolotherapy may be performed on all PAVMs that can be selectively cannulated. Embolotherapy catheters are ideally placed distal to branches supplying normal lung and as close as possible to the neck of the PAVM (**Figs. 9.6, 9.7**). Reperfusion of embolized PAVMs is reported.

Suggested Reading

1. González SB, Busquets JC, Figueiras RG, et al. Imaging arteriovenous fistulas. AJR Am J Roentgenol 2009;193(5): 1425–1433

2. Jaskolka J, Wu L, Chan RP, Faughnan ME. Imaging of hereditary hemorrhagic telangiectasia. AJR Am J Roentgenol 2004;183(2):307–314

3. Pelage JP, El Hajjam M, Lagrange C, et al. Pulmonary artery interventions: an overview. Radiographics 2005;25(6): 1653–1667

4. Schneider G, Uder M, Koehler M, et al. MR angiography for detection of pulmonary arteriovenous malformations in patients with hereditary hemorrhagic telangiectasia. AJR Am J Roentgenol 2008;190(4):892–901

CASE 10

■ Clinical Presentation

36-year-old woman with cough and fever

■ Radiologic Findings

Coned-down PA chest radiograph (**Fig. 10.1**) demonstrates an abnormal contour of the left superior mediastinum (*arrow*). Coronal (**Fig. 10.2**) and axial (**Figs. 10.3, 10.4**) contrast-enhanced chest CT (mediastinal window) demonstrates the anomalous course of the left superior pulmonary vein (*arrowhead*) (**Fig. 10.2**), which anastomoses with a vertical left superior mediastinal vein (*arrow*) (**Fig. 10.3**), which drains into the left brachiocephalic vein (*double asterisk*). Note the absence of the left superior pulmonary vein from its normal anatomic position posterior to the left atrial appendage (*asterisk*) (**Fig. 10.4**) and dilatation of the superior vena cava (**Fig. 10.2**).

■ Diagnosis

Partial Anomalous Pulmonary Venous Return; Left Upper Lobe

■ Differential Diagnosis

• Persistent Left Superior Vena Cava

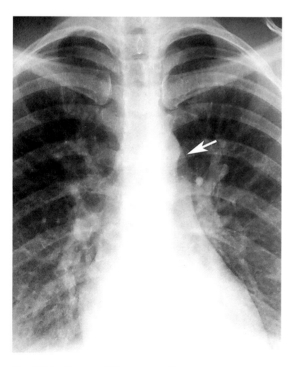

Fig. 10.1 (*Image 10.1 courtesy of Maysiang Lesar, MD, National Naval Medical Center, Bethesda, Maryland.*)

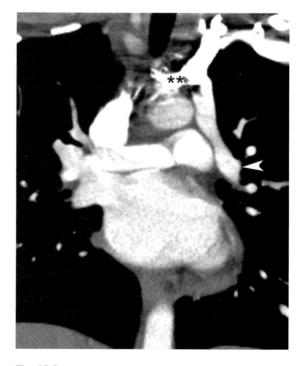

Fig. 10.2

98

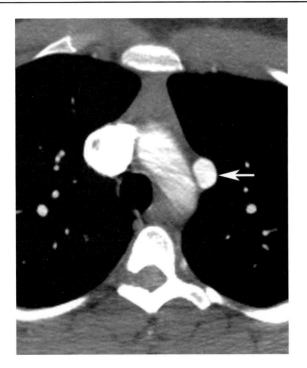

Fig. 10.3

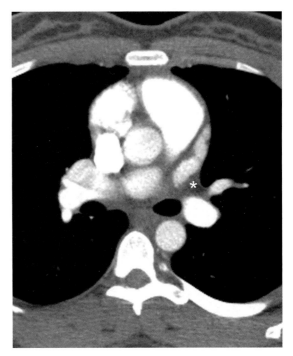

Fig.10.4

■ Discussion

Background

Anomalous pulmonary venous connections are congenital anomalies in which one or more pulmonary veins drain into the right-sided circulation with a resultant left-to-right shunt. These anomalous connections may be total (the entire pulmonary venous return) or partial. Partial anomalous pulmonary venous connections may affect left or right pulmonary veins and are reported in up to 0.7% of autopsies and in approximately 0.2% of adults studied with CT.

Etiology

The primitive common pulmonary vein begins to drain into the heart early in embryogenesis by joining the pulmonary portion of the splanchnic plexus. Partial anomalous pulmonary venous return is thought to result from premature atresia of the right or left primitive pulmonary veins while there are still primitive pulmonary-systemic connections.

Clinical Findings

Patients with partial anomalous pulmonary venous return and a significant left-to-right shunt present with symptoms. Symptomatic patients are typically children and adolescents who are usually males and in whom the anomalous venous return is right-sided (superior vena cava or right atrium). Up to 90% of these patients have an associated sinus venosus atrial septal defect and up to 15% have an associated ostium primum atrial septal defect. These patients may present with fatigue, exertional dyspnea, and heart failure. Asymptomatic patients are usually adults without known atrial septal defect, are more frequently female, characteristically have left-sided anomalous venous drainage, and are often diagnosed incidentally with chest CT.

Imaging Findings

Radiography

- Abnormal left superior mediastinal contour (**Fig. 10.1**)
- Abnormal/anomalous course of pulmonary veins

MDCT/MRI

- Demonstration of anomalous pulmonary vein (**Fig. 10.2**)
- Demonstration of anomalous vascular connections
  - Left upper lobe anomalous pulmonary vein drainage into a vertical vein (**Figs. 10.2, 10.3**) which drains into a dilated left brachiocephalic vein (**Fig. 10.2**); absence of left superior pulmonary vein from its normal location anterior to the left mainstem bronchus and posterior to the left atrial appendage (**Fig. 10.4**)
  - Right upper lobe anomalous pulmonary venous drainage into the superior vena cava, azygos vein, or right atrium; may exhibit absence of right upper lobe pulmonary vein from its normal location
- Identification of associated sinus venosus atrial septal defect

Management

- Surgical repair of partial anomalous venous connection when ratio of pulmonary-to-systemic shunt exceeds 1.5:1
- Surgical repair of associated anomalies, such as atrial septal defect

Prognosis

- Excellent in patients without associated anomalies
- Dependent on severity and number of associated conditions in patients with congenital heart disease

Suggested Reading

1. Demos TC, Posniak HV, Pierce KL, Olson MC, Muscato M. Venous anomalies of the thorax. AJR Am J Roentgenol 2004;182(5):1139–1150

2. Dillman JR, Yarram SG, Hernandez RJ. Imaging of pulmonary venous developmental anomalies. AJR Am J Roentgenol 2009;192(5):1272–1285

3. Haramati LB, Moche IE, Rivera VT, et al. Computed tomography of partial anomalous pulmonary venous connection in adults. J Comput Assist Tomogr 2003;27(5):743–749

4. Ho ML, Bhalla S, Bierhals A, Gutierrez F. MDCT of partial anomalous pulmonary venous return (PAPVR) in adults. J Thorac Imaging 2009;24(2):89–95

CASE 11

■ Clinical Presentation

Asymptomatic 29-year-old woman

■ Radiologic Findings

PA (**Fig. 11.1**) chest X-ray demonstrates a small right lung with ipsilateral mediastinal shift and arcuate tubular opacities that course toward the right cardiophrenic angle. Note that the right bronchus is hyparterial (**Fig. 11.1**). Contrast-enhanced chest CT (lung window) (**Fig. 11.2**) demonstrates the small volume of the bilobed right lung. Contrast-enhanced chest CT (mediastinal window) (**Figs. 11.3, 11.4**) demonstrates paired anomalous pulmonary veins (**Fig. 11.3**) that drain into the inferior vena cava (**Fig. 11.4**).

■ Diagnosis

Scimitar Syndrome

■ Differential Diagnosis

- Arteriovenous Malformation
- Pulmonary Varix
- Intralobar Sequestration
- Mucoid Impaction/Bronchial Atresia

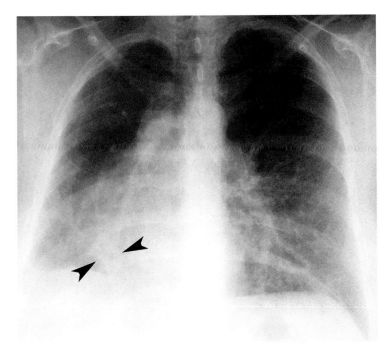

Fig. 11.1

101

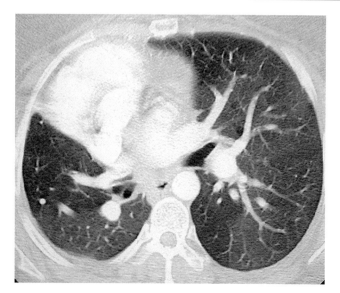

Fig. 11.2

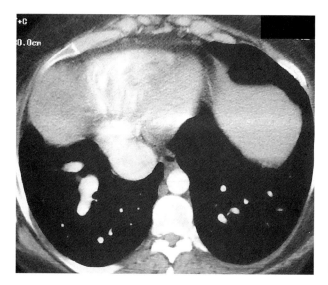

Fig. 11.3

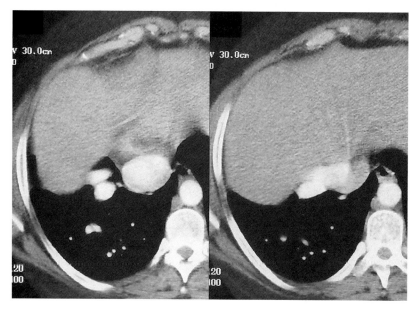

Fig. 11.4

■ Discussion

Background

Scimitar syndrome is a complex disorder also known as pulmonary venolobar syndrome and hypogenetic lung syndrome. It characteristically affects the right lung and manifests with a variety of cardiopulmonary anomalies. The term *scimitar* refers to the arcuate course followed by the anomalous pulmonary vein, which resembles the shape of a scimitar (a Turkish sword). The anomalous vein(s) may affect all or part of the right lung and typically drains into the inferior vena cava, hepatic/portal circulation, azygos vein, coronary sinus, or right atrium. Associated findings include aplasia/hypoplasia of the right pulmonary artery, systemic blood supply to the right lung, interruption of the inferior vena cava, duplication, eventration or partial absence of the right hemidiaphragm, tracheal trifurcation, esophageal/gastric communication with the lung, and horseshoe lung. The hypogenetic right lung may exhibit anomalous segmentation, lobation, and/or bronchial branching

Etiology

Scimitar syndrome is a rare congenital anomaly of the right lung and pulmonary vasculature of unknown etiology.

Clinical Findings

Patients with scimitar syndrome may be diagnosed as infants or neonates because of associated symptomatic congenital cardiovascular disease (in approximately 25–50%). Associated congenital cardiac anomalies include: secundum atrial septal defect, ventricular septal defect, patent ductus arteriosus, tetralogy of Fallot, coarctation of the aorta, hypoplastic left heart, double-outlet right ventricle, double-chambered right ventricle, endocardial cushion defect, and pulmonary arterial hypertension. Patients with significant left-to-right shunts (typically 2:1 or greater) may present with fatigue and dyspnea. Patients may also present with hemoptysis and/or recurrent pulmonary infection. Approximately 50% of patients are asymptomatic and diagnosed incidentally on chest radiography. Pulmonary artery pressures are normal or slightly elevated in the majority of patients who present as adults. Women are slightly more commonly affected, with a female-to-male ratio of 1.4:1.

Imaging Findings

Radiography

- Small right lung and hemithorax (**Figs. 11.1**), mediastinal shift to the right (dextroposition of the heart) (**Fig. 11.1**), indistinct right cardiac border (**Fig. 11.1**), increased right lung opacity (**Fig. 11.1**), right apical pleural cap (**Fig. 11.1**)
- Blunt costophrenic angle (**Fig. 11.1**)
- Vertically oriented curved tubular opacity (anomalous draining vein) in right inferior hemithorax coursing toward right cardiophrenic angle (**Figs. 11.1, 11.5**); may be obscured by the heart in cases with pronounced cardiac dextroposition (**Fig. 11.1**)
- Diminished right pulmonary vascularity (**Fig. 11.1**)
- Broad retrosternal band-like opacity on lateral radiography

MDCT/MRI

- Small right lung; mediastinal shift to the right (**Fig. 11.2**)
- Optimal visualization of anomalous vessel (variable size and number), its course and drainage into inferior vena cava (**Figs. 11.3, 11.4, 11.6**), right atrium, coronary sinus, or hepatic circulation
- Evaluation/identification of other components of the syndrome (**Fig. 11.6**)
- Non-invasive assessment of left-to-right shunt with velocity-encoded cine MRI

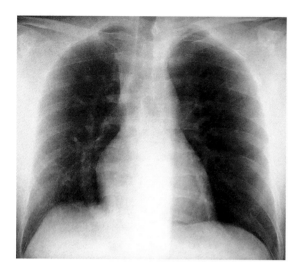

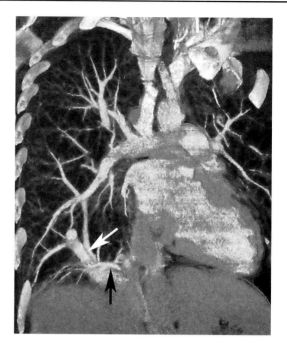

Fig. 11.5 PA chest radiograph of an asymptomatic 22-year-old man demonstrates the *scimitar sign* in association with mild right pulmonary hypoplasia.

Fig. 11.6 Coronal contrast-enhanced volume rendered chest CT image of an asymptomatic 19-year-old man with chest pain and scimitar syndrome demonstrates the course of the anomalous vein (*white arrow*). Note the systemic arterial supply to the right lower lobe (*black arrow*) that arose from the celiac axis.

Management

- Observation of asymptomatic patients without associated anomalies
- Surgical correction, ligation, or coil embolization for symptomatic patients with significant shunts
- Lung resection for patients with recurrent hemoptysis and/or pulmonary infection
- Correction of significant associated congenital cardiovascular disease

Prognosis

- Excellent in the absence of associated anomalies
- Related to associated congenital heart disease and its severity

PEARLS

- Most frequent anomalies in patients with pulmonary venolobar (scimitar) syndrome are hypogenetic right lung and partial anomalous pulmonary venous return.
- Radiographic visualization of the anomalous pulmonary (scimitar) vein with its typical curved configuration is known as the *scimitar sign* (**Figs. 11.1, 11.5**).
- Partial anomalous pulmonary venous return occurs in up to 0.7% of patients with congenital heart disease. It is most commonly associated with atrial septal defect (ASD). ASD occurs in approximately 90% of patients with partial anomalous pulmonary venous return to the superior vena cava or right atrium, and in only 15% of patients with anomalous drainage to the inferior vena cava.
- Some investigators classify cases of scimitar syndrome with abnormal right bronchial communications and systemic blood supply to the right lung as variants of intralobar sequestration. There are also reports of pulmonary venolobar syndrome in association with extralobar sequestration. In some cases of scimitar syndrome, there is systemic blood supply to the hypogenetic lung without other typical features of pulmonary sequestration (**Fig. 11.6**).

Suggested Reading

1. Cirillo RL Jr. The scimitar sign. Radiology 1998;206(3):623–624

2. Ferguson EC, Krishnamurthy R, Oldham SAA. Classic imaging signs of congenital cardiovascular abnormalities. Radiographics 2007;27(5):1323–1334

3. Konen E, Raviv-Zilka L, Cohen RA, et al. Congenital pulmonary venolobar syndrome: spectrum of helical CT findings with emphasis on computerized reformatting. Radiographics 2003;23(5):1175–1184

4. Mulligan ME. History of scimitar syndrome. Radiology 1999;210(1):288–290

5. Woodring JH, Howard TA, Kanga JF. Congenital pulmonary venolobar syndrome revisited. Radiographics 1994;14(2): 349–369

CASE 12

■ Clinical Presentation

65-year-old woman with chest pain

■ Radiologic Findings

PA (**Fig. 12.1**) and lateral (**Fig. 12.2**) chest radiographs demonstrate a multi-lobular soft-tissue mass that projects over the right hilum (**Fig. 12.1**) and focal enlargement of the superior aspect of the left atrium (**Fig. 12.2**). Nodular upper lobe parenchymal opacities represented remote granulomatous infection. Contrast-enhanced chest CT (**Figs. 12.3, 12.4**) shows that the lobular opacities seen on radiography correspond to focal dilatation of the pulmonary veins as they enter an enlarged left atrium.

■ Diagnosis

Pulmonary Varix

■ Differential Diagnosis

- Indeterminate Pulmonary Nodule/Mass

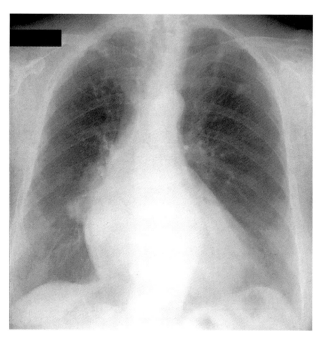

Fig. 12.1

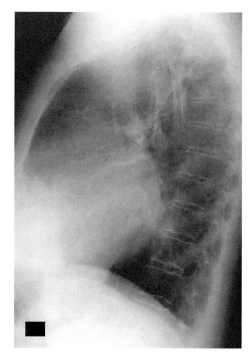

Fig. 12.2

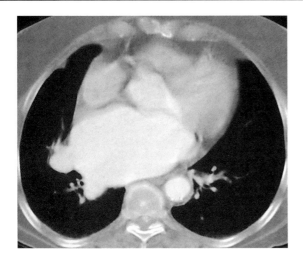

Fig. 12.3

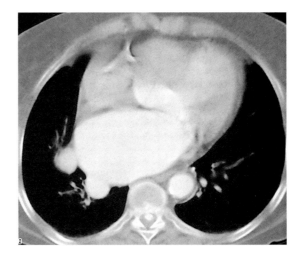

Fig. 12.4

■ Discussion

Background

Pulmonary varix is a rare lesion characterized by focal non-obstructive aneurysmal enlargement of one or more pulmonary veins prior to entering the left atrium.

Etiology

Both acquired and congenital etiologies of pulmonary varix have been proposed. Pulmonary varix is typically associated with mitral valve dysfunction, particularly insufficiency. In these cases, the right pulmonary veins are typically affected.

Clinical Findings

Affected patients are often asymptomatic and are diagnosed incidentally because of a radiographic abnormality. Some patients present with symptoms related to mitral valve disease. Hemoptysis and chronic lobar collapse are reported. Rarely, patients present with systemic embolization of associated endoluminal thrombus.

Imaging Findings

Radiography

- Single/multiple rounded or ovoid lobular mass/nodule (**Fig. 12.1**) projecting over the medial lower lobe; may be visible on only one radiographic projection (PA or lateral)
- Round mass/nodule related to the left atrium on lateral radiography (**Fig. 12.2**)
- May enlarge with onset of pulmonary venous hypertension
- Cardiomegaly; left atrial enlargement (**Figs. 12.1, 12.2**)

MDCT/MRI

- Demonstration of vascular nature of the nodule/mass seen on radiography (**Figs. 12.3, 12.4**)
- Demonstration of communication with the left atrium (**Figs. 12.3, 12.4**)
- Prompt (**Figs. 12.3, 12.4**) and delayed vascular enhancement reported
- Left atrial enlargement related to mitral valve disease (**Figs. 12.3, 12.4**)

Management

- Awareness of vascular nature of radiographic abnormality
- Management of mitral valve dysfunction in symptomatic patients

Prognosis

- Good
- Death rarely reported from associated hemoptysis

PEARLS

- Pulmonary varix typically affects the right inferior pulmonary or the lingular vein.
- Pulmonary varix is also known as hilar pseudotumor. Imaging abnormalities typically relate to enlargement of the right venous confluence.
- Peripheral pulmonary varix may mimic arteriovenous malformation.

Suggested Reading

1. Abujudeh H. Pulmonary varix: blood flow is essential in the diagnosis. Pediatr Radiol 2004;34(7):567–569

2. Cole TJ, Henry DA, Jolles H, Proto AV. Normal and abnormal vascular structures that simulate neoplasms on chest radiographs: clues to the diagnosis. Radiographics 1995;15(4):867–891

3. Gaeta M, Volta S, Vallone A. Hilar pseudonodule due to varix of the inferior pulmonary vein. AJR Am J Roentgenol 1995;165(5):1305

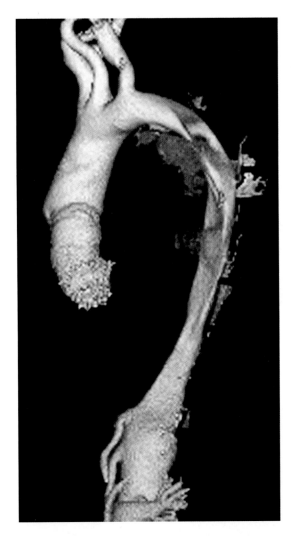

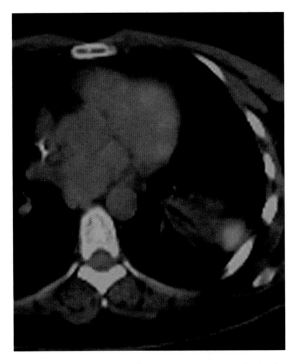

Fig. 82.6B FDG PET-CT shows intense FDG uptake in the lesion.

Figs. 6.4B The ascending aortic repair and the morphology of the true lumen of the descending aorta are shown on the oblique sagittal volume-rendered CT aortogram.

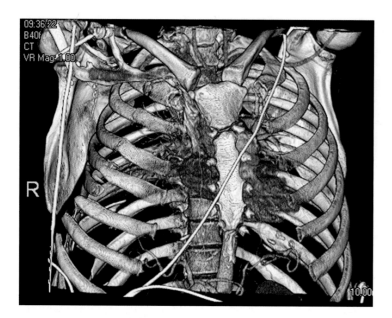

Fig. 95.1B 3-D CT reconstruction illustrates the acutely fractured first through eighth anterior and more inferiorly displaced posterior rib fractures to better advantage.

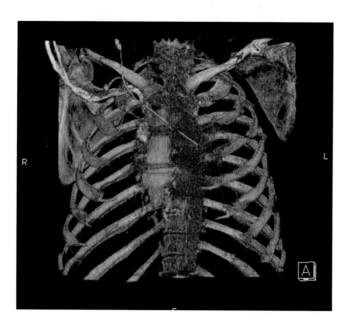

Fig. 97.3E 3-D volume-rendered reconstruction demonstrates marked separation of the left scapula from the chest wall. The scapulothoracic ratio (i.e., thoracic spinous process-medial scapular border distance) is 1.8. Compare the relationship of the left and right scapula to the thoracic cage on the 3-D images.

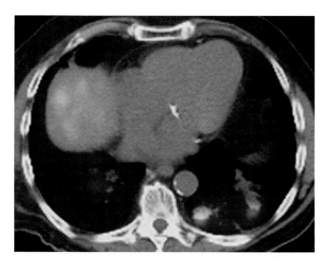

Fig. 113.2C Fused transverse PET/CT images show focal increased uptake of ^{18}F-FDG in the areas of basilar disease incorrectly suggesting neoplasia.

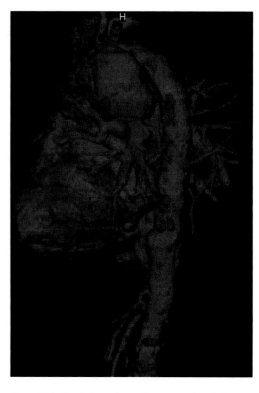

Fig. 135.1E 3-D color volume-rendered image confirms the mediastinal mass is a large saccular aneurysm off the transverse aorta.

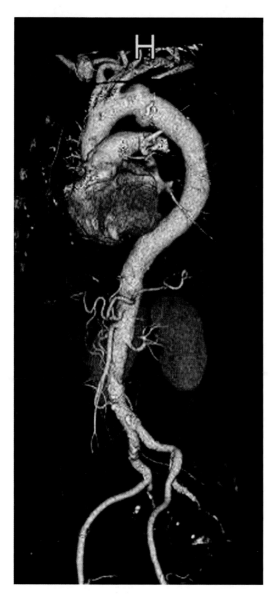

Fig. 135.5C The TAA and its great vessel relationships are nicely depicted on the 3-D volume-rendered CTA.

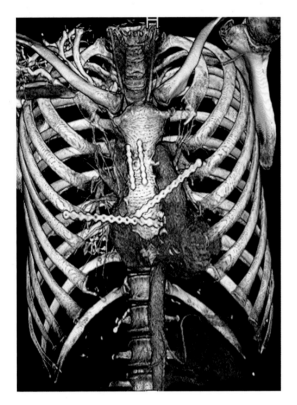

Fig. 183.2C Metallic bands and bars extend along and across the sternum, respectively; the bars connect to the anterior aspect of adjacent ribs. The 3-D volume-rendered image shows the post-surgical changes to better advantage.

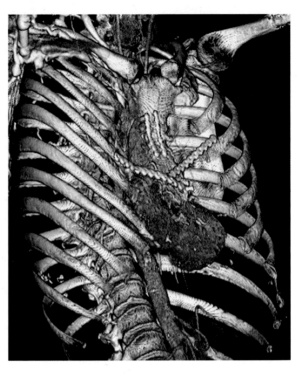

Fig. 183.2D Metallic bands and bars extend along and across the sternum, respectively; the bars connect to the anterior aspect of adjacent ribs. The 3-D volume-rendered image shows the post-surgical changes to better advantage.

CASE 13

■ Clinical Presentation

68-year-old woman admitted for pacemaker placement

■ Radiologic Findings

PA chest radiograph (**Fig. 13.1**) demonstrates cardiomegaly, marked enlargement of the azygos arch and vein, and bilateral hyparterial bronchi. Contrast-enhanced CT (mediastinal window) (**Figs. 13.2, 13.3, 13.4**) demonstrates bilateral hyparterial bronchi (**Fig. 13.3**), enlargement of the azygos arch (*a*) (**Fig. 13.2**), and descending azygos vein (*arrowhead*) (**Figs. 13.3, 13.4**), consistent with azygos continuation of the inferior vena cava and multiple left-sided spleens (polysplenia) (**Fig. 13.4**).

■ Diagnosis

Heterotaxy Syndrome: Polysplenia, Azygos Continuation of the Inferior Vena Cava

■ Differential Diagnosis

• Azygos Continuation of the Inferior Vena Cava with Situs Solitus

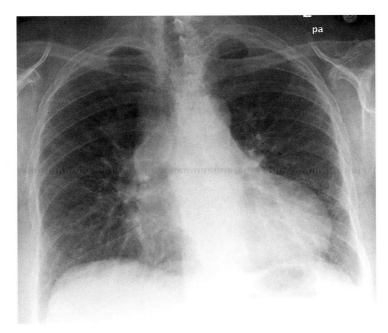

Fig. 13.1

109

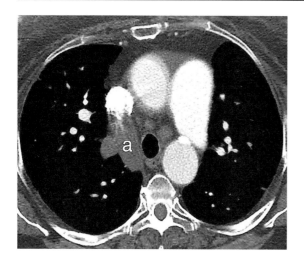

Fig. 13.2

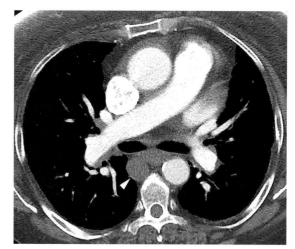

Fig. 13.3

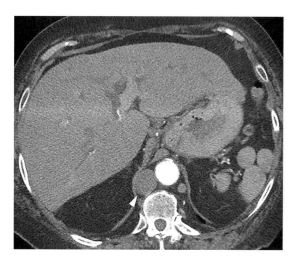

Fig. 13.4

■ Discussion

Background

Visceroatrial situs (location, position) refers to the location of the atria with respect to the midline and to other organs. The majority of the population exhibit normal visceroatrial situs (situs solitus) characterized by a morphologic right (systemic) atrium on the right side and a contralateral morphologic left (pulmonary) atrium. The pulmonary anatomy is characterized by a tri-lobed right lung with ipsilateral liver, gallbladder, and inferior vena cava and a bi-lobed left lung with ipsilateral stomach, single spleen, and aortic arch. The incidence of congenital heart disease in patients with situs solitus is approximately 0.8%. Approximately 0.1% of the population exhibit situs inversus, characterized by mirror image location of the atria, major vessels, and abdominal structures. These patients have a 3–5% incidence of congenital heart disease. The terms *heterotaxy, isomerism,* and *situs ambiguous* refer to absence of an orderly arrangement of visceroatrial morphology (in one or the other side of the body). Patients with heterotaxy or situs ambiguous have a high incidence (50–100%) of congenital heart disease. Tracheobronchial situs is characteristically concordant with visceroatrial situs. However, tracheobronchial situs is not necessarily concordant with situs of the cardiac apex, ventricles, or great vessels.

Etiology

The primitive heart and its vascular connections form early in embryogenesis (between 20 and 30 days of gestation). The cardiac atria retain their situs during embryologic development of the heart. Failure of normal lateralization results in duplication of left- or right-sided structures and, therefore, situs ambiguous or indeterminate situs. The major types of situs ambiguous are asplenia and polysplenia. The latter is associated with absence of, or less severe, congenital heart disease.

Clinical Findings

Polysplenia more commonly affects women than men. Affected patients may be diagnosed as infants or neonates because of associated symptomatic (typically non-cyanotic) congenital cardiovascular disease, including endocardial cushion defects, double-outlet right ventricle, aortic coarctation, and atrial septal defect. Approximately 25% of patients with polysplenia have no significant congenital heart disease. These patients are asymptomatic and are diagnosed incidentally. Associated abnormalities include interruption of the intrahepatic inferior vena cava with azygos continuation, duplication of the superior vena cava, and partial anomalous pulmonary venous return. Patients with *asplenia* typically present in infancy with symptoms of cyanosis and respiratory distress from severe complex cyanotic congenital heart disease, usually total anomalous pulmonary venous return, common atrioventricular canal, and univentricular heart. They may also present with symptoms of immune deficiency related to absence of the spleen.

Abdominal abnormalities in patients with heterotaxy include multiple spleens (polysplenia), absence of the spleen (asplenia), bowel malrotation, midline liver and gallbladder, truncated pancreas, and biliary atresia. Thus, affected patients may present with symptoms related to abdominal situs abnormalities.

Imaging Findings

Radiography

- Bilateral hyparterial bronchi (**Fig. 13.1**)
- Variable position of the heart (dextrocardia in up to 50%), aortic arch, and stomach
- Enlarged azygos arch and visualization of enlarged azygos vein (with associated azygos continuation of the inferior vena cava) (**Fig. 13.1**)

MDCT/MRI

- Demonstration of bilateral hyparterial bronchial morphology (**Figs. 13.3, 13.5**); bilateral bi-lobed lungs on CT
- Variable position of the heart
- Multiple spleens or single multi-lobate spleen (**Figs. 13.4, 13.6, 13.7**)
- Variable positions of spleen(s), stomach, liver, and gallbladder (**Fig. 13.7**)
- Demonstration of azygos (**Figs. 13.2, 13.3, 13.4, 13.6**) or hemiazygos continuation of the inferior vena cava; hepatic vein drainage into atrium
- Demonstration of atrial morphology through evaluation of atrial appendage morphology on MRI; morphologic left atrial appendages have a tubular shape and a curved downward apex
- Evaluation of associated cardiac anomalies

Management

- Awareness of abnormalities and associations in asymptomatic patients
- Surgical correction of symptomatic/significant congenital heart disease and associated conditions

Prognosis

- Polysplenia: Excellent without associated anomalies; high mortality with associated biliary atresia
- Asplenia: Poor; death in the first year of life in up to 80% of affected patients

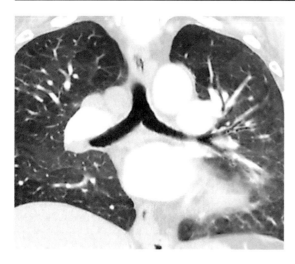

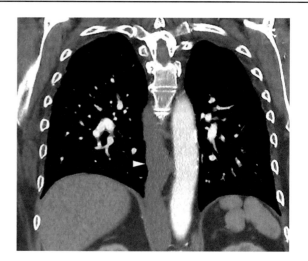

Fig. 13.5 Coronal contrast-enhanced chest CT (lung and mediastinal window) of a patient with polysplenia demonstrates bilateral hyparterial bronchi (**Fig. 13.5**), an enlarged azygos vein (*arrowhead*), and multiple left-sided spleens (**Fig. 13.6**).

Fig. 13.6

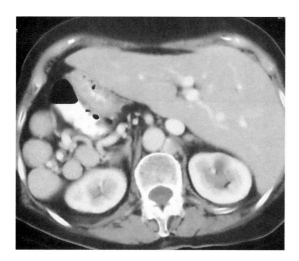

Fig. 13.7 Contrast-enhanced abdominal CT of a patient with polysplenia (soft-tissue window) demonstrates a left-sided liver, a right-sided stomach, and multiple right-sided spleens. This patient also had dextrocardia.

PEARLS

- Morphology of the tracheobronchial tree is a reliable indicator of underlying atrial morphology. An *eparterial* bronchus exists when the main bronchus is superior to the ipsilateral pulmonary artery, and a *hyparterial* bronchus exists when the main bronchus is inferior to the ipsilateral pulmonary artery. The morphologic right (systemic) atrium is usually ipsilateral to an eparterial bronchus while the morphologic left (pulmonary) atrium is usually ispilateral to a hyparterial bronchus.
- Identification of situs is the first step in the assessment of patients with complex congenital heart disease.

Suggested Reading

1. Applegate KE, Goske MJ, Pierce G, Murphy D. Situs revisited: imaging of the heterotaxy syndrome. Radiographics 1999;19(4):837–852, discussion 853–854

2. Ghosh S, Yarmish G, Godelman A, Haramati LB, Spindola-Franco H. Anomalies of visceroatrial situs. AJR Am J Roentgenol 2009;193(4):1107–1117

3. Lapierre C, Déry J, Guérin R, Viremouneix L, Dubois J, Garel L. Segmental approach to imaging of congenital heart disease. Radiographics 2010;30(2):397–411

4. Maldjian PD, Saric M. Approach to dextrocardia in adults: review. AJR Am J Roentgenol 2007;188(6, Suppl):S39–S49, quiz S35–S38

CASE 14

■ Clinical Presentation

35-year-old man evaluated for a murmur found on a routine physical examination

■ Radiologic Findings

PA (**Fig. 14.1**) and lateral (**Fig. 14.2**) chest radiographs demonstrate cardiomegaly and over-circulation. Note the enlarged central and peripheral pulmonary arteries.

■ Diagnosis

Atrial Septal Defect

■ Differential Diagnosis

- Other Left-to-Right Shunts; Ventricular Septal Defect; Patent Ductus Arteriosus
- Pulmonary Arterial Hypertension

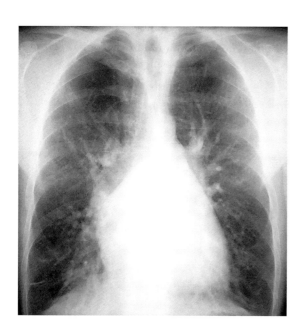

Fig. 14.1

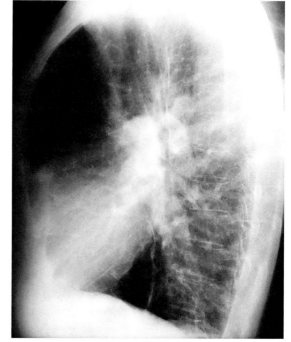

Fig. 14.2

■ Discussion

Background

Atrial septal defect (ASD) accounts for approximately 10% of congenital heart disease and is a common congenital cardiac lesion among those that initially manifest in adulthood. It represents approximately 30% of all congenital cardiac lesions in patients over the age of 40 years. ASD may be an isolated condition or may be associated with other cardiovascular anomalies.

Etiology

Atrial septal defect represents a congenital defect in the interatrial septum that results in communication between the two atria. ASD is classified based on anatomic location (**Fig. 14.3**). *Ostium secundum* ASD is the most common type, located at the fossa ovalis; *ostium primum* ASD is rare but represents the second most common ASD, is located in the inferior atrial septum, and is associated with partial atrioventricular septal defect (including a cleft mitral valve); *sinus venosus* ASD is rare, is located at the superior aspect of the septum near the orifice of the superior vena cava, and is associated with anomalous pulmonary venous drainage in up to 90% of cases; *coronary sinus* ASD represents unroofing of the coronary sinus with resultant interatrial communication and is associated with persistent left superior vena cava, partial anomalous pulmonary venous connections, and mitral valve prolapse.

Clinical Findings

Patients with ostium secundum ASD may remain asymptomatic until the second or third decade of life. Women are more commonly affected than men, with a 3:2 female-to-male ratio. Some patients are diagnosed incidentally because of a left sternal murmur, which is typically systolic with a split fixed second heart sound. Approximately half of patients over the age of 40 years are symptomatic and present with exertional dyspnea, fatigue, chest pain from atrial flutter/fibrillation, fever from infective endocarditis, paradoxical emboli, clinical right heart failure, and/or pulmonary hypertension. Palpitations and recurrent pulmonary infections are also reported. Approximately 15% of affected patients also have mitral insufficiency. ASD is described as part of the autosomal dominant Holt-Oram syndrome

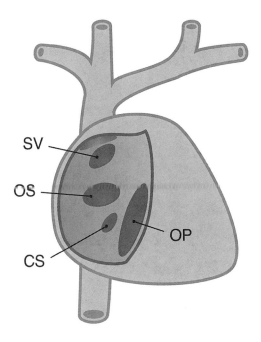

Fig. 14.3 Artist's illustration of the different types of ASD and their locations within the atrial septum. The most common is the ostium secundum (*OS*) type of ASD. The sinus venosus (*SV*) type of ASD occurs superiorly near the orifice of the superior vena cava, and the ostium primum (*OP*) type occurs inferiorly. The coronary sinus (*CS*) type of ASD occurs near the ostium of the coronary sinus.

Imaging Findings

Radiography

- Cardiomegaly (**Figs. 14.1, 14.4, 14.5**)
- Right atrial and ventricular enlargement with filling of retrosternal space
- Enlargement of central and peripheral pulmonary arteries from shunt circulation (**Fig. 14.1**)
- Pulmonary arterial hypertension (untreated patients) and Eisenmenger physiology
  - Enlargement of central pulmonary arteries and pulmonary trunk (**Figs. 14.4, 14.5**)
  - Decreased visualization ("pruning") of peripheral pulmonary arteries (**Figs. 14.4, 14.5**)
  - Calcification of central pulmonary arteries (with sustained pulmonary hypertension) (**Fig. 14.5**)
- Normal or small left atrium, normal pulmonary valve
- Left atrial enlargement and pulmonary venous hypertension in older adults with ASD
- Visualization of post-treatment changes (**Figs. 14.7, 14.8**)

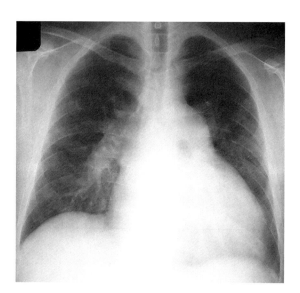

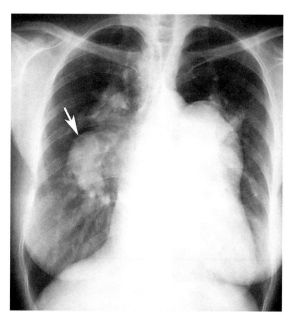

Fig. 14.4 PA chest radiograph of a 33 year old man with ASD and Eisenmenger physiology who presented with a brain abscess following an episode of bacteremia demonstrates cardiomegaly and marked enlargement of the central pulmonary arteries. Note the poor visualization of peripheral pulmonary arteries.

Fig. 14.5 PA chest radiograph of a 45-year-old woman with an ASD and Eisenmenger physiology demonstrates findings consistent with long-standing pulmonary arterial hypertension: cardiomegaly, massive enlargement and mural calcification (*arrow*) of the central pulmonary arteries, and vascular pruning.

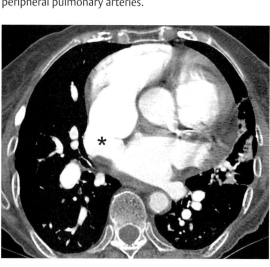

Fig. 14.6 Contrast-enhanced chest CT (mediastinal window) of a patient with an ASD demonstrates discontinuity of the atrial septum at the site of the ASD (*asterisk*). (*Image courtesy of Diane C. Strollo, MD, University of Pittsburgh Medical Center, Pittsburgh, Pennsylvania.*)

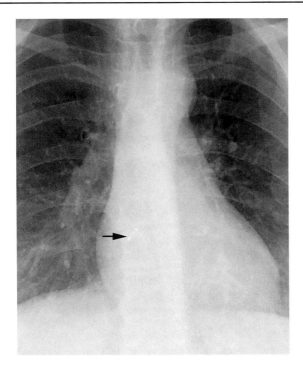

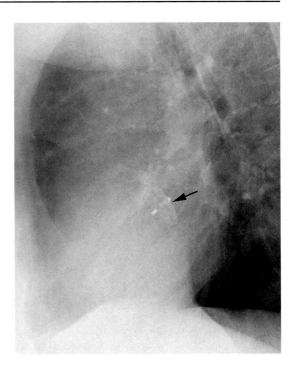

Fig. 14.7   Coned-down PA (**Fig. 14.7**) and lateral (**Fig. 14.8**) chest radiographs of a 35-year-old woman who was treated for a secundum ASD demonstrate the radio-opaque portions of an atrial septal closure device (*arrows*). Contrast-enhanced chest CT (mediastinal window) (**Fig. 14.9**) demonstrates the metallic portion of the atrial septal device (*arrow*) used for treatment of an ASD.

Fig. 14.8

Ultrasound

- Demonstration and evaluation of ASD
- Evaluation of associated valvular dysfunction
- Measurement of defect and chamber size

MRI/MDCT

- Demonstration of ASD (**Fig. 14.6**); visualization of defect at two adjacent anatomic levels on MR
- Gradual pulmonary artery enhancement during bolus tracking on contrast-enhanced CT pulmonary angiography related to left-to-right intracardiac shunt
- Demonstration of anomalous right superior pulmonary vein
- Measurement of size of shunt with velocity-encoded cine MR
- Flow turbulence in pulmonary arteries in patients with pulmonary arterial hypertension
- Visualization of post-treatment changes (**Fig. 14.9**)

Management

- Spontaneous closure reported in secundum ASD within the first year of life
- Transcatheter closure of selected secundum ASD with prosthetic closure device
- Elective surgical repair (closure) for children with ASD and persistent left-to-right shunt greater than 50% between ages 2 and 4 years
- Surgical repair for adults without severe pulmonary arterial hypertension
- Surgical repair of sinus venosus, ostium primum, and coronary sinus ASD

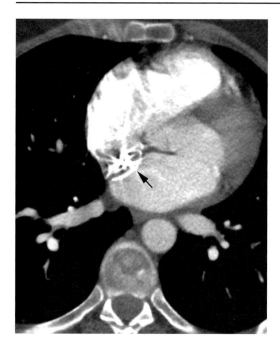

Fig. 14.9 Contrast-enhanced chest CT (mediastinal window) of the same patient illustrated in **Figs. 14.7** and **14.8** demonstrates the metallic portion of the atrial septal device (*arrow*) used for treatment of an ASD.

Prognosis

- Good for surgically treated patients; 95% 10-year survival
- Relates to degree of mitral valve dysfunction and associated dysrhythmias in patients with ostium secundum ASD
- Unknown long-term outcome for transcatheter closure devices

PEARLS

- Echocardiography with color flow Doppler is the modality of choice for evaluation of ASD.
- Lung perfusion scintigraphy may establish the presence of a shunt.
- Surgery for correction of ASD is not indicated before the age of 1 year, as many times the ASD will close spontaneously.

Suggested Reading

1. Cook AL, Hurwitz LM, Valente AM, Herlong JR. Right heart dilatation in adults: congenital causes. AJR Am J Roentgenol 2007;189(3):592–601

2. Gaca AM, Jaggers JJ, Dudley LT, Bisset GS III. Repair of congenital heart disease: a primer—Part 2. Radiology 2008; 248(1):44–60

3. Ko SF, Liang CD, Yip HK, et al. Amplatzer septal occluder closure of atrial septal defect: evaluation of transthoracic echocardiography, cardiac CT, and transesophageal echocardiography. AJR Am J Roentgenol 2009;193(6): 1522–1529

4. Tsai IC, Lee T, Chen MC, et al. Gradual pulmonary artery enhancement: new sign of septal defects on CT. AJR Am J Roentgenol 2007;188(6):1660–1664

CASE 15

■ Clinical Presentation

22-year-old man evaluated for newly diagnosed leukemia

■ Radiologic Findings

PA (**Fig. 15.1**) and lateral (**Fig. 15.2**) chest radiographs demonstrate enlargement of the main pulmonary artery. The heart and peripheral pulmonary vasculature are normal. Note the central venous catheter with its tip in the superior vena cava. Contrast-enhanced chest CT (mediastinal window) (**Figs. 15.3, 15.4**) demonstrates marked enlargement of the pulmonary trunk and the left pulmonary artery with a normal right pulmonary artery (**Fig. 15.4**)

■ Diagnosis

Pulmonic Stenosis

■ Differential Diagnosis

- Patent Ductus Arteriosus
- Pulmonary Artery Hypertension

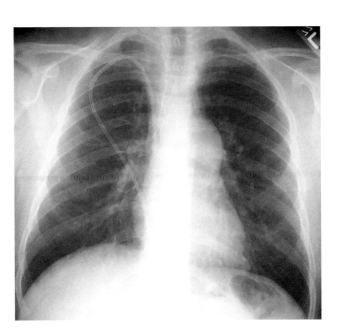

Fig. 15.1

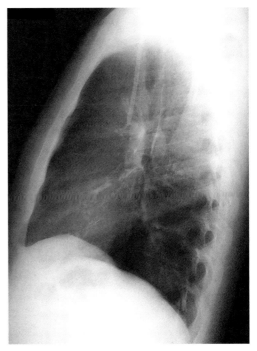

Fig. 15.2

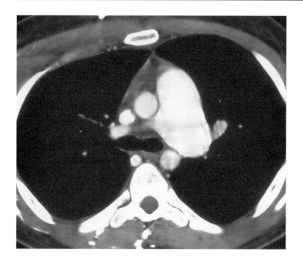

Fig. 15.3

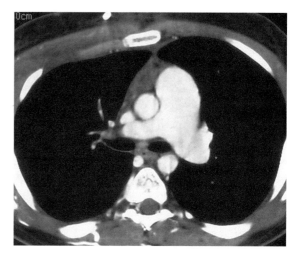

Fig. 15.4 (*Images courtesy of Diane C. Strollo, MD, University of Pittsburgh Medical Center, Pittsburgh, Pennsylvania.*)

■ Discussion

Background

Pulmonic stenosis is the most common anomaly that produces obstruction of the right ventricular outflow tract. It occurs as an isolated anomaly in up to 7% of patients with congenital heart disease. It is a common congenital cardiac lesion among those that initially manifest in adulthood. Pulmonic stenosis may be associated with other congenital heart lesions and is a component of tetralogy of Fallot.

Etiology

Pulmonic stenosis is a congenital malformation of the pulmonary valve. Stenosis may be related to fused valve commissures, dome-shaped stenosis, and bicuspid or dysplastic morphology. Stenosis may be valvular, subvalvular, or supravalvular. Acquired pulmonic stenosis is rare and can be related to rheumatic heart disease or carcinoid syndrome.

Clinical Findings

Patients with pulmonic stenosis are acyanotic. Many are entirely asymptomatic and most present in the third or fourth decade of life. Physical examination typically reveals a harsh long (diamond-shaped) systolic ejection murmur. Patients with severe obstruction from pulmonic stenosis may present in childhood with easy fatigability and right ventricular failure.

Imaging Findings

Radiography

- Mild to moderate pulmonary trunk enlargement (**Figs. 15.1, 15.5**)
- Left pulmonary artery enlargement (**Figs. 15.1, 15.5**)
- Normal right pulmonary artery, peripheral pulmonary arteries, and pulmonary veins (**Figs. 15.1, 15.2, 15.5**)
- Normal heart size (**Figs. 15.1, 15.2, 15.5**); right ventricular enlargement in cases of right ventricular failure
- Left lung may appear oligemic relative to the right.

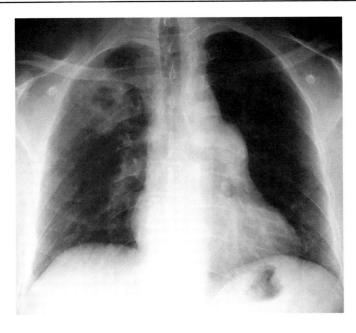

Fig. 15.5 PA chest radiograph of a young man with post-primary tuberculosis and asymptomatic pulmonic stenosis demonstrates a cavitary lesion of the right upper lobe and enlargement of the pulmonary trunk (initially thought to represent lymphadenopathy).

MDCT/MRI

- Pulmonary trunk and left pulmonary artery enlargement (**Figs. 15.3, 15.4, 15.6**)
- Rarely pulmonic valve calcification
- Normal right pulmonary artery (**Figs. 15.4, 15.6**)
- Right ventricular hypertrophy
- Bowing of interventricular septum to the left
- Velocity-encoded cine MR imaging; demonstration of differential blood flow in the pulmonary arteries, estimation of gradient across stenotic valve, and assessment of valve motion
- Turbulent flow on gradient-echo cine sequences
- Left lung may appear oligemic relative to the right.

Management

- Balloon dilatation for reduction of transvalvular gradient
- Repeat dilatation or open surgical correction (valve replacement) in approximately 20% of patients

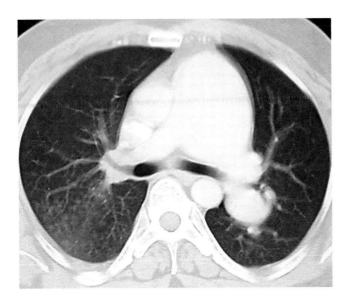

Fig. 15.6 Chest CT (lung window) demonstrates marked enlargement of the pulmonary trunk and the left pulmonary artery. Note the normal right pulmonary artery and the tree-in-bud opacities in the right lung secondary to transbronchial dissemination of tuberculosis.

Prognosis

- Good with appropriate treatment
- Survival beyond 50 years unusual in untreated patients
- Mortality and morbidity from infective endocarditis

PEARLS

- Pulmonary artery enlargement in pulmonic stenosis results from post-stenotic dilatation secondary to the high-velocity jet of blood forced through the stenotic valve, but the degree of dilatation is not related to the severity of the obstruction.
- Pulmonic stenosis and pulmonary arterial hypertension may both manifest with pulmonary artery enlargement. The two conditions are differentiated based on the fact that the right pulmonary artery is normal in pulmonic stenosis and enlarged in pulmonary arterial hypertension. The right pulmonary artery originates at a 90° angle from the pulmonary trunk, is not affected by the turbulent jet, and does not dilate.
- Trilogy of Fallot refers to pulmonic stenosis complicated by right ventricular hypertrophy and a right-to-left shunt through an incompetent foramen ovale.

Suggested Reading

1. Chen JJ, Manning MA, Frazier AA, Jeudy J, White CS. CT angiography of the cardiac valves: normal, diseased, and post-operative appearances. Radiographics 2009;29(5):1393–1412

2. Ryan R, Abbara S, Colen RR, et al. Cardiac valve disease: spectrum of findings on cardiac 64-MDCT. AJR Am J Roentgenol 2008;190(5):W294–W303

3. Steiner RM, Reddy GP, Flicker S. Congenital cardiovascular disease in the adult patient: imaging update. J Thorac Imaging 2002;17(1):1–17

CASE 16

■ Clinical Presentation

50-year-old man evaluated for chest and abdominal pain

■ Radiologic Findings

Coned-down PA chest radiograph (**Fig. 16.1**) demonstrates enlargement of the azygos arch, a right eparterial bronchus, and a left hyparterial bronchus. Axial (**Figs. 16.2, 16.3**) and coronal (**Fig. 16.4**) contrast-enhanced chest CT (mediastinal and lung windows) show enlargement of the azygos arch (*a*) and azygos vein (*arrowhead*). Note right eparterial and left hyparterial bronchi consistent with situs solitus (**Fig. 16.4**).

■ Diagnosis

Interruption of the Inferior Vena Cava with Azygos Continuation

■ Differential Diagnosis

- Lymphadenopathy
- Situs Ambiguous

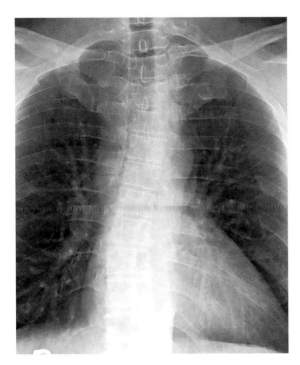

Fig. 16.1

123

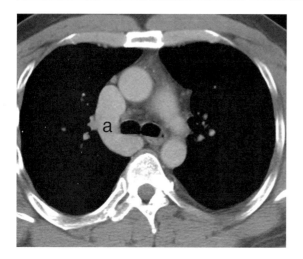

Fig.16.2

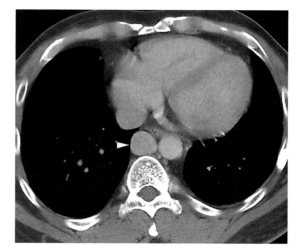

Fig.16.3

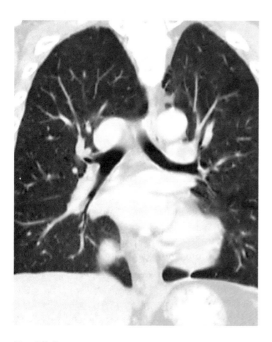

Fig. 16.4

■ Discussion

Background

Interruption of the inferior vena cava (IVC) is a congenital anomaly characterized by absence or hypoplasia of the hepatic IVC, with blood from the infrarenal and renal IVC draining into the azygos or hemiazygos system to reach the superior vena cava. Associated conditions include congenital heart disease, left-sided or duplicated IVC, and situs ambiguous (specifically left isomerism).

Etiology

Interruption of the inferior vena cava with azygos (or hemiazygos) continuation results from malformation of the right subcardinal-phrenic vascular anastomosis with resultant subcardinal (suprarenal) inferior vena cava atrophy.

Clinical Findings

Patients with interruption of the IVC and azygos (or hemiazygos) continuation may be entirely asymptomatic. Patients with associated anomalies may have symptoms referable to these associated conditions.

Imaging Findings

Radiography

- Dilatation of the azygos arch (**Fig. 16.1**)
- Dilatation of the azygos (or hemiazygos) vein and the superior vena cava
- Normal tracheobronchial morphology (**Fig. 16.1**)

MDCT/MRI

- Enlarged azygos arch (**Fig. 16.2**)
- Enlarged azygos/hemiazygos vein (**Figs. 16.3, 16.5**)
- Visualization of normal tracheobronchial morphology (**Fig. 16.4**)
- Absence or hypoplasia of hepatic segment of IVC with hepatic veins draining into the right atrium via suprahepatic IVC
- Left-sided (**Figs. 16.6, 16.7**) or duplicated IVC
- Visualization of hemiazygos and/or azygos enlargement; enlargement of hemiazygos and accessory hemiazygos systems draining into a persistent left SVC, enlarged hemiazygos vein draining into the accessory hemiazygos, the left superior intercostal vein, and the left brachiocephalic vein

Management

- Awareness of interruption of the IVC in patients undergoing venous catheterization

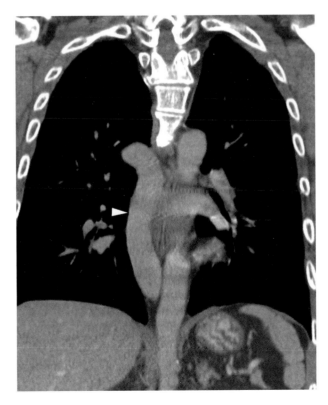

Fig. 16.5 Coronal contrast-enhanced chest CT demonstrates an enlarged azygos vein (*arrowhead*).

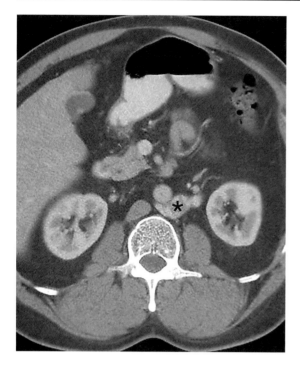 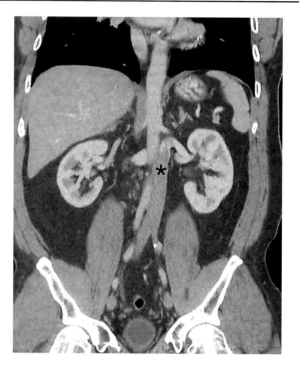

Fig. 16.6 Axial (**Fig. 16.6**) and coronal (**Fig. 16.7**) contrast-enhanced abdomen CT (soft-tissue window) demonstrate absence of the normal right-sided IVC. The renal veins drain into a left-sided IVC (*asterisk*).

Fig. 16.7

Prognosis

- Excellent in the absence of associated congenital anomalies

PEARLS

- Diagnosis of interruption of the IVC and azygos continuation is particularly important in patients undergoing cardiac catheterization or cardiopulmonary bypass surgery.
- Identification of the dilated azygos vein as a right paramediastinal interface is helpful in avoiding the pitfall of confusing this entity with mediastinal lymphadenopathy.

Suggested Reading

1. Demos TC, Posniak HV, Pierce KL, Olson MC, Muscato M. Venous anomalies of the thorax. AJR Am J Roentgenol 2004;182(5):1139–1150

2. Kandpal H, Sharma R, Gamangatti S, Srivastava DN, Vashisht S. Imaging the inferior vena cava: a road less traveled. Radiographics 2008;28(3):669–689

3. Sheth S, Fishman EK. Imaging of the inferior vena cava with MDCT. AJR Am J Roentgenol 2007;189(5): 1243–1251

Section III

Airways Disease

OVERVIEW OF AIRWAYS DISEASE

The airways may be affected by a variety of congenital and acquired conditions. These include infectious and inflammatory lesions, benign and malignant neoplasms, and various idiopathic disease entities.

Airways disease is categorized in terms of the size of the affected airways. The *large airways* include the trachea and most bronchi. *Small airways* are those measuring 2 mm or less, most of which are bronchioles, although the designation does include the smallest of bronchi. Bronchioles are also distinguished by their lack of cartilage and submucosal glands—features characteristic of bronchi.

Large airway diseases can be categorized as *focal* or *diffuse*. Most neoplasms, for example, result in *focal* tracheobronchial abnormalities, whereas inflammatory diseases are generally *diffuse* (e.g., relapsing polychondritis). Some disease may produce both patterns of involvement. Wegener granulomatosis, for example, may manifest as focal lesions in the large airways but may also produce multifocal lesions with tracheobronchial wall thickening and stenosis.

The posterior wall of the trachea is *membranous*; the remainder of the tracheal wall is composed of incomplete cartilaginous rings. The membranous wall extends inferiorly into the mainstem bronchi and large central airways (e.g., bronchus intermedius). Diseases that affect the central airways may be categorized by their propensity to involve or spare the membranous wall. For example, relapsing polychondritis and tracheobronchopathia osteochondroplastica characteristically spare the posterior wall, whereas amyloidosis, Wegener granulomatosis, and infectious tracheobronchitis often involve the membranous tracheal wall.

Bronchiectasis occurs in a spectrum of pulmonary diseases, most commonly as a sequela of previous infection or inflammatory disease. Other diseases within this spectrum may have distinguishing patterns of distribution and associated clinical findings that help to narrow the imaging differential diagnosis.

The *small airways* are not normally visible on MDCT/HRCT. Small airway disease can be categorized as *proliferative* (cellular) or *fibrotic* (constrictive), and may manifest with direct or indirect imaging signs, respectively. The *direct* imaging signs of small airway disease are bronchiolectasis and centrilobular nodules. Bronchiolectasis may be detected in the extreme lung periphery in the setting of chronic fibrosis but is an uncommon finding. Centrilobular nodules may be solid (soft tissue) nodular opacities, appear as branching (tree-in-bud) opacities, or be of ground-glass attenuation.

Indirect signs of small airway disease include mosaic attenuation and air trapping, demonstrated on inspiratory and expiratory MDCT/HRCT imaging, respectively. Mosaic attenuation manifests on MDCT/HRCT as a patchwork of regions of differing attenuation, with borders that often follow the outlines of the underlying secondary pulmonary lobules. Mosaic attenuation may indicate the presence of obliterative (constrictive) small airways disease, patchy interstitial disease, or occlusive vascular disease.

Air trapping manifests on expiratory MDCT/HRCT as sharply defined "geographic" areas of low attenuation. These areas often follow the outlines of underlying secondary pulmonary lobules.

The cases in this section illustrate the range of imaging findings that may be encountered in large and small airways.

Suggested Reading

1. Hansell DM, Lynch DA, McAdams HP, Bankier AA. Diseases of the airways. In: Hansell DM, Lynch DA, McAdams HP, Bankier AA, eds. Imaging of Diseases of the Chest, 5th ed. Philadelphia: Mosby Elsevier; 2010:715–785

2. Abbott GF, Rosado-de-Christenson ML, Rossi SE, Suster S. Imaging of small airways disease. J Thorac Imaging 2009;24(4):285–290

CASE 17

■ Clinical Presentation

34-year-old man with stridor that developed six months after prolonged tracheostomy

■ Radiologic Findings

Coned-down PA chest radiograph (**Fig. 17.1A**) demonstrates symmetric narrowing of the tracheal lumen. Chest CT (lung window) with axial and coronal reformation (**Figs. 17.1B, 17.1C**) demonstrates tracheal narrowing with a reduced coronal diameter and anterior luminal tapering. Surface rendered 3-D image (**Fig. 17.1D**) of tracheal and central airways shows a tapered area of stenosis in the upper trachea at the level of previous tracheostomy.

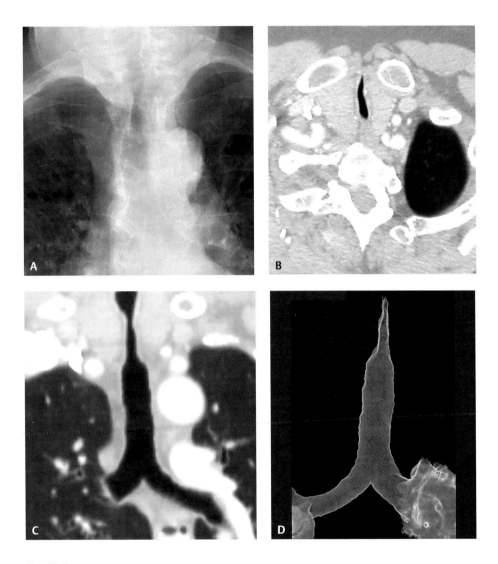

Fig. 17.1

■ Diagnosis

Tracheal Stenosis; Post-Intubation Injury

■ Differential Diagnosis

- Benign and Malignant Tracheal Neoplasm
- Wegener Granulomatosis
- Amyloidosis

■ Discussion

Background

Tracheal stenosis is defined as narrowing of the tracheal lumen by more than 10% of its normal diameter. It is a relatively uncommon condition with a frequently insidious onset. Early signs and symptoms may be disregarded or confused with other disorders.

Etiology

Congenital tracheal stenosis manifests during infancy. The most common cause of benign tracheal stenosis in adults is trauma, usually related to endotracheal intubation or tracheostomy. Stricture typically occurs at the site of an inflatable endotracheal tube cuff but may also develop at the site of a tracheotomy stoma. The portions of the trachea most susceptible to stenosis are those where mucosa overlies the cartilaginous rings. Inflation of the endotracheal tube cuff to pressures exceeding 20 mm Hg (the mean capillary pressure in the tracheal mucosa) may obstruct blood flow and cause ischemic necrosis and subsequent fibrosis. Strictures may occur as early as 36 hours post-intubation. Use of endotracheal tubes with low-pressure cuffs has reduced the prevalence of tracheal stenosis to less than 1%, as compared with a prevalence of 20% when high-pressure cuffs were in use. Tracheal stenosis may also result from direct blunt trauma to the trachea.

Clinical Findings

Affected patients may present with dyspnea on exertion, stridor, and wheezing. Stridor typically develops five weeks or more after extubation.

Imaging Features

Chest Radiography

- Circumferential, symmetric, or eccentric tracheal narrowing; often with an hourglass configuration (**Fig. 17.1A**)
- Narrowed segment is typically less than 2 cm in length (**Fig. 17.1A**)
- Typical location above thoracic inlet (**Fig. 17.1A**)

MDCT

- Circumferential or eccentric tracheal narrowing (**Figs. 17.1B, 17.1C, 17.1D, 17.2**)
- Variable tracheal wall thickness (**Figs. 17.1B, 17.1C, 17.1D, 17.2**)

Management

- Surgical excision of stenotic segment and reconstruction
- Endoscopic mechanical dilatation
- Tracheal stenting
- Laser photoablation for focal mucosal lesions

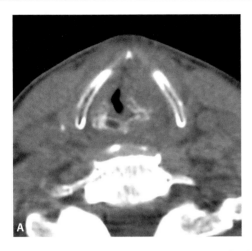
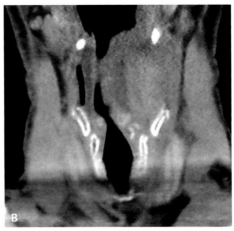

Fig. 17.2 Unenhanced axial **(A)** with coronal reformation **(B)** chest CT (mediastinal window) of a 42-year-old man with acute stridor after receiving blunt trauma to the trachea during a barroom fight demonstrates a longitudinal fracture through the left thyroid cartilage with adjacent hematoma narrowing the tracheal lumen.

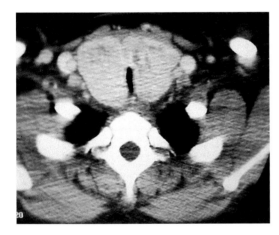

Fig. 17.3 Contrast-enhanced chest CT (mediastinal window) of a 39-year-old woman with goiter demonstrates diffuse enlargement of the thyroid gland, which produces extrinsic mass effect on the trachea, with resultant luminal narrowing.

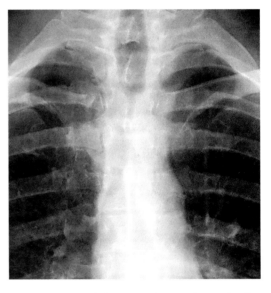

Fig. 17.4 Coned-down PA chest radiograph of a 62-year-old man with squamous cell carcinoma of the trachea demonstrates severe narrowing of the tracheal lumen.

Prognosis

- Excellent; sleeve resection curative in 91% of patients

PEARLS

- Tracheal stenosis may result from granuloma formation caused by surgical sutures related to tracheostomy and may mimic an endoluminal tracheal neoplasm.
- Tracheomalacia results from an abnormal degree of compliance of the tracheal wall and its supporting cartilage.

- Tracheomalacia and/or ulcerative tracheoesophageal fistula may occur as sequelae of endotracheal intubation.
- Tracheal stenosis may result from extrinsic compression by vascular anomalies (aberrant right subclavian artery, double aortic arch, pulmonary artery sling) or thyroid enlargement related to goiter or neoplasia (**Figs. 17.3, 17.4**).

Suggested Reading

1. Grenier PA, Beigelman-Aubry C, Brillet PY. Nonneoplastic tracheal and bronchial stenoses. Radiol Clin North Am 2009;47(2):243–260

2. Grenier PA, Beigelman-Aubry C, Fetita C, Martin-Bouyer Y. Multidetector-row CT of the airways. Semin Roentgenol 2003;38(2):146–157

3. Lee KS, Yoon JH, Kim TK, Kim JS, Chung MP, Kwon OJ. Evaluation of tracheobronchial disease with helical CT with multiplanar and three-dimensional reconstruction: correlation with bronchoscopy. Radiographics 1997;17(3):555–567, discussion 568–570

4. Grillo HC, Donahue DM. Postintubation tracheal stenosis. Chest Surg Clin N Am 1996;6(4):725–731

5. Stark P. Imaging of tracheobronchial injuries. J Thorac Imaging 1995;10(3):206–219

CASE 18

■ Clinical Presentation

62-year-old man with chronic obstructive pulmonary disease

■ Radiologic Findings

Coned-down PA chest radiograph (**Fig. 18.1A**) demonstrates narrowing of the tracheal coronal diameter. Contrast-enhanced chest CT (mediastinal window) demonstrates normal tracheal morphology at the level of the thoracic inlet (**Fig. 18.1B**) and deformity of the tracheal lumen below that level (**Fig. 18.1C**). The tracheal wall is of normal thickness. The cross-sectional morphology of the tracheal lumen resembles that of a saber sheath.

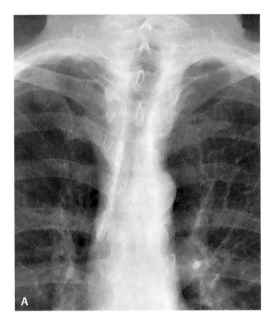

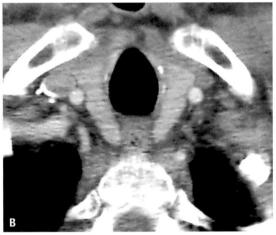

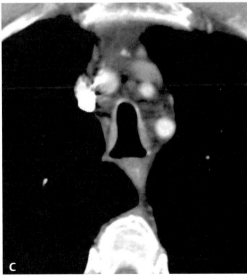

Fig. 18.1

135

■ Diagnosis

Saber Sheath Trachea

■ Differential Diagnosis

- Tracheal Stricture
- Relapsing Polychondritis
- Amyloidosis
- Tracheobronchopathia Osteochondroplastica

■ Discussion

Background

Saber sheath trachea is defined as a tracheal deformity in which the coronal tracheal diameter is equal to or less than one-half the sagittal diameter, measured 1 cm above the superior aspect of the aortic arch. The deformity begins at the thoracic inlet, affects only the intrathoracic trachea, and is a manifestation of chronic obstructive pulmonary disease.

Etiology

Saber sheath trachea is thought to result from repeated coughing and abnormal intrathoracic pressures, which may cause tracheal collapse and fixed coronal narrowing.

Clinical Findings

Most individuals with saber sheath trachea have chronic obstructive pulmonary disease and may have chronic cough. Affected patients are typically older men with emphysema. There are no specific symptoms associated with saber sheath trachea. Correlative studies of radiographic findings and CT determinations of tracheal size and morphology along with pulmonary function testing have shown that saber sheath tracheal deformity is basically a sign of thoracic hyperinflation.

Imaging Features

Chest Radiography

- Abrupt coronal narrowing of the intrathoracic tracheal diameter on frontal radiography (**Fig. 18.1A**)

MDCT

- Characteristic "saber sheath" intrathoracic tracheal deformity; narrow coronal diameter (**Fig. 18.1C**), widened sagittal diameter (**Fig. 18.1C**)
- Normal tracheal wall thickness (**Fig. 18.1C**)
- Smooth (**Fig. 18.1C**), irregular, or nodular inner tracheal margins
- Calcification of cartilaginous tracheal rings

Management

- None

Prognosis

- Good

PEARLS

- Chest CT of patients with saber sheath trachea, when performed during forced expiration, may show further tracheal narrowing or tracheomalacia.

Suggested Reading

1. Hansell DM, Lynch DA, McAdams HP, Bankier AA. Diseases of the airways. In: Hansell DM, Lynch DA, McAdams HP, Bankier AA, eds. Imaging of Diseases of the Chest, 5th ed. Philadelphia: Mosby Elsevier; 2010:715–785

2. Boiselle PM, Lee KS, Ernst A. Multidetector CT of the central airways. J Thorac Imaging 2005;20(3):186–195

3. Webb EM, Elicker BM, Webb WR. Using CT to diagnose nonneoplastic tracheal abnormalities: appearance of the tracheal wall. AJR Am J Roentgenol 2000;174(5):1315–1321

4. Trigaux JP, Hermes G, Dubois P, Van Beers B, Delaunois L, Jamart J. CT of saber-sheath trachea. Correlation with clinical, chest radiographic and functional findings. Acta Radiol 1994;35(3):247–250

CASE 19

■ Clinical Presentation

38-year-old woman with recurrent respiratory infections

■ Radiologic Findings

Coned-down PA (**Fig. 19.1A**) and lateral (**Fig. 19.1B**) chest radiographs demonstrate enlargement of the tracheal lumen and bilateral central thin-walled pulmonary cystic lesions. HRCT (lung window) (**Figs. 19.1C, 19.1D**) demonstrates marked tracheal enlargement involving the origins of the mainstem bronchi. Note the corrugated contour of the tracheal wall and bilateral branching thin-walled cystic lesions located centrally in the lung, consistent with bronchiectasis.

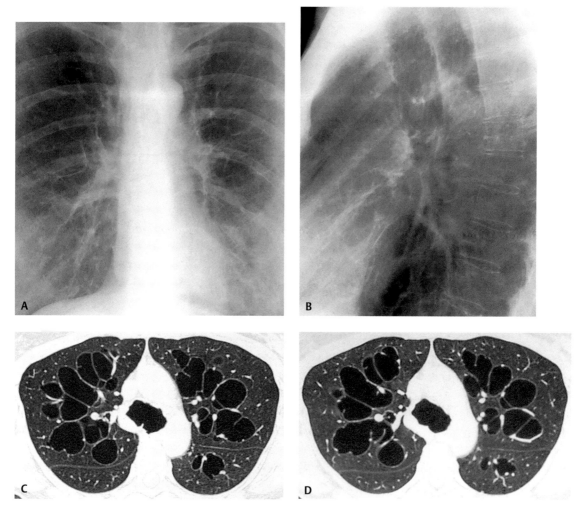

Fig. 19.1

138

■ Diagnosis

Tracheobronchomegaly; Mounier-Kuhn Syndrome

■ Differential Diagnosis

- Bronchiectasis
- Williams-Campbell Syndrome
- Chronic Airway Inflammation/Infection with Tracheobronchomalacia
- Allergic Bronchopulmonary Fungal Disease

■ Discussion

Background

Tracheobronchomegaly or Mounier-Kuhn syndrome is a rare condition also known as tracheal diverticulosis and tracheobronchiectasis.

Etiology

The etiology of tracheobronchomegaly is unknown. Some authors have postulated a *congenital etiology* related to connective tissue disease because of associated conditions, such as Ehlers-Danlos syndrome in affected adults and cutis laxa in affected children, with reported associations with double carina, tracheal trifurcation, and congenitally short right upper lobe bronchus. A familial form of the disease with autosomal recessive inheritance has also been reported. Other authors postulate an *acquired etiology*, as the disease has been reported in infants after intensive ventilatory support. Cigarette smoking may also be implicated in the development of the disease. Tracheobronchomegaly is thought to result from weakness of cartilaginous and membranous components of the trachea and main bronchi.

Clinical Findings

Affected patients are often adult men who are diagnosed in the third to fifth decades of life. Most affected adults present with recurrent pulmonary infection and marked sputum production, but symptoms usually date back to childhood. These patients may develop dyspnea on exertion and respiratory failure. Hemoptysis may occur. Spontaneous pneumothorax and digital clubbing have also been described. Some patients are entirely asymptomatic and are diagnosed incidentally.

Imaging Findings

Chest Radiography

- Dilatation of trachea and main bronchi (**Figs. 19.1A, 19.1B**); may be limited to the trachea

MDCT

- Dilatation of trachea and main bronchi (**Figs. 19.1C, 19.1D, 19.2A, 19.2B**)
- Diameter of trachea, right main bronchus, or left main bronchus exceeding 30 mm, 24 mm, and 23 mm, respectively (**Figs. 19.1C, 19.1D, 19.2A, 19.2B**)
- Corrugated appearance of airway walls due to mucosal prolapse through adjacent cartilaginous rings (**Figs. 19.1C, 19.1D**)
- Perihilar cystic spaces representing bronchial diverticulosis (**Figs. 19.1C, 19.1D, 19.2A, 19.2B**)
- Proximal airway collapse on expiration due to tracheobronchomalacia

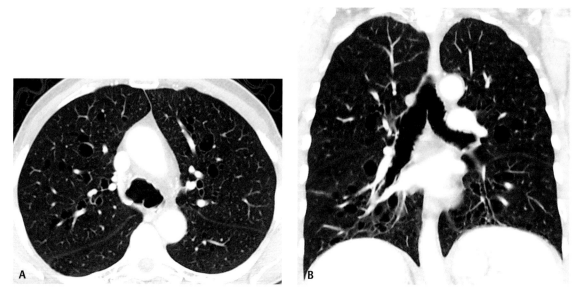

Fig.19.2   Chest CT (lung window) of a 38-year old man with tracheobronchomegaly demonstrates tracheal enlargement involving the origins of the mainstem bronchi. Note the corrugated contour of the tracheal and mainstem bronchial walls and bilateral bronchiectasis located centrally in the lungs.

Management

- Antibiotics
- Postural drainage
- Bronchoscopy for clearance of secretions
- Tracheostomy/tracheal stenting
- Lung transplantation

Prognosis

- Recurrent lower respiratory tract infections
- Affected patients develop dyspnea and respiratory failure as the lungs become progressively damaged

PEARLS

- Williams-Campbell syndrome results from absence of cartilage rings beyond the first and second bronchial divisions, with resultant bronchiectasis that typically affects the fourth- to sixth-order bronchi (**Figs. 19.3A, 19.3B**). Affected patients have normal-caliber trachea and central bronchi.

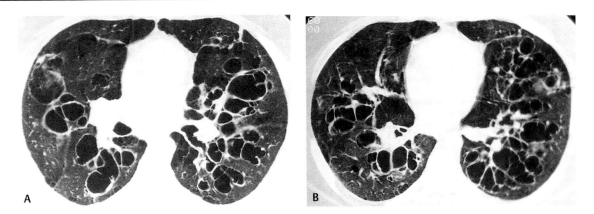

Fig.19.3 Unenhanced chest CT (lung window) of a 27-year-old man with recurrent pulmonary infection and Williams-Campbell syndrome demonstrates extensive bronchiectasis. The central bronchi (not shown) were of normal caliber. (*Images courtesy of H. Page McAdams, MD, Duke University Medical Center, Durham, North Carolina.*)

Suggested Reading

1. Hansell DM, Lynch DA, McAdams HP, Bankier AA. Diseases of the airways. In: Hansell DM, Lynch DA, McAdams HP, Bankier AA, eds. Imaging of Diseases of the Chest, 5th ed. Philadelphia: Mosby Elsevier; 2010:715–785

2. Kwong JS, Müller NL, Miller RR. Diseases of the trachea and main-stem bronchi: correlation of CT with pathologic findings. Radiographics 1992;12(4):645–657

3. Marom EM, Goodman PC, McAdams HP. Diffuse abnormalities of the trachea and main bronchi. AJR Am J Roentgenol 2001;176(3):713–717

4. Lazzarini-de-Oliveira LC, Costa de Barros Franco CA, Gomes de Salles CL, de Oliveira AC Jr. A 38-year-old man with tracheomegaly, tracheal diverticulosis, and bronchiectasis. Chest 2001;120(3):1018–1020

5. Blake MA, Clarke PD, Fenlon HM. Thoracic case of the day. Mounier-Kuhn syndrome (tracheobronchomegaly). AJR Am J Roentgenol 1999;173(3):822, 824–825

CASE 20

■ Clinical Presentation

64-year-old man presenting with chronic cough and recurrent respiratory infections

■ Radiologic Findings

Paired end-inspiratory (**Fig. 20.1**) and dynamic-expiratory (**Fig. 20.2**) chest CT (lung windows) acquired at the aortic arch. End-inspiratory CT (**Fig. 20.1**) shows a slightly dilated, ovoid tracheal morphology. Dynamic-expiratory CT (**Fig. 20.2**) reveals near total collapse of the trachea with a crescentic frown-like appearance (*frown sign*)

■ Diagnosis

Tracheomalacia; confirmed at bronchoscopy

■ Differential Diagnosis

None

■ Discussion

Background

Tracheomalacia (TM) is undetectable and therefore under-diagnosed on routine end-inspiratory imaging. The normally more compliant posterior membranous tracheal wall is displaced to a greater degree than the less compliant cartilaginous anterolateral walls during forced expiration or coughing. TM is characterized

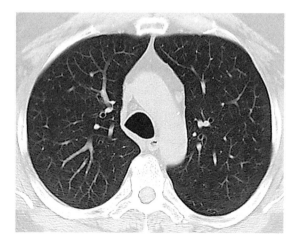

Fig. 20.1

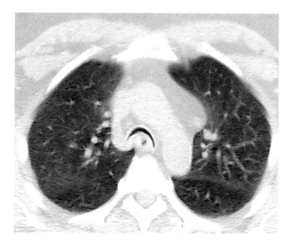

Fig. 20.2 (*Images courtesy of Philip Boiselle, MD, Harvard Medical School and Beth Israel Deaconess Medical Center, Boston, Massachusetts.*)

by excessive expiratory collapse of the tracheal walls and/or supporting cartilage and is an important cause of airway obstruction, chronic cough, recurrent lung infection, and other respiratory symptoms. Although most cases of *acquired TM* diffusely involve the intrathoracic trachea, TM may also be localized. If the main-stem bronchi are also involved, the term *tracheobronchomalacia* (TBM) is used. Bronchomalacia (BM) is iso-lated weakness and collapsibility of one or both mainstem bronchi without tracheal involvement and is less common.

Etiology

TM is divided into *congenital (primary)* and *acquired (secondary)* forms of disease. TM is the most com-mon congenital anomaly of the trachea. It can occur as an isolated finding in healthy infants, but is more commonly seen in premature infants as a consequence of immature tracheobronchial cartilage. *Primary TM* may also be associated with tracheoesophageal fistula and vascular rings. Other forms of *primary disease* result from an abnormal tracheal cartilaginous matrix and include polychondritis, chon-dromalacia, and various mucopolysaccharidoses (e.g., Hunter and Hurler syndrome). Further discussion of *congenital* or *primary TM* is beyond the scope of this textbook. An additional congenital condition, although some authorities contend it is acquired, found in adults, is tracheomegaly (aka Mounier-Kuhn syndrome). This rare condition is characterized by atrophy of longitudinal elastic fibers and thinning of the muscularis mucosa (see Case 19). *Acquired* or *secondary TM* is more common than *congenital TM* and caused by degeneration of normal cartilaginous support. A variety of entities can cause *secondary TM* in adults, including prior prolonged intubation, tracheotomy, tracheostomy, antecedent tracheal surgery, lung transplantation, recurrent tracheobronchitis, external tracheal compression from various struc-tures (e.g., thyroid mass or goiter, aberrant vasculature, aneurysmal dilatation of great vessels, left atrial and/or left atrial appendage enlargement, mediastinal tumors), mediastinal radiation therapy, chest wall musculoskeletal deformities (e.g., scoliosis, pectus excavatum), severe emphysema, etc. Antecedent tra-cheostomy or endotracheal tube intubation is the most common cause of *secondary TM*. Additionally, chronic inflammation and irritants, such as cigarette smoke, are important contributors to the develop-ment of TM.

Clinical Findings

Acquired TM is a disease of the middle-aged and elderly, and most commonly seen in men over 40 years of age. Symptoms are nonspecific and include productive cough, dyspnea, and hemoptysis, which are often attributed to tobacco abuse and/or coexistent asthma, chronic bronchitis, or emphysema. Patients may also exhibit a "barking" cough, inspiratory wheezing, stridor, recurrent lung infections, and upper airway collapse during forced exhalation. Some patients are asymptomatic until physically stressed by an infection (e.g., bronchitis, pneumonia). TM may not be clinically evident in intubated patients as airway patency is maintained by the positive pressure. Following extubation, affected patients may ex-perience respiratory distress, wheezing, and stridor, necessitating reintubation. PFTs commonly reveal a decreased FEV_1 and a low peak flow rate with a rapid decrease in flow. Airway resistance is almost always elevated. A characteristic pattern is seen on forced expiratory spirograms with near complete absence of the usual sloping phase of the mid-portion of the curve and a "break" or "notch" in the expiratory phase of the flow-volume loop. Bronchoscopic visualization of dynamic tracheal or bronchial collapse is the "gold standard" for diagnosing TM. On direct visualization, the membranous trachea appears widened or redundant. Airway collapse is seen with forced exhalation or coughing and can be graded based on its severity. In *mild TM*, airway collapse is one-half the lumen diameter; in *moderate TM*, airway collapse is three-quarters the lumen diameter; in *severe TM*, the posterior membranous wall touches the anterior cartilaginous wall.

Imaging Findings

Radiography

- Often unrevealing, even when inspiratory-expiratory views acquired

MDCT

- Paired end-inspiratory–dynamic-expiratory MDCT is an effective, noninvasive method for diagnosing TM, TMB, BM (**Figs. 20.1, 20.2**)
- Percentage of luminal collapse between end inspiration and expiration is calculated as follows: $LC = 100 \cdot [1 - (LA_{ee}/LA_{ei})]$
  - LC = percentage of luminal collapse
  - LA_{ee} = luminal area at end expiration (mm^2)
  - LA_{ei} = luminal area at end inspiration (mm^2)
- ≥70% luminal narrowing on forced expiration is the diagnostic threshold for TM
- Visual assessment and classification of tracheal shape 1 cm above the aortic arch at end-inspiration and dynamic expiration
  - *Normal inspiratory trachea shape classifications* (**Fig. 20.1**)
    - Round (circular with equivalent coronal and sagittal diameters)
    - Oval (elliptical with nonequivalent coronal and sagittal diameters)
    - Horseshoe (rounded anterior contour and flattened posterior membranous wall resembling a horseshoe)
    - Inverted pear (bulbous, rounded anterior wall with smaller, rounded posterior wall; contour resembles an upside-down pear)
  - *Abnormal inspiratory trachea shape classifications*
    - Saber sheath (sagittal-to-coronal ratio >2)
    - Lunate (coronal-to-sagittal ratio >1)
  - *Expiratory trachea shape classifications*
    - Expiratory-1 (relative flattening of posterior membranous wall with slight anterior bowing)
    - Expiratory-2 (mild to moderate anterior bowing of posterior membranous wall with a broad anterior convexity)
    - Expiratory-3 (mild to moderate anterior bowing of posterior membranous wall with a narrow anterior convexity)
    - Frown configuration (marked anterior bowing of posterior membranous wall with close apposition to anterior wall, forming an upside-down smile) (**Fig. 20.2**)
- Multiplanar paired end-inspiratory and dynamic-expiratory sagittal reformations can display the craniocaudal extent of excessive tracheal collapse at end expiration
- Data can be reconstructed into 2-D and 3-D images, including virtual bronchoscopy
- Air trapping seen at a higher frequency (TM patients, 100%; control subjects, 60%) and is more severe in patients with TM

Management

Asymptomatic (incidental) TM and TBM

- No therapy necessary

Symptomatic TM and TBM

- Initial conservative therapy preferred: treatment of respiratory infections, humidified oxygen, and pulmonary physiotherapy

Conservative Management Failure/Progressive Symptomatic TM and TBM

- Continuous positive airway pressure (CPAP)
- Surgical intervention in select patients
  - Tracheostomy tube bypasses malacic segment or serves to splint the airway open
  - External surgical stent supports for the pars membranacea
    - Bone graft
    - Various prosthetic and autologous materials
  - Biocompatible ceramic rings
  - Plication of posterior wall of trachea with crystalline polypropylene and high-density polyethylene mesh
  - Resection and reconstruction for focal TM
- Array of endoluminal stents (e.g., silicone, metal, hybrid, biodegradable) used to mechanically maintain airway patency

Prognosis

- Majority of healthy and premature infants with *primary TM* unassociated with other diseases or syndromes outgrow the condition by 2 years of age
- Other forms of *primary TM* in patients with connective tissue disorders and congenital syndromes; often unrecognized or misdiagnosed as asthma; substantial morbidity and mortality (up to 80%)
- Although *acquired TM* may remain stable, it may progress into *acquired TBM* in some patients, and *acquired BM* may progress to *acquired TBM*

PEARLS

- Inspiratory tracheal morphology is almost always normal in patients with tracheomalacia; a lunate configuration is rarely observed.
- Frown-like expiratory tracheal configuration is closely associated with true tracheomalacia.
- Unexplained extubation failure should prompt evaluation for TM.
- >50% luminal narrowing has been widely used as both a bronchoscopic and CT criterion for TM. However, the trachea of some healthy individuals may exceed this level of collapse. If a lower threshold is used, CT results should be correlated with clinical symptoms, PFT results, and appropriate risk factors, to avoid a false-positive diagnosis of tracheomalacia.

Suggested Reading

1. Boiselle PM, O'Donnell CR, Bankier AA, et al. Tracheal collapsibility in healthy volunteers during forced expiration: assessment with multidetector CT. Radiology 2009;252(1):255–262

2. Boiselle PM, Ernst A. Tracheal morphology in patients with tracheomalacia: prevalence of inspiratory lunate and expiratory "frown" shapes. J Thorac Imaging 2006;21(3):190–196

3. Boiselle PM, Lee KS, Lin S, Raptopoulos V. Cine CT during coughing for assessment of tracheomalacia: preliminary experience with 64-MDCT. AJR Am J Roentgenol 2006;187(2):W175–W177

4. Carden KA, Boiselle PM, Waltz DA, Ernst A. Tracheomalacia and tracheobronchomalacia in children and adults: an in-depth review. Chest 2005;127(3):984–1005

5. Kandaswamy C, Balasubramanian V. Review of adult tracheomalacia and its relationship with chronic obstructive pulmonary disease. Curr Opin Pulm Med 2009;15(2):113–119

CASE 21

■ Clinical Presentation

37-year-old man with cough after swallowing

■ Radiologic Findings

Coned-down PA chest radiograph (**Fig. 21.1A**) demonstrates a tracheostomy tube in place; the tube was removed 6 weeks later. Coned-down AP chest radiograph (**Fig. 21.1B**) obtained one week after tracheostomy tube removal demonstrates air distension of the esophagus that overlies the normal tracheal air column. Coned-done oblique (RPO) radiograph (**Fig. 21.1C**) obtained during Gastrografin swallow demonstrates a fistulous communication between the posterior wall of the trachea and the esophagus at the level of a replaced tracheostomy tube. Contrast material opacifies the esophagus, trachea, tracheostomy stoma, and both mainstem bronchi (**Fig. 21.1C**).

■ Diagnosis

Tracheoesophageal Fistula; Complication of Prolonged Tracheostomy Tube Placement

■ Differential Diagnosis

None

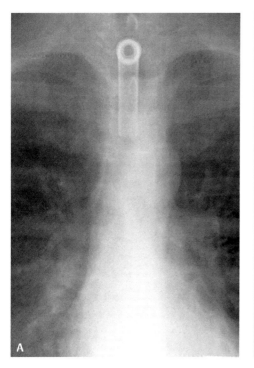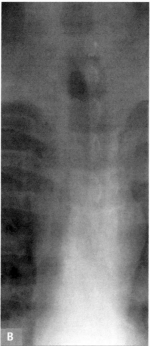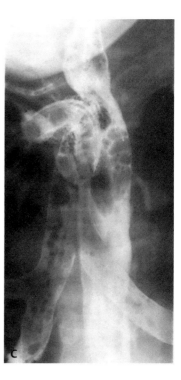

Fig. 21.1

■ Discussion

Background

Most tracheoesophageal fistulas in adults are acquired lesions. In the pediatric population, they are most commonly associated with congenital lesions (e.g., esophageal atresia). Tracheoesophageal fistula (TEF) should be excluded in all patients with a history of penetrating trauma to the mediastinum or neck.

Etiology

TEF may occur as a complication of intrathoracic malignancy (60%), prolonged tracheal intubation, esophageal instrumentation, infection, or trauma. TEF occurs in 5–10% of patients with advanced esophageal cancer and is more prevalent in those who have had prior irradiation. The diagnosis is usually made with a fluoroscopic contrast esophagogram. CT may demonstrate an occult TEF in patients at risk who have a normal esophagogram.

Clinical Findings

Symptoms related to TEF vary depending on the fistula size. Affected patients may cough after swallowing or may present with indirect signs related to the fistula such as pneumonia, gaseous distension of the esophagus, pneumomediastinum, and subcutaneous air.

Imaging Features

Chest Radiography

- Normal chest radiographs
- Pneumomediastinum (common)
- Pneumothorax
- Consolidation related to aspiration
- Air-distended esophagus (**Fig. 21.1B**)
- Airway opacification on contrast esophagography (**Fig. 21.1C**)

MDCT/3-D Reformations

- Direct visualization of fistula
- Assessment of fistula size and location
- Pneumomediastinum
- Pneumothorax
- Consolidation
- Air-distended esophagus

Management

- Esophageal stenting
- Surgical repair

Prognosis

- Favorable with prompt stenting or repair
- Morbidity and mortality from secondary infection

PEARLS

- When the esophagus and trachea are injured simultaneously, failure to recognize TEF may jeopardize surgical airway repair, as contamination with saliva may persist from an unrecognized esophageal communication.
- Endotracheal cuff-related tracheal injury is the most common cause of non-malignant TEF.
- TEF secondary to malignancy has a bleak prognosis, but improved survival and quality of life may be gained by prompt esophageal bypass or stenting.

Suggested Reading

1. Giménez A, Franquet T, Erasmus JJ, Martínez S, Estrada P. Thoracic complications of esophageal disorders. Radiographics 2002;22(Spec No):S247–S258
2. Kanne JP, Stern EJ, Pohlman TH. Trauma cases from Harborview Medical Center. Tracheoesophageal fistula from a gunshot wound to the neck. AJR Am J Roentgenol 2003;180(1):212
3. Reed MF, Mathisen DJ. Tracheoesophageal fistula. Chest Surg Clin N Am 2003;13(2):271–289

CASE 22

■ Clinical Presentation

56-year-old woman with cough

■ Radiologic Findings

Contrast-enhanced chest CT (mediastinal window) (**Figs. 22.1A, 22.1B**) demonstrates abnormal soft tissue extending anterolaterally along the tracheal wall and narrowing the lumen. Note the absence of soft-tissue infiltration/obliteration of peritracheal tissue planes.

■ Diagnosis

Tracheobronchial Amyloidosis

■ Differential Diagnosis

- Primary and Secondary Neoplasia (e.g., adenoid cystic carcinoma, tracheal metastases)
- Wegener Granulomatosis
- Tracheobronchopathia Osteochondroplastica

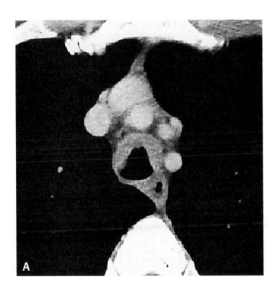 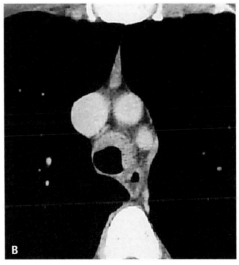

Fig. 22.1

■ Discussion

Background

Amyloidosis is a rare disease that may affect the lung or tracheobronchial tree. It may occur as a *primary lesion* or as *secondary amyloid deposition* in association with chronic disease. Tracheobronchial involvement is the most common and severe form of thoracic amyloidosis. Primary tracheal amyloidosis is rare and usually involves the trachea in a slow and indolent manner.

Etiology

The etiology of tracheobronchial amyloidosis is unknown. Chronic diseases associated with secondary amyloidosis include rheumatoid arthritis, Crohn disease, ankylosing spondylitis, tuberculosis, bronchiectasis, and familial Mediterranean fever.

Clinical Findings

Affected patients may be asymptomatic or may present with dyspnea, cough, hemoptysis, and/or hoarseness. Patients with severe proximal disease may have significantly decreased air flow, air trapping, and fixed upper airway obstruction on pulmonary function tests. Symptoms may develop over a period of months or years.

Imaging Features

Chest Radiography

- Nodular, irregular, or smooth narrowing of tracheal lumen
- Lobar/segmental atelectasis/consolidation from endobronchial obstruction

MDCT

- Nodular or plaque-like (**Figs. 22.1A, 22.1B, 22.2**) thickening of the airway wall; focal or circumferential
- Irregular narrowing/occlusion of airway lumen (**Figs. 22.1A, 22.1B, 22.2**)
- Calcification within areas of mural thickening or masses (**Fig. 22.2**)
- Associated paratracheal/peribronchial lymphadenopathy; may calcify

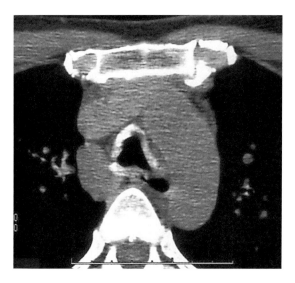

Fig. 22.2 Unenhanced chest CT (mediastinal window) of a patient with tracheal amyloidosis shows extensive circumferential thickening with calcification within the tracheal wall; note the involvement of the posterior membranous tracheal wall.

Management

- Bronchoscopic recanalization (laser resection, stent placement)
- External radiation
- Systemic therapy (melphalan, corticosteroids, colchicines)

Prognosis

- Unpredictable; severe morbidity/mortality with increasing airway obstruction; 30% mortality within 7–12 years post diagnosis in one study
- Common recurrences; may require repeated bronchoscopic re-canalization; airway compromise may persist post treatment

PEARLS

- Serial pulmonary function tests and CT may offer the best assessment of airway involvement and disease progression in patients with tracheobronchial amyloidosis.
- *Tracheobronchial amyloidosis* may involve the posterior tracheal membrane (unlike tracheobronchopathia osteochondroplastica and relapsing polychondritis) and is not associated with tracheomalacia on expiratory imaging.
- *Relapsing polychondritis* may diffusely involve the large airways, but typically spares the membranous posterior tracheal wall (**Fig. 22.3**).
- *Tracheobronchopathia osteochondroplastica* typically manifests on HRCT as small multifocal mural nodules in the trachea and proximal bronchi, with calcification of some or all nodules; characteristically spares the membranous posterior tracheal wall (**Fig. 22.4**).

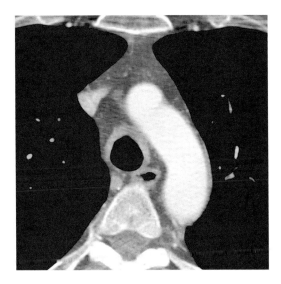

Fig. 22.3 Contrast-enhanced chest CT (mediastinal window) of a patient with relapsing polychondritis demonstrates mild thickening along the anterolateral tracheal wall, with sparing of the posterior membranous wall.

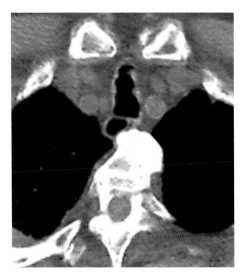

Fig. 22.4 Unenhanced chest CT of a patient with tracheobronchopathia osteochondroplastica demonstrates small mural nodules in the trachea, some of which appear partially calcified, with sparing of the membranous posterior tracheal wall.

Suggested Reading

1. Prince JS, Duhamel DR, Levin DL, Harrell JH, Friedman PJ. Nonneoplastic lesions of the tracheobronchial wall: radiologic findings with bronchoscopic correlation. Radiographics 2002;22(Spec No):S215–S230

2. Capizzi SA, Betancourt E, Prakash UB. Tracheobronchial amyloidosis. Mayo Clin Proc 2000;75(11):1148–1152

3. Kim HY, Im JG, Song KS, et al. Localized amyloidosis of the respiratory system: CT features. J Comput Assist Tomogr 1999;23(4):627–631

4. Lechner GL, Jantsch HS, Greene RE. Radiology of the trachea. In: Taveras JM, Ferrucci JT, eds. Radiology: Diagnosis-Imaging-Intervention, vol. I. Philadelphia: JB Lippincott; 1998:1–31

5. Travis WD, Colby TV, Koss MN, Rosado-de-Christenson ML, Müller NL, King TE Jr. Miscellaneous diseases of uncertain etiology. In: King DW, ed. Atlas of Nontumor Pathology: Non-Neoplastic Disorders of the Lower Respiratory Tract. First Series. Fascicle 2. Washington, DC: The American Registry of Pathology; 2002:857–900

CASE 23

■ Clinical Presentation

27-year-old man with fever and malaise and known tracheobronchial papillomatosis

■ Radiologic Findings

PA chest radiograph (**Fig. 23.1A**) demonstrates right lower lobe consolidation and bilateral irregular cystic lung lesions more numerous in the right lung. Unenhanced chest CT (lung window) (**Figs. 23.1B, 23.1C, 23.1D**) demonstrates multifocal thin-walled cystic lung lesions with variable shapes and endobronchial soft-tissue masses affecting the carina, right mainstem bronchus, and bronchus intermedius (**Figs. 23.1B, 23.1C**). Note also the near complete obstruction and circumferential thickening of the bronchus intermedius by an endobronchial papilloma (**Fig. 23.1C**) and right lower lobe consolidation and infrahilar mass (**Fig. 23.1D**). At endoscopy, squamous cell carcinoma was diagnosed.

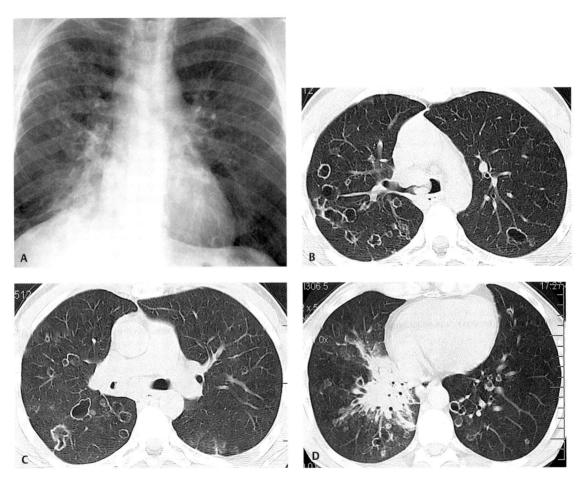

Fig. 23.1

153

■ Diagnosis

Tracheobronchial Papillomatosis; Complicating Squamous Cell Carcinoma

■ Differential Diagnosis

- Pulmonary Metastases
- Multifocal Cavitary Primary Lung Cancer
- Langerhans Cell Histiocytosis
- *Pneumocystis carinii* Pneumonia
- Vasculitis

■ Discussion

Background

Papillomas are the most common laryngeal tumor of young children. Tracheobronchial papillomatosis is a pre-malignant condition that results from tracheobronchial dissemination of laryngeal papillomas. It is also known as recurrent respiratory papillomatosis. The lesions typically involve the larynx but extend into the trachea and proximal bronchi in 5% of cases and into the small airways and lung parenchyma in less than 1%.

Etiology

Tracheobronchial papillomatosis is caused by infection with the human papilloma virus, typically HPV types 6 and 11. The infection may be transmitted to the newborn during passage through a birth canal previously colonized by the papilloma virus. Papillomas typically affect the larynx but may extend distally to the tracheobronchial tree and lung parenchyma, particularly after treatment with laser or endoscopic fulguration or after local resection or tracheostomy. The mechanism of distal dissemination is thought to relate to aspiration of infected fragments or multicentric infection. Distal dissemination of papillomas typically occurs approximately 10 years following laryngeal involvement. Malignant transformation is thought to be associated with HPV types 16 and 18.

Clinical Findings

Tracheobronchial papillomatosis usually affects young children, and males are more frequently affected than females. Hoarseness is a common initial symptom of laryngeal involvement. Patients with pulmonary disease may present with recurrent infection, hemoptysis or obstructive effects of endoluminal papillomas, such as wheezing and atelectasis. These patients are at risk of malignant degeneration of papillomas into squamous cell carcinoma.

Imaging Findings

Chest Radiography

- Multiple endoluminal airway nodules or irregular airway walls; may be limited to the trachea or main bronchi
- Multiple bilateral pulmonary nodules/masses/thin-walled cavitary nodules/masses
- Atelectasis, consolidation (**Fig. 23.1A**), bronchiectasis from obstructing endobronchial papillomas
- Consolidation or mass related to malignant degeneration (**Fig. 23.1A**)

MDCT

- Multifocal pulmonary nodules (**Figs. 23.1B, 23.1C, 23.1D, 23.2B**)
- Multifocal thick- and thin-walled cavitary pulmonary nodules/masses (**Figs. 23.1B, 23.1C, 23.1D, 23.2B, 23.2C, 23.3**)

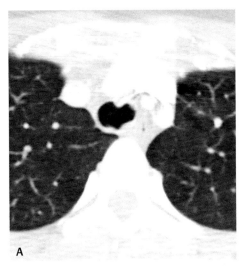
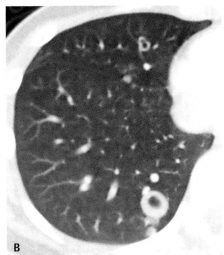
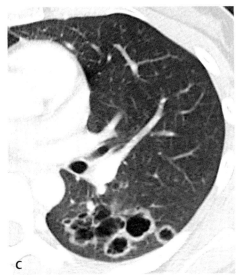

Fig. 23.2 Contrast-enhanced chest CT (lung window) **(A,B)** of a 27-year-old woman with tracheobronchial papillomatosis demonstrates an endoluminal soft-tissue nodule within the trachea **(A)** and multiple thick-walled **(B)** and thin-walled **(C)** cavitary pulmonary nodules. Note the predominance of findings in posterior aspects of both lungs.

- Endoluminal soft-tissue nodules/masses of variable size (**Figs. 23.1B, 23.1C, 23.2A**); may significantly occlude airway lumen
- Post-obstructive atelectasis/consolidation (**Fig. 23.1D**)
- Enlarging consolidation (**Fig. 23.1D**); mass (**Fig. 23.1D**) in cases of malignant transformation to squamous cell carcinoma (**Figs. 23.1D**)
- Predominance of findings in posterior aspects of both lungs

Management

- Antibiotics
- Clearance of secretions with postural drainage/bronchoscopy
- Laser/endoscopic fulguration of papillomas
- Tracheostomy/tracheal stenting
- Lung transplantation

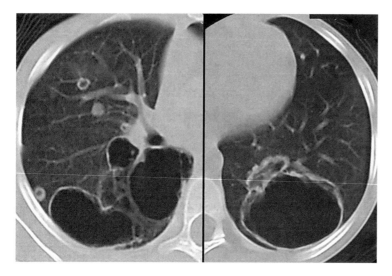

Fig. 23.3 Composite chest CT (modified lung window) of a 22-year-old man with tracheobronchial papillomatosis shows bilateral thin-walled cavitary lung nodules. Note the predominance of findings in the posterior aspects of both lungs.

PEARLS

- An increase in size or change in morphology of a pulmonary lesion in a patient with known papillomatosis requires further imaging and/or tissue sampling to exclude malignant degeneration.

Suggested Reading

1. Hansell DM, Lynch DA, McAdams HP, Bankier AA. Diseases of the airways. In: Hansell DM, Lynch DA, McAdams HP, Bankier AA, eds. Imaging of Diseases of the Chest, 5th ed. Philadelphia: Mosby Elsevier; 2010:715–785

2. Prince JS, Duhamel DR, Levin DL, Harrell JH, Friedman PJ. Nonneoplastic lesions of the tracheobronchial wall: radiologic findings with bronchoscopic correlation. Radiographics 2002;22(Spec No):S215–S230

3. Kotylak TB, Barrie JR, Raymond GS. Answer to case of the month #81. Tracheobronchial papillomatosis with spread to pulmonary parenchyma and the development of squamous cell carcinoma. Can Assoc Radiol J 2001;52(2):126–128

4. Gruden JF, Webb WR, Sides DM. Adult-onset disseminated tracheobronchial papillomatosis: CT features. J Comput Assist Tomogr 1994;18(4):640–642

5. Rady PL, Schnadig VJ, Weiss RL, Hughes TK, Tyring SK. Malignant transformation of recurrent respiratory papillomatosis associated with integrated human papillomavirus type 11 DNA and mutation of p53. Laryngoscope 1998;108(5):735–740

CASE 24

■ Clinical Presentation

30-year-old woman with cough and stridor

■ Radiologic Findings

Coned-down PA (**Fig. 24.1A**) and coned-down lateral (**Fig. 24.1B**) chest radiographs demonstrate a well-defined ovoid mass within the distal tracheal lumen. Unenhanced chest CT (mediastinal [**Fig. 24.1C**] and lung [**Fig. 24.1D**] windows) demonstrates an endoluminal spherical soft-tissue mass arising from the posterolateral tracheal wall that almost completely obstructs the airway lumen. There is circumferential tracheal wall thickening that suggests local invasion.

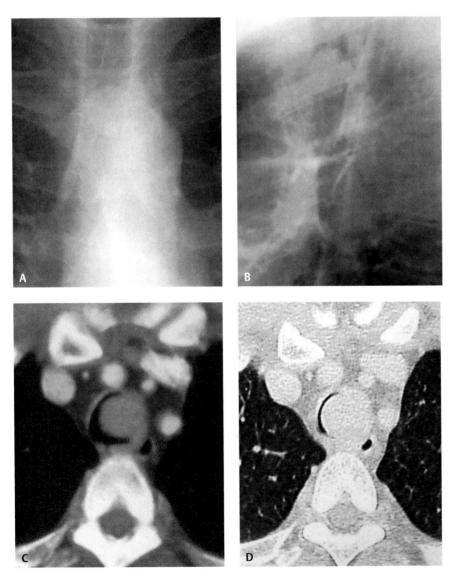

Fig. 24.1

157

■ Diagnosis

Adenoid Cystic Carcinoma

■ Differential Diagnosis

- Mucoepidermoid Carcinoma
- Carcinoid
- Squamous Cell Carcinoma
- Other Mesenchymal Neoplasms (benign or malignant)

■ Discussion

Background

Primary tracheal tumors are rare and occur much less frequently than bronchial tumors. Adenoid cystic carcinoma represents the second most common primary malignant neoplasm of the trachea after squamous cell carcinoma, although some argue that it may be the most common. Adenoid cystic carcinoma and mucoepidermoid carcinoma (another malignant neoplasm that typically affects the proximal bronchi) are primary malignancies of the airway that exhibit histologic features identical to those of primary salivary gland neoplasms of the same name. Adenoid cystic carcinoma may spread into the adjacent mediastinum or neck and may involve regional cervical and mediastinal lymph nodes. Metastases to distant extrathoracic sites are less common.

Etiology

Adenoid cystic carcinoma and mucoepidermoid carcinoma are malignant neoplasms of unknown etiology thought to originate from the submucosal bronchial glands. A relationship between cigarette smoking and these neoplasms has not been identified.

Clinical Findings

Patients with adenoid cystic carcinoma are usually young adults who are typically symptomatic and present with clinical features of airway obstruction, including cough, hemoptysis, and respiratory infection. Rarely, affected patients may present because of symptoms related to distant metastases.

Imaging Findings

Chest Radiography

- Focal endoluminal nodule/mass (**Figs. 24.1A, 24.1B**)
- Focal circumferential airway narrowing
- Secondary obstruction; atelectasis; consolidation

MDCT/MRI

- Well-defined endoluminal nodule/mass (**Figs. 24.1C, 24.1D, 24.2A, 24.2B**)
- May extend longitudinally or circumferentially along airway wall (**Figs. 24.2A, 24.2B**)
- May invade peritracheal soft tissues

Management

- Complete excision, which may be difficult in cases of locally invasive tumors
- Lung-sparing excision (sleeve resection) if tumor-free margins can be attained
- Radiation therapy is utilized for unresectable adenoid cystic carcinoma

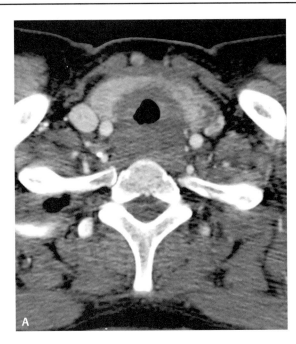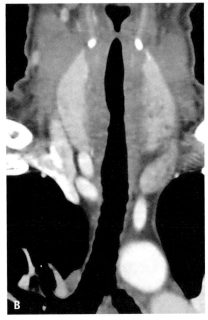

Fig. 24.2   **(A)** Contrast-enhanced chest CT (mediastinal window) of a patient with adenoid cystic carcinoma demonstrates circumferential tumor with an annular growth pattern that narrows the tracheal lumen. **(B)** CT coronal reformation demonstrates the longitudinal extent of airway involvement by tumor.

Prognosis

- Guarded because of local recurrence and distant metastases
- Best for completely excised localized tumors

PEARLS

- Tracheal masses may become quite large before the onset of symptoms. Silent growth of an endotracheal lesion may produce compromise of up to 75% of the airway lumen (**Figs. 24.1C, 24.1D, 24.3, 24.4, 24.5**).
- Axial CT imaging tends to underestimate the longitudinal extent of the tumor; multi-planar coronal, sagittal, and 3-D volume-rendered reconstructions are more accurate.
- *Squamous cell carcinoma of the trachea* (**Fig. 24.3**) is considered in some reports the most frequent primary tracheal malignancy and may account for approximately 45% of tracheal neoplasms. Affected patients are typically men (male-to-female ratio of 4:1) and are usually cigarette smokers. These lesions are exophytic ulcerative endoluminal nodules/masses. Imaging studies demonstrate endoluminal nodules (**Fig. 24.3**), masses, and/or annular constriction of the trachea with or without local mediastinal invasion.
- *Mucoepidermoid carcinoma* (**Fig. 24.4**) consists of mucin-secreting, squamous, and intermediate cells with little mitotic activity or necrosis. It is a polypoid, well-defined endoluminal nodule typically found in the central bronchi. Patients with mucoepidermoid carcinoma are usually young adults and children who present with cough, hemoptysis and/or wheezing. Imaging studies demonstrate a well-defined ovoid or lobular endoluminal mass that parallels the orientation of the airway in which it originates (**Fig. 24.4**). Intrinsic foci of high attenuation or calcification are described. Associated mucoid impaction, bronchial dilatation, air trapping, consolidation (**Fig. 24.4**), and/or atelectasis may be seen.
- *Metastatic tumors* may mimic primary tracheal lesions. Primary malignant tumors that most commonly occur as endobronchial and/or tracheal metastases include melanoma (**Fig. 24.5**), renal cell carcinoma, breast and colon cancer.

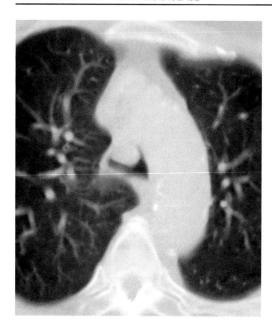

Fig. 24.3 Unenhanced chest CT (lung window) of a 56-year-old man with stridor and squamous cell tracheal carcinoma demonstrates an endoluminal tumor nodule arising from the anterior tracheal wall.

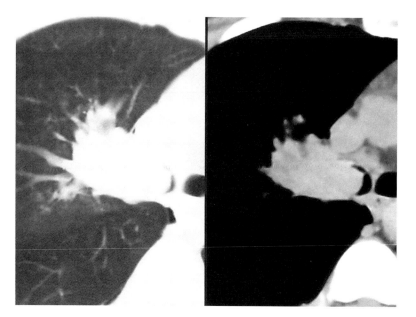

Fig. 24.4 Composite contrast-enhanced chest CT (lung and mediastinal windows) of a 9-year-old boy with wheezing and mucoepidermoid carcinoma reveals an endoluminal ovoid mass within the right mainstem bronchus. Note the well-defined margin of the lesion, the linear orientation of the mass along the bronchial lumen, and early post-obstructive effects.

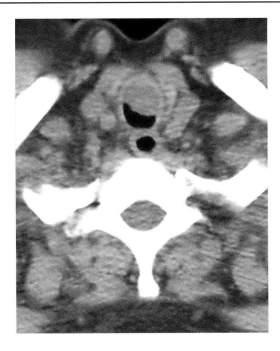

Fig. 24.5 Unenhanced chest CT (mediastinal window) of a 46-year-old man with stridor and metastatic melanoma demonstrates an endoluminal tumor nodule arising from the anterior tracheal wall.

Suggested Readings

1. Kwak SH, Lee KS, Chung MJ, Jeong YJ, Kim GY, Kwon OJ. Adenoid cystic carcinoma of the airways: helical CT and histopathologic correlation. AJR Am J Roentgenol 2004;183(2):277–281

2. Kim TS, Lee KS, Han J, et al. Mucoepidermoid carcinoma of the tracheobronchial tree: radiographic and CT findings in 12 patients. Radiology 1999;212(3):643–648

3. Gaissert HA. Primary tracheal tumors. Chest Surg Clin N Am 2003;13(2):247–256

4. McCarthy MJ, Rosado-de-Christenson ML. Tumors of the trachea. J Thorac Imaging 1995;10(3):180–198

5. Colby T, Koss M, Travis WD. Tumors of salivary gland type. In: Colby T, Koss M, Travis WD, eds. Atlas of Tumor Pathology: Tumors of the Lower Respiratory Tract, fasc 13, ser 3. Washington, DC: Armed Forces Institute of Pathology; 1995:65–89

CASE 25

■ Clinical Presentation

36-year-old man with chronic productive cough and recurrent pneumonia

■ Radiologic Findings

Coned-down PA (**Fig. 25.1A**) and lateral (**Fig. 25.1B**) chest radiographs demonstrate central coarse linear and interstitial opacities with ring-like and cystic morphology and a bronchial distribution affecting the middle lobe and right lower lobe. Unenhanced chest CT (lung window) (**Fig. 25.1C**) targeted at the lower right lung demonstrates areas of moderate and severe bronchiectasis with bronchial wall thickening. Note the varied morphology of the bronchiectatic airways, including cylindrical, varicoid, and saccular (cystic) forms (**Figs. 25.1C, 25.2**). Multiple areas of mucoid impaction and endoluminal air-fluid levels are seen in the right lower lobe (**Fig. 25.1C**).

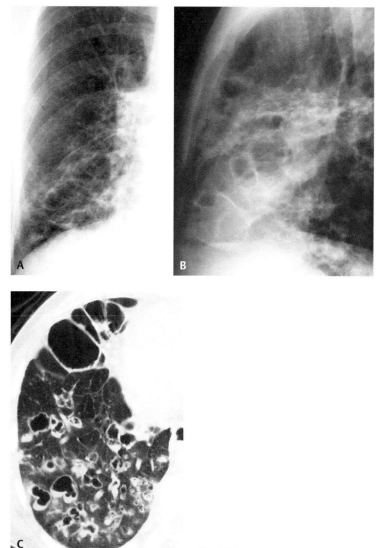

Fig. 25.1

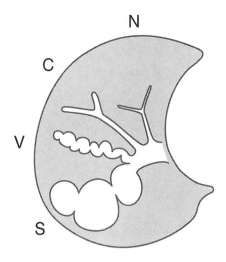

Fig. 25.2   Artist's illustration depicts a normal bronchus (*N*) and the three grades of severity of bronchiectasis: cylindrical (*C*), varicose (*V*), and saccular (cystic) (*S*).

■ Diagnosis

Bronchiectasis with Mucous Plugging; Secondary Superinfection

■ Differential Diagnosis

None

■ Discussion

Background

Bronchiectasis is defined as chronic irreversible bronchial dilatation and may be secondary to a variety of inflammatory and destructive bronchial wall disorders. It is typically graded according to its severity as mild, moderate, and severe forms, respectively termed cylindrical, varicose, and saccular (cystic) (**Fig. 25.2**). *Cylindrical bronchiectasis* is characterized by mild bronchial dilatation with preservation of bronchial morphology (**Figs. 25.2, 25.3, 25.4, 25.6**). *Varicose bronchiectasis* is characterized by areas of bronchial dilatation alternating with foci of luminal constriction that result in a beaded bronchial morphology (**Figs. 25.1C, 25.2, 25.4, 25.6**). The most severe form of bronchiectasis is characterized by *cystic* or *saccular* bronchial dilatation measuring over 1.0 cm in diameter (**Figs. 25.1A, 25.1B, 25.1C, 25.2, 25.7**). All forms of bronchiectasis are associated with bronchial wall thickening.

Etiology

The underlying mechanism behind most forms of bronchiectasis is bronchial wall injury. Etiologies include childhood viral and bacterial infections, cystic fibrosis, ciliary dyskinesia syndromes, immunodeficiency disorders, allergic bronchopulmonary fungal disease, and lung and bone marrow transplantation. Pulmonary fibrosis may cause bronchiectasis by retraction of peribronchial fibrous tissue (traction bronchiectasis) and is usually a localized process (e.g., tuberculosis, sarcoidosis, pulmonary fibrosis, radiation therapy).

Clinical Findings

Affected patients are often symptomatic, with cough, purulent sputum, fever, dyspnea, and hemoptysis (which may be severe), and many have coexisting sinusitis. Patients commonly experience recurrent acute pneumonia and exacerbations of bronchitis. Until the mid-twentieth century, most cases of bronchiectasis were related to post-infectious bronchial damage. Since the advent of antibiotic therapy, there has been a marked decline in the incidence of bronchiectasis in developed countries. However, bronchiectasis remains a significant health problem in developing countries.

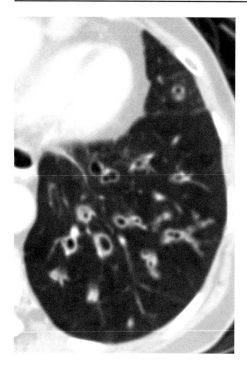

Fig. 25.3 Unenhanced chest CT (lung window) of a 55-year-old man with recurrent pneumonia demonstrates cylindrical bronchiectasis in the lingula and left lower lobes. The dilated airways are larger than their respective adjacent pulmonary arteries and exhibit the "signet ring" sign of bronchiectasis. Some of the dilated airways have mildly thickened walls.

Imaging Features

Chest Radiography

- Visible bronchial walls (**Figs. 25.1A, 25.1B**)
  - Single or parallel "tram track" lines (thickened airway walls seen longitudinally)
  - Poorly defined ring-like/curvilinear opacities (thickened airway walls seen on-end or obliquely)
- Variable lung volume (atelectasis or hyperinflation)
  - Round, oval, or tubular Y- or V-shaped opacities (dilated airways filled with secretions, mucoid impaction)
- Multiple thin-walled ring-like opacities in cystic bronchiectasis, often with air-fluid levels (**Figs. 25.1A, 25.1B**)
- Normal chest radiograph in 7% of affected patients

MDCT/HRCT

- Absence of normal distal tapering of bronchial lumen (**Figs. 25.2, 25.3, 25.4, 25.5, 25.6, 25.7**)
- Internal diameter of bronchial lumen greater than that of adjacent pulmonary artery (i.e., *signet ring* sign) (**Figs. 25.3, 25.5**)
- Visible bronchi within 1.0 cm of costal pleura or abutting mediastinal pleura (**Figs. 25.1C, 25.4, 25.7**)
- Mucus-filled dilated bronchi (**Figs. 25.1C, 25.3, 25.4, 25.5**)
- Associated bronchiolitis in 75% of patients (decreased lung attenuation and vascularity, bronchiolectasis, and centrilobular tree-in-bud opacities) (**Fig. 25.4**)

Management

- Antibiotics
- Treatment of underlying condition
- Surgical excision: localized disease and recurrent or severe persistent symptoms
- Lung transplantation for selected patients with severe, diffuse, advanced disease
- Bronchial artery embolization or surgery in patients with severe hemoptysis

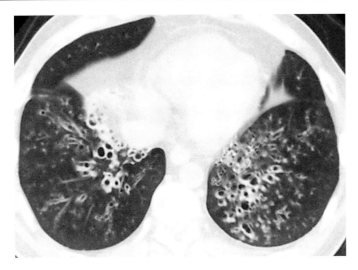

Fig. 25.4 Unenhanced chest CT (lung window) of a 35-year-old man with primary ciliary dyskinesia (PCD) referred for lung transplantation demonstrates diffuse cylindrical and varicose bronchiectasis, nodular opacities representing mucus-filled dilated bronchi, and centrilobular opacities consistent with bronchiolitis.

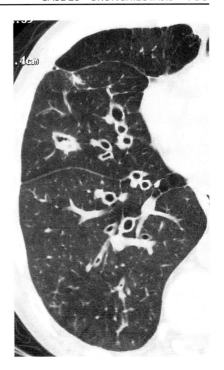

Fig. 25.5 Unenhanced chest CT (lung window) targeted at the right mid- and lower lung of a 49-year-old HIV-positive man demonstrates cylindrical bronchiectasis and bronchial wall thickening. Similar findings were present in the left lung (not shown).

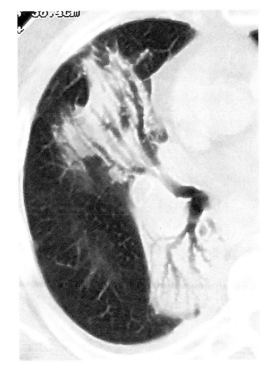

Fig. 25.6 Unenhanced chest CT (lung window) of a 45-year-old man who received radiation therapy for lung cancer demonstrates parenchymal fibrosis and atelectasis with internal cylindrical and varicose (traction) bronchiectasis.

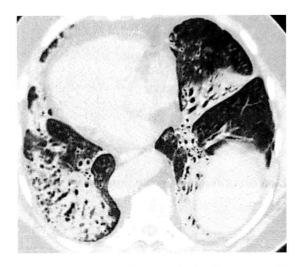

Fig. 25.7 Chest CT (lung window) of a 47-year-old woman with Kartagener syndrome demonstrates situs inversus and extensive cystic (saccular) bronchiectasis that predominantly involves the lower lung zones.

Prognosis

- Good; response to conservative treatment in mild cases
- Reported mortality rate: 19% during a 14-year follow-up period; mean age at death 54 years
- Progression of disease in some patients who undergo surgical excision of localized post-infectious bronchiectasis

PEARLS

- Reversible bronchial dilatation may occur in patients with pneumonia, and typically resolves within 4–6 months. This is not considered "true" bronchiectasis.
- HRCT: "gold standard" for the diagnosis and characterization of bronchiectasis (sensitivity 98%). Distinctive patterns of bronchiectasis in specific clinical settings may be recognized, including allergic bronchopulmonary aspergillosis (ABPA), atypical mycobacterial infection (e.g., MAC, MAI), AIDS, and cystic fibrosis.
- Bronchiectasis may occur in the setting of radiation pneumonitis and is secondary to surrounding pulmonary fibrosis. Radiation fibrosis typically manifests with dense consolidation and volume loss with internal traction bronchiectasis (**Figs. 25.6**). These abnormalities typically conform to the expected radiation port.
- *Kartagener syndrome* is a variant of *primary ciliary dyskinesia* (PCD) characterized by bronchiectasis (**Fig. 25.7**), chronic sinusitis, and situs inversus. Only 50% of patients with PCD have situs inversus (**Fig. 25.7**). PCD is associated with male infertility, a distinguishing clinical feature that may be useful in the differential diagnosis of patients with bronchiectasis. The disorder results from an abnormality in the cilia although these disorders have been described in patients with structurally normal cilia.

PITFALLS

- Pulsation ("star") artifact commonly occurs at the left lung base on CT/HRCT and produces thin streaks that radiate from the edges of vessels, simulating bronchiectasis.
- Doubling artifact on CT/HRCT causes fissures, vessels, and airways to be seen as duplicated structures due to cardiac pulsation or respiration. The resultant imaging findings may mimic bronchiectasis. Doubling artifact may be reduced by utilizing ECG gating, very rapid scan times, and/or spirometrically controlled respiration.

Suggested Reading

1. Hansell DM, Lynch DA, McAdams HP, Bankier AA. Diseases of the airways. In: Hansell DM, Lynch DA, McAdams HP, Bankier AA, eds. Imaging of Diseases of the Chest, 5th ed. Philadelphia: Mosby Elsevier; 2010:715–785
2. Barker AF. Bronchiectasis. N Engl J Med 2002;346(18):1383–1393
3. Kumar NA, Nguyen B, Maki D. Bronchiectasis: current clinical and imaging concepts. Semin Roentgenol 2001;36(1): 41–50
4. McGuinness G, Naidich DP. CT of airways disease and bronchiectasis. Radiol Clin North Am 2002;40(1):1–19
5. Grenier PA, Beigelman-Aubry C, Fetita C, Martin-Bouyer Y. Multidetector-row CT of the airways. Semin Roentgenol 2003;38(2):146–157

CASE 26

■ Clinical Presentation

33-year-old man with wheezing, dyspnea and productive cough

■ Radiologic Findings

Coned-down composite PA chest radiograph (**Fig. 26.1A**) reveals extensive bilateral bronchiectasis manifesting as ring, tram track, nodular and reticular opacities most severe in the upper lungs. Unenhanced chest CT (lung window) coronal reformation (**Fig. 26.1B**) and axial images (**Figs. 26.1C, 26.1D**) demonstrate increased lung volumes (**Fig. 26.1B**) and extensive bronchiectasis in both lungs that predominantly involves the upper lobes; focal nodular and tubular opacities represent mucoid impaction (**Figs. 26.1B, 26.1C, 26.1D**). Note subtle parenchymal heterogeneity (mosaic attenuation) (**Figs. 26.1B, 26.1C, 26.1D**).

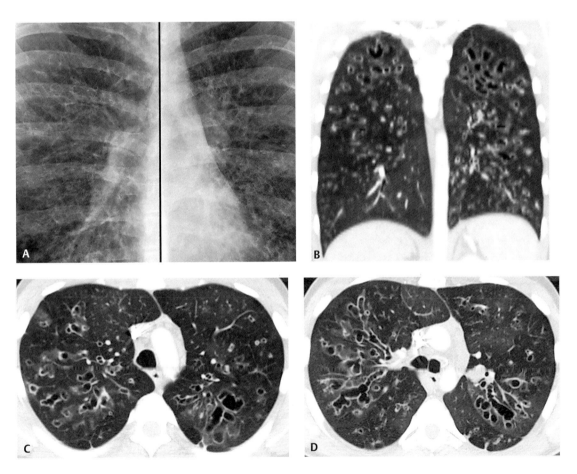

Fig. 26.1

167

■ Diagnosis

Cystic Fibrosis

■ Differential Diagnosis

- Williams-Campbell Syndrome
- Allergic Bronchopulmonary Aspergillosis (ABPA)
- Other Causes of Bronchiectasis (e.g., chronic aspiration, healed tuberculosis)

■ Discussion

Background

Cystic fibrosis is a hereditary, multi-system, genetically transmitted disease that affects exocrine tissues in the lung, pancreas, gastrointestinal tract, liver, salivary glands, and the male reproductive system.

Etiology

Cystic fibrosis is transmitted as an autosomal recessive trait. The responsible gene is located on the long arm of chromosome 7. The protein product of the cystic fibrosis transmembrane conductance regulator (CFTR) gene may undergo many different mutations that can lead to cystic fibrosis. Phenotypic variations occur in the magnitude of sweat chloride elevation, the presence and degree of pancreatic insufficiency, the age of onset, and the severity of pulmonary disease. In the lung, dysfunction of an amino acid protein impairs the ability of airway epithelial cells to secrete salt (and thus water), with resultant excessive reabsorption of salt and water. This leads to dessication of luminal secretions with mucous plugging. Mucociliary clearance decreases, predisposing to colonization by bacteria and recurrent infection.

Clinical Findings

Patients with cystic fibrosis may present during infancy (meconium ileus) or as young adults, reflecting variations in underlying genetic factors. Patients with thoracic involvement present with recurrent infections with associated wheezing, dyspnea, productive cough, and/or hemoptysis. Recurrent infection is associated with malnutrition and protein depletion. Common complications include hemoptysis, pneumothorax, and asthma, with an increased prevalence of allergic bronchopulmonary aspergillosis. Many patients with cystic fibrosis now survive into adulthood.

Imaging Features

Chest Radiography

- Large lung volumes (**Fig. 26.1A**)
- Atelectasis with or without mucous plugging
- Widespread bronchiectasis most severe in the upper lobes (**Fig. 26.1A**)
- Nodular or tubular opacities (mucoid impaction)
- Recurrent consolidation
- Lymphadenopathy
- Advanced disease
  - Pulmonary arterial hypertension
  - Cardiomegaly (cor pulmonale)

MDCT/HRCT

- Bronchiectasis; cylindrical, diffuse, bilateral with preferential upper lobe involvement (**Figs. 26.1B, 26.1C, 26.1D, 26.2, 26.3, 26.4A, 26.4B**)
- Airway wall thickening (**Figs. 26.1B, 26.1C, 26.1D, 26.2, 26.3, 26.4A, 26.4B**)

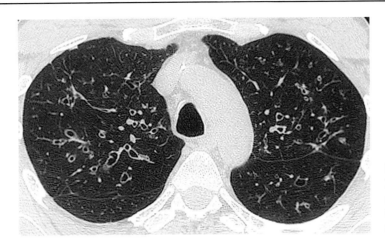

Fig. 26.2 Unenhanced chest CT of a 27-year-old woman with cystic fibrosis demonstrates cylindrical bronchiectasis, airway wall thickening, and nodular areas of mucous plugging.

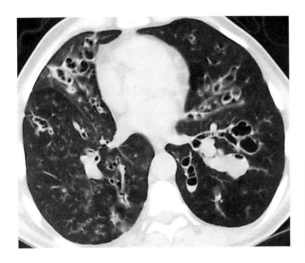

Fig. 26.3 Unenhanced chest CT of a 34-year-old man with cystic fibrosis demonstrates cylindrical, varicose, and saccular (cystic) bronchiectasis; airway wall thickening; tubular and nodular areas of mucous plugging; and scattered centrilobular nodules and associated linear opacities with "tree-in-bud" morphology.

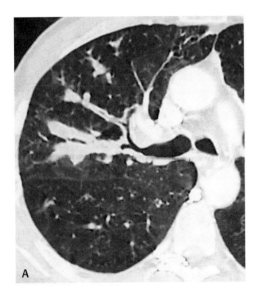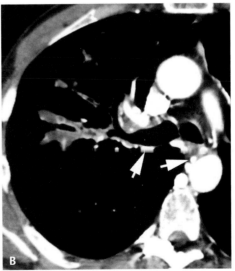

Fig. 26.4 Contrast-enhanced chest CT (lung **[A]** and mediastinal **[B]** windows) of a 29-year-old man with cystic fibrosis demonstrates bronchiectasis and mucous plugging that predominantly involve the upper lobes. The mucous plugs manifest as low-attenuation material within dilated bronchi **(B)**. Note the numerous dilated bronchial arteries (*arrows*) **(B)**, a common finding in patients with advanced cystic fibrosis.

- Centrilobular nodules and associated linear opacities with "tree-in-bud" morphology (**Fig. 26.3**)
- Geographic lung attenuation (**Figs. 26.1B, 26.1C, 26.1D, 26.2, 26.3**)
- Air-trapping
- Mucus plugs within dilated airways (**Figs. 26.2, 26.3, 26.4A, 26.4B**)

Management

- Maintenance of airway clearance (chest physiotherapy)
- Antibiotics for treatment of secondary infection
- Nutritional support
- Lung transplantation in selected cases

Prognosis

- Variable; depends on clinical severity
- Significantly increased life expectancy in recent decades; predicted mean life expectancy of 40 years

PEARLS

- Hilar enlargement in patients with cystic fibrosis may be due to lymphadenopathy (30–50% of adults) or central pulmonary artery enlargement from pulmonary arterial hypertension.
- HRCT is the imaging modality of choice for diagnosing bronchiectasis and is more sensitive than radiography in detecting early disease in patients with cystic fibrosis.
- Upper lobe predominance of bronchiectasis in cystic fibrosis is a distinguishing imaging feature from bronchiectasis secondary to impaired mucociliary clearance, which has a lower lobe predominance.
- Allergic bronchopulmonary aspergillosis (ABPA) is a hypersensitivity reaction to *Aspergillus fumigatus* that occurs most often in asthmatics, but also occurs in patients with cystic fibrosis (see Case 27).

Suggested Reading

1. Hansell DM, Lynch DA, McAdams HP, Bankier AA. Diseases of the airways. In: Hansell DM, Lynch DA, McAdams HP, Bankier AA, eds. Imaging of Diseases of the Chest, 5th ed. Philadelphia: Mosby Elsevier; 2010:715–785

2. Saavedra MT, Lynch DA. Emerging roles for CT imaging in cystic fibrosis. Radiology 2009;252(2):327–329

3. McDermott S, Barry SC, Judge EE, et al. Tracheomalacia in adults with cystic fibrosis: determination of prevalence and severity with dynamic cine CT. Radiology 2009;252(2):577–586

4. Brody AS, Klein JS, Molina PL, Quan J, Bean JA, Wilmott RW. High-resolution computed tomography in young patients with cystic fibrosis: distribution of abnormalities and correlation with pulmonary function tests. J Pediatr 2004;145(1):32–38

5. Stevens DA, Moss RB, Kurup VP, et al; Participants in the Cystic Fibrosis Foundation Consensus Conference. Allergic bronchopulmonary aspergillosis in cystic fibrosis—state of the art: Cystic Fibrosis Foundation Consensus Conference. Clin Infect Dis 2003;37(Suppl 3):S225–S264

CASE 27

■ Clinical Presentation

57-year-old woman with a long history of asthma

■ Radiologic Findings

Coned-down PA (**Fig. 27.1A**) and lateral (**Fig. 27.1B**) chest radiographs demonstrate ring-like opacities in the perihilar regions and upper lobes and a left upper lobe tubular opacity that appears to emanate from the hilum. Unenhanced chest CT (lung window) (**Figs. 27.1C, 27.1D**) demonstrates cystic bronchiectasis that predominantly involves the central aspects of the lungs with relative sparing of the lung periphery. Well-defined soft-tissue upper lobe nodules (**Fig. 27.1C**) represent mucoid impaction within dilated bronchi.

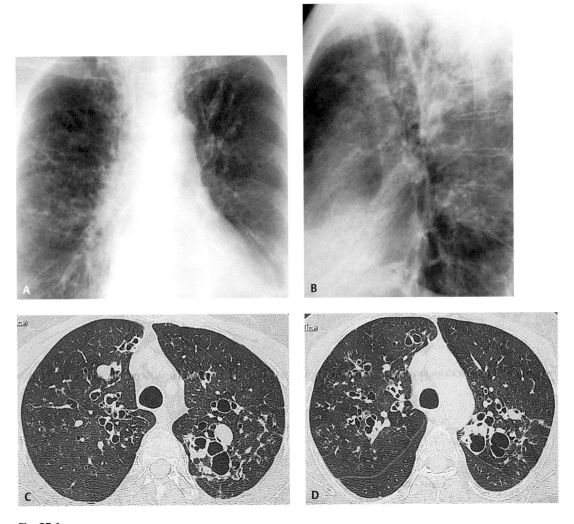

Fig. 27.1

171

■ Diagnosis

Allergic Bronchopulmonary Aspergillosis (ABPA)

■ Differential Diagnosis

- Bronchiectasis of Other Etiologies

■ Discussion

Background

Allergic bronchopulmonary aspergillosis (ABPA) is also known as allergic bronchopulmonary fungal disease, since species other than *Aspergillus* are sometimes implicated. Typically, *Aspergillus fumigatus* colonizes the airway lumen in patients with asthma. The retained bronchial secretions initiate immune complex and complement formation with resultant tissue injury. Acutely, the injury may manifest as transient subsegmental or lobar consolidation. Chronic changes damage the larger bronchi and produce central bronchiectasis, which is the imaging hallmark of ABPA. In asthmatic patients, CT detection of bronchiectasis involving three or more lobes, combined with findings of centrilobular nodules and mucoid impaction, is highly suggestive of ABPA. Affected patients typically have diffuse disease at the time of diagnosis, manifesting as central cystic and/or varicose bronchiectasis involving both lungs.

Etiology

ABPA is caused by type I and type III (IgE and IgG) immunologic responses to the fungal (usually *Aspergillus*) species in the airway lumen. Excessive mucus production and abnormal ciliary function result in mucoid impaction.

Clinical Findings

Affected patients may present with recurrent wheezing, malaise, low-grade fever, cough, sputum production, and chest pain. ABPA typically affects patients with asthma but also occurs in 2–5% of patients with cystic fibrosis. Patients with ABPA characteristically have blood and sputum eosinophilia and elevated total serum IgE. Serum levels of IgE may be used to confirm the diagnosis and acute exacerbations of the disease.

Imaging Features

Radiography

- Central (proximal) bronchiectasis predominantly involving the upper lobes (**Figs. 27.1A, 27.1B**)
- Parallel linear opacities and ring shadows (central and upper zone predominance) (**Figs. 27.1A, 27.1B**)
- Tubular opacities from mucoid impaction (**Figs. 27.1A, 27.1B**)
- Atelectasis in 50% of patients (single lobe, multiple lobes, entire lung)

MDCT/HRCT

- Central bronchiectasis, often severe and widespread (**Figs. 27.1C, 27.1D, 27.2A, 27.2B, 27.3, 27.4**)
- Mucoid impaction (**Figs. 27.1C, 27.1D, 27.4**); may exhibit high-attenuation mucus (30%) and occasional calcification
- Bronchial wall thickening (**Figs. 27.1C, 27.1D, 27.2B, 27.3, 27.4**)
- Linear or branching centrilobular opacities (tree-in-bud) (**Fig. 27.1D**)
- Air-fluid levels within dilated bronchi; may indicate infection
- Peripheral consolidation or diffuse ground-glass opacity (subacute)
- Atelectasis (**Fig. 27.3**)
- Air trapping on expiration

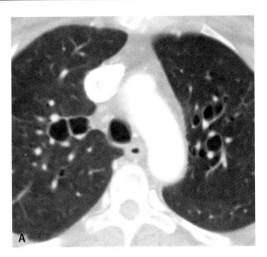 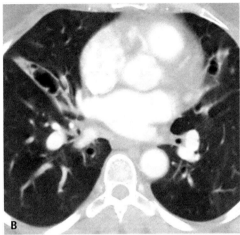

Fig. 27.2 Contrast-enhanced chest CT (lung window) of a 38-year-old man with asthma and ABPA demonstrates **(A)** central cystic and **(B)** varicoid bronchiectasis.

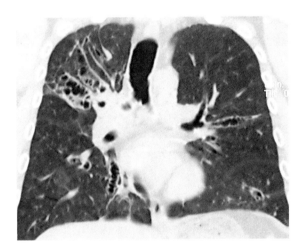

Fig. 27.3 Unenhanced chest CT (lung window, coronal reformation) demonstrates central varicoid bronchiectasis emanating from both hila, with mild loss of volume in the right upper lobe. The findings involved all five pulmonary lobes.

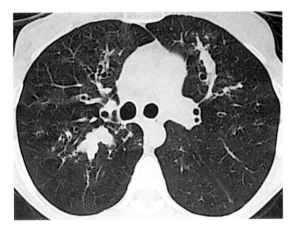

Fig. 27.4 Unenhanced chest CT (lung window) of a 44-year-old man with asthma and ABPA demonstrates central bronchiectasis involving both lungs, with tubular opacities emanating from both hila representing mucoid impaction.

Management

- Corticosteroids

Prognosis

- Resolution of acute disease
- Prevention of disease progression with corticosteroid therapy
- Recurrence
- Progression to diffuse pulmonary fibrosis
- Steroid dependence

PEARLS

- Chest CT in patients with *asthma* may be normal or may demonstrate bronchial wall thickening that extends to the centrilobular structures. Expiratory chest CT may demonstrate a mosaic pattern of attenuation from air trapping with focal or diffuse hyperlucency interposed with areas of normally aerated and perfused lung. Central pulmonary arteries may undergo irreversible enlargement.
- Patients with *ABPA* typically have cystic bronchiectasis, in comparison to patients with *cystic fibrosis*, who often have diffuse cylindrical bronchiectasis.

Suggested Reading

1. Franquet T, Müller NL, Oikonomou A, Flint JD. Aspergillus infection of the airways: computed tomography and pathologic findings. J Comput Assist Tomogr 2004;28(1):10–16

2. Kumar R. Mild, moderate, and severe forms of allergic bronchopulmonary aspergillosis: a clinical and serologic evaluation. Chest 2003;124(3):890–892

3. Mitchell TA, Hamilos DL, Lynch DA, Newell JD. Distribution and severity of bronchiectasis in allergic bronchopulmonary aspergillosis (ABPA). J Asthma 2000;37(1):65–72

4. Ward S, Heyneman L, Lee MJ, Leung AN, Hansell DM, Müller NL. Accuracy of CT in the diagnosis of allergic bronchopulmonary aspergillosis in asthmatic patients. AJR Am J Roentgenol 1999;173(4):937–942

5. McGuinness G, Naidich DP. CT of airways disease and bronchiectasis. Radiol Clin North Am 2002;40(1):1–19

CASE 28

■ Clinical Presentation

62-year-old woman with dyspnea and a 30-pack-year history of cigarette smoking

■ Radiologic Findings

Unenhanced axial chest CT (lung window) (**Figs. 28.1A, 28.1B**) demonstrates abnormal centrilobular areas of low attenuation with imperceptible walls. CT coronal reformation (**Fig. 28.1C**) shows the upper lobe distribution of disease.

■ Diagnosis

Proximal Acinar Emphysema (syn. Centrilobular, Centriacinar)

■ Differential Diagnosis

None

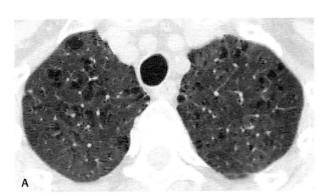
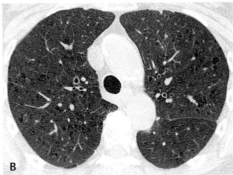

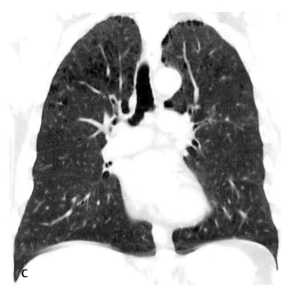

Fig. 28.1

■ Discussion

Background

Emphysema is defined as abnormal permanent enlargement of the airspaces distal to the terminal bronchiole accompanied by destruction of their walls with minimal or absent fibrosis. Emphysema is categorized according to the affected part of the pulmonary acinus. Proximal acinar (syn. centrilobular, centriacinar) emphysema involves the proximal aspect of the acinus with distension and destruction that primarily affects the respiratory bronchioles (**Fig. 28.2**).

Etiology

Proximal acinar (centrilobular) emphysema occurs primarily in cigarette smokers and is related to an imbalance between elastolytic and anti-elastolytic processes in the lung. Cigarette smoke impairs α-1-antiprotease's inhibitory function, resulting in increased elastolytic activity with subsequent loss of the connective tissue attachments of the terminal bronchiole and damage to the lung's elastic framework. These changes are responsible for terminal bronchiolar collapse and resultant airflow obstruction.

Clinical Findings

Patients with proximal acinar (centrilobular) emphysema are typically adults between the ages of 55 and 75 years. They present with dyspnea and less commonly with cough. These patients may be thin and appear to be in respiratory distress. They exhibit prolonged expiration, breathe with pursed lips, and may sit leaning forward. Pulmonary function tests are characterized by increased total lung capacity (TLC) and residual volume (RV) and decreased diffusing capacity.

Imaging Features

Radiography

- Increased lung volumes or lung height (measured ≥30 cm from right first rib tubercle to diaphragm dome)
- Diaphragmatic flattening (highest level of diaphragmatic contour is <1.5 cm above a line connecting the costophrenic and vertebrophrenic junctions on PA view or a line connecting the sternophrenic and posterior costophrenic angles on lateral view)
- Enlarged retrosternal clear space (horizontal distance between sternum and anterior margin ascending aorta >2.5 cm on lateral view)
- Abnormal lucency in the upper lung zones
- Reduction in number and caliber of pulmonary vessels; vessels may be displaced by bullae or emphysematous spaces; may exhibit widened branching angles with loss of side branches
- Crowding of vessels in mid and lower lungs in moderate and severe emphysema
- Focal lucencies, decreased vascularity and bullae
- Normal in mild cases

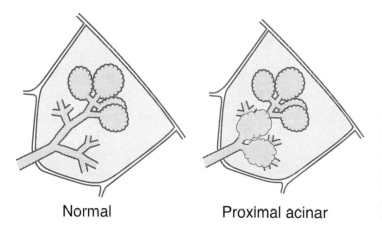

Normal   Proximal acinar

Fig. 28.2 Artist's illustration (*left*) depicts a normal pulmonary acinus contained within a secondary pulmonary lobule. Each acinus is comprised of respiratory bronchioles, alveolar ducts, and alveolar sacs. Proximal acinar emphysema (*right*) predominantly affects the proximal elements of the pulmonary acinus.

MDCT/HRCT

- Focal areas (3–10 mm) of centrilobular low attenuation with imperceptible walls (**Figs. 28.1A, 28.1B, 28.1C, 28.3A, 28.3B, 28.3C, 28.5**)
- Central nodular opacity (centrilobular arteriole) within an area of low attenuation (**Figs. 28.3A, 28.3B, 28.3C**)
- More severe involvement of upper lobes and superior segments of lower lobes (**Figs. 28.1C, 28.3B, 28.5**)
- Large confluent areas of emphysema may progress to panlobular involvement (**Figs. 28.3A, 28.3B, 28.5**)
- Associated paraseptal emphysema and/or bullae (**Figs. 28.3A, 28.3B, 28.5**)

Management

- Cessation of smoking
- Lung volume reduction surgery in selected patients
- Lung transplantation in end-stage disease

Prognosis

- Poor; progressive, disabling dyspnea
- Reports of improvements in lung function, exercise tolerance, and quality of life following lung volume reduction surgery (see Case 188)

PEARLS

- Thin-section CT and HRCT: useful in detection of early proximal acinar emphysema and in assessment of severity and extent of disease in patients undergoing evaluation for lung volume reduction surgery.

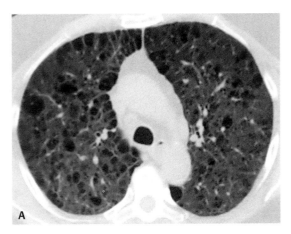
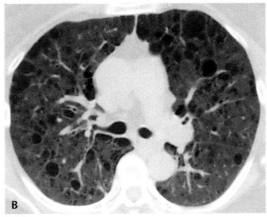
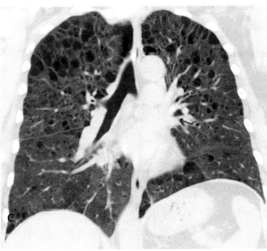

Fig. 28.3   (A,B) Unenhanced axial chest CT (lung window) of a 61-year-old man with advanced emphysema demonstrates scattered areas of proximal acinar emphysema in both upper lobes, distal acinar (paraseptal) emphysema in the subpleural right upper lobe, and confluent panacinar (panlobular) areas of parenchymal destruction. **(C)** Coronal reformatted CT demonstrates the predominant distribution of findings in the upper lung zones.

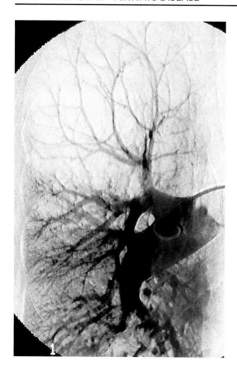

Fig. 28.4 Selective right pulmonary arteriogram of a 61-year-old woman with marked upper lobe emphysema demonstrates straightening and separation of pulmonary arteries in the upper lung with associated crowding of vessels (passive atelectasis) in the middle and lower lung zones.

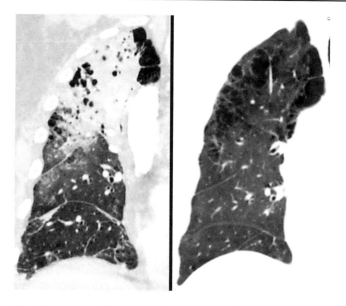

Fig. 28.5 Chest CT (lung window, coronal reformation) (*left*) of a 58-year-old man with emphysema and pneumonia demonstrates areas of lucency within right upper lobe consolidation that represent numerous foci of emphysema, resulting in a "Swiss cheese" appearance. Follow-up CT performed two months later, after antibiotic therapy (*right*), shows the underlying marked emphysematous and bullous changes in the right upper lobe.

- Bullae are emphysematous spaces in the lung that measure over 1 cm in diameter. They may occur in association with any type of emphysema but are most common in patients with distal acinar (paraseptal) and proximal acinar (centrilobular) emphysema.
- Upper zone predominance of proximal acinar emphysema may be related to several factors, including a slower transit time of neutrophils in the upper as compared with the lower lungs, decreased perfusion of the upper as compared with lower zones (gravity related), and increased mechanical stress in the upper lungs caused by more negative pleural pressures and relative hyperinflation (**Fig. 28.4**).
- Emphysema may affect the imaging manifestations of other lung diseases. Vascular findings of pulmonary edema are more prominent in the mid- and lower lungs than in the upper lungs in patients with moderate or severe emphysema. Pneumonia may exhibit atypical appearances with foci of low attenuation (emphysematous lung) within areas of confluent opacity (pneumonia) in a pattern sometimes referred to as *Swiss cheese lung* (**Fig. 28.5**).
- Combined pulmonary fibrosis and emphysema (CPFE) is a recently defined syndrome in which centrilobar and/or paraseptal emphysema in upper lung zones coexist with pulmonary fibrosis in lower lobes. Affected patients have a characteristic lung function profile, with unexpected subnormal dynamic and static lung volumes, significant reduction of carbon monoxide transfer (DL_{CO}), and exercise hypoxemia. Pulmonary hypertension is highly prevalent and is the leading cause of death in these patients.

Suggested Reading

1. Hansell DM, Lynch DA, McAdams HP, Bankier AA. Diseases of the airways. In: Hansell DM, Lynch DA, McAdams HP, Bankier AA, eds. Imaging of Diseases of the Chest, 5th ed. Philadelphia: Mosby Elsevier; 2010:715–785

2. Copley SJ, Wells AU, Müller NL, et al. Thin-section CT in obstructive pulmonary disease: discriminatory value. Radiology 2002;223(3):812–819

3. Wright JL, Churg A. Advances in the pathology of COPD. Histopathology 2006;49(1):1–9

4. Collins J. CT signs and patterns of lung disease. Radiol Clin North Am 2001;39(6):1115–1135

5. Webb WR, Müller NL, Naidich DP. Diseases characterized primarily by cysts and emphysema In: Webb WR, Müller NL, Naidich DP, eds. High-Resolution CT of the Lung, 3rd ed. Philadelphia: Lippincott Williams and Wilkins; 2001:421–466

6. Matthew DJ, Rounds SIS. Cmbined pulmonary fibrosis and emphysema: A review. Chest 2012;141(1):222–231

CASE 29

■ Clinical Presentation

72-year-old woman with exertional dyspnea

■ Radiologic Findings

Unenhanced chest CT (lung window) (**Figs. 29.1A, 29.1B, 29.1C, 29.1D**) demonstrates bilateral decreased attenuation throughout both lungs with simplification of lung architecture and diffuse hypovascularity.

■ Diagnosis

Panacinar (Panlobular) Emphysema

■ Differential Diagnosis

- α-1-Antiprotease (Antitrypsin) Deficiency

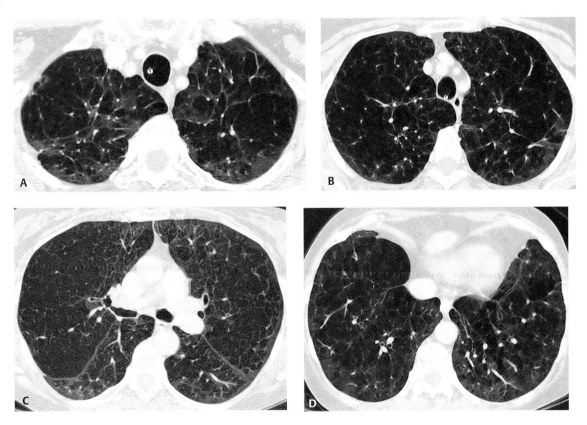

Fig. 29.1

■ Discussion

Background

Panacinar (syn. panlobular) emphysema affects each acinus in its entirety and all acini within the secondary pulmonary lobule (**Fig. 29.2**, right). It is the characteristic finding in patients with α-1-antiprotease deficiency. While panacinar emphysema may involve the lung diffusely, predominant lower lung involvement is characteristic. This is in contradistinction to proximal acinar emphysema, which predominantly involves the upper lungs. Panacinar emphysema is less common than proximal acinar (centrilobular) emphysema.

Etiology

The familial form of panacinar emphysema is seen in association with α-1-antiprotease deficiency. Panacinar emphysema also occurs as a result of intravenous drug abuse (e.g., talc, Ritalin [Novartis, New York]) and in segments of lung affected by congenital bronchial atresia.

Clinical Findings

The clinical manifestations of panacinar emphysema are similar to those of proximal acinar emphysema. Affected patients may present with nonproductive cough and progressive exertional dyspnea. The degree of disability relates to the severity of the emphysema.

Imaging Features

Radiography

- Large lung volumes (**Fig. 29.3**)
- Decreased pulmonary vascularity (**Fig. 29.3**)
- Predominant lower lobe involvement (**Fig. 29.3**)

MDCT/HRCT

- Extensive areas of abnormal low attenuation (**Figs. 29.1A, 29.1B, 29.1C, 29.1D, 29.4A, 29.4B, 29.4C**)
- Paucity of vasculature (**Figs. 29.1A, 29.1B, 29.1C, 29.1D, 29.4A, 29.4B, 29.4C**)
- Involvement of entire secondary pulmonary lobule (**Figs. 29.1A, 29.1B, 29.1C, 29.1D, 29.4A, 29.4B, 29.4C**)
- Diffuse (**Figs. 29.1A, 29.1B, 29.1C, 29.1D**) or lower lobe predominance (**Figs. 29.4A, 29.4B, 29.4C**)
- Absence of focal lucencies or bullae (**Figs. 29.4A, 29.4B, 29.4C**)

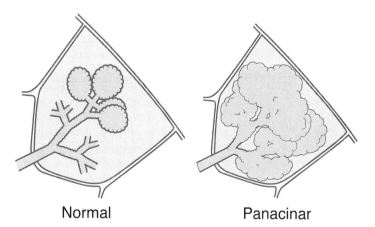

Normal   Panacinar

Fig. 29.2 Artist's illustration (*left*) depicts a normal pulmonary acinus contained within a secondary pulmonary lobule. Each acinus is comprised of respiratory bronchioles, alveolar ducts, and alveolar sacs. Panacinar emphysema (*right*) destroys the entire acinus and all acini within the secondary pulmonary lobule.

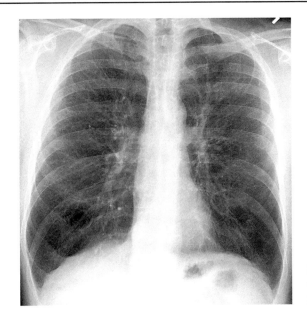

Fig. 29.3 PA chest radiograph demonstrates increased lung volumes, decreased pulmonary vascularity, and predominance of lower lobe involvement.

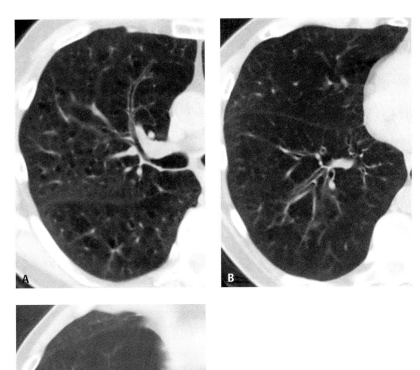

Fig. 29.4 Unenhanced chest CT (lung window) of the right lung demonstrates decreased attenuation affecting the lower lobes with simplification of lung architecture and hypovascularity.

Management

- Supportive
- Replacement therapy with α-1-antiprotease inhibitor purified from human blood

Prognosis

- Dependent on pulmonary function
- Variable disease progression; worse prognosis in patients with α-1-antiprotease deficiency who are also cigarette smokers

PEARLS

- α-1-antiprotease deficiency, the most common cause of panacinar emphysema, is an autosomal co-dominant genetic disorder in which reduced levels of α-1-antiprotease allow neutrophil elastase to damage pulmonary elastic fibers and other connective tissues, with resultant emphysema. Symptoms occur at an earlier age (third or fourth decade of life) and are exacerbated in those patients who also smoke.

Suggested Readings

1. Copley SJ, Wells AU, Müller NL, et al. Thin-section CT in obstructive pulmonary disease: discriminatory value. Radiology 2002;223(3):812–819

2. Hansell DM, Lynch DA, McAdams HP, Bankier AA. Diseases of the airways. In: Hansell DM, Lynch DA, McAdams HP, Bankier AA, eds. Imaging of Diseases of the Chest, 5th ed. Philadelphia: Mosby Elsevier; 2010:715–785

3. Spouge D, Mayo JR, Cardoso W, Müller NL. Panacinar emphysema: CT and pathologic findings. J Comput Assist Tomogr 1993;17(5):710–713

4. Travis WD, Colby TV, Koss MN, et al. Obstructive pulmonary diseases. In: King DW, ed. Atlas of Nontumor Pathology: Non-Neoplastic Disorders of the Lower Respiratory Tract. First Series. Fascicle 2. Washington, DC: The American Registry of Pathology; 2002:435–471

5. Webb WR, Müller NL, Naidich DP. Diseases characterized primarily by cysts and emphysema. In: Webb WR, Müller NL, Naidich DP, eds. High-Resolution CT of the Lung, 3rd ed. Philadelphia: Lippincott Williams and Wilkins; 2001:421–466

CASE 30

■ Clinical Presentation

46-year-old man with dyspnea

■ Radiologic Findings

PA chest radiograph (**Fig. 30.1A**) demonstrates hyperinflation with bilateral upper lobe hyperlucency secondary to bilateral large apical bullae that compress adjacent lung. Bands of atelectasis are demonstrated at both lung bases. High-resolution CT (lung window) (**Figs. 30.1B, 30.1C, 30.1D**) demonstrates bilateral large bullae that preferentially affect the right lung and produce mediastinal shift to the left. Scattered areas of proximal acinar emphysema and a single subpleural arcade of distal acinar emphysema are demonstrated in the left upper lobe (**Fig. 30.1D**).

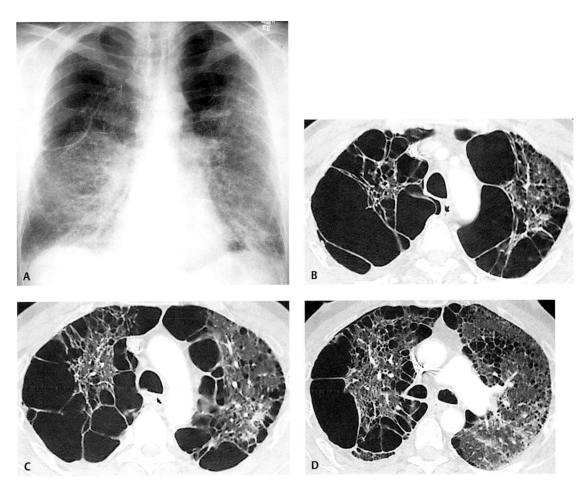

Fig. 30.1

■ Diagnosis

Bullous Lung Disease and Distal Acinar Emphysema

■ Differential Diagnosis

None

■ Discussion

Background

Distal acinar (paraseptal) emphysema is the least common type of emphysema and, together with proximal acinar emphysema, is frequently associated with the formation of bullae. It affects the periphery of the acinus (**Fig. 30.2**) adjacent to the subpleural upper lobe interlobular septa and is usually an incidental imaging finding. Adjacent foci of paraseptal emphysema may coalesce to form bullae. A bulla is defined as a sharply demarcated air-containing space measuring 1.0 cm in diameter or more in the distended state. Bullae are characteristically thin-walled (1 mm) and may be unilocular or compartmentalized by thin septa. Bullae may be solitary or multiple and most commonly occur in the lung apex. Multiple adjacent subpleural bullae may mimic distal acinar emphysema. The term *giant bullous emphysema* refers to bullae that occupy at least one-third of a hemithorax.

Etiology

The pathogenesis of distal acinar emphysema is uncertain but is probably related to a relative paucity of vascular and elastic fibers in subpleural pulmonary lobules.

Clinical Findings

Bullous lung disease is most commonly detected in patients who have concomitant emphysema but also occurs in patients with connective-tissue diseases, such as Marfan syndrome and Ehlers-Danlos syndrome. Affected patients may be asymptomatic but commonly complain of dyspnea on exertion. Distal acinar emphysema rarely causes functional abnormalities. Rupture of subpleural bullae may result in primary spontaneous pneumothorax in tall, asthenic individuals.

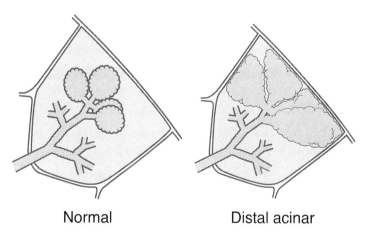

Normal   Distal acinar

Fig. 30.2 Artist's illustration (*left*) depicts a normal pulmonary acinus contained within a secondary pulmonary lobule. Each acinus is comprised of respiratory bronchioles, alveolar ducts, and alveolar sacs. Distal acinar emphysema destroys the distal portion of the acinus in the periphery of the secondary pulmonary lobule (*right*).

Imaging Features

Chest Radiography

- Thin-walled, well-defined avascular areas in lung parenchyma (bullae) (**Fig. 30.1A**)
- Mass effect on adjacent lung (**Fig. 30.1A**)
- Air-fluid levels within secondarily infected bullae
- Associated pneumothorax

MDCT/HRCT

- Many of the same features seen on chest radiography
- Focal subpleural cystic areas near interlobular septa, large vessels, and bronchi (**Figs. 30.1B, 30.1C, 30.1D, 30.3, 30.4, 30.5**)
- Frequent associated proximal acinar emphysema (**Figs. 30.1D, 30.4**)
- Large bullae, usually between 2–8 cm in diameter (giant bullous emphysema) (**Figs. 30.4, 30.5**)

Management

- Smoking cessation and preoperative pulmonary rehabilitation
- Surgical resection of affected lobe for patients with incapacitating dyspnea and large bullae that fill more than 30% of the affected hemithorax, and for patients with recurrent infection/pneumothorax

Prognosis

- Good

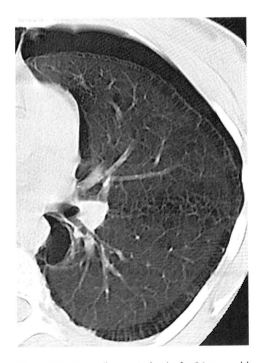

Fig. 30.3 HRCT (lung window) of a 21-year-old woman with 14 pack-years of cigarette smoking demonstrates distal acinar (paraseptal) emphysema forming a single tier along the subpleural lung parenchyma in the left upper lobe and a primary spontaneous pneumothorax.

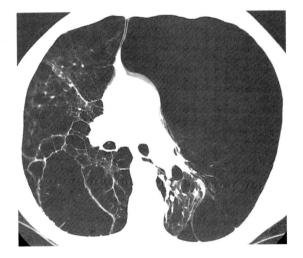

Fig. 30.4 HRCT (lung window) of a 67-year-old man with giant bullous lung disease demonstrates bilateral giant bullae that produce mediastinal shift to the right.

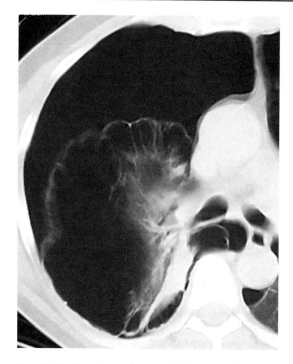

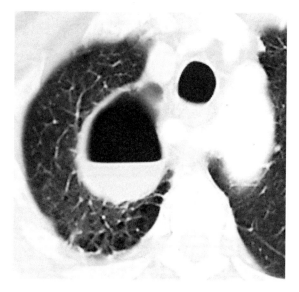

Fig. 30.5 Unenhanced chest CT (lung window) of a 51-year-old man with giant bullous lung disease demonstrates giant bullae in the right lung and a primary spontaneous pneumothorax.

Fig. 30.6 Chest CT (lung window) of a 47-year-old man with bullous lung disease demonstrates an air-fluid level within an infected bulla in the right lung apex.

PEARLS

- Bullae typically increase progressively in size, but may also become infected and subsequently disappear (**Fig. 30.6**).
- Patient selection remains one of the most important aspects of successful surgery for bullous lung disease. Compressed, atelectatic lung may re-expand following resection of bullae.
- Distal acinar emphysema may be an isolated finding or may be associated with chronic bronchitis and chronic airflow obstruction.

Suggested Reading

1. Hansell DM, Lynch DA, McAdams HP, et al. Diseases of the airways. In: Hansell DM, Lynch DA, McAdams HP, Bankier AA, eds. Imaging of Diseases of the Chest, 5th ed. Philadelphia: Mosby Elsevier; 2010:715–785

2. Copley SJ, Wells AU, Müller NL, et al. Thin-section CT in obstructive pulmonary disease: discriminatory value. Radiology 2002;223(3):812–819

3. Greenberg JA, Singhal S, Kaiser LR. Giant bullous lung disease: evaluation, selection, techniques, and outcomes. Chest Surg Clin N Am 2003;13(4):631–649

4. Travis WD, Colby TV, Koss MN, et al. Obstructive pulmonary diseases. In: King DW, ed. Atlas of Nontumor Pathology: Non-Neoplastic Disorders of the Lower Respiratory Tract. First Series. Fascicle 2. Washington, DC: The American Registry of Pathology; 2002:435–471

5. Webb WR, Müller NL, Naidich DP. Diseases characterized primarily by cysts and emphysema. In: Webb WR, Müller NL, Naidich DP, eds. High-Resolution CT of the Lung, 3rd edition. Philadelphia: Lippincott Williams and Wilkins; 2001:421–466

CASE 31

■ Clinical Presentation

32-year-old woman with cough and dyspnea six months after being trapped in a burning house

■ Radiologic Findings

Inspiratory high-resolution chest CT (lung window) (**Figs. 31.1A, 31.1B**) demonstrates heterogeneous lung attenuation with geographic areas of low attenuation and intervening normal lung. Vessels within the areas of low attenuation appear reduced in caliber. Expiratory high-resolution CT (lung window) (**Figs. 31.1C, 31.1D**) shows accentuation of lung heterogeneity and increased contrast between the geographic areas of increased and decreased attenuation.

■ Diagnosis

Bronchiolitis Obliterans

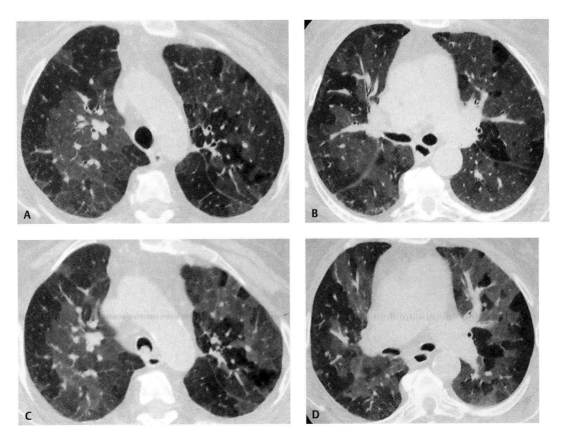

Fig. 31.1

187

■ Differential Diagnosis

- Hypersensitivity Pneumonitis (syn. Extrinsic Allergic Alveolitis)
- Infection
- Hemorrhage
- Chronic Pulmonary Arterial Hypertension

■ Discussion

Background

The term *bronchiolitis* refers to a spectrum of inflammatory and fibrotic pulmonary diseases centered on the small conducting airways. Bronchiolitis obliterans (BO) (syn. constrictive bronchiolitis) is a clinical syndrome caused by air flow obstruction and air trapping as a result of concentric peribronchiolar inflammation and fibrosis involving the small airways (i.e., terminal bronchioles, respiratory bronchioles, and alveolar ducts). It is a nonspecific reaction to a variety of insults.

Etiology

Bronchiolitis obliterans may be idiopathic or related to a variety of disorders, including infection, collagen vascular diseases (e.g., rheumatoid arthritis), toxic gas inhalation, graft-versus-host disease (e.g., from heart-lung or bone marrow transplantation), and drug-induced disease. Damage to bronchiolar epithelium results in peribronchiolar inflammation and fibrosis in the airway wall, airway lumen, or both.

Clinical Findings

Affected patients typically present with subacute or chronic symptoms of dyspnea, malaise, fatigue, chronic cough, and occasional wheezing. In some cases, the symptoms follow a lower respiratory tract infection.

Imaging Features

Radiography

- Often normal
- Mild hyperinflation
- Subtle peripheral attenuation of vascular markings

MDCT/HRCT

- Mosaic perfusion (air trapping and oligemia); typical patchy distribution (**Figs. 31.1A, 31.1B, 31.1C, 31.1D**)
- Air trapping on expiration (**Figs. 31.1C, 31.1D**); may occur in conjunction with normal inspiratory scans
- Bronchiectasis/bronchiolectasis

Management

- Corticosteroids

Prognosis

- Poor prognosis in bronchiolitis obliterans related to connective tissue disease
- Potentially fatal in heart-lung, lung, or bone marrow transplantation

PEARLS

- HRCT findings in bronchiolitis obliterans are similar regardless of the underlying cause of the disease.
- Mosaic attenuation may also occur in patients with occlusive vascular disease and in association with infiltrative lung disease. Mild mosaic attenuation and air trapping on expiratory CT have also been described in normal, healthy subjects.
- Bronchiolitis obliterans should be distinguished from cryptogenic organizing pneumonia (previously known as bronchiolitis obliterans organizing pneumonia). The former typically manifests with mosaic attenuation and air trapping, while the latter is characterized by multifocal consolidation, nodules, or masses.

Suggested Reading

1. Abbott GF, Rosado-de-Christenson ML, Rossi SE, Suster S. Imaging of small airways disease. J Thorac Imaging 2009; 24(4):285–298

2. Lynch DA. Imaging of small airways disease and chronic obstructive pulmonary disease. Clin Chest Med 2008;29(1): 165–179, vii

3. Visscher DW, Myers JL. Bronchiolitis: the pathologist's perspective. Proc Am Thorac Soc 2006;3(1):41–47

4. Boehler A, Kesten S, Weder W, Speich R. Bronchiolitis obliterans after lung transplantation: a review. Chest 1998; 114(5):1411–1426

5. Webb WR, Müller NL, Naidich DP. Airways disease. In: Webb WR, Müller NL, Naidich DP, eds. High-Resolution CT of the Lung, 3rd ed. Philadelphia: Lippincott Williams and Wilkins; 2001:467–546

CASE 32

■ Clinical Presentation

Young adult woman presenting with the fourth episode of recurrent pneumonia over the past 18 months

■ Radiologic Findings

PA (**Fig. 32.1A**) and lateral (**Fig. 32.1B**) chest radiographs demonstrate central perihilar bronchial wall thickening and air space disease in the retrocardiac region left lower lobe and right middle lobe, the latter associated with some volume loss. Chest CT (**Figs. 32.1C, 32.1D, 32.1E, 32.1F**) (lung window) shows left lower lobe consolidation, bronchial dilatation, and bronchiectasis. Similar changes are seen to a lesser degree in the right middle lobe, with associated volume loss. There are areas of scarring in the right middle and lower lobe, scattered air space, and centrilobular nodules. Bronchiectatic airways parallel the right inferior pulmonary vein (**Fig. 32.1E**). Contrast-enhanced chest CT (**Figs. 32.1G, 32.1H, 32.1I**) (mediastinal window) reveals anterior mediastinal and left subpectoral lymphadenopathy (**Fig. 32.1G**), right hilar and subcarinal lymphadenopathy (**Fig. 32.1H**), and subdiaphragmatic lymphadenopathy and splenomegaly (**Fig. 32.1I**). Residual thymus tissue is seen (**Fig. 32.1H**).

■ Diagnosis

Common Variable Immune Deficiency Syndrome with Community-Acquired Pneumonia

■ Differential Diagnosis

*   Severe Combined Immunodeficiency Syndrome
*   Transient Hypogammaglobulinemia Secondary to Infection
*   X-linked Agammaglobulinemia (XLA)

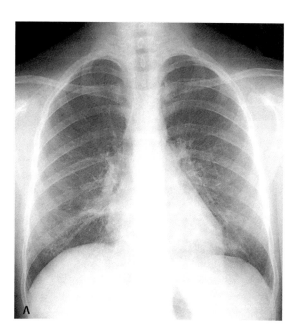

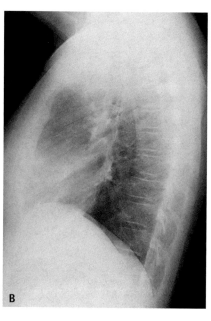

A   B   Fig. 32.1

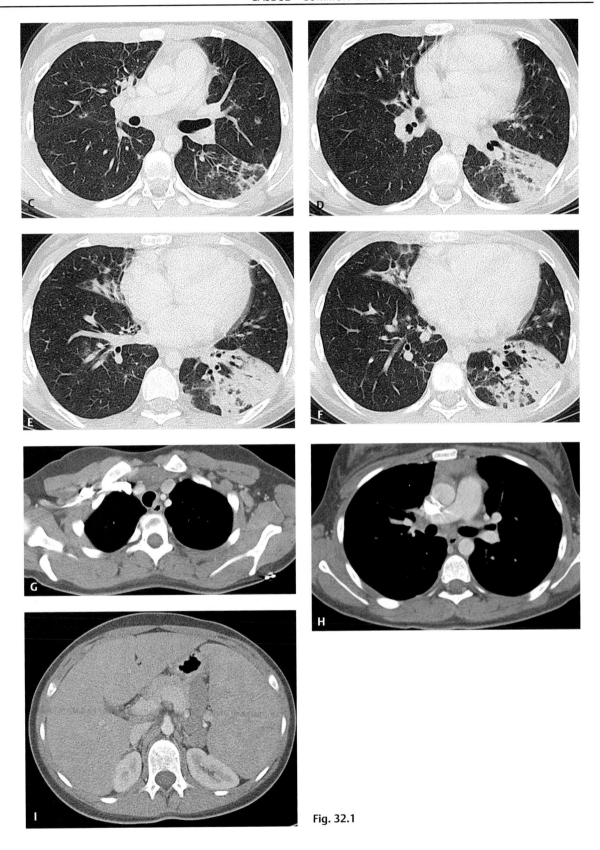

Fig. 32.1

■ Discussion

Background

Common variable immune deficiency syndrome (CVID), also called hypo-gammaglobulinemia or adult-onset hypo-gammaglobulinemia, is a relatively common primary immune deficiency. CVID is characterized by low levels of most or all immunoglobulins, lack of B-lymphocytes or plasma cells capable of producing antibodies, and recurrent bacterial infections. Both humoral and cell-mediated lymphocytic responses are affected.

Etiology

The etiology of CVID is unknown. Most patients present sporadically, although up to 20% of patients have a first-degree relative with selective IgA deficiency. CVID is also reportedly associated with the use of various antirheumatic (e.g., sulfasalazine) or antiepileptic (e.g., hydantoin, carbamazepine) drugs.

Clinical Findings

The estimated prevalence of CVID is approximately 1 case per 50,000 population. Most patients develop the disorder between 20 and 50 years of age. Only approximately 20% of patients are diagnosed during childhood. There is no sexual predilection. Nearly all patients have recurrent symptoms or bronchitis and to a lesser extent sinusitis, usually secondary to *Haemophilus influenzae*, and less often pneumococcus, *Moraxella catarrhalis*, or mycoplasma. Prior to the advent of immunoglobulin (Ig) replacement therapy, most patients died of complications of bronchiectasis. Even today, most patients continue to suffer from recurrent bouts of infectious bronchitis and require prophylactic antibiotics to prevent bronchiectasis and its sequelae. Inflammatory bowel disease is common, with approximately 30% of CVID patients suffering from chronic diarrhea. Granuloma formation is a unique feature and can mimic sarcoidosis in the lung. Infiltration of the spleen occurs in 20% of affected patients and can extend to the liver, resulting in presinusoidal venous congestion, esophageal varices, cirrhosis, and liver failure. Cutaneous granulomas can appear as a maculopapular rash, erythematous papules, plaques, excoriated papules, and ulcers. Autoimmune diseases affect 10% of patients, most commonly hemolytic anemia, immune thrombocytopenia (ITP), neutropenia, rheumatoid arthritis, autoimmune hepatitis, and sprue-like intestinal malabsorption disorders. Five percent of patients develop mycoplasma infections of the urinary tract and joints. Decreased serum levels of immunoglobulin G (IgG) and immunoglobulin A (IgA) are characteristic of CVID. Approximately 50% of patients may also have diminished serum immunoglobulin M (IgM) levels and T-lymphocyte dysfunction.

Imaging Findings

Radiography

- May be normal
- Bronchial wall thickening/peribronchial cuffing (**Figs. 32.1A, 32.1B**)
- Bronchiectasis
- Air space disease (**Figs. 32.1A, 32.1B**)
- Partial or complete lobar collapse (**Figs. 32.1A, 32.1B**)
- Pleural thickening

MDCT/HRCT

- May be normal
- Bronchial wall thickening/peribronchial cuffing (**Figs. 32.1C, 32.1D, 32.1E, 32.1F**)
- Bronchiectasis (**Figs. 32.1C, 32.1D, 32.1E, 32.1F**)
- Air space disease (**Figs. 32.1C, 32.1D, 32.1E, 32.1F**)
- Partial or complete lobar collapse (**Figs. 32.1E, 32.1F**)
- Mediastinal/hilar lymphadenopathy (**Figs. 32.1G, 32.1H**)
- Fibrosis (**Figs. 32.1C, 32.1D**)
- Pleural thickening
- Emphysema
- ± Abdominal lymphadenopathy/splenomegaly (**Fig. 32.1I**)
- ± Hepatomegaly

CVID Systemic Granulomatous Disease–Associated Interstitial Lung Disease (10%)

- Diffuse bronchial wall thickening
- Bronchiectasis
- Widespread pulmonary micronodules (<10 mm); lower lobe predominance (80%)
- Smooth interlobular septal thickening; mid-lower lung zone predominance (20%)
- Diffuse reticulation (septal and non-septal linear opacities)/scarring
- Mediastinal and/or hilar lymphadenopathy
- Air trapping

Management

- Mainstay: Ig replacement therapy (stops cycle of recurrent infections)
- Antimicrobial therapy: initiated at first sign of infection
- Annual thyroid examination and thyroid function testing
- Periodic CBC and differential WBC counts to detect complicating lymphoma
- Biopsy to exclude infection or malignancy in enlarging lymph nodes
- Individuals with bronchiectasis: Avoid contact with peat or other sources of *Aspergillus*
- HRCT scan every 2–3 years to follow progression of lung disease
- Role of lung transplantation in CVID patients with respiratory failure: limited long-term follow-up studies

Prognosis

- 20-year survival rate: 64% (males), 67% (females)
- Factors associated with mortality: low IgG levels, poor T-cell response to antigens, low percentage of peripheral B-cells
- Common cause of death in CVID: lymphoma (NHL > HL)
- Increased incidence of other malignancies, including breast, prostate, actinic keratosis, and squamous cell carcinoma, melanoma, and basal cell carcinoma
- Other causes of morbidity and mortality include cor pulmonale (secondary to chronic pulmonary infection), liver failure (caused by viral or autoimmune hepatitis), malnutrition (resulting from GI tract disease), and other viral infections

PEARLS

- Most patients with CVID have recurrent sinopulmonary infections.
- Recurrent pulmonary infection may be complicated by bronchiectasis.
- Risk of certain malignancies, especially lymphomas, is high.

Suggested Reading

1. Cunningham-Rundles C, Bodian C. Common variable immunodeficiency: clinical and immunological features of 248 patients. Clin Immunol 1999;92(1):34–48
2. Hammarström L, Vorechovsky I, Webster D. Selective IgA deficiency (SIgAD) and common variable immunodeficiency (CVID). Clin Exp Immunol 2000;120(2):225–231
3. Thickett KM, Kumararatne DS, Banerjee AK, Dudley R, Stableforth DE. Common variable immune deficiency: respiratory manifestations, pulmonary function and high-resolution CT scan findings. QJM 2002;95(10):655–662
4. Torigian DA, LaRosa DF, Levinson AI, Litzky LA, Miller WT Jr. Granulomatous-lymphocytic interstitial lung disease associated with common variable immunodeficiency: CT findings. J Thorac Imaging 2008;23(3):162–169

Section IV

Atelectasis

OVERVIEW OF MECHANISMS OF ATELECTASIS

The word *atelectasis* is derived from the Greek words *ateles*, meaning "incomplete," and *ektasis*, for "expansion." Thus atelectasis means "incomplete expansion." This incomplete expansion may involve only a portion of the lung, as with segmental or lobar collapse, or it can affect the entire lung, as with a mainstem obstruction or bronchial atresia. Atelectasis is the antithesis of consolidation. That is, atelectasis is an *air-losing process*. The "lost air" is not replaced. Thus, the imaging hallmark of atelectasis is "volume loss." Alternatively, consolidation is an *air space replacing process*. The air within alveoli is replaced by something else, such as pus (e.g., pneumonia), fluid (e.g., edema), blood (e.g., alveolar hemorrhage), or cells (e.g., primary pulmonary lymphoma or adenocarcinoma in situ, formerly known as bronchioloalveolar cell carcinoma). Because there is an equal exchange of air for one of these four other products, the lung volumes are preserved on imaging studies.

There are four basic pathophysiologic mechanisms of atelectasis. One mechanism is *obstructive* (i.e., resorption atelectasis) and three are *non-obstructive* and include relaxation or passive atelectasis, adhesive atelectasis, and cicatrization atelectasis. These mechanisms and some of the more commonly encountered clinical causes for each are summarized in **Table IV.1**.

Table IV.1   Pulmonary Atelectasis: Mechanism and Etiology

Resorption	Relaxation	Cicatrization	Adhesive
Malpositioned ETT	Pneumothorax	Granulomatous infection/insult	Respiratory distress syndrome
Foreign body	Pleural effusion	Interstitial fibrosis	Radiation pneumonitis
Mucoid impaction	Bulla	Radiation therapy	ARDS
Primary/secondary neoplasia	Mass(es)	Necrotizing pneumonia	Post-operative CABG
Strictures and stenoses	Chest wall mass or deformity	Pneumoconiosis	Uremia
RML syndrome	Subdiaphragmatic disease		Inhalation injury
Lymphadenopathy			Pulmonary hemorrhage

CASE 33

■ Clinical Presentation

25-year-old woman, status post conversion of pre-existing endotracheal tube to a tracheostomy device, with an abrupt decrease in oxygen saturations and increased work of breathing immediately following the procedure

■ Radiologic Findings

AP chest radiograph (**Fig. 33.1**) demonstrates opacification of the upper one-third of the right hemithorax without air bronchograms. The horizontal fissure (*arrow*) is displaced cephalad. Various life support tubes and lines are appropriately positioned. Free air beneath the left diaphragm is related to the concurrent recent PEG placement.

■ Diagnosis

Right Upper Lobe Atelectasis (Resorption); Endobronchial Mucus Plug

■ Differential Diagnosis

- Acute Lobar Collapse of Other Etiologies
  - Aspirated or Dislodged Foreign Body (e.g., tooth, dental amalgam)
  - Aspirated Peri-operative Blood/Endobronchial Clot

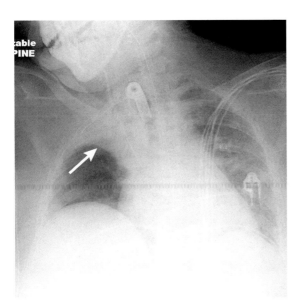

Fig. 33.1

199

■ Discussion

Background

Resorption atelectasis is the most common and complex mechanism of volume loss and results from obstruction in airflow somewhere between the trachea and alveoli. In acute endobronchial obstruction, the partial pressure of gases in mixed venous blood (Pp mixed venous blood) becomes less than that in alveolar air (Pp alveolar air). As blood passes through alveolar capillaries, the partial pressures of gases (Pp gases) equilibrate and oxygen (O_2) diffuses into the capillary bed. Alveoli diminish in volume in proportion to the quantity of O_2 absorbed. The partial pressures of alveolar carbon dioxide (Pp CO_2) and nitrogen (Pp N_2) then increase relative to those in the capillary bed. These gases also diffuse into the capillary bed to maintain gaseous equilibrium, with a proportional decrease in alveolar volume. The partial pressure of alveolar oxygen (Pp alveolar O_2) then increases relative to the capillary bed. Oxygen again diffuses into the capillary bed to maintain equilibrium, with a resultant proportional decrease in alveolar volume. This cycle repeats over and over until eventually all alveolar gas is absorbed and the alveoli are completely collapsed (**Fig. 33.2**).

Clinical Findings

Complete lobar collapse may occur in 18–24 hours while breathing room air. Because oxygen is absorbed 60 times more rapidly than nitrogen, resorption atelectasis is expedited when breathing 100% oxygen, and total collapse may then occur in less than 1 hour. Some studies even report this occurring in as little as 5 minutes. These latter situations may occur in intubated acute trauma patients, ICU ventilator-dependent patients, and surgical patients in the operating room under general anesthesia. Confirmation of appropriate ET tube positioning is critical in such patients (**Fig. 33.3**).

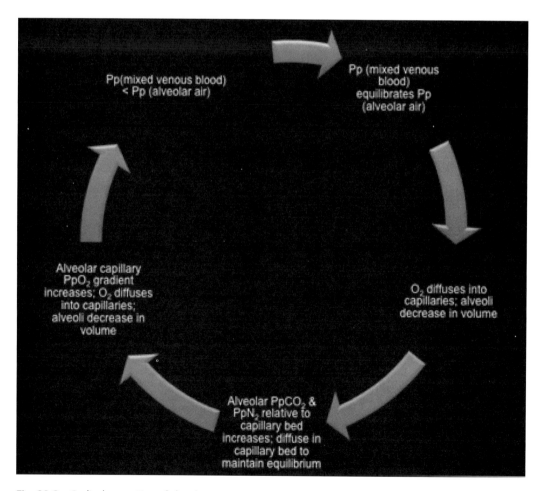

Fig. 33.2   Cyclical resorption of alveolar gases.

Acute resorption atelectasis may occur in trauma victims with aspirated foreign bodies (e.g., teeth, tooth fragments [**Fig. 33.4**], dental amalgam, tongue rings, windshield glass fragments, etc.) as well as patients with an acute bronchial fracture. More insidious resorption atelectasis occurs with primary (**Figs. 33.5A, 33.5B**) and secondary endobronchial neoplasms, airway strictures or stenosis (e.g., granulomatous diseases, Wegener granulomatosis), and exobronchial lesions that extrinsically compromise the bronchus over time, such as the bulky lymphadenopathy associated with sarcoidosis or lymphoma.

Imaging Findings

Radiography/MDCT

- Acute development of segmental, lobar, or total lung collapse (**Figs. 33.1, 33.3, 33.4**)
- Absent air bronchograms (**Figs. 33.1, 33.3, 33.4, 33.5**)
- Identify cause of the obstruction (**Figs. 33.1, 33.3, 33.4, 33.5**)
- Rapid re-expansion of affected lung following relief of obstruction when possible

Management

- Respiratory physiotherapy (chest wall percussion and vibration), bronchiolytics, postural drainage, and bronchodilators
- Bronchoscopy in selected cases
- Relief of obstructing medical device (e.g., malpositioned endotracheal tube) or foreign body where appropriate
- *N*-acetylcysteine aerosols
- Nebulized or direct tracheal application of DNase may reduce viscoelastic properties of purulent airway secretions, reducing the viscosity and allowing easier clearance
- Endobronchial laser and stents in complicated cases

Prognosis

- Lung returns to normal after relief of obstruction and resolution of post-obstructive pneumonia in un-complicated cases
- Untreated or unrecognized resorption atelectasis stemming from endobronchial obstruction may be complicated by
  ○ Persistent obstruction/infection
  ○ Bronchiectasis with recurrent infection and/or hemoptysis
  ○ Fibrosis

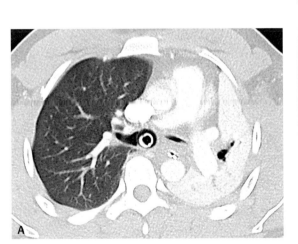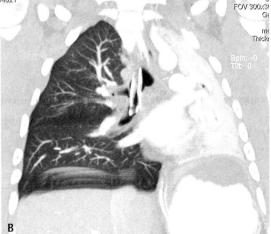

Fig. 33.3 **(A)** Chest CT axial and **(B)** coronal MIP (lung windows) of a 25 year old man involved in a motor vehicle collision with absent left breath sounds shows a malpositioned ET tube coursing deep into the right mainstem bronchus occluding airflow to the left lung with total collapse of that lung. Note the leftward mediastinal shift and left diaphragmatic elevation.

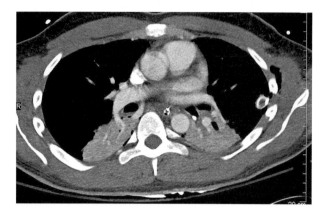

Fig. 33.4 Contrast-enhanced chest CT (mediastinal window) of a 23-year-old un-helmeted man involved in a motorcycle collision with maxillofacial trauma reveals a high-attenuation obstructing foreign body occluding the proximal left lower lobe bronchus. Bronchoscopy removed a dominant tooth fragment. Right lower lobe resorption atelectasis was secondary to bronchorrhea, which also improved following bronchoscopy.

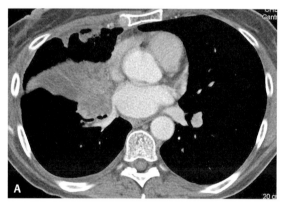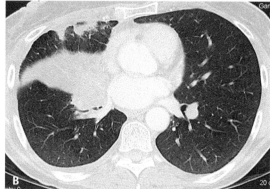

Fig. 33.5 **(A)** Contrast-enhanced chest CT (mediastinal windows) and **(B)** (lung windows) in a 49-year-old woman with a long-standing cough shows a "drowned" right middle lobe from a slow-growing airflow-obstructing endobronchial squamous cell cancer.

PEARLS

- In children, obstruction is often due to a mucus plug or aspirated foreign body.
- In young adults (<35 years), obstruction is often due to a mucus plug, foreign body, or benign neoplasm.
- In older adults, primary and secondary endobronchial neoplasms must be excluded (see Section VI).

Suggested Reading

1. Demir A, Olcmen A, Kara HV, Dincer SI. Delayed diagnosis of a complete bronchial rupture after blunt thoracic trauma. Thorac Cardiovasc Surg 2006;54(8):560–562

2. Fraser RS, Müller NL, Colman N, Paré PD. Atelectasis. In: Fraser and Paré's Diagnosis of Diseases of the Chest, 4th ed. Philadelphia: Saunders; 1999:513–517

3. Peroni DG, Boner AL. Atelectasis: mechanisms, diagnosis and management. Paediatr Respir Rev 2000;1(3): 274–278

4. Woodring JH, Reed JC. Types and mechanisms of pulmonary atelectasis. J Thorac Imaging 1996;11(2):92–108

CASE 34

■ Clinical Presentation

72-year-old man with long-standing history of chronic obstructive lung disease presents to his physician with progressive dyspnea over the last several weeks and left-sided pleuritic chest pain

■ Radiologic Findings

PA (**Fig. 34.1A**) and lateral (**Fig. 34.1B**) chest X-rays show opacification of nearly two-thirds of the left hemithorax. Note the airless left mid- and lower thorax and contralateral mediastinal shift from this pleural space-occupying process. The lateral exam (**Fig. 34.1B**) also demonstrates a *positive spine sign* characterized by increased opacity over the lower thoracic spine and obscuration of the left diaphragm.

■ Diagnosis

Relaxation Atelectasis Lingula and Left Lower Lobe; Left Pleural Effusion (Empyema)

■ Differential Diagnosis

- Atelectasis
- Parenchymal Consolidation

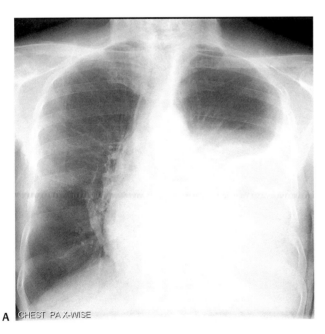 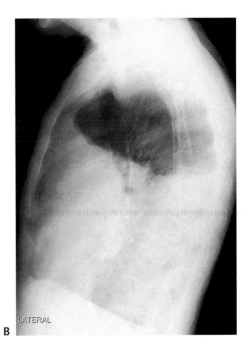

Fig. 34.1

■ Discussion

Background

Relaxation (passive) atelectasis occurs when there is loss of contact between the visceral and parietal pleurae by a space-occupying process (e.g., pleural effusion, pneumothorax) exerting *extrinsic* pressure on the parenchyma. The elastic recoil properties of the lung preserve its shape as it loses volume. In the absence of pleural adhesions, the degree of atelectasis is proportional to the volume of fluid (**Fig. 34.2C**) or air (**Fig. 34.3**) in the pleural space. *Mantle* or *compressive atelectasis* is a subtype of relaxation atelectasis resulting from a space-occupying lesion exerting *intrinsic* pressure on the lung, forcing air out of the alveoli (**Fig. 34.4**). Mantle atelectasis may occur in response to large bullous lesions (**Fig. 34.4**) as well as from dominant intraparenchymal lung masses, loculated pleural fluid collections, chest wall–based lesions, and subdiaphragmatic disease (e.g., massive ascites).

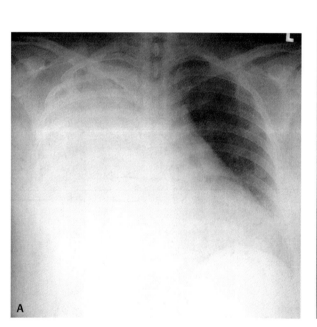

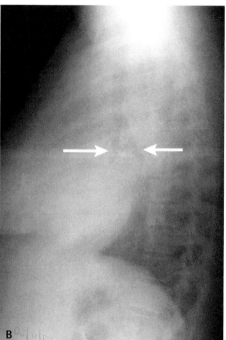

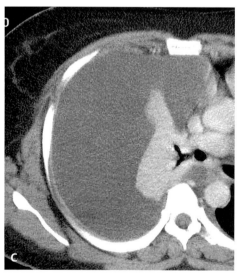

Fig. 34.2   (A) PA and **(B)** lateral chest X-rays of a 42-year-old woman 1-year status post total abdominal hysterectomy for ovarian carcinoma now complaining of progressive dyspnea demonstrate an opaque right hemithorax and contralateral mediastinal shift. Note the posterior displacement of the bronchi (*arrows*) on the lateral exam **(B)**. **(C)** Contrast-enhanced chest CT (mediastinal window) reveals a massive right hydrothorax, right lung relaxation atelectasis, and contralateral mediastinal shift. The collapsed right lung maintains its normal shape but has decreased in volume in proportion to the volume of fluid in the pleural space.

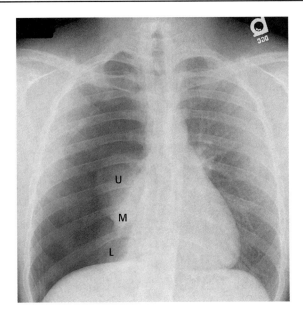

Fig. 34.3 PA chest radiograph of a 20-year-old man presenting with primary spontaneous right-sided tension pneumothorax. The mediastinum is displaced leftward. The individual collapsed upper (*U*), middle (*M*), and lower (*L*) lobes can be delineated and maintain their normal shape, but have markedly decreased in volume in proportion to the volume of air in the pleural space.

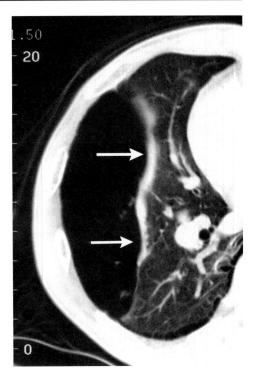

Fig. 34.4 Chest CT (lung window) of a 62-year-old man with dyspnea reveals a large bullous lesion in the peripheral right lung with adjacent mantle atelectasis (*arrows*).

Clinical Findings

If atelectasis is secondary to massive pleural effusion, as in this case, the affected hemithorax is dull to percussion with diminished breath sounds on auscultation. The severity of dyspnea depends on the patient's underlying respiratory reserve and the rate at which the fluid accumulated. The gradual accumulation of fluid over time allows the patient to accommodate for the volume loss. Such patients may be less symptomatic.

Imaging Findings

- Upper lobes demonstrate greater degree of relaxation atelectasis with pneumothorax
- Lower lobes exhibit greater degree of relaxation atelectasis with pleural effusion (**Figs. 34.1A, 34.1B**)
- Cartilaginous support of lobar and segmental bronchi allows them to resist collapse, remain air-filled, and manifest as air bronchograms (**Fig. 34.2B**)

Management

- Directed toward underlying disease process and evacuation of pleural fluid or air when necessary

Prognosis

- In the absence of pleural adhesions, once the pleural air or fluid collection is evacuated, the elastic recoil properties of the chest wall and affected lung allow it to re-expand and function normally

PEARLS

- Endobronchial tumor must be excluded if air bronchograms are absent.
- Mantle atelectasis from dominant bullous lesion(s): Elastic recoil properties of the lung allow the lung to re-expand and function once the bulla(e) have been excised. This is the rationale behind lung volume reduction surgery (LVRS) (see Section XIII, Case 188).

Suggested Reading

1. Fraser RS, Müller NL, Colman N, Paré PD. Atelectasis. In: Fraser and Paré's Diagnosis of Diseases of the Chest, 4th ed. Philadelphia: Saunders; 1999:513–517
2. Stark P, Leung A. Effects of lobar atelectasis on the distribution of pleural effusion and pneumothorax. J Thorac Imaging 1996;11(2):145–149
3. Woodring JH, Reed JC. Types and mechanisms of pulmonary atelectasis. J Thorac Imaging 1996;11(2):92–108

CASE 35

■ Clinical Presentation

51-year-old man who is now five months status post mantle radiation therapy for unresectable adenocarcinoma of the lung

■ Radiologic Findings

PA (**Fig. 35.1A**) and lateral (**Fig. 35.1B**) chest radiographs demonstrate well-defined opacities with sharp borders involving the superior mediastinum and paramediastinal lung zones. The bronchi within the affected lung are distorted and dilated. Note the hilar retraction, diaphragmatic elevation, and compensatory overinflation of the uninvolved lower lungs. Chest CT (lung window) (**Fig. 35.1C**) reveals sharply demarcated bands of increased attenuation in the medial anterior and posterior paramediastinal lung zones. Note the traction bronchiectasis and bronchovascular reorientation in the affected lung.

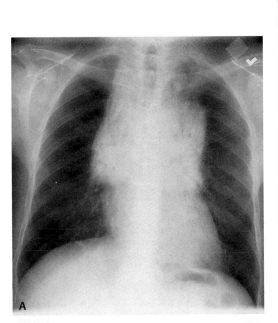

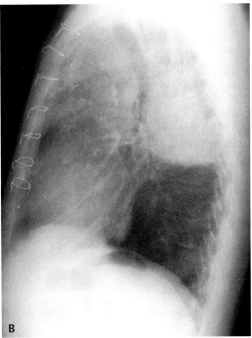

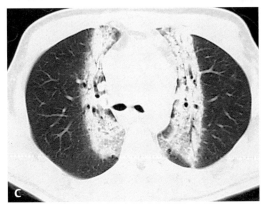

Fig. 35.1

207

■ Diagnosis

Cicatrization Atelectasis: Iatrogenic Radiation-Therapy Induced; Corresponding to the Radiation Therapy Portal

■ Differential Diagnosis

None

■ Discussion

Background

Localized cicatrization atelectasis is a fibrotic process associated with irreversible volume loss (**Figs. 35.1A, 35.1B, 35.1C**). The prototypical example is fibrosis secondary to chronic infection (e.g., long-standing tuberculosis) and necrotizing pneumonia. Idiopathic pulmonary fibrosis (IPF) and other chronic infiltrative lung diseases (see Section VIII) are associated with a more *generalized* but also irreversible form of cicatrization atelectasis.

Clinical Findings

Chronic radiation damage begins 3–4 months following initiation of therapy. The fibrosis and volume loss develop gradually and stabilize 9–12 months after completion of therapy. Many patients are asymptomatic. Symptoms, when present, may be insidious and include cough and dyspnea. Forced vital capacity and diffusion capacity may be reduced. The associated lung fibrosis on imaging correlates with the expected location of the radiation therapy port (**Figs. 35.1A, 35.1B, 35.1C**). For example, paramediastinal cicatrization atelectasis occurs in patients who have received mantle radiation (e.g., lymphoma and other mediastinal malignancies) whereas cicatrization atelectasis and bronchovascular reorientation occur in the peripheral upper and middle lobes in patients receiving chest wall radiation (e.g., breast cancer).

Imaging Findings

- Parenchymal opacity with loss of lung volume (**Figs. 35.1A, 35.1B, 35.1C**)
- Parenchymal opacity conforming to the radiation portal (**Fig. 35.1A, 35.1B, 35.1C**)
- Affected lung occupies a smaller volume than normal, appears dense and heterogeneous because of architectural distortion, dilated bronchi, and bronchioles (**Figs. 35.1A, 35.1B, 35.1C**)
- Compensatory signs of chronic volume loss are usually evident (e.g., localized mediastinal shift, compensatory overinflation of unaffected lung) (**Figs. 35.1A, 35.1B, 35.1C**)

Management

- Observation
- Supportive with supplemental oxygen
- Corticosteroids in select cases

Prognosis

- Irreversible
- Dependent on the underlying disease process

PEARLS

- Cicatrization atelectasis is the only form of pulmonary atelectasis that is irreversible.
- Late complications of radiation therapy also include pericardial effusion, pericardial calcification, accelerated atherosclerosis, airway strictures, and osseous demineralization.

Suggested Readings

1. Fraser RS, Müller NL, Colman N, Paré PD. Atelectasis In: Fraser and Paré's Diagnosis of Diseases of the Chest, 4th ed. Philadelphia: Saunders; 1999:522–525
2. Fraser RS, Müller NL, Colman N, Paré PD. Irradiation. In: Fraser and Paré's Diagnosis of Diseases of the Chest, 4th ed. Philadelphia: Saunders; 1999:2595–2606
3. Westcott JL, Cole SR. Traction bronchiectasis in end-stage pulmonary fibrosis. Radiology 1986;161(3):665–669
4. Woodring JH, Reed JC. Types and mechanisms of pulmonary atelectasis. J Thorac Imaging 1996;11(2):92–108

CASE 36

■ Clinical Presentation

1,260 g girl born at 30 weeks' gestation presenting with retractions, grunting, and poor air movement and requiring oxygen; has received one dose of surfactant, with some clinical improvement

■ Radiologic Findings

AP chest radiograph (**Fig. 36.1**) shows bilateral, symmetrical, perihilar opacities with a fine granular pattern and associated air bronchograms. The lung volumes are diminished bilaterally. Note the endotracheal tube, enteric tube, umbilical arterial and umbilical venous catheters.

■ Diagnosis

Adhesive Atelectasis: Respiratory Distress Syndrome (RDS) of the Newborn

■ Differential Diagnosis

- Pneumonia
- Volume overload or heart failure
- Massive aspiration
- Pulmonary hemorrhage

■ Discussion

Background

The pressure-volume relationships of the lung depend on forces acting at the air-tissue interface of the alveolar wall. These forces are further understood by applying Laplace's law $(p = 2T/r)$, where p represents pressure, T the surface tension at the air-tissue interface, and r the radius of a sphere, which in this case represents the alveoli. As alveoli diminish in volume, the surface tension of the interface is diminished by surfactant (phos-

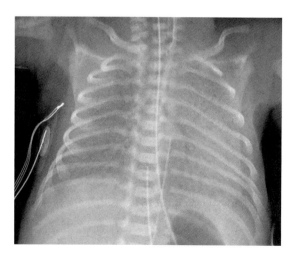

Fig. 36.1 (*Image Courtesy of Stephanie E. Spottswood, M.D., MSPH, Vanderbilt Children's Hospital, Nashville, Tennessee.*)

pholipid dipalmitoyl phosphatidylcholine). The production of abnormal or insufficient surfactant results in increased surface tension within the alveoli and widespread alveolar collapse (e.g., microatelectasis) despite patent airways. Once collapsed, alveolar walls tend to adhere (hence the term adhesive atelectasis), making re-expansion difficult. Adhesive atelectasis may produce significant arteriovenous shunting in spite of a relatively normal chest radiograph.

Clinical Findings

The best examples of adhesive atelectasis are RDS of the newborn (**Fig. 36.1**) and acute radiation pneumonitis. Adhesive atelectasis may also occur with acute respiratory distress syndrome (ARDS) of adults, smoke inhalation, bronchopneumonia, uremia, prolonged shallow breathing associated with surgery, cardiac bypass surgery, pulmonary contusions and other causes of pulmonary hemorrhage, and acute pulmonary thromboembolic disease. Adhesive atelectasis tends to be more widespread with both newborn and adult forms of ARDS and smoke inhalation, whereas it is limited to the radiation port or its outer margins with acute radiation pneumonitis. In pulmonary embolism, focal ischemia distal to the embolus can result in a marked reduction in surfactant levels, leading to subsegmental or even segmental atelectasis.

Imaging Findings

- Chest radiography may be relatively normal
- Ground-glass opacities and/or consolidation with associated volume loss (**Fig. 36.1**)
- Subsegmental or even segmental atelectasis
- Patent bronchi and bronchioles may manifest as air bronchograms (i.e., nonobstructive atelectasis) (**Fig. 36.1**)

Management

- Directed toward underlying cause
- Supportive; supplemental oxygen and mechanical ventilation (positive end-expiratory pressure) as needed
- Surfactant (Curosurf [Poractant Alpha] [Chiesi Farmaceutici, Parma, Italy]) administration

Prognosis

- Variable
- Curosurf improves oxygenation and lung compliance and reduces mortality and pneumothoraces associated with RDS

PEARLS

- Prototypical examples of adhesive atelectasis include respiratory distress syndrome of the newborn and acute radiation pneumonitis.

Suggested Readings

1. Fraser RS, Müller NL, Colman N, Paré PD. Atelectasis. In: Fraser and Paré's Diagnosis of Diseases of the Chest, 4th ed. Philadelphia: Saunders; 1999:522

2. Plavka R, Kopecký P, Sebron V, et al. Early versus delayed surfactant administration in extremely premature neonates with respiratory distress syndrome ventilated by high-frequency oscillatory ventilation. Intensive Care Med 2002;28(10):1483–1490

3. Schindler MB. Treatment of atelectasis: where is the evidence? Crit Care 2005;9(4):341–342

4. Wilcox P, Baile EM, Hards J, et al. Phrenic nerve function and its relationship to atelectasis after coronary artery bypass surgery. Chest 1988;93(4):693–698

5. Woodring JH, Reed JC. Types and mechanisms of pulmonary atelectasis. J Thorac Imaging 1996;11(2):92–108

OVERVIEW OF RADIOLOGIC SIGNS OF ATELECTASIS

Radiologic signs of atelectasis or lobar collapse may be classified into *direct* and *indirect* signs (**Table IV.2**). *Direct* signs of volume loss include displacement of interlobar fissures, crowding of vessels and bronchi, and a focal increase in radio-opacity. Displacement of interlobar fissures is one of the most dependable and easily recognized *direct* signs. Interlobar fissures are formed by visceral pleura that invest each pulmonary lobe. Thus, as a particular lobe loses volume, the local fissures move in concert with the deflating lobe in a predictable manner. At the same time, bronchovascular structures supplying the involved lobe will approximate and may appear "crowded" on the chest radiograph or CT. As there is less air per unit lung volume in the collapsed lobe, there will often be a localized increase in radio-opacity. The major *indirect* radiologic signs of atelectasis are related to mechanisms compensating for a reduction in intrapleural pressure. Some signs occur more often than others, and are more reliable indicators of atelectasis. For example, hilar displacement is the most reliable *indirect* sign. Other signs are unique in their own right (e.g., Luftsichel sign) and serve as reliable indicators of volume loss that may otherwise go unrecognized. The cases that follow in this section demonstrate various patterns of lobar and multilobar atelectasis and illustrate many of the direct and indirect signs of volume loss listed in **Table IV.2**. Once the radiologic findings of lobar or multilobar atelectasis have been observed, the potential etiologies for such must be investigated (see **Table IV.2**). This may necessitate further evaluation with sputum analysis, CT, or even bronchoscopy.

Table IV.2   Radiologic Signs of Atelectasis

Direct Signs	Indirect Signs
Displacement of interlobar fissures	Hilar displacement
Crowding of vessels and bronchi	Reorientation of normal vascular structures
Focal increase in radio-opacity	Mediastinal shift or displacement
	Compensatory overinflation
	Ipsilateral diaphragmatic elevation
	"Luftsichel" sign
	Absence of air bronchograms
	Absence of interlobar artery visibility
	Juxtaphrenic peak
	"Pseudomass" sign
	Shifting granuloma
	Rib approximation
	"Flat-waist" sign
	"Top of the aortic knob" sign

CASE 37

■ Clinical Presentation

38-year-old man status post recent abdominal surgery requiring ventilator support with an abrupt drop in oxygen saturations and decreased breath sounds over the upper right thorax

■ Radiologic Findings

AP chest radiograph (**Fig. 37.1**) shows cephalad displacement of the horizontal fissure (*arrow*) and elevation of the right hilum (*asterisk*) and diaphragm. Note the decrease in volume of the right hemithorax and the ipsilateral mediastinal shift.

■ Diagnosis

Right Upper Lobe Atelectasis; Obstructing Mucus Plug

■ Differential Diagnosis

•   Aspirated Foreign Body (e.g., tooth)

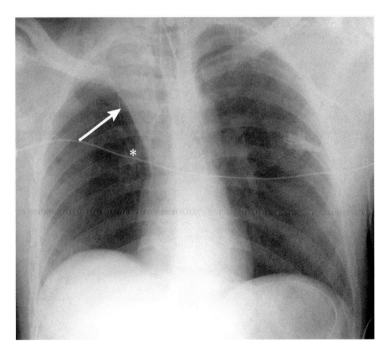

Fig. 37.1

213

■ Discussion

Background

The horizontal fissure and upper half of the oblique fissure approximate by shifting upward and forward, respectively (**Fig. 37.2**). On lateral chest radiography, both fissures appear gently curved. The horizontal fissure assumes a concave configuration inferiorly, whereas the oblique fissure may appear convex, concave, or flat (**Fig. 37.2**). On frontal radiography, the horizontal fissure maintains a superiorly convex morphology. With increased volume loss, the horizontal fissure continues to move up, over the apex of the thorax, and the collapsed lobe becomes contiguous with the superior mediastinum. In total lobar atelectasis, the volume of the collapsed right upper lobe may be so small that the atelectatic lobe mimics superior mediastinal widening on the frontal chest exam (**Figs. 37.2, 37.3**). On lateral radiography, the completely collapsed upper lobe may be obscured by the overlying shoulders and upper arms. When conspicuous, the collapsed upper lobe appears as a distinct wedge-shaped triangular mediastinal opacity with its apex directed toward the hilum and its base contiguous with the parietal pleura posterior to the apex of the hemithorax.

Hilar displacement is an *indirect* sign of volume loss. In 97% of individuals, the left hilum is higher than the right. In 3% of individuals, the hila lie at approximately the same level. The normal left hilum never lies lower than the normal right hilum. An alteration in normal hilar relationships is the most reliable *indirect* sign of atelectasis. Hilar shift is more common in upper lobe than in lower lobe collapse, and is usually more marked in cases of chronic volume loss.

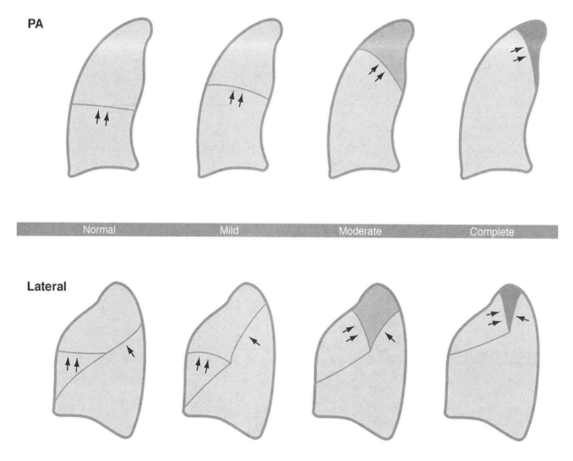

Fig. 37.2 Artist's illustration demonstrating the normal anatomic positions of both the horizontal and oblique fissures and their gradual displacement with progressive degrees of mild, moderate, and complete right upper lobe volume loss in the frontal and lateral radiographic planes. See description in text.

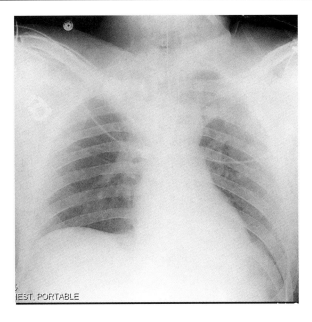

Fig. 37.3 AP chest radiograph of a 31-year-old trauma victim with bronchorrhea and near total right upper lobe collapse. Complete right upper lobe atelectasis may simulate superior mediastinal widening. Observation of additional indirect signs of volume loss, in this case hilar displacement and ipsilateral diaphragmatic elevation, establish the correct diagnosis.

Clinical Findings

Affected patients may exhibit an abrupt drop in oxygen saturations, altered A-a gradient, and diminished breath sounds over the affected region.

Imaging Findings

- Alteration in normal hilar relationships (**Figs. 37.1, 37.3, 37.4A, 37.4B. 37.4C**)
- Alteration of normal course and position of interlobar fissures (**Figs. 37.1, 37.2, 37.3, 37.4**)
- Increased opacity of affected lung parenchyma (**Figs. 37.1, 37.2, 37.3, 37.4**)
- Ipsilateral mediastinal shift (**Figs. 37.1, 37.4**)
- Ipsilateral diaphragmatic elevation (**Figs. 37.1, 37.3, 37.4A, 37.4B**)
- Juxtaphrenic peak

Management

- Respiratory physiotherapy (chest wall percussion and vibration), bronchiolytics, postural drainage, and bronchodilators
- Bronchoscopic aspiration of bronchial secretions or mucus plugs in selected cases
- *N*-acetylcysteine aerosols
- Nebulized or direct tracheal application of DNase may reduce viscoelastic properties of purulent airway secretions, reducing viscosity of secretions and facilitating clearance

Prognosis

- Good if recognized and treated early
- Delayed recognition and treatment may result in secondary bacterial infection

PEARLS

- Because the normal right hilum lies lower than the left, downward displacement of the right hilum in lower lobe collapse is more difficult to recognize radiographically than downward displacement of the left hilum. Recognition of concomitant indirect signs is therefore even more critical to make the correct diagnosis.

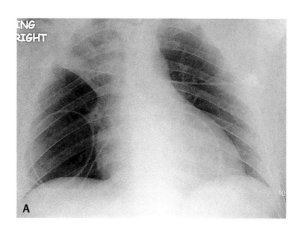

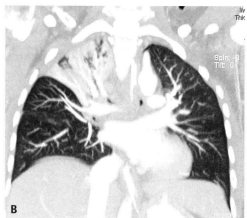

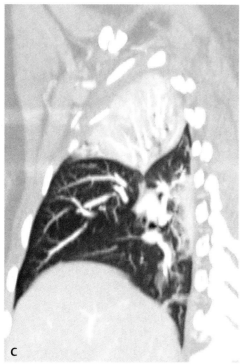

Fig. 37.4 **(A)** AP chest radiograph of a 30-year-old victim of an inhalation injury following a house fire with bronchorrhea shows classic radiographic signs of right upper lobe atelectasis. Note the cephalad displacement of the right hilum and horizontal fissure as well as rightward shift of the tracheal air column. **(B)** Chest CT coronal and **(C)** sagittal MIP images (lung windows) illustrate the expected displacement of the horizontal and oblique fissures. Correlate with **Fig. 37.2**.

Suggested Reading

1. Felson B. The lobes. In: Felson B, ed. Chest Roentgenology. Philadelphia: WB Saunders; 1973:92–133
2. Fraser RS, Müller NL, Colman N, Paré PD. Atelectasis. In: Fraser and Paré's Diagnosis of Diseases of the Chest, 4th ed. Philadelphia: Saunders; 1999:532–533
3. Gurney JW. Atypical manifestations of pulmonary atelectasis. J Thorac Imaging 1996;11(3):165–175
4. Kreider ME, Lipson DA. Bronchoscopy for atelectasis in the ICU: a case report and review of the literature. Chest 2003;124(1):344–350

CASE 38

■ Clinical Presentation

27-year-old woman complains of non-productive cough and weight loss over the last several months

■ Radiologic Findings

PA (**Fig. 38.1A**) and lateral (**Fig. 38.1B**) chest X-rays reveal reduction in volume of the right hemithorax, right hemidiaphragm elevation, and a "peaked" appearance (i.e., juxtaphrenic peak) of the superomedial hemidiaphragm. The trachea is minimally displaced to the right. On the frontal exam (**Fig. 38.1A**), the horizontal fissure is displaced cephalad. A mass-like convex-appearing bulge is present in the inferior and medial portion of the fissure. The lateral aspect of the fissure is concave superiorly. The configuration creates a "reverse S-shaped" morphology to the fissure. The lateral exam (**Fig. 38.1B**) reveals displacement of both the horizontal and oblique fissures and an indistinct wedge-shaped triangular mediastinal opacity with its apex directed toward the hilum and its base contiguous with the parietal pleura posterior to the apex of the hemithorax.

■ Diagnosis

Complicated Right Upper Lobe Atelectasis; Lymphoma with "Reverse 'S' Sign of Golden"

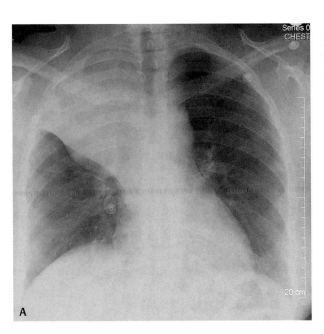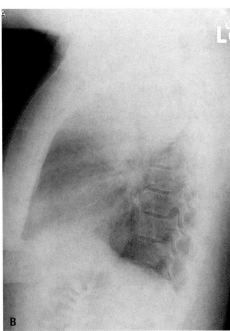

Fig. 38.1

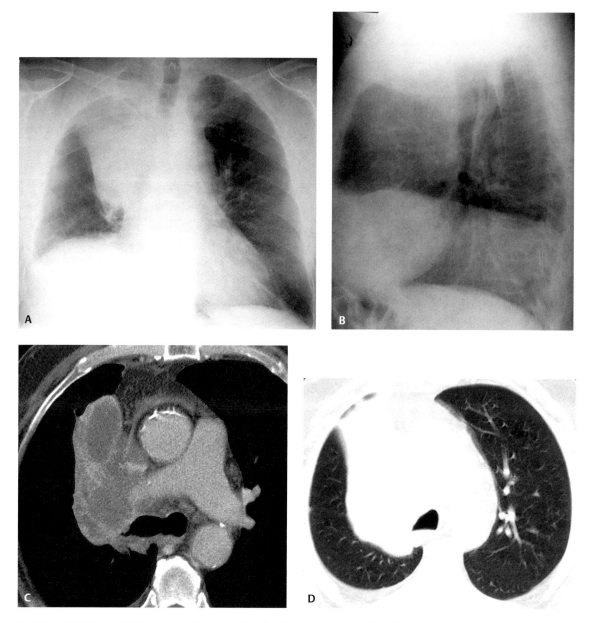

Fig.38.2 **(A)** PA and **(B)** lateral chest radiographs of a 58-year-old man with a long history of tobacco abuse, worsening cough, and recent episode of hemoptysis show a mass-like opacity involving the anterior-superior right hemithorax with well-defined borders. A focal convex bulge is seen in the medial portion of the horizontal fissure at the bronchus intermedius. The right hemidiaphragm is elevated. **(C)** Contrast-enhanced chest CT, **(D)** mediastinal window, and lung window reveals an encased right upper lobe bronchus with associated post-obstructive changes, volume loss, and ipsilateral mediastinal shift. Note the upward and medial displacement of the horizontal fissure and the upward and forward displacement of the oblique fissure. Diagnosis: small cell lung cancer.

■ Differential Diagnosis

- Post-Obstructive Upper Lobe Atelectasis from an Endobronchial Mass (e.g., primary and secondary neoplasia)
- Post-Obstructive Upper Lobe Atelectasis from Extrinsic Bronchial Compression by Reactive or Neoplastic Lymphadenopathy

■ Discussion

Background

In *non-complicated* right upper lobe atelectasis, the inferior border of the horizontal fissure should be *concave* on frontal and lateral radiography (**Figs. 37.1, 37.2, 37.4**). *Complicated* right upper lobe atelectasis caused by a hilar mass (e.g., small cell cancer, squamous cell cancer, lymphoma, lymphadenopathy) is often associated with a *convex* bulge in the medial aspect of the fissure (**Fig. 38.1A,B; 38.2A, B**). The lateral aspect of the fissure is appropriately concave. The result is a "reverse S-shaped" configuration to the horizontal fissure (i.e., *reverse "S" sign of Golden*), a sign highly suggestive of a central neoplasm causing the atelectasis.

Clinical Findings

Affected patients may present with cough, weight loss, hypoxemia, progressive dyspnea, hemoptysis, diminished or absent breath sounds over the affected area, and various paraneoplastic syndromes (see Section VI).

Imaging Findings

- Opaque right upper thorax (**Figs. 38.1, 38.2**)
- Direct and indirect signs of right hemithoracic volume loss (**Figs. 38.1, 38.2**)
- Convex bulge at medial aspect of displaced horizontal fissure (**Figs. 38.1, 38.2**)
- Central hilar mass lesion or extrinsic bronchial compression by lymphadenopathy (**Figs. 38.1, 38.2**)

Management

- Prompt bronchoscopic evaluation and biopsy to determine etiology of the complicated lobar atelectasis and establish a tissue diagnosis
- Surgical resection when possible
- Endobronchial stent deployment in select cases
- Palliative chemotherapy and/or radiation therapy in unresectable cases (see Section VI)

Prognosis

- Dependent on the stage at presentation in cases of neoplasia (see Section VI)

PEARLS

- *Reverse "S" sign of Golden* is highly suggestive of a central bronchogenic cancer as the cause of atelectasis on both radiography and CT. Its presence on chest X-ray should always prompt further investigation with bronchoscopy and/or CT.
- Although initially described for right upper lobe atelectasis, the sign is applicable to atelectasis of any lobe (see Case 39).

Suggested Reading

1. Golden R. The effect of bronchostenosis upon the roentgen-ray shadows in carcinoma of the bronchus. Am J Roentgenol 1925;13:21–30
2. Proto AV, Tocino I. Radiographic manifestations of lobar collapse. Semin Roentgenol 1980;15(2):117–173
3. Reinig JW, Ross P. Computed tomography appearance of Golden's "S" sign. J Comput Tomogr 1984;8(3):219–223
4. Woodring JH, Reed JC. Types and mechanisms of pulmonary atelectasis. J Thorac Imaging 1996;11(2):92–108

CASE 39

■ Clinical Presentation

37-year-old woman with new onset of seizures and brain metastases

■ Radiologic Findings

PA (**Fig. 39.1A**) and lateral (**Fig. 39.1B**) chest radiographs show a convex perihilar mass (*arrow*) medial to the bronchus intermedius obliterating the right lower lobe bronchus origin. There is inferior displacement of the right hilum and oblique fissure. The right interlobar artery and proximal lower lobe bronchus are inconspicuous. A *positive spine sign* is present on the lateral exam manifest by increased opacity over the lower thoracic spine which silhouettes the posterior right diaphragm. Note the right diaphragm elevation on both frontal and lateral chest radiography. Contrast-enhanced chest CT (**Fig. 39.1C**, mediastinal window, and **Fig. 39.1D**, lung window) demonstrates a heterogeneous subcarinal and right infra-hilar mass encasing the bronchus intermedius (*arrow*) and interlobar artery. The middle lobe bronchi are narrowed but patent. There is obliteration of the lower lobe bronchi with distal atelectasis and consolidation as well as inferior, medial, and posterior displacement of the oblique fissure.

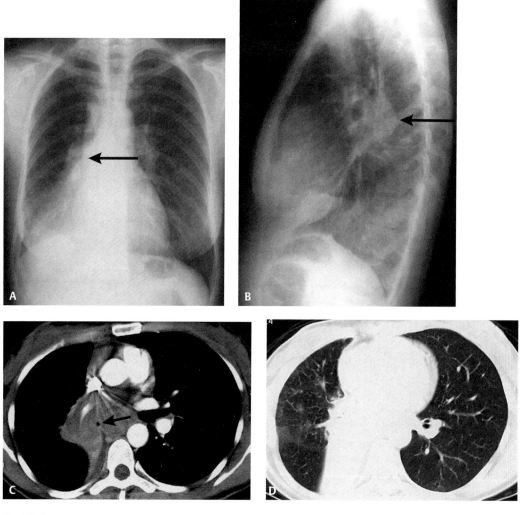

Fig. 39.1

220

■ Diagnosis

Right Lower Lobe Atelectasis; Obstructing Small Cell Lung Cancer

■ Differential Diagnosis

- Post-Obstructive Lower Lobe Atelectasis from an Endobronchial Mass (e.g., primary and secondary neoplasia)
- Post-Obstructive Lower Lobe Atelectasis from Extrinsic Bronchial Compression by Reactive or Neoplastic Lymphadenopathy

■ Discussion

Background

The right and left lower lobe demonstrate similar patterns of lobar collapse on imaging. The *triangular* versus *rounded* configuration assumed by the atelectatic lower lobe is related to the fulcrum-like effect exerted on the lung by the hilum and the integrity of the pulmonary ligament. When the pulmonary ligament is *complete*, the lower lobe is tethered to the mediastinum and hemidiaphragm and maintains a close relationship to both structures, assuming a *triangular* configuration as it loses volume (**Fig. 39.2**). Alternatively, when the pulmonary ligament is *incomplete*, the lung base is not adherent to the ipsilateral hemidiaphragm. As the lower lobe looses volume, the resultant shape depends primarily on its mediastinal attachment and the collapsed lobe assumes a more *rounded* morphology (**Fig. 39.3**).

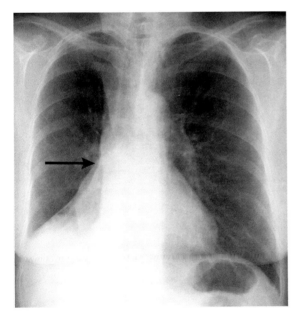

Fig. 39.2 PA chest radiograph of a 52-year-old woman with a long history of tobacco abuse and now with progressive cough and fatigue demonstrates caudal displacement of the oblique fissure and right hilum. Note the convex bulge in the medial aspect of the displaced oblique fissure (i.e., *reverse "S" sign of Golden* [*arrow*]). A triangular right basilar opacity obscures part of the hemidiaphragm. Diagnosis: complicated right lower lobe atelectasis from obstructing non–small cell lung cancer.

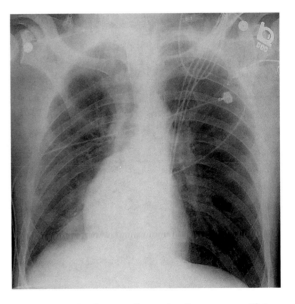

Fig. 39.3 AP chest radiograph of young ventilator-dependent trauma patient in the rehabilitation unit who experienced an acute onset of increased work of breathing reveals right lower lobe atelectasis characterized by ipsilateral mediastinal and tracheal shift and diaphragmatic elevation. Note the downward displacement of the oblique fissure. The atelectatic lower lobe assumes a more rounded morphology with an incomplete pulmonary ligament. Diagnosis: mucus plug.

As the lower lobes lose volume, the fissures approximate one another as the *upper half* of the oblique fissure moves *downward* and the *lower half* moves *backward* (**Fig. 39.4**, mild). This is best appreciated on lateral exams when the lobe is only partially collapsed and the oblique fissure is tangential to the X-ray beam. At the same time, the *upper half* of the oblique fissure may become conspicuous on the frontal radiograph as a well-defined fissural interface extending obliquely down from the hilum (**Fig. 39.4**, mild). With progressive volume loss, the lower lobe continues to move *posteriorly* and *medially* and occupies the posterior costophrenic gutter and medial costovertebral angle (**Fig. 39.4**, moderate). With complete lower lobe collapse, the only abnormality seen on the lateral view may be subtle increased opacity over the normally radiolucent lower thoracic spine (i.e., *positive spine* sign) (**Fig. 39.4**, complete). On frontal radiography, the atelectatic lobe appears as a small triangular or rounded opacity in the medial cardiophrenic angle (**Fig. 39.4**, complete). The interlobar artery is not seen, and the ipsilateral hilum will appear small or will be non-apparent because of obscuration by the surrounding airless lung.

Clinical Findings

Affected patients may present with cough, weight loss, hypoxemia, progressive dyspnea, hemoptysis, diminished or absent breath sounds over the affected area, and various paraneoplastic syndromes (see Section VI).

Imaging Findings

- Upper half of oblique fissure shifts inferiorly and lower half posteriorly (**Figs. 39.1, 39.2, 39.3, 39.4**)
- Horizontal fissure may or may not shift inferiorly (**Fig. 39.4**)

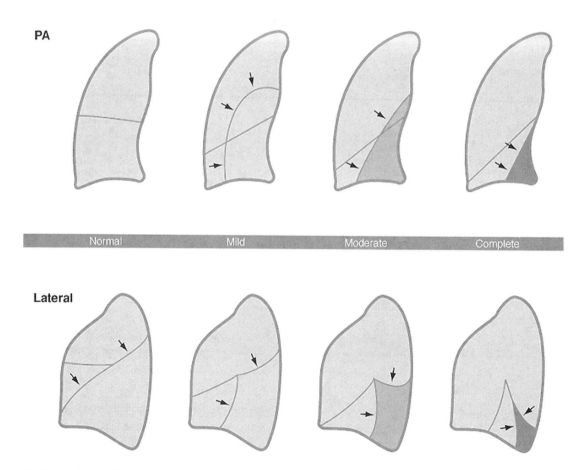

Fig. 39.4 Artist's illustration demonstrating the normal anatomic position of both the horizontal and oblique fissures and their gradual displacement with progressive degrees of mild, moderate, and complete right lower lobe volume loss in the frontal and lateral radiographic planes. See description in text.

- Atelectatic right lower lobe obscures the hemidiaphragm, paraspinal interface, and inferior vena cava; right heart border remains visible (**Figs. 39.1, 39.2, 39.3**)
- Other radiologic features include
  - Inferior and medial displacement of ipsilateral hilum and mainstem bronchus (**Figs. 39.1, 39.2, 39.3**)
  - Reorientation of mainstem and lower lobe bronchi into a more vertical plane (**Figs. 39.1, 39.2, 39.3**)
  - Narrowing of the normal carinal angle (**Figs. 39.1, 39.2, 39.3**)
  - Interlobar pulmonary artery is incorporated into atelectatic lower lobe, becoming inconspicuous, and ipsilateral hilum appears small (**Figs. 39.1, 39.2, 39.3**)
- As the degree of lower lobe atelectasis progresses
  - Opaque atelectatic lobe assumes "triangular" or "rounded" morphology (**Figs. 39.1, 39.2, 39.3, 39.4**)
  - Apex of "triangular" or "rounded" opacity is directed toward the hilum, and base abuts the hemidiaphragm (**Figs. 39.1, 39.2, 39.3, 39.4**)

Management

- Prompt bronchoscopic evaluation and biopsy to determine etiology of the complicated lobar atelectasis and establish a tissue diagnosis
- Surgical resection when possible
- Endobronchial stent deployment in select cases
- Palliative chemotherapy and/or radiation therapy, unresectable cases (see Section VI)

Prognosis

- Dependent on the stage at presentation in cases of neoplasia (see Section VI)

PEARLS

- Loss of definition of the interlobar artery and/or a small or non-apparent ipsilateral hilum is a *cardinal sign* of lower lobe atelectasis.
- Because both lower lobes are large in volume, compensatory signs of volume loss are present, and their recognition may prevent the misdiagnosis of pleural effusion.
- A localized convex bulge in the expected location of the interlobar artery suggests the presence of an underlying central obstructing mass (**Figs. 39.1, 39.2**).

Suggested Reading

1. Fraser RS, Müller NL, Colman N, Paré PD. Atelectasis. In: Fraser and Paré's Diagnosis of Diseases of the Chest, 4th ed. Philadelphia: Saunders; 1999:552
2. Mintzer RA, Sakowicz BA, Blonder JA. Lobar collapse. Usual and unusual forms. Chest 1988;94(3):615–620
3. Woodring JH, Reed JC. Radiographic manifestations of lobar atelectasis. J Thorac Imaging 1996;11(2):109–144
4. Woodring JH. Right hilar pseudomass due to partial right lower lobe atelectasis. J Thorac Imaging 2001;16(3):170–173

CASE 40

■ Clinical Presentation

68-year-old man with a long history of tobacco abuse experiencing a recent change in the nature of his pre-existing chronic "smoker's" cough

■ Radiologic Findings

PA (**Fig. 40.1A**) chest radiograph reveals an ill-defined right perihilar opacity that partially obscures the right heart border and contains no air bronchograms. On the coned-down lateral radiograph (**Fig. 40.1B**), there is a corresponding triangular opacity with its base abutting the sternum and its apex directed toward the hilum. Note the anterior displacement of the oblique fissure (*arrow*) and elevation of the right hemidiaphragm.

■ Diagnosis

Right Middle Lobe Atelectasis; Occult Endobronchial Squamous Cell Cancer

■ Differential Diagnosis

- Uncomplicated Right Middle Lobe Atelectasis (e.g., mucus plug)
- Complicated Right Middle Lobe Atelectasis from Other Primary or Secondary Endobronchial Neoplasms
- Right Middle Lobe Syndrome
- Right Middle Lobe Pneumonia

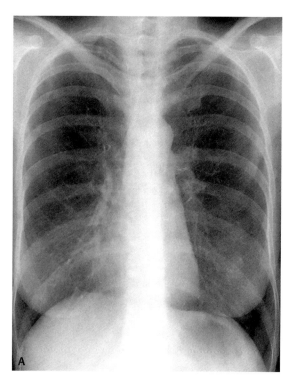 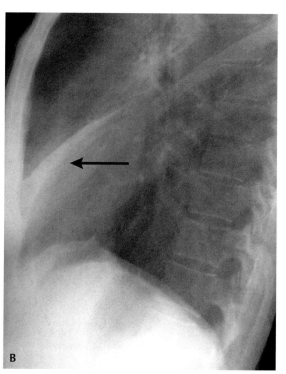

Fig. 40.1

224

■ Discussion

Background

Right middle lobe atelectasis is one of the easiest diagnoses to make on lateral chest radiography (**Figs. 40.1B, 40.2B**) but one of the most difficult on frontal chest exams (**Figs. 40.1A, 40.2A**). As the middle lobe loses volume, the horizontal fissure and the lower half of the oblique fissure approximate, forming a "triangular" opacity with its apex at the hilum and its base against the parietal pleura behind the sternum. These fissures almost contact one another, with complete lobar collapse manifesting as a thin, almost imperceptible retrosternal triangular opacity (**Fig. 40.3**). On frontal exams, there may be no obvious increase in radio-opacity. The only radiologic sign of middle lobe volume loss may be a partial silhouette of the right heart border due to the contiguity of the medial segment of the middle lobe with the right atrium (**Figs. 40.1A, 40.4A**).

Air bronchograms are a reliable sign that a process is parenchymal. The most common causes are pneumonia and pulmonary edema. Air bronchograms may also be seen in atelectatic lobes if the airway is patent. Compensatory *indirect* signs of volume loss may be absent as collapse is prevented by accumulation of fluid and alveolar macrophages within distal air spaces, and by chronic inflammatory cells and fibrous tissue within the interstitium (e.g., obstructive pneumonitis). Resorption atelectasis is excluded if air is visible within the bronchial tree. If the obstruction is severe enough to cause absorption of air from the affected lobe, it must also result in absorption of gas from the airways. The normal right diaphragm is 1–2 cm higher than the left. In 2% of individuals it may be 3.0 cm higher or more. In 9% of individuals, the two hemidiaphragms lie at the same level, or the left diaphragm will even be slightly higher. Diaphragmatic elevation is more often seen in acute as opposed to chronic atelectasis and is more often an *indirect* sign of lower lobe than of upper lobe atelectasis.

Clinical Findings

Affected patients may be asymptomatic. Others present with cough, weight loss, hypoxemia, progressive dyspnea, hemoptysis, diminished or absent breath sounds over the affected area, and various paraneoplastic syndromes (see Section VI).

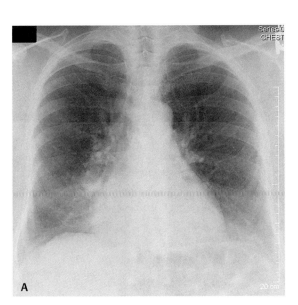
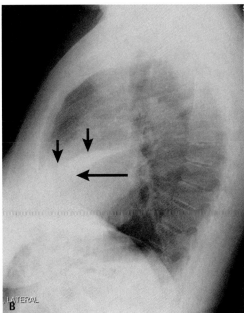

Fig. 40.2   **(A)** PA and **(B)** lateral chest X-rays of a 59-year-old man with uncomplicated right middle lobe atelectasis and bronchorrhea admitted with acute chest pain after snorting heroin. The frontal exam **(A)** shows ill-defined right perihilar opacity that partially obscures the right heart border. Note the lack of air bronchograms. The lateral exam **(B)** reveals a well-defined sharply delineated triangular opacity, the base of which abuts the sternum and the apex of which is directed toward the hilum. Note the downward displacement of the horizontal fissure (*short arrows*) and the anterior displacement of the oblique fissure (*long arrow*).

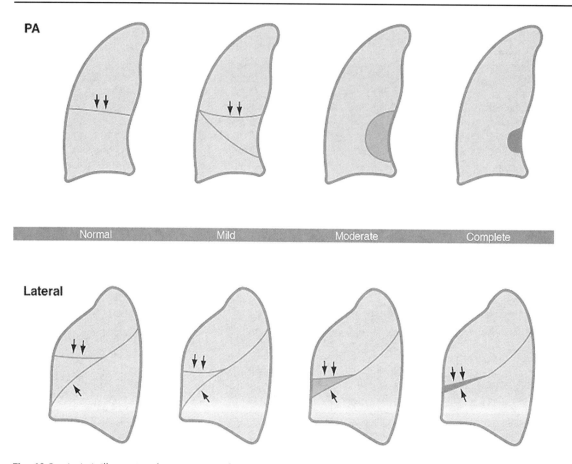

Fig. 40.3 Artist's illustration demonstrating the normal anatomic position of both the horizontal and oblique fissures and their gradual displacement with progressive degrees of mild, moderate, and complete right middle lobe volume loss in the frontal and lateral radiographic planes. See description in text.

Imaging Findings

Radiography

Frontal Radiography

- No discernible increase in opacity
- Obscuration (silhouette) of right heart border (**Figs. 40.1A, 40.2A, 40.3, 40.4A**)

Lateral Radiography

- Well-defined, curved triangular opacity bordered by the oblique and horizontal fissures, extending anteriorly and inferiorly from the hilum toward the sternum (**Figs. 40.1B, 40.2B, 40.3, 40.4B**)
- Collapsed lobe may be very thin and misinterpreted as a thickened fissure (**Figs. 40.1B, 40.2B, 40.3, 40.4B**)

MDCT

- Characteristic broad triangular or trapezoidal opacity with apex directed toward the hilum (**Figs. 40.5A, 40.5B**)
- Anterior margin of atelectatic lobe retracts toward the hilum (**Figs. 40.5A, 40.5B**)
- Overinflated upper lobe intrudes anteriorly and medially (**Figs. 40.5A, 40.5B**)
- Horizontal and oblique fissures move toward each other with progressive volume loss (**Figs. 40.5A, 40.5B**)
- Posterior border of atelectatic middle lobe is usually well defined because oblique fissure is perpendicular to plane of sectioning (**Figs. 40.5A, 40.5B**)
- Interface between right middle and upper lobes is often indistinct because of the dome-shaped contour of the horizontal fissure (**Figs. 40.5A, 40.5B**)

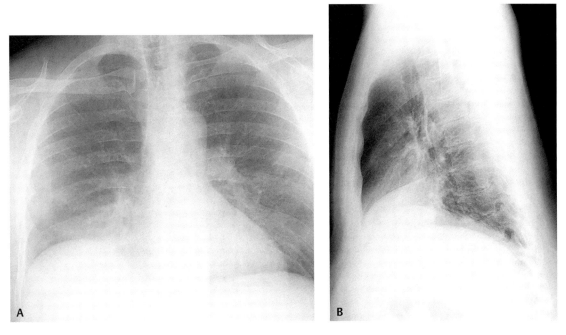

Fig. 40.4 **(A)** PA and **(B)** lateral chest exams of a 52-year-old man with alcoholic cirrhosis shows a subtle silhouette of the right atrial border on the frontal exam **(A)**. The lateral exam confirms this is the result of middle lobe atelectasis **(B)**.

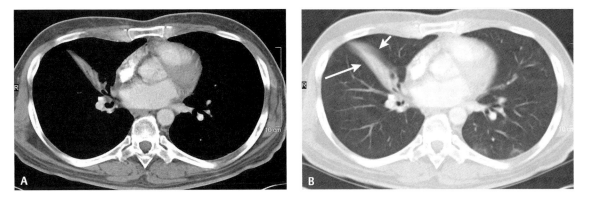

Fig. 40.5 Contrast-enhanced chest CT (**A**, mediastinal window; **B**, lung window) of a 50-year-old man with hepatocellular carcinoma demonstrates characteristic imaging features of right middle lobe atelectasis. Note the anterior displacement of the oblique fissure (*long arrow*) and posterior displacement of the horizontal fissure (*short arrow*).

Management

- Prompt bronchoscopic evaluation and biopsy to determine etiology of the complicated lobar atelectasis and establish a tissue diagnosis
- Surgical resection when possible
- Endobronchial stent deployment in select cases
- Palliative chemotherapy and/or radiation therapy, unresectable cases (see Section VI)

Prognosis

- Dependent on the stage at presentation in cases of neoplasia (see Section VI)

PEARLS

- In the absence of air bronchograms, an underlying occult endobronchial lesion must be excluded.
- Acute confluent pneumonia (e.g., *Staphylococcus aureus*) with homogeneous opacification of a lobe or segment and bronchi filled with inflammatory exudate may also result in absent air bronchograms.
- Collapsed middle lobe is obliquely oriented on CT; thus only a small portion of the atelectatic lobe may be conspicuous.
- Lingular atelectasis resembles middle lobe atelectasis (**Figs. 40.6A, 40.6B**).
- *Nordenstrom's sign*—presence of subsegmental lingula atelectasis associated with left lower collapse.

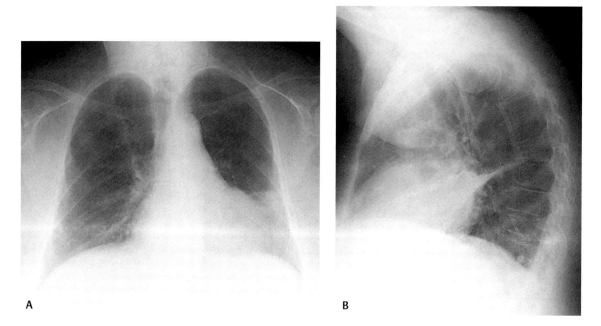

A   **B**

Fig. 40.6 Isolated lingular atelectasis. Note the radiographic resemblance to right middle lobe atelectasis. **(A)** Frontal chest X-ray shows obscuration of the left heart border. **(B)** Lateral chest exam reveals a thin triangular opaque band extending from the hilum to the retrosternum. Because of the relatively small size of the lingula, mediastinal shift and signs of compensatory overinflation are absent.

Suggested Reading

1. Fraser RS, Müller NL, Colman N, Paré PD. Atelectasis. In: Fraser and Paré's Diagnosis of Diseases of the Chest, 4th ed. Philadelphia: Saunders; 1999:552

2. Mintzer RA, Sakowicz BA, Blonder JA. Lobar collapse. Usual and unusual forms. Chest 1988;94(3):615–620

3. Woodring JH, Reed JC. Radiographic manifestations of lobar atelectasis. J Thorac Imaging 1996;11(2):109–144

CASE 41

■ Clinical Presentation

An elderly woman with persistent cough and wheezing

■ Radiologic Findings

PA (**Fig. 41.1A**) chest exam demonstrates a vague opacity in the lower right thorax that obscures the heart border. The horizontal fissure is inferiorly displaced and the ipsilateral diaphragm is elevated. Subtle bronchiectasis is seen in the infrahilar region paralleling the right heart border. The cardiac silhouette is poorly defined on the lateral exam (**Fig. 41.1B**). A small pleural effusion blunts the posterolateral sulcus. The lungs are hyperexpanded, consistent with underlying obstructive lung disease. PA (**Fig. 41.1C**) and lateral (**Fig. 41.1D**) chest radiographs from two years earlier demonstrate similar imaging findings with respect to the right thorax. Contrast-enhanced chest CT (**Figs. 41.1E, 41.1F, 41.1G**; mediastinal window) reveal a triangular focal area of consolidated lung in the right middle lobe. The proximal bronchi are patent but irregular and distorted. The visualized middle lobe segmental bronchi are also bronchiectatic.

■ Diagnosis

Right Middle Lobe Syndrome (RMLS)
Synonyms
- Brock Syndrome
- Middle Lobe Syndrome
- Shrunken Middle Lobe

■ Differential Diagnosis

- Middle Lobe Pneumonia
- Middle Lobe Obstruction Secondary to Primary or Secondary Endobronchial Neoplasia

■ Discussion

Background

Middle lobe syndrome is an uncommon lung disorder associated with recurrent atelectasis, pneumonias, or bronchiectasis of the right middle lobe, lingula, or both. It was originally thought that bronchial compression by inflamed peribronchial lymph nodes (e.g., tuberculous lymphadenitis) was responsible for the development of this syndrome. That theory has since been rejected. Most authors now believe this syndrome is related to relative *isolation* of the middle lobe from the remainder of the lung, especially in patients with a *complete* horizontal fissure. This isolation prevents collateral air flow from reaching the middle lobe and impairs clearance of retained bronchial secretions. Benign inflammatory disease is the most common etiological factor (62%), with bronchiectasis responsible for at least a quarter of affected patients. Early studies suggested that cancer rarely originates in the right middle lobe; however, in 1983, Wagner and Johnston reported 22% of patients reviewed had malignant tumors as a cause of the syndrome. Bronchoscopy and CT are vital in the evaluation of patients with this syndrome. Severe stenosis of the middle lobe bronchus or tumor is seen endoscopically in up to 40% of patients. Bronchoscopy and CT with multiplanar or volume rendered images may demonstrate anatomical airway abnormalities in more than 70% of cases.

229

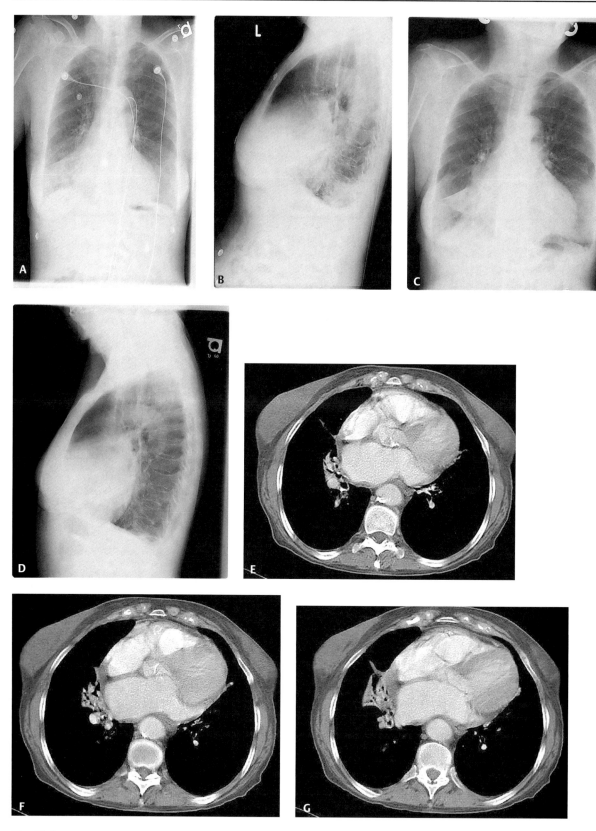

Fig. 41.1

Clinical Findings

The most common symptoms include persistent or recurrent cough, recurrent or chronic pneumonia, intermittent wheezing, and dyspnea. Less common symptoms include hemoptysis, low-grade fever, chest pain, and weight loss. Rales, fine wheezes, or diffuse rhonchi may occasionally be heard on auscultation. Some patients are asymptomatic and only come to clinical evaluation following recognition of the radiologic abnormality on chest studies acquired for unrelated reasons. Serial chest radiography, especially when studies are available for several years demonstrating chronicity of the middle lobe disease, is extremely helpful in establishing the diagnosis.

Imaging Findings

Radiography

- Frontal chest radiography
  - Obscuration of right heart border (**Figs. 41.1A, 41.1C**); right middle lobe collapse
  - Obscuration of left heart border with lingular collapse
  - Consolidation and/or volume loss in middle lobe and/or lingula (**Figs. 41.1A, 41.1C**)
  - Downward displacement of horizontal fissure in select cases (**Figs. 41.1A, 41.1C**)
  - Elevation of ipsilateral hemidiaphragm in select cases (**Figs. 41.1A, 41.1C**)
  - Middle lobe bronchiectasis may or may not be conspicuous (**Figs. 41.1A, 41.1C**)
- Lateral chest radiography
  - Poor definition or obscuration of heart border (**Figs. 41.1B, 41.1D**)
  - Well-defined, curved opacity bordered by oblique and horizontal fissures and extending anteriorly and inferiorly from the hilum (**Fig. 41.2**)
  - Consolidation and/or volume loss in middle lobe and/or lingula
  - Middle lobe/lingular bronchiectasis

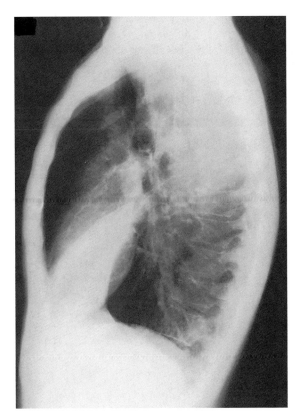

Fig. 41.2 Lateral chest radiograph on a 48-year-old man with long history of tobacco abuse and chronic cough with right middle lobe syndrome demonstrates a retrosternal triangular opacity with its base against the sternum and apex directed toward the hilum bordered superiorly by the inferiorly displaced horizontal fissure and inferiorly by the anteriorly displaced oblique fissure.

MDCT

- "Triangular" opacity bounded posteriorly by oblique fissure, medially by mediastinum (i.e., right atrium), and anteriorly by horizontal fissure (**Figs. 41.1E, 41.1F, 41.1G**)
- Middle lobe bronchus enters posteromedial corner of the triangular opacity
- Consolidation and/or volume loss in middle lobe (**Figs. 41.1E, 41.1F, 41.1G**) and/or lingula
- Middle lobe (**Figs. 41.1E, 41.1F, 41.1G**) and lingular bronchiectasis seen to better advantage than with radiography

Management

- Directed toward underlying cause
- Respiratory therapy, bronchodilators, mucolytics, and postural drainage
- Antibiotics
- Lobectomy indicated in cases of malignancy, bronchial stenosis, and recurrent infection or hemoptysis refractory to medical management
- 22% of patients require lobectomy

Prognosis

- Resolution in one-third of pediatric patients after bronchoscopy
- Resolution in one-third of patients with medical management alone

PEARLS

- Serial radiographs demonstrating chronic right middle lobe and/or lingular volume loss are critical to making the correct diagnosis.
- Evaluation with CT and/or bronchoscopy is indicated to assess for abnormalities of the airway and to exclude potential neoplasia.

Suggested Reading

1. Ayed AK. Resection of the right middle lobe and lingula in children for middle lobe/lingula syndrome. Chest 2004; 125(1):38–42
2. Culiner MM. The right middle lobe syndrome, a non-obstructive complex. Dis Chest 1966;50(1):57–66
3. De Boeck K, Willems T, Van Gysel D, Corbeel L, Eeckels R. Outcome after right middle lobe syndrome. Chest 1995; 108(1):150–152
4. Gudmundsson G, Gross TJ. Middle lobe syndrome. Am Fam Physician 1996;53(8):2547–2550
5. Kawamura M, Arai Y, Tani M. Improvement in right lung atelectasis (middle lobe syndrome) following administration of low-dose roxithromycin. Respiration 2001;68(2):210–214
6. Wagner RB, Johnston MR. Middle lobe syndrome. Ann Thorac Surg 1983;35(6):679–686

CASE 42

■ Clinical Presentation

42-year-old man with complaints of cough, fever, and shortness of breath

■ Radiologic Findings

PA (**Fig. 42.1A**) chest radiograph shows an ill-defined left perihilar and upper lobe opacity without perceptible air bronchograms that partially silhouettes the upper left heart border. The left thorax appears smaller than the right. The left diaphragm is elevated. A hyperlucent crescent (*arrow*) insinuates between the perihilar opacity and the transverse aorta and outlines the aortic arch. The lateral exam (**Fig. 42.1B**) demonstrates a retrosternal sigmoid band of increased opacity and marked anterior displacement of the oblique fissure (*arrows*).

■ Diagnosis

Left Upper Lobe Atelectasis; Endobronchial Carcinoid Tumor

■ Differential Diagnosis

- Uncomplicated Upper Lobe Atelectasis (e.g., obstructing mucus plug, foreign body)
- Complicated Upper Lobe Atelectasis
    - Endobronchial Mass (e.g., primary and secondary neoplasia)
    - Extrinsic Bronchial Compression by Reactive or Neoplastic Lymphadenopathy

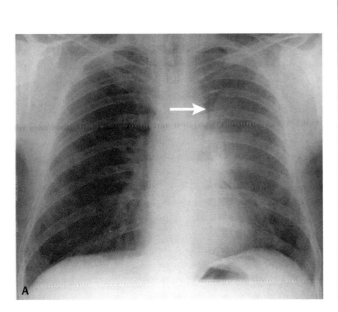 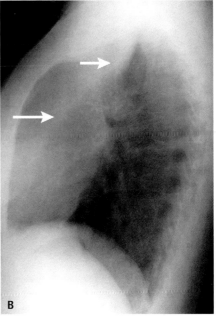

Fig. 42.1

■ Discussion

Background

The major difference between atelectasis of the left and right upper lobes is the absence of a horizontal fissure in the left thorax. Thus, all lung tissue anterior to the oblique fissure is involved. On lateral chest radiography, the oblique fissure shifts *forward* in a plane roughly parallel to the anterior chest wall (**Fig. 42.2**). As volume loss increases, the fissure moves further *anteriorly* and *medially*, until the opacity of the collapsed lobe is no more than a broad linear opacity contiguous and parallel to the anterior chest wall (**Figs. 42.1B, 42.2, 42.3B**). On frontal chest radiography, contiguity of the atelectatic upper lobe with the anterior mediastinum obliterates the upper left cardiac border (*silhouette sign*) (**Figs. 42.1A, 42.2, 42.3A**). As the apical segment collapses, the space it vacates becomes "filled in" by compensatory overinflation of the left lower lobe superior segment. The apex of the thorax will contain aerated lung which can mimic an apical pneumothorax. The overinflated superior segment may also insinuate between the collapsed upper lobe and mediastinum, sharply delineating the aortic arch by a hyperlucent air crescent (*Luftsichel sign*) (**Figs. 42.1A, 42.3A**).

On CT, the atelectatic upper lobe will abut the anterior chest wall and mediastinum (**Figs. 42.3C, 42.3D, 42.3E, 42.3F**). The oblique fissure will be displaced cephalad and anteriorly (**Figs. 42.3C, 42.3D**). An aerated portion of the superior segment of the lower lobe medial to the pleural reflection will outline the aorta and create the radiographic *Luftsichel sign* (**Fig. 42.3C**). The posterior surface of the collapsed upper lobe assumes a V-shaped morphology that results from tethering of the oblique fissure by the hilum (**Figs. 42.3C, 42.3D**).

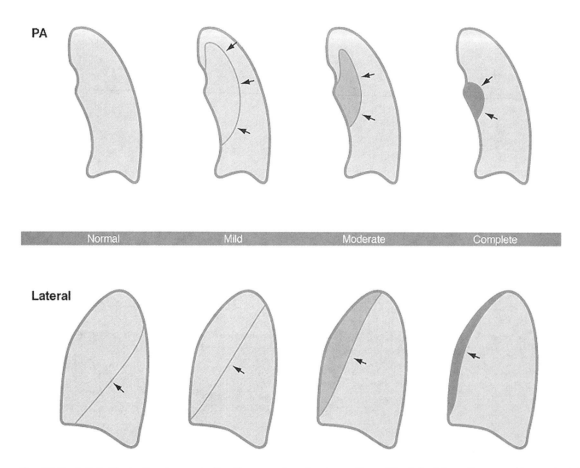

Fig. 42.2 Artist's illustration demonstrating the normal anatomic position of the left oblique fissure and its gradual displacement with progressive degrees of mild, moderate, and complete left upper lobe volume loss in the frontal and lateral radiographic planes. See description in text.

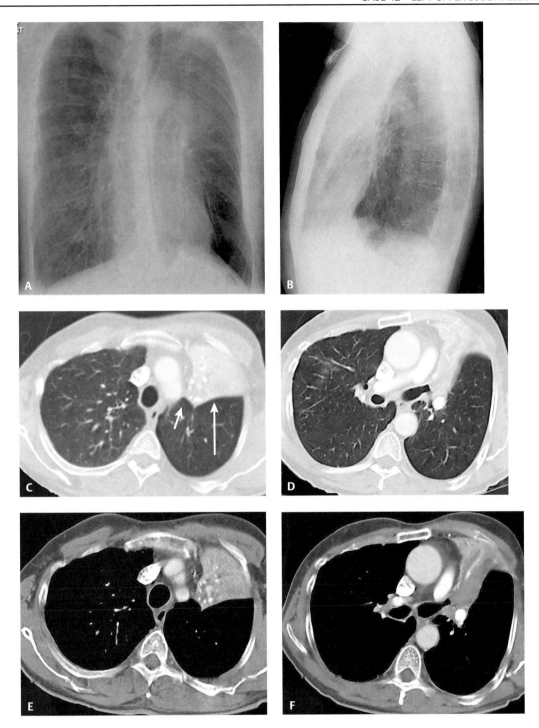

Fig. 42.3 A 55-year-old man with an endobronchial hamartoma presented with low-grade fever, cough, and shortness of breath. **(A)** Slightly rotated PA view shows an ill-defined left perihilar opacity silhouetting the upper left heart border. The left thorax appears smaller than the right, and the left diaphragm is elevated. A *Luftsichel sign* is present, seen as a hyperlucent crescent between the collapsed upper lobe and the aorta. **(B)** The lateral view reveals a retrosternal sigmoid opacity and anterior displacement of the fissure. Contrast-enhanced chest CT (**C, D**, lung window; **E, F**, mediastinal window) illustrate the collapsed left upper lobe. Note the collapsed lobe abuts both the anterior chest wall and mediastinum. There is anterior and cephalad displacement of the oblique fissure (*long arrow*). The aerated superior segment of the lower lobe medial to the pleural reflection outlines the aorta, creating the *Luftsichel sign* (**C**, *short arrow*). Also note the V-shaped morphology the posterior surface of the collapsed upper lobe assumes where the fissure is tethered by the hilum. An obstructing endobronchial lesion is seen in the upper lobe bronchial orifice (**D, F**).

Clinical Findings

The majority of central carcinoid tumors give rise to symptoms as a result of bronchial obstruction. Affected patients may present with cough, fever, and chest pain. Hemoptysis occurs in 30–50% of patients. Some patients may be misdiagnosed with asthma. Physical signs depend upon lesion size, diameter of the affected bronchus, and whether or not post-obstructive infection has occurred. Uncommonly, a small tumor is associated with a paraneoplastic syndrome, most often Cushing syndrome (see Section VI).

Imaging Findings

Radiography

- Frontal chest radiography
  - Left parahilar opacity without a distinct fissural edge; partially silhouettes the upper left cardiac border (*silhouette sign*) (**Figs. 42.1A, 42.2, 42.3A**)
  - Absent air bronchograms (**Figs. 42.1A, 42.3A**)
  - Elevation of left hilum (**Figs. 42.1A, 42.3A**)
  - More horizontal lie of the left mainstem bronchus (**Figs. 42.1A, 42.3A**)
  - Superior displacement of lower lobe bronchus and descending pulmonary artery (**Figs. 42.1A, 42.3A**)
  - Crowding of bronchovascular markings may be an early sign
  - Lucent ipsilateral apex and sharply demarcated transverse aorta (*Luftsichel sign*) (**Figs. 42.1A, 42.3A**)
  - Smaller-volume left thorax (**Figs. 42.1A, 42.3A**)
  - Elevation of left diaphragm (**Figs. 42.1A, 42.3A**)
- Lateral chest radiography
  - Anterior displacement oblique fissure (**Figs. 42.1B, 42.2, 42.3B**)
  - As volume loss progresses, anteriorly displaced oblique fissure is seen as an arcuate interface between the opaque, collapsed upper lobe and the lucent, over-expanded lower lobe (**Figs. 42.1B, 42.2, 42.3B**)
  - Retrosternal sigmoid band of increased opacity (**Figs. 42.1B, 42.2, 42.3B**)
  - Ipsilateral diaphragmatic elevation

MDCT

- Atelectatic upper lobe abuts anterior chest wall and mediastinum (**Figs. 42.3C, 42.3D, 42.3E, 42.3F**)
- Oblique fissure displaced cephalad and anteriorly (**Figs. 42.3C, 42.3D**)
- Posterior surface of collapsed upper lobe assumes V-shaped morphology from tethering of the oblique fissure by the hilum (**Figs. 42.3C, 42.3D**)
- Offending lesion may be visualized (**Figs. 42.3D, 42.3F**)

Management

- Surgical excision; typically lobectomy or pneumonectomy
- Tracheobronchial sleeve resection
- See Section VI

Prognosis

- Typical bronchial carcinoid; excellent, with 92% five-year survival
- See Section VI

PEARLS

- Radiologist must be careful not to misinterpret the *Luftsichel sign* as right upper lobe herniation across the midline or as a left apical pneumothorax.
- *Luftsichel sign* is rarely seen in right upper lobe collapse.

Suggested Readings

1. Blankenbaker DG. The Luftsichel sign. Radiology 1998;208(2):319–320

2. Fraser RS, Müller NL, Colman N, Paré PD. Atelectasis. In: Fraser and Paré's Diagnosis of Diseases of the Chest, 4th ed. Philadelphia: Saunders; 1999:529–532

3. Isbell D, Grinnan D, Patel MR. Luftsichel sign upper-lobe collapse. Am J Med 2002;112(8):676–677

4. Woodring JH, Reed JC. Radiographic manifestations of lobar atelectasis. J Thorac Imaging 1996;11(2):109–144

CASE 43

■ Clinical Presentation

65-year-old woman with a long history of tobacco abuse has developed intermittent hemoptysis and progressive cough

■ Radiologic Findings

PA (**Fig. 43.1A**) and lateral (**Fig. 43.1B**) chest exams reveal a relatively small left thorax, leftward mediastinal shift, and increased opacity in the lower left lung silhouetting the diaphragm. A localized basilar opacity overlies the lower thoracic spine (*positive spine sign*) and silhouettes the posterior-lateral diaphragm. There is loss of definition of the left hilum and the interlobar pulmonary artery is inconspicuous. Note the focal convexity in the medial aspect of the displaced oblique fissure (*reverse "S" sign of Golden*) (*arrow*) indicating the presence of an obstructing central hilar mass.

■ Diagnosis

Left Lower Lobe Atelectasis; Obstructing Small Cell Lung Cancer

■ Differential Diagnosis

- Post-Obstructive Lower Lobe Atelectasis from an Endobronchial Mass (e.g., primary and secondary neoplasia)
- Post-Obstructive Lower Lobe Atelectasis from Extrinsic Bronchial Compression by Reactive or Neoplastic Lymphadenopathy

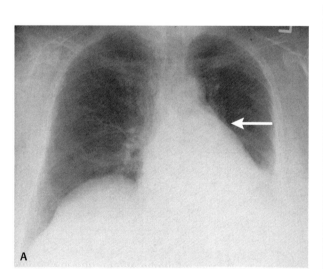 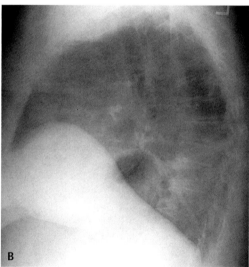

Fig. 43.1

■ Discussion

Background

The right and left lower lobes demonstrate similar patterns of lobar collapse on imaging. The *triangular* versus *rounded* configuration assumed by the atelectatic lower lobe is related to the fulcrum-like effect exerted on the lung by the hilum and the integrity of the pulmonary ligament. When the pulmonary ligament is *complete*, the lower lobe is tethered to the mediastinum and hemidiaphragm and maintains a close relationship to both structures, assuming a *triangular* configuration as it loses volume (**Figs. 43.2, 43.3**). Alternatively, when the pulmonary ligament is *incomplete*, the lung base is not adherent to the diaphragm. When the lower lobe loses volume, its shape depends primarily on its mediastinal attachment and the collapsed lobe assumes a more *rounded* morphology, often creating an apparent left-sided paraspinal mass (*pseudomass sign*).

As the left lower lobe loses volume, the cephalad and caudal aspects of the oblique fissure shift backward and downward, approximating one another. This is best appreciated on lateral chest studies (**Fig. 43.4**). With increased volume loss, the atelectatic lobe may silhouette the posterior diaphragm, adding to the density of the lower thoracic spine (*positive spine sign*). Total lower lobe collapse may be difficult to appreciate, manifesting as subtle obscuration of the posterolateral sulcus (**Fig. 43.4**). Left lower lobe atelectasis can be overlooked on frontal chest exams when the collapsed lobe is silhouetted by the heart. Increased retrocardiac opacity may silhouette the lower lobe pulmonary artery. Thus, a small or non-apparent interlobar pulmonary artery is a sign of lower lobe atelectasis on frontal chest exams (**Figs. 43.2, 43.3, 43.4**). The lower thoracic aorta stripe and paraspinal line may also become obscured by the collapsed lobe (**Figs. 43.2, 43.3, 43.4**).

Clinical Findings

Affected patients may present with cough, weight loss, hypoxemia, progressive dyspnea, hemoptysis, diminished or absent breath sounds over the affected area, and various paraneoplastic syndromes (see Section VI).

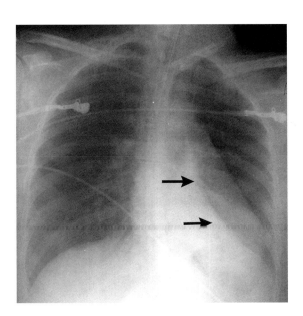

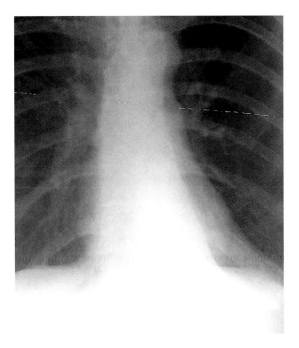

Fig.43.2 AP chest radiograph of a 28-year-old man recently involved in a motor vehicle collision with bronchorrhea and no audible breath sounds at the left lung base. The collapsed lower lobe demonstrates a *triangular* morphology (*arrows*) because of the presence of a *complete* pulmonary ligament.

Fig. 43.3 Coned-down PA chest of a 43-year-old woman with recurrent pneumonia and lower lobe bronchiectasis reveals chronic left lower lobe collapse manifesting as a triangular retrocardiac opacity silhouetting the descending thoracic aorta stripe and left paraspinal line. The apex of the opacity is directed toward the hilum and its base against the diaphragm. Note the small left hilum and inconspicuous interlobar pulmonary artery.

Imaging Findings

Radiography

- Frontal radiography
  - ○ Hilar structures shift downward (**Figs. 43.1A, 43.2, 43.3**)
  - ○ Small or non-apparent hilum (**Figs. 43.1A, 43.2, 43.3**)
  - ○ Loss of conspicuity of interlobar pulmonary artery (**Figs. 43.1A, 43.2, 43.3**)
  - ○ Rotation of heart produces flattening of the cardiac waist, simulating a right anterior oblique (RAO) projection (*flat waist sign*) (**Figs. 43.1A, 43.2, 43.3**)
  - ○ Superior mediastinum may shift and silhouette the aortic arch (*"top of the aortic knob" sign*)
  - ○ Lower thoracic aorta stripe and left paraspinal line may become silhouetted by the collapsed lower lobe (**Figs. 43.2, 43.3**)
- Lateral radiography
  - ○ Cephalad and caudal aspects of the oblique fissure shift posteriorly and inferiorly, approximating one another (**Fig. 43.4**)
  - ○ With increased volume loss, the atelectatic lower lobe silhouettes the posterior diaphragm, adding to the density of the lower thoracic spine (*positive spine sign*) (**Figs. 43.1B, 43.4**)
  - ○ Total collapse may be difficult to appreciate, manifesting by subtle obscuration of the posterolateral sulcus (**Fig. 43.4**)

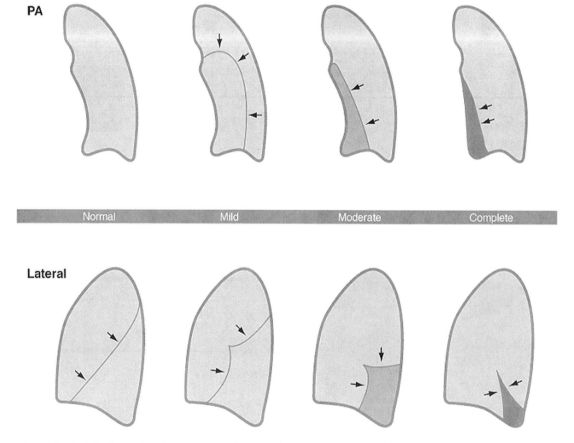

Fig. 43.4 Artist's illustration demonstrating the normal anatomic position of the left oblique fissure and its gradual displacement with progressive degrees of mild, moderate, and complete left lower lobe volume loss in the frontal and lateral radiographic planes. See description in text.

Management

- Prompt bronchoscopic evaluation and biopsy to determine cause of the complicated lobar atelectasis and establish a tissue diagnosis
- Surgical resection when possible
- Endobronchial stent deployment in select cases
- Palliative chemotherapy and/or radiation therapy in unresectable cases (see Section VI)

Prognosis

- Dependent on stage at presentation (i.e., limited versus extensive) (see Section VI)

PEARLS

- Loss of definition of the interlobar artery and a small or non-apparent ipsilateral hilum represent *cardinal signs* of lower lobe atelectasis.
- Because both lower lobes are large in volume, compensatory signs of volume loss are usually present; their recognition may prevent the misdiagnosis of pleural effusion.
- A localized convex bulge in the expected location of the interlobar artery suggests an underlying central obstructing mass.

Suggested Reading

1. Fraser RS, Müller NL, Colman N, Paré PD. Atelectasis. In: Fraser and Paré's Diagnosis of Diseases of the Chest, 4th ed. Philadelphia: Saunders; 1999:552

2. Kattan KR, Wlot JF. Cardiac rotation in left lower lobe collapse. "The flat waist sign." Radiology 1976;118(2): 275–279

3. Mintzer RA, Sakowicz BA, Blonder JA. Lobar collapse. Usual and unusual forms. Chest 1988;94(3):615–620

4. Woodring JH, Reed JC. Radiographic manifestations of lobar atelectasis. J Thorac Imaging 1996;11(2):109–144

5. Woodring JH. Right hilar pseudomass due to partial right lower lobe atelectasis. J Thorac Imaging 2001;16(3): 170–173

CASE 44

■ Clinical Presentation

42-year-old man with an acute asthma exacerbation, chest pain, and shortness of breath

■ Radiologic Findings

PA (**Fig. 44.1**) chest radiograph shows inferior displacement of the oblique (*short arrow*) and horizontal fissures (*long arrow*). A radio-opacity silhouettes both the right heart border and the right diaphragm. This opacity extends to but does not blunt the lateral sulcus. Note the discrepancy in volume between the right and left thorax and the rightward mediastinal shift.

■ Diagnosis

Combined Right Middle and Lower Lobe Atelectasis; Mucus Plug Bronchus Intermedius

■ Differential Diagnosis

• Isolated Right Lower Lobe Atelectasis
• Right Subpulmonic Pleural Effusion
• Large Right Pleural Effusion

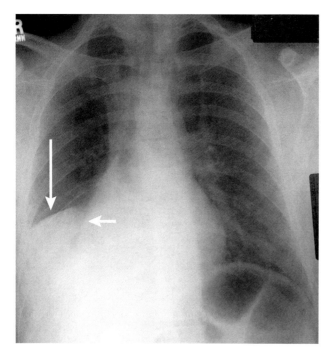

Fig. 44.1

■ Discussion

Background

Simultaneous right middle and lower lobe collapse localizes the obstructing lesion to the bronchus intermedius. This combination of bilobar atelectasis may be misinterpreted as *isolated right lower lobe collapse* on frontal chest exams and as *subpulmonic effusion* on lateral X-rays. Extension of the increased opacity to the lateral costophrenic angle on the frontal exam supports the diagnosis of bilobar collapse. On lateral chest exams, the upper border of a subpulmonic effusion is usually flat superiorly and appears to terminate at the oblique fissure anteriorly (*"rock of Gibraltar" sign*) (see Section XII, Case 171). Alternatively, the opacity created by bilobar atelectasis extends from the front to the back of the chest (**Fig. 44.2**).

Clinical Findings

Affected patients may exhibit an abrupt drop in oxygen saturations, altered A-a gradient, and diminished breath sounds over the affected region.

Imaging Findings

Radiography

- Frontal radiography
  - Silhouette of right atrial border (atelectatic middle lobe) (**Figs. 44.1, 44.3**)
  - Silhouette of right hemidiaphragm (atelectatic lower lobe) (**Figs. 44.1, 44.3**)
  - Oblique fissure displaced inferiorly and medially but maintains a convex lateral border (**Figs. 44.1, 44.3**)
  - Horizontal fissure displaced inferiorly (**Figs. 44.1, 44.3**)
  - Ipsilateral mediastinal shift (**Figs. 44.1, 44.3**)
- Lateral radiography
  - Bilobar atelectatic lobes create an opacity over the inferior hemithorax extending from the anterior to posterior chest wall (**Fig. 44.2**)
  - Radio-opacity may demonstrate either a convex or concave superior border that can be misinterpreted as a subpulmonic effusion

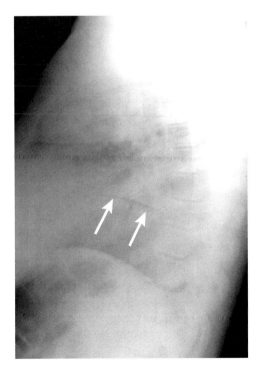

Fig. 44.2 Lateral chest radiograph of 47-year-old woman following recent hysterectomy with new onset of tachypnea and diminished breath sounds on the right revealed bilobar collapse of the middle and lower lobe from a mucus plug on the frontal exam (not illustrated). The lateral exam reveals increased opacity over the inferior third of the hemithorax, extending from the front to the back of the chest and silhouetting the ipsilateral diaphragm. Postoperative pneumoperitoneum outlines the undersurface of the right diaphragm (*arrows*).

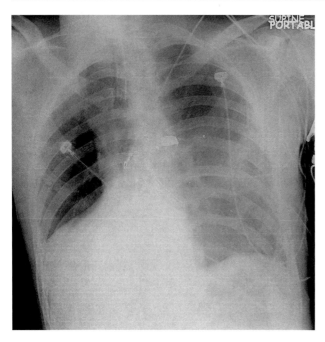

Fig. 44.3 AP chest radiograph of a young man status post multiple gunshot wounds to the chest and head with an inability to clear secretions and experiencing increased work of breathing. There is combined right middle and lower lobe collapse from a mucus plug. Note the downward displacement of the horizontal fissure and the inferior and medial displacement of the oblique fissure. Both the right heart border and ipsilateral diaphragm are silhouetted.

MDCT

- Combined atelectatic middle and lower lobes occupy the lower hemithorax (**Figs. 44.4A, 44.4B, 44.4C, 44.4D**)
- Bilobar collapsed lobes abut right cardiac border medially (**Figs. 44.4A, 44.4B, 44.4C, 44.4D**)
- Bilobar collapsed lobes abut right hemidiaphragm inferiorly (**Figs. 44.4A, 44.4B, 44.4C, 44.4D**)
- Oblique fissure borders lateral margin of atelectatic lobes (**Figs. 44.4A, 44.4B, 44.4C, 44.4D**)
- Horizontal fissure borders anteromedial margin of atelectatic lobes (**Figs. 44.4A, 44.4B, 44.4C, 44.4D**)

Management

- Respiratory physiotherapy (chest wall percussion and vibration), bronchiolytics, postural drainage, and bronchodilators
- Bronchoscopic aspiration of bronchial secretions or mucus plugs in select cases
- *N*-acetylcysteine aerosols
- Nebulized or direct tracheal application of DNase

Prognosis

- Good if recognized and treated early
- Delayed recognition and treatment may result in secondary bacterial infection

PEARLS

- Combination of right middle and lower lobe atelectasis may be misinterpreted as isolated right lower lobe collapse.
- Extension of the radio-opacity to the lateral costophrenic angle favors combined bilobar collapse.
- Visualization of the horizontal fissure in its normal anatomic position favors isolated right lower lobe atelectasis.
- Identification of standard fissures in their normal anatomic position is the most useful radiologic sign differentiating subpulmonic effusion from bilobar atelectasis.
- Reversal of normal bronchoarterial relationships at the lung base may indicate combined bilobar collapse.

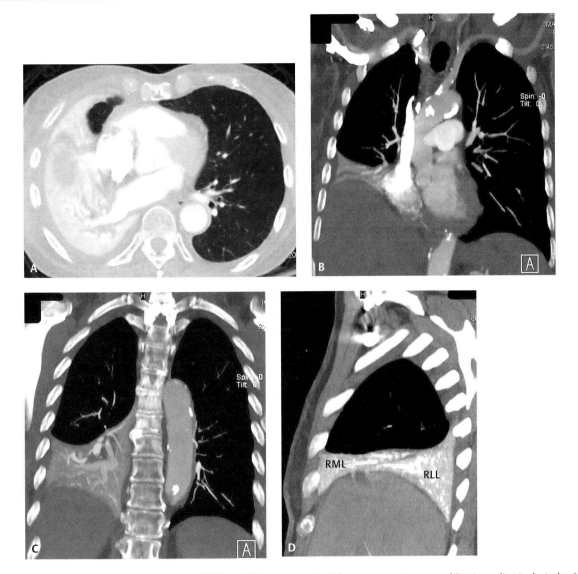

Fig. 44.4   Contrast-enhanced chest CT (**A**, axial, lung window) with accompanying coronal (**B, C**, mediastinal window) and sagittal (**D**, mediastinal window) maximum-intensity projection images show bilobar atelectasis in a young trauma victim with bronchorrhea. Note the relationship of the bilobar collapse to the right heart border and hemidiaphragm in all three imaging planes. The coronal images **(B,C)** also illustrate concomitant elevation of the right diaphragm. The sagittal image **(D)** also shows the extension of the bilobar collapse from the anterior to posterior chest wall typically seen on lateral chest radiography. (*RML*, collapsed right middle lobe; *RLL*, collapsed right lower lobe.)

Suggested Reading

1. Fraser RS, Müller NL, Colman N, Paré PD. Atelectasis. In: Fraser and Paré's Diagnosis of Diseases of the Chest, 4th ed. Philadelphia: Saunders; 1999:554

2. Mintzer RA, Sakowicz BA, Blonder JA. Lobar collapse. Usual and unusual forms. Chest 1988;94(3):615–620

3. Saida Y, Itai Y, Kujiraoka Y, Tohno E, Shimizu HT. Bronchoarterial inversion: radiographic-CT correlation in combined right middle and lower lobe collapse. J Thorac Imaging 1997;12(1):59–63

4. Woodring JH, Reed JC. Radiographic manifestations of lobar atelectasis. J Thorac Imaging 1996;11(2):109–144

CASE 45

■ Clinical Presentation

62-year-old woman with cough, weight loss, and generalized fatigue

■ Radiologic Findings

PA (**Fig. 45.1A**) and lateral (**Fig. 45.1B**) chest radiographs demonstrate opacification of the upper half of the right chest with cephalad displacement of the hilum and silhouetting of the ascending aorta and right heart border. A *juxtaphrenic peak* (*arrow*) is created by tethering of the inferior accessory fissure. The lateral exam also reveals marked anterior displacement of the oblique fissure. The displaced fissure is convex posteriorly. The right diaphragm is elevated and the mediastinum is shifted rightward.

■ Diagnosis

Combined Right Upper and Middle Lobe Atelectasis; Small Cell Lung Cancer

■ Differential Diagnosis

- Mucus Plug
- Primary Lung Cancer
- Carcinoid Tumor
- Metastatic Tumors
- Neoplastic or Reactive Lymphadenopathy
- Inflammatory Disease

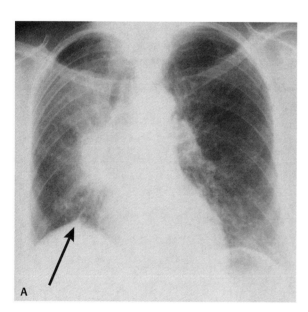
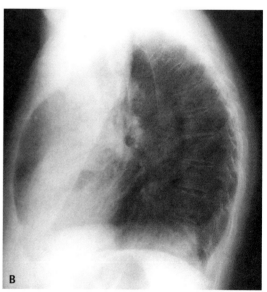

Fig. 45.1

■ Discussion

Background

Combined simultaneous collapse of the right upper and middle lobes is uncommon because of the disparate location of their lobar bronchi. Thus, two different diseases or a single disease simultaneously involving these two separate bronchi must be considered. Bilobar collapse is most often described in the setting of mucus plugs with concomitant primary lung cancer, primary lung cancer with associated reactive or neoplastic lymphadenopathy, metastatic disease, carcinoid tumors, or inflammatory strictures.

Clinical Findings

Affected patients may present with cough, weight loss, hypoxemia, progressive dyspnea, hemoptysis, diminished or absent breath sounds over the affected area, and various paraneoplastic syndromes (see Section VI).

Imaging Findings

Radiography

- Frontal radiography
    - Radiographic findings mirror left upper lobe atelectasis (see Case 42).
    - Radio-opacity silhouettes normal superior mediastinal borders, lines, stripes, and interfaces (**Fig. 45.1A**)
    - Radio-opacity appears denser medially but fades laterally (**Fig. 45.1A**)
    - Cephalad and lateral displacement and rotation of ipsilateral hilar vessels (**Fig. 45.1A**)
    - Silhouette of ascending aorta and right atrium (**Fig. 45.1A**)
    - Ipsilateral mediastinal shift (**Fig. 45.1A**)
    - Ipsilateral diaphragmatic elevation (**Fig. 45.1A**)
- Lateral radiography
    - Opacification of upper half of the chest (**Fig. 45.1B**)
    - Displacement of oblique fissure anteriorly (**Fig. 45.1B**)
    - Displaced oblique fissure may appear straight or convex anteriorly or convex posteriorly (**Fig. 45.1B**)

MDCT

- Anterior displacement of oblique fissure
- Hyperexpanded lower lobe occupies most of affected hemithorax
- Collapsed lobes create a wedge-shaped opacity that abuts the chest wall anteriorly and ascending aorta and right heart medially

Management

- Prompt bronchoscopic evaluation and potential biopsy to determine etiology of the bilobar atelectasis and establish a tissue diagnosis where appropriate
- Surgical resection if applicable when possible
- Endobronchial stent deployment in select cases
- Palliative chemotherapy and/or radiation therapy in unresectable cases (see Section VI)

Prognosis

- Dependent on stage at presentation (i.e., limited versus extensive) (see Section VI).

PEARLS

- Two different diseases or a single disease simultaneously involving two separate bronchi must be considered in such cases of bilobar atelectasis.
- Radiographic findings are similar to those of left upper lobe atelectasis.

Suggested Reading

1. Fraser RS, Müller NL, Colman N, Paré PD. Atelectasis. In: Fraser and Paré's Diagnosis of Diseases of the Chest, 4th ed. Philadelphia: Saunders; 1999:554

2. Lee KS, Logan PM, Primack SL, Müller NL. Combined lobar atelectasis of the right lung: imaging findings. AJR Am J Roentgenol 1994;163(1):43–47

3. Mintzer RA, Sakowicz BA, Blonder JA. Lobar collapse. Usual and unusual forms. Chest 1988;94(3):615–620

4. Saterfiel JL, Virapongse C, Clore FC. Computed tomography of combined right upper and middle lobe collapse. J Comput Assist Tomogr 1988;12(3):383–387

5. Woodring JH, Reed JC. Radiographic manifestations of lobar atelectasis. J Thorac Imaging 1996;11(2):109–144

CASE 46

■ Clinical Presentation

Asthmatic child with an acute exacerbation

■ Radiologic Findings

PA (**Fig. 46.1A**) and lateral (**Fig. 46.1B**) chest radiographs reveal abnormal opacities in each hemithorax. The frontal exam (**Fig. 46.1**) demonstrates an ill-defined left parahilar opacity silhouetting the upper left heart border. Note the absence of air bronchograms, ipsilateral mediastinal shift, and juxtaphrenic peak. This exam also shows a triangular opacity silhouetting the right heart border. The apex of this opacity is directed away from the hilum. The upper thorax on the lateral exam (**Fig. 46.2**) demonstrates a triangular opacity with its apex at the hilum and its base contiguous with the parietal pleura posterior to the extreme apex of the hemithorax (*mediastinal wedge*). Note the anterior displacement of the left oblique fissure. More inferiorly, a thin triangular opacity extends from the retrosternum toward the hilum. The horizontal fissure is displaced inferiorly and the right oblique fissure anteriorly

■ Diagnosis

Combined Right Middle Lobe and Left Upper Lobe Atelectasis; Mucus Plugs

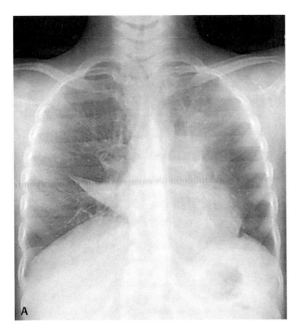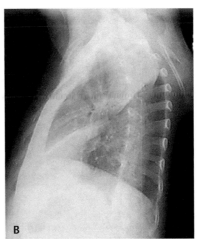

Fig. 46.1 (*Images courtesy of Lakshmana Das Narla, MD, VCU Medical Center; Richmond, Virginia.*)

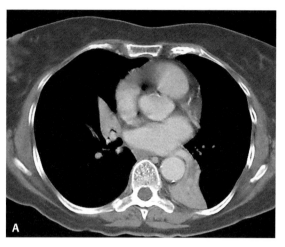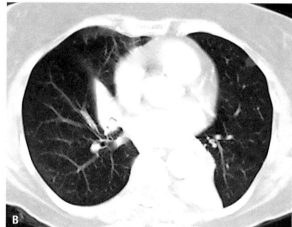

Fig. 46.2 Contrast-enhanced chest CT (**A**, mediastinal window; **B**, lung window) of a 68-year-old woman with asthma, chronic cough, and allergic bronchopulmonary aspergillosis (ABPA) reveals total collapse of the right middle and left lower lobes. Note the mucus-filled bronchi in the collapsed left lower lobe. Affected patients may suffer from asthma and often present with bronchospasm, initially episodic but later becoming more chronic. (*Images courtesy of Malcolm K. Sydnor, MD, VCU Medical Center; Richmond, Virginia.*)

■ Differential Diagnosis

- Non-Neoplastic Causes of Multi-Lobar Collapse
  - ○ Mucus Plugs
  - ○ Aspirated Foreign Bodies
  - ○ Post-Infectious or Post-Inflammatory Strictures
- Neoplastic Disease

■ Discussion

Background

The *double lesion* sign was originally described by Felson. The basic premise is, if a single endobronchial lesion cannot explain the collapse of multiple lobes or segments, then one has a reasonable level of confidence in excluding neoplasia. For example, because of the independent anatomic relationship of the right upper and middle lobe bronchi, it would be unusual for a single endobronchial lesion to cause simultaneous collapse of both lobes. However, many cases do indeed prove to be the result of malignancy. A single endobronchial lesion in the bronchus intermedius could explain combined middle and lower lobe collapse. However, neoplastic disease is unlikely to be responsible for combined collapse of the left lower lobe and any one segment of the upper lobe. Similarly, simultaneous collapse of lobes or segments in different lungs, as in this case, will invariably be the result of non-neoplastic disease (**Figs. 46.1, 46.2**).

Combined right middle and left upper lobe atelectasis demonstrates the expected radiographic features of both right middle and left upper lobe atelectasis occurring in isolation. This case also illustrates the *tipped-up* pattern of right middle lobe atelectasis. Severe right middle lobe atelectasis may result in a *tipped-down* pattern of collapse in which the atelectatic lobe creates a radiographic opacity insufficiently thick to create a perceptible opacity on frontal chest exams (**Figs. 40.1A, 40.3, 40.4A**). Alternatively, when the downward displaced horizontal fissure becomes oriented in a plane *parallel* to the X-ray beam, the collapsed middle lobe appears as a thin, triangular, sail-like opacity on frontal X-rays (**Fig. 46.1A**). This *tipped-up* pattern of middle lobe collapse is characterized by an opacity, the apex of which is directed away from the hilum and the base of which abuts the right heart border, and can be misinterpreted as anterior segmental disease of the right upper lobe.

Clinical Findings

Atelectasis is a common complication of asthma, often due to mucus plugging of bronchi. Asthma is characterized by recurrent episodes of wheezing, shortness of breath, chest tightness, and cough with associated airflow obstruction. Exacerbations frequently begin with an unproductive cough and rapidly progressive dyspnea. Respiratory rate may not increase but expiration becomes prolonged and labored, and wheezing may be heard. Affected patients may profusely sweat. Breathing may be accompanied by coarse rales. Mucus plugging may temporarily cause localized loss of breath sounds.

Asthma commonly begins in childhood and adolescence, but may occur anytime in life. Allergens often play a role in adult-onset asthma. These individuals often have concomitant nasal polyps, sinusitis, and hypersensitivity to aspirin or other non-steroidal anti-inflammatory drugs (NSAIDs). Occupational exposure to various workplace materials can cause airway inflammation and bronchial hyper-responsiveness.

Imaging Findings

Each individual collapsed lobe or segment demonstrates its own typical radiographic pattern of volume loss (**Figs. 46.1, 46.2**) (also see Cases 37–43)

Management

- Persistent asthma requires long-term medications to maintain control of disease
- Appropriate quick-relief medications to manage exacerbations
    - β-adrenoceptor agonist (provides prompt relief of airflow obstruction)
    - Systemic corticosteroids (suppress and reverse airway inflammation)
    - Oxygen (relieves hypoxemia)
- Short-acting β-2-agonists: therapy of choice for relief of acute symptoms and prevention of exercise-induced asthma
- Most effective medications for long-term control
    - Anti-inflammatory effects (e.g., inhaled corticosteroids)
    - Long-acting β-2-agonists, especially for control of nocturnal symptoms
    - Cromones (potent mast cell stabilizers)
    - Sustained-release theophylline (mild to moderate bronchodilators)
    - Leukotriene modifiers: alternative to low doses of inhaled corticosteroids or cromolyn for mild persistent asthma

Prognosis

- Acute attacks represent medical emergencies; may have fatal outcome
- Most patients have good prognosis with appropriate management
- Bronchiectasis and pneumonia may occur as sequelae

PEARLS

- Each individual lobe or segment demonstrates its own predictable radiographic pattern of collapse.
- *Double lesion sign* does not always invalidate primary lung neoplasia as the cause of multi-lobar collapse. Combined right upper and middle lobe collapse may occur with tumor infiltration of both lobar bronchi. Tumor may obstruct one bronchus and metastatic lymphadenopathy may obstruct the other. It is also possible to have simultaneous multicentric neoplasms or a benign lesion affecting one bronchus (e.g., tuberculosis) and malignancy affecting the second bronchus.
- Consider ABPA in asthmatic patients with no other explanation for lobar collapse.

Suggested Reading

1. Felson B. The lobes. In: Felson B, ed. Chest Roentgenology. Philadelphia: WB Saunders; 1973:128–133

2. Franquet T, Müller NL, Giménez A, Guembe P, de La Torre J, Bagué S. Spectrum of pulmonary aspergillosis: histologic, clinical, and radiologic findings. Radiographics 2001;21(4):825–837

3. Fraser RS, Müller NL, Colman N, Paré PD. Atelectasis. In: Fraser and Paré's Diagnosis of Diseases of the Chest, 4th ed. Philadelphia: Saunders; 1999:539–554

4. Gotway MB, Dawn SK, Caoili EM, Reddy GP, Araoz PA, Webb WR. The radiologic spectrum of pulmonary *Aspergillus* infections. J Comput Assist Tomogr 2002;26(2):159–173

5. Travis WD, Colby TV, Koss MN, Rosado-de-Christenson ML, Müller NL, King TE Jr. Obstructive pulmonary disorders. In: King DW, ed. Atlas of Nontumor Pathology: Non-Neoplastic Disorders of the Lower Respiratory Tract, first series, fascicle 2. Washington, DC: American Registry of Pathology; 2002:457–465

CASE 47

■ Clinical Presentation

Pediatric burn victim with an acute onset of respiratory distress and oxygen desaturation

■ Radiologic Findings

AP chest radiograph (**Fig. 47.1**) demonstrates an opaque left thorax with marked overinflation of the right lung and ipsilateral mediastinal shift. The endotracheal tube is malpositioned, with the tip in the right mainstem bronchus.

■ Diagnosis

Total Atelectasis Left Lung; Inadvertent Right Mainstem Bronchial Intubation

■ Differential Diagnosis

- Post-Pneumonectomy
- Massive Hydrothorax
- Extensive Pneumonia

■ Discussion

Background

Atelectasis of an entire lung is common and more often affects the left lung. Mainstem bronchus obstruction from any etiology may produce ipsilateral collapse. Complete atelectasis of either lung is usually associated with complete opacification of affected thorax, ipsilateral mediastinal shift, diaphragmatic elevation, and compensatory overinflation of the contralateral lung, and may be misinterpreted as massive unilateral

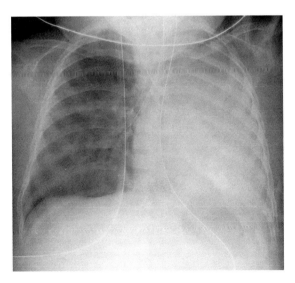

Fig. 47.1

253

pleural effusion or extensive pneumonia. Massive unilateral pleural effusion behaves as a space-occupying lesion and enlarges the affected hemithorax. Thus, the ipsilateral diaphragm is depressed or inverted, and the mediastinum shifts to the contralateral side. Diffuse unilateral pneumonia may completely opacify the thorax and silhouettes the ipsilateral diaphragm and mediastinal borders, but the lung volume remains the same and signs of atelectasis are absent.

Clinical Findings

Complete atelectasis of a lung is associated with diminished or absent breath sounds in the affected thorax. Patients may experience tachypnea, tachycardia, and an abrupt drop in oxygen saturations.

Imaging Findings

- Opacification of affected thorax (**Fig. 47.1**)
- Ipsilateral mediastinal shift (**Fig. 47.1**)
- Ipsilateral diaphragmatic elevation (**Fig. 47.1**)
- Compensatory overinflation of contralateral lung (**Fig. 47.1**)

Management

- Relieve mainstem bronchial obstruction
- Correction of malpositioned endotracheal tube

Prognosis

- Good if recognized early and promptly treated
- Delayed recognition and treatment may be complicated by barotrauma (e.g., pulmonary interstitial emphysema, pneumomediastinum, spontaneous pneumothorax) as aerated lung is subjected to the tidal volume delivery for two lungs rather than one

PEARLS

- Entire lung atelectasis is usually secondary to complete obstruction of a main bronchus.
- Malpositioned ET tube should be excluded in critical care patients with isolated upper lobe or complete lung atelectasis; atelectasis occurs rapidly in such settings.
- Understanding *direct* and *indirect signs* of volume loss allows the radiologist to exclude massive unilateral effusion or diffuse unilateral pneumonia.

Suggested Reading

1. Fraser RS, Müller NL, Colman N, Paré PD. Atelectasis. In: Fraser and Paré's Diagnosis of Diseases of the Chest, 4th ed. Philadelphia: Saunders; 1999:517–539

2. Proto AV, Tocino I. Radiographic manifestations of lobar collapse. Semin Roentgenol 1980;15(2):117–173

3. Woodring JH, Reed JC. Radiographic manifestations of lobar atelectasis. J Thorac Imaging 1996;11(2):109–144

CASE 48

■ Clinical Presentation

77-year-old man formerly employed as a construction site foreman with long-standing history of tobacco abuse complains of chronic cough

■ Radiologic Findings

PA (**Fig. 48.1A**) and lateral (**Fig. 48.1B**) chest radiographs show a 3.0 cm mass in the retrocardiac region of the left lower lobe. On the coned-down frontal exam (**Fig. 48.1C**), the margins of the mass are poorly defined, suggesting it is pleural based. The coned-down lateral exam (**Fig. 48.1D**) shows adjacent vessels and bronchi curving into the medial edge of this mass. Note the adjacent pleural thickening.

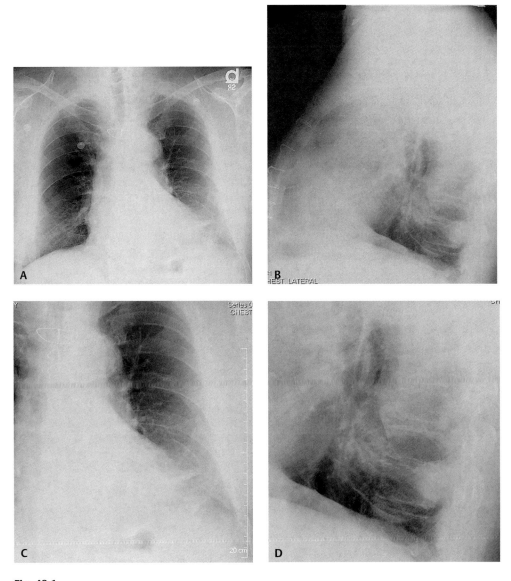

Fig. 48.1

■ Diagnosis

Rounded Atelectasis
Synonyms
- Round Atelectasis
- Folded Lung
- Asbestos Pseudotumor

■ Differential Diagnosis

- Primary Lung Cancer
- Secondary Lung Cancer
- Pneumonia

■ Discussion

Background

Rounded atelectasis is a distinct form of relaxation atelectasis seen in association with focal pleural thickening. Decortication of the adjacent pleura is often associated with re-expansion of this focally atelectatic lung. Two hypotheses have been proposed for the development of rounded atelectasis. The *first* is predicated on a pre-existent pleural effusion (**Fig. 48.2A**). The effusion causes the adjacent lower lobe to float upward and compresses the lung. A cleft or fold then occurs in the visceral pleura (**Fig. 48.2B**). The lung then begins to tilt and curl on itself in a concentric fashion along this cleft (**Fig. 48.2C**). Fibrinous adhesions along this cleft suspend the atelectatic segment (**Fig. 48.2C**). As the effusion resorbs, aerated lung fills in the space around the focal "rounded" atelectatic lung. Organization of the fibrinous exudate and fibrous contraction cause the affected lung to remain "balled up" as a mass-like lesion (**Fig. 48.2C**). The *second* hypothesis suggests an irritant (e.g., asbestos) induces a local pleuritis, causing the pleura to thicken and contract. The adjacent lung "shrinks," and the atelectasis develops in a rounded mass-like configuration.

Clinical Findings

Most cases of rounded atelectasis occur in patients with a history of asbestos exposure. Other manifestations of asbestos exposure may be observed in such patients (e.g., pleural plaques) (**Figs. 48.3A, 48.3B**). However, rounded atelectasis has also been described in association with pleural effusions of tuberculous and non-

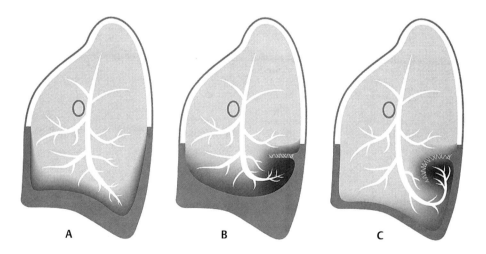

A   B   C

Fig. 48.2 Artist's illustration demonstrating the evolution of rounded atelectasis in the setting of a pre-existing pleural effusion. See description in text.

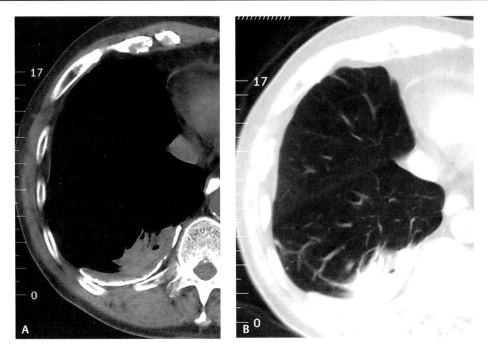

Fig. 48.3   Unenhanced chest CT (**A**, mediastinal window; **B**, lung window) of a 63-year-old man employed as a construction worker reveals an ovoid soft-tissue attenuation mass in the medial posterior basal segment right lower lobe abutting the costovertebral pleura. The mass contains air bronchograms and the adjacent vasculature is drawn in toward its medial margin. Note the pleural thickening and calcified pleural plaque (**A**) adjacent to the rounded atelectasis.

tuberculous etiologies, pulmonary infarction, iatrogenic pneumothorax, heart failure, coronary artery revascularization, talc pleurodesis, malignant pleural disease, etc. Most patients are asymptomatic and the lesion is often an incidental radiologic finding. Rounded atelectasis most frequently occurs in the lower lobes (55% of cases). Less frequent presentations occur in the middle lobe and lingula (39% of cases) and in the upper lobes (6% of cases).

Imaging Findings

Radiography

- 2–8 cm diameter focal juxtapleural mass with adjacent pleural thickening in posterolateral or posteromedial aspect of lower lobes (**Figs. 48.1A, 48.1B, 48.1C**)
- Adjacent bronchovascular bundles drawn together in curvilinear fashion toward medial margin of the mass (**Figs. 48.1B, 48.2**)
- Adjacent lung overexpands; often appears oligemic
- Lesion/mass remains relatively stable in size and shape over time

MDCT

- Ovoid or rounded parenchymal lesion ranging from 2 to 8 cm in diameter (**Figs. 48.3, 48.4**)
- Adjacent pleural thickening and hypertrophy of subcostal fat (**Figs. 48.3A, 48.4A, 48.4B**)
- Adjacent bronchi and vessels tethered together; converge on medial margin of mass creating *parachute cord* or *comet tail sign* (**Figs. 48.3B, 48.4C, 48.4D**) or *hurricane sign* (**Fig. 48.5**)
- Central or hilar aspect of mass is often *ill defined* where vessels are drawn together; lateral margin of mass is *better defined* (**Figs. 48.3B, 48.4C, 48.4D**)
- Air bronchograms visualized in approximately 18% of lesions (**Fig. 48.3B**)
- Additional signs of asbestos exposure (e.g., plaques) observed in 20–60% of cases (**Figs. 48.3A, 48.4A, 48.4B**)

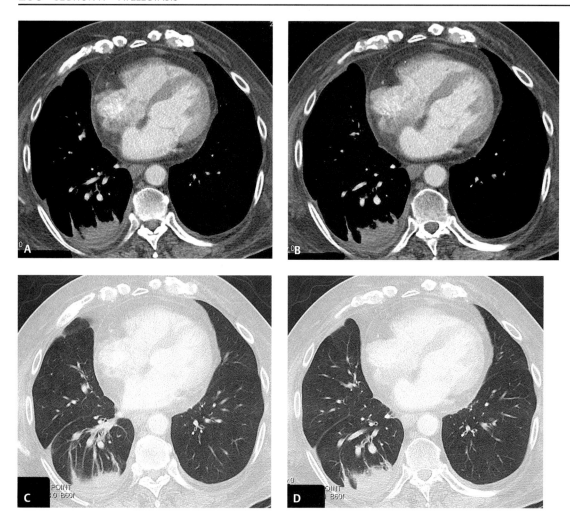

Fig. 48.4 Contrast-enhanced chest CT (**A**, **B**, mediastinal window; **C**, **D**, lung window) of an asymptomatic 63-year-old man with remote history of asbestos exposure and abnormal chest radiograph (not illustrated) reveals an ovoid soft-tissue attenuation mass in the posterior basal segment of the lower lobe abutting thickened costovertebral pleura. Note preservation and hypertrophy of the underlying subcostal fat and contralateral non-calcified costovertebral pleural plaques **(A,B)**. CT lung windows **(C,D)** show the adjacent bronchi and vessels tethered together and converging on the medial margin of the mass, creating the *parachute cord* or *comet tail sign*.

MR

- T1-weighted images
  - Signal intensity of rounded atelectasis higher than muscle and lower than fat
- T2-weighted images
  - Signal intensity of rounded atelectasis similar to, or lower than, fat
  - Rounded atelectasis and thickened pleura often more clearly separated on T2-weighted images compared with CT
- Post gadopentetate dimeglumine administration (Gd-DTPA)
  - Atelectatic mass homogeneously enhances
  - Structures within and surrounding the rounded atelectasis clearly depicted
  - Pulmonary vessels and bronchi converge toward the area of atelectasis (*comet tail sign*); better demonstrated on sagittal or oblique sagittal planes
  - Infolded visceral pleura may be seen as a low-signal-intensity line
  - Small amount of entrapped pleural effusion may be noted in select cases

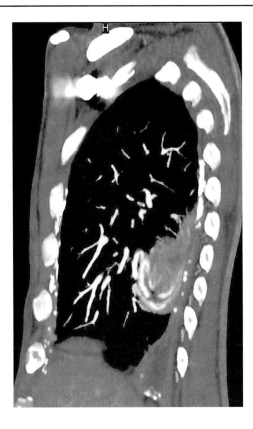

Fig. 48.5 Contrast-enhanced sagittal MIP chest CT of a 55-year-old man status post remote talc pleurodesis shows a focal dominant 5.0 cm right lower lobe mass. The adjacent blood vessels converge medially and are drawn into the folded lung in a "swirling" manner likened to the appearance of a hurricane, forming the *hurricane sign*. Note the ipsilateral pleural thickening and high-attenuation talc precipitates.

PET

- Rounded atelectasis is metabolically "inactive"

Management

- Affected patients with typical imaging findings and negative bronchoscopy may be followed prospectively without surgical intervention
- Affected patients with atypical imaging findings often undergo surgical excision to exclude neoplasia
- Pleural decortication may be performed for patients with restrictive symptoms

Prognosis

- Good, benign process with no malignant potential
- Majority of lesions remain stable for years
  - On occasion, the region of "folded" lung may slightly decrease or increase in size
  - Total regression sometimes occurs; unusual in patients with asbestos-related pleural disease
- Recurrences not a problem in patients managed with surgical excision

PEARLS

- Although most cases occur in patients with a history of asbestos exposure, rounded atelectasis is not pathognomonic of such, and may result from a variety of pleural and parenchymal insults.
- PET imaging may be necessary to differentiate rounded atelectasis from lung cancer in problematic cases demonstrating atypical imaging features.

Suggested Readings

1. Gilkeson RC, Adler LP. Rounded atelectasis. Evaluation with (18) PET scan. Clin Positron Imaging 1998;1(4): 229–232

2. Kiryu T, Ohashi N, Matsui E, Hoshi H, Iwata H, Shimokawa K. Rounded atelectasis: delineation of enfolded visceral pleura by MRI. J Comput Assist Tomogr 2002;26(1):37–38

3. McHugh K, Blaquiere RM. CT features of rounded atelectasis. AJR Am J Roentgenol 1989;153(2):257–260

4. Travis WD, Colby TV, Koss MN, Rosado-de-Christenson ML, Müller NL, King TE Jr. Occupational lung diseases and pneumoconioses. In: King DW, ed. Atlas of Nontumor Pathology: Non-Neoplastic Disorders of the Lower Respiratory Tract, first series, fascicle 2. Washington, DC: American Registry of Pathology; 2002:827–828

5. Yamaguchi T, Hayashi K, Ashizawa K, et al. Magnetic resonance imaging of rounded atelectasis. J Thorac Imaging 1997;12(3):188–194

Section V

Pulmonary Infections and Aspiration Pneumonia

OVERVIEW OF COMMON BACTERIAL PNEUMONIAS

Bacterial pneumonia is an inflammatory process that usually affects the distal air spaces (e.g., respiratory bronchioles, alveolar ducts, and alveoli) but may also involve the trachea, bronchi, and larynx. *Primary bacterial pneumonia* can be caused by inhalation of aerosolized organisms (e.g., *M. tuberculosis, L. pneumophila*) or can result from aspiration of contaminated oropharyngeal secretions. *Secondary bacterial pneumonia* results from hematogenous dissemination of infection from one organ to another—for example, endocarditis leading to staphylococcal lung abscesses. The upper respiratory tract is the source of both most *community-acquired* and *nosocomial pneumonias*. The most common causes of *community-acquired pneumonia* in *non-hospitalized patients* include *M. pneumoniae, C. pneumoniae*, and various viruses (**Table V.1**). Those organisms causing more severe illness, often requiring hospitalization, include *S. pneumoniae, S, aureus, H. influenza, M. pneumoniae, C. pneumoniae, L. pneumophila, Klebsiella pneumoniae*, and the influenza virus (**Table V.1**). *Nosocomial pneumonias* are most often associated with methicillin-resistant *S. aureus* (MRSA), *P. aeruginosa*, enteric Gram-negative bacilli, anaerobes, and *A. baumannii* (**Table V.1**). Potential risk factors for nosocomial pneumonia include advanced age, immunosuppression, altered states of consciousness or neurologic insults predisposing to aspiration, and colonization and contamination of respiratory and other medical equipment, which is especially prevalent in many ICUs. Many patients with underlying chronic diseases, especially chronic lung diseases, and other particular risk factors or behaviors, are also prone to bacterial pneumonias often associated with specific organisms. These are summarized in **Table V.2**.

Bacterial pneumonia may be broadly classified into two categories based on the anatomic distribution in the lung. *Lobar pneumonia* is best exemplified by pneumococcal pneumonia (*S. pneumoniae*). Infection begins in the distal air spaces, edema fluid rapidly accumulates, and the inflammatory exudate spreads contiguously and centrifugally from acinus to acinus across segmental boundaries, resulting in confluent air space consolidation involving the entire lobe and confined only by the pleural surface and fissural borders. Because alveolar air is replaced by exudate, there is little volume loss and air bronchograms may be seen. *Lobular pneumonia* (bronchopneumonia) is characterized by centrilobular inflammation. The inflammatory exudate begins around the respiratory bronchioles and spreads to the alveolar ducts and alveolar spaces and eventually fills the large airways following the course of the tracheobronchial tree. The consolidation is usually segmental, characterized by volume loss and no air bronchograms. Advanced cases of lobular pneumonia may be difficult to differentiate from lobar pneumonia. The cases that follow in this section initially focus on the common bacterial pneumonias (**Table V.1, Table V.2**).

Table V.1 Most Common Causes of Community-Acquired and Nosocomial Bacterial Pneumonia

Community-Acquired	Nosocomial
S. pneumoniae	*S. aureus*/MRSA
M. pneumoniae	*P. aeruginosa*
H. influenzae	Enteric Gram-negative bacilli
L. pneumophila	Various anaerobes
C. pneumoniae	*A. baumannii*
Various anaerobes	

Modified from Johnson CC, Finegold SM. Pyogenic bacterial pneumonia, lung abscess and empyema. In: Murray JF, Nadel JA, eds. Textbook of Respiratory Medicine, 2nd ed. Philadelphia: WB Saunders; 1994:1036–1093.

Table V.2 Underlying Chronic Processes and Risk Factors Associated with Various Bacterial Pneumonias

Disease Process or Risk Factor	Responsible Bacterium
Alcoholism	*S. pneumoniae* *K. pneumoniae* *H. influenzae* Anaerobes
Altered states of consciousness	Anaerobes *S. aureus* Gram-negative bacilli
Cell-mediated immune deficiency	*Legionella* sp. *Nocardia* sp.
Chronic obstructive lung disease (COPD)	*S. pneumoniae* *H. influenzae* *M. catarrhalis*
Cystic fibrosis	*P. aeruginosa* *S. aureus* *B. cepacia*
HIV-AIDS	*S. pneumoniae* *H. influenzae* *S. aureus* *R. equi*
Intravenous drug abuse (IVDA)	*S. aureus*
Neutropenia (granulocytes <1,000/µL)	*P. aeruginosa* *S. aureus* Enteric Gram-negative bacilli
Pulmonary alveolar proteinosis	*Nocardia* sp.

Modified from Johnson CC, Finegold SM. Pyogenic bacterial pneumonia, lung abscess and empyema. In: Murray JF, Nadel JA, eds. Textbook of Respiratory Medicine, 2nd ed. Philadelphia: W.B. Saunders; 1994:1036–1093.

Suggested Readings

1. Herold CJ, Sailer JG. Community-acquired and nosocomial pneumonia. Eur Radiol 2004;14(Suppl 3):E2–E20

2. Johnson CC, Finegold SM. Pyogenic bacterial pneumonia, lung abscess and empyema. In: Murray JF, Nadel JA, eds. Textbook of Respiratory Medicine, 2nd ed. Philadelphia: WB Saunders; 1994:1036-1093

3. Katz DS, Leung AN. Radiology of pneumonia. Clin Chest Med 1999;20(3):549–562

4. Travis WD, Colby TV, Koss MN, Rosado-de-Christenson ML, Müller NL, King TE Jr. Lung infections. In: King DW, ed. Atlas of Nontumor Pathology: Non-Neoplastic Disorders of the Lower Respiratory Tract, first series, fascicle 2. Washington, DC: American Registry of Pathology; 2002:827–828

5. Van Mieghem IM, De Wever WF, Verschakelen JA. Lung infection in radiology: a summary of frequently depicted signs. JBR-BTR 2005;88(2):66–71

6. Vilar J, Domingo ML, Soto C, Cogollos J. Radiology of bacterial pneumonia. Eur J Radiol 2004;51(2):102–113

CASE 49

■ Clinical Presentation

59-year-old man with high fever and cough productive of rusty, blood-streaked sputum

■ Radiologic Findings

PA (**Fig. 49.1A**) and lateral (**Fig. 49.1B**) chest X-rays reveal dense, non-segmental homogeneous lobar consolidation that partially silhouettes the right heart border (**Fig. 49.1A**) and is bordered by the horizontal and oblique fissure (**Fig. 49.1B**). No associated volume loss. A small ipsilateral pleural effusion blunts the posterior sulcus (**Fig. 49.1B**).

■ Diagnosis

Pneumococcal Pneumonia; Right Middle Lobe

■ Differential Diagnosis

• Other Community-Acquired Pneumonias

■ Discussion

Background

Most pneumococcal infections occur in the winter and early spring. The organism is acquired through person-to-person transmission by inhalation of aerosolized droplets, physical contact, or both. *Risk factors* for infection include very young or advanced age, chronic heart and/or lung disease, alcoholism and/or cirrhosis,

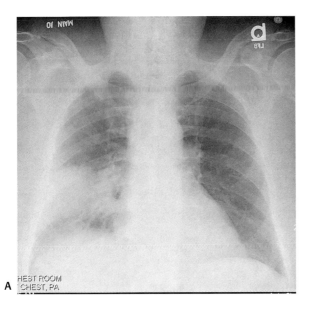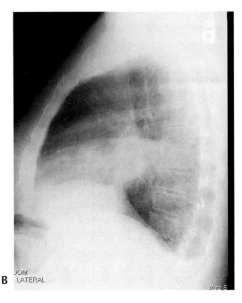

Fig. 49.1

sickle cell anemia, lymphoma, leukemia, multiple myeloma, HIV-AIDS, intravenous drug abuse (IVDA), and prior splenectomy.

Etiology

Pneumococcal pneumonia is caused by the Gram-positive, diplococcal bacterium *Streptococcus pneumoniae*. This bacterium is responsible for at least half of all cases of community-acquired pneumonia and is also the *most common cause* of community-acquired pneumonia resulting in hospital admission. Pneumococci colonize the upper respiratory tract of 5–60% of the general population.

Clinical Findings

Pneumococcal pneumonia is the *most common* bacterial pneumonia to follow influenza pneumonia infection. Additionally, up to 70% of patients with pneumococcal pneumonia have had a recent upper respiratory tract infection (URI). Affected patients often have an abrupt onset of rigors, followed by fever, cough productive of rusty sputum, and dyspnea. Pleuritic chest pain is common, experienced in up to 75% of patients. Leukocytosis is usually present (WBC 15,000–25,000), but severe infection may be associated with white blood cell counts of less than 3,000/mm^3.

Complications

- Metastatic infection (e.g., endocarditis, meningitis, arthritis)
- Pericarditis
- Rarely empyema
- Pneumatoceles; more common in children

Imaging Findings

Chest Radiography

- Homogeneous, non-segmental, parenchymal consolidation involving one lobe; multi-lobar involvement less common (**Figs. 49.1, 49.2A, 49.4**)
- Air space disease abuts surrounding visceral pleura of fissural surfaces (**Figs. 49.1, 49.4**)
- Predilection for lower lobes or posterior segments of upper lobes (**Figs. 49.4, 49.5**)
- Minimal volume loss (**Figs. 49.1, 49.2A, 49.4, 49.5**)
- Air bronchograms common (**Fig. 49.4**)
- Rare cavitation
- Mass-like rounded consolidation (i.e., round pneumonia) infrequent in adults; more common in children (**Figs. 49.5A, 49.5B**)
- Pleural effusion common (60%); empyema unusual

MDCT

- Homogeneous, non-segmental, parenchymal consolidation involving one lobe; multi-lobar involvement less common (**Figs. 49.2B, 49.3B**)
- Air space disease abuts visceral pleura of fissural surfaces (**Figs. 49.2B, 49.3B**)
- Predilection for lower lobes or posterior segments of upper lobes (**Figs. 49.3A, 49.3B**)
- Minimal volume loss (**Figs. 49.2B, 49.3B**)
- Air bronchograms common (**Figs. 49.2B, 49.2C , 40.2D, 49.2E**)
- Rare cavitation; CT more sensitive than conventional radiography
- Pleural effusion common (60%); empyema unusual; CT more sensitive than conventional radiography (**Figs. 49.6A, 49.6B**)
- Lymphadenopathy common in hospitalized patients
  - Ipsilateral to pneumonia in most affected patients
- Bronchopneumonia pattern characterized by peribronchial and peribronchiolar consolidation affecting one or more lobes (**Figs. 49.7A, 49.7B**)
  - Air space nodules 4–10 mm in diameter
  - Opacification of entire secondary pulmonary lobule (**Fig. 49.7B**)

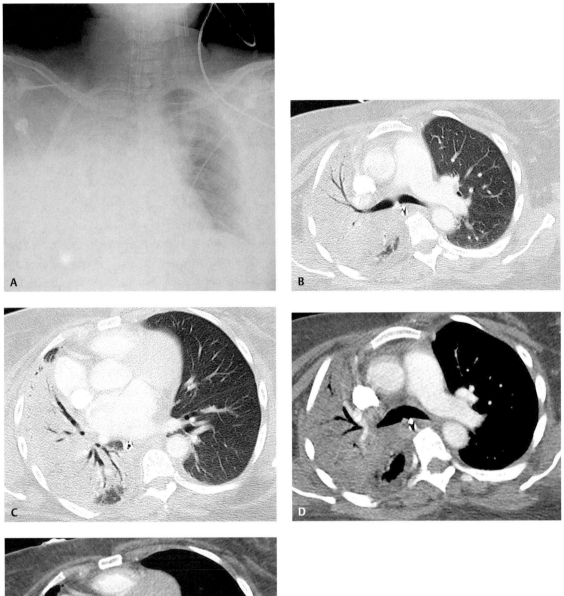

Fig. 49.2 **(A)** AP chest radiograph of a 45-year-old HIV-positive woman with high fever, dyspnea, and respiratory failure requiring intubation shows extensive homogeneous air space consolidation involving most of the right lung. Contrast-enhanced chest CT (**B**, **C**, lung window; **D**, **E**, mediastinal window) through the upper and lower lobes reveals extensive dense air space consolidations extending out to the pleura. Note the air bronchograms.

Management

- Penicillin is antibiotic of choice
- Vancomycin is antibiotic of choice for penicillin-resistant strains (30% of isolates)
- Pneumococcal polysaccharide vaccine encouraged for high-risk patient populations

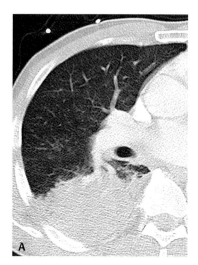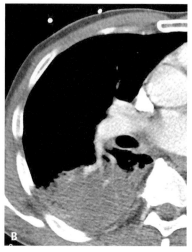

Fig. 49.3 Coned-down contrast-enhanced chest CT (**A**, lung window; **B**, mediastinal window) through the right lower lobe of a 55-year-old man with 104°F fever and rusty sputum production demonstrates extensive air space consolidation extending out to the pleural surface bordered by the oblique fissure.

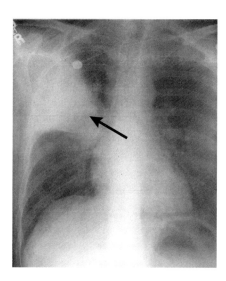

Fig. 49.4 AP chest radiograph of a 38-year-old man with fever and cough productive of rusty blood-streaked sputum shows dense, non-segmental homogeneous right upper lobe consolidation abutting the horizontal fissure. Note the subtle air bronchograms medially (*arrow*).

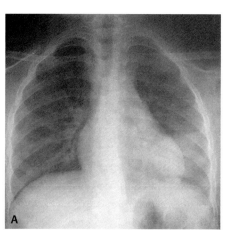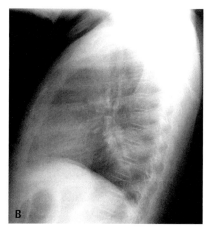

Fig. 49.5 (**A**) PA and (**B**) lateral chest radiographs of a 5-year-old with round (pneumococcal) pneumonia reveals a homogeneous, ovoid opacity that partially silhouettes the left heart border and the T8–T10 vertebrae (*positive spine sign*). Subtle air bronchograms are present, but there is no volume loss.

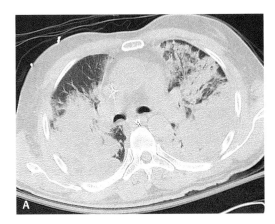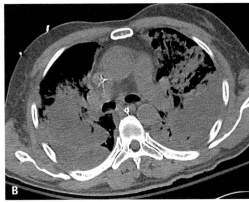

Fig. 49.6 Unenhanced chest CT (**A**, lung window; **B**, mediastinal window) of an alcoholic with pneumococcal pneumonia complicated by bilateral multi-loculated pleural fluid collections (i.e., empyema). The left upper lobe air space disease extends from the hilum to the pleural surface. Air bronchograms are present. The volume of the upper lobe is maintained.

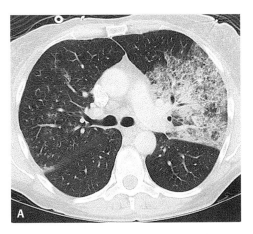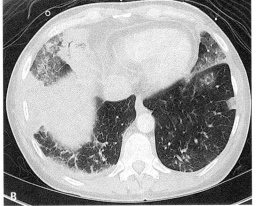

Fig. 49.7 Chest CT (lung window) of a patient with multi-lobar pneumococcal bronchopneumonia shows peribronchiolar left upper lobe air space disease extending from the hilum to the pleural surface and peribronchiolar consolidation in the right middle lobe. Subtle nodules are present in the right upper lobe and complete opacification of a secondary pulmonary lobule in the left lower lobe.

Prognosis

- Onset of recovery within 24–48 hours of antibiotic therapy; resolution after two weeks
- Slow clearance in elderly, those requiring hospitalization, smokers, and patients with underlying lung disease and bacteremia; 4–8-week disease course in these cases
- Increased mortality in patients >50 years and those with cirrhosis, cardiac and/or chronic pulmonary disease, asplenia, leukopenia (<4,000 cells/mm³), leukocytosis (>20,000 cells/mm³), malignancy, multi-lobar involvement, hypoxemia, bacteremia, and penicillin-resistant disease

PEARLS

- Absence of air bronchograms argues against the diagnosis.
- Round pneumonias are more frequently seen in children <8 years of age, but may be seen in adults. Adult infection rapidly progresses to more typical lobar pneumonia. Failure to do so suggests underlying neoplasia.

- Necrotizing pneumonia most often occurs with polymicrobial infections.
- Lymphadenopathy is common on CT in hospitalized patients. Thus, when a patient with pneumococcal pneumonia has lymphadenopathy identified on CT, other etiologies for the lymphadenopathy need not be suspected.

Suggested Reading

1. Fraser RS, Müller NL, Colman N, Paré PD. Pulmonary infection. In: Fraser and Paré's Diagnosis of Diseases of the Chest, 4th ed. Philadelphia: Saunders; 1999:736–743

2. Reimer LG. Community-acquired bacterial pneumonias. Semin Respir Infect 2000;15(2):95–100

3. Stein DL, Haramati LB, Spindola-Franco H, Friedman J, Klapper PJ. Intrathoracic lymphadenopathy in hospitalized patients with pneumococcal pneumonia. Chest 2005;127(4):1271–1275

4. Travis WD, Colby TV, Koss MN, Rosado-de-Christenson ML, Müller NL, King TE Jr. Lung infections. In: King DW, ed. Atlas of Nontumor Pathology: Non-Neoplastic Disorders of the Lower Respiratory Tract. First Series. Fascicle 2. Washington, DC: The American Registry of Pathology; 2002:541–544

5. Wagner AL, Szabunio M, Hazlett KS, Wagner SG. Radiologic manifestations of round pneumonia in adults. AJR Am J Roentgenol 1999;172(2):549–550

CASE 50

■ Clinical Presentation

26-year-old man with fever, cough productive of purulent sputum, and hemoptysis

■ Radiologic Findings

PA (**Fig. 50.1A**) and lateral (**Fig. 50.1B**) chest radiographs demonstrate a patchy area of consolidation with associated cavitation and surrounding ground glass in the superior segment right lower lobe. Contrast-enhanced chest CT (**Fig. 50.1C,** lung window; **Fig. 50.1D,** mediastinal window) shows a corresponding focus of ill-defined parenchymal consolidation with surrounding ground glass and adjacent pleural thickening. Note the low-attenuation areas (**Fig. 50.1D**), reflecting regions of necrosis and the cavitation. Paraseptal emphysema parallels the costovertebral pleura (**Fig. 50.1C**).

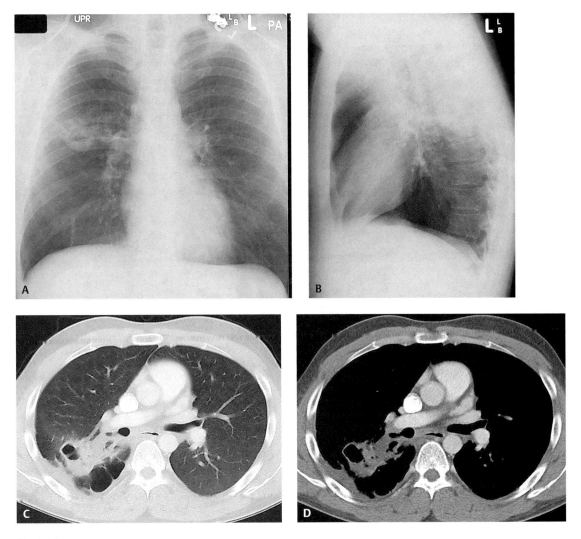

Fig. 50.1

271

■ Diagnosis

Staphylococcal Pneumonia; Superior Segment Right Lower Lobe

■ Differential Diagnosis

• Other Community-Acquired Bronchopneumonias

■ Discussion

Background

Pulmonary infection occurs through hematogenous spread or aspiration of contaminated oral secretions. Twenty to 40% of older children and adults, and more than 50% of health care workers, are nasal carriers of staphylococci. *S. aureus* causes less than 5% of community-acquired pneumonias, but is responsible for more than 10% of hospital-acquired pneumonias. Staphylococcal pneumonia often complicates viral pneumonias (e.g., influenza) in adults (**Fig. 50.2**) and measles in children. Aspiration can lead to pneumonia in intubated patients and in those with underlying COPD or lung cancer. Patients with contaminated vascular catheters and those with endocarditis (**Fig. 50.3**) or intravenous drug abuse (IVDA) history (**Figs. 50.4A, 50.4B**) may have hematogenous spread to the lungs.

Etiology

Staphylococcal pneumonia is caused by the Gram-positive bacteria *Staphylococcus* sp. *S. aureus* is responsible for most cases of staphylococcal bronchopneumonia. Staphylococci produce toxins causing significant tissue destruction and lung abscesses (**Figs. 50.1A, 50.3, 50.4. 50.5, 50.6**). The inflammatory exudate is multifocal and fills the large airways, following the course of the tracheobronchial tree. Consolidation is usually segmental and is characterized by segmental volume loss and the absence of air bronchograms.

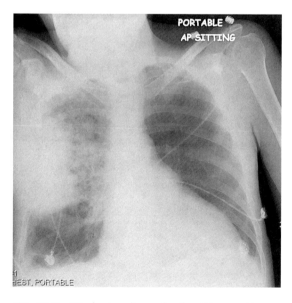

Fig. 50.2 AP chest radiograph of a 57-year-old man with methicillin-resistant *Staphylococcus aureus* (MRSA) pneumonia complicating recent influenza reveals an ill-defined right perihilar bronchopneumonia with peripheral air space consolidation. A small ipsilateral pleural effusion is present.

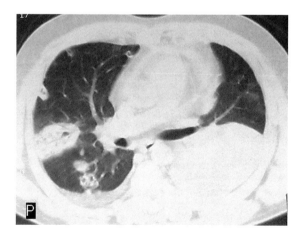

Fig. 50.3 Chest CT (lung window) of a 41-year-old patient with tricuspid valve murmur, fever, and *S. aureus* endocarditis shows multiple intraparenchymal and juxta-pleural nodules, and consolidations of variable size consistent with septic emboli. Many lesions are cavitated, and some exhibit associated feeding vessels supporting a hematogenous route of dissemination.

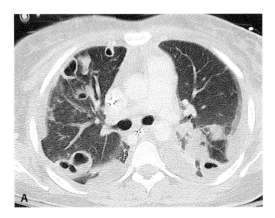
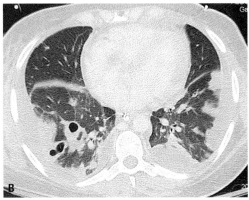

Fig. 50.4   Chest CT (lung window) through the **(A)** upper and **(B)** lower lung zones of a 29-year-old heroin intravenous drug user with fever and septic pulmonary emboli from *S. aureus* reveals multiple variable-sized, primarily peripheral and juxtapleural cavitary lesions throughout both lungs and frank parenchymal consolidations. Many cavitary lung abscesses have varying wall thickness and internal septations. Note the loculated pleural fluid collections bilaterally.

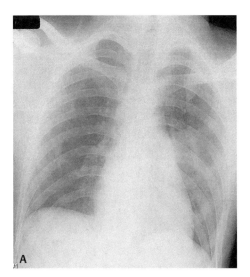
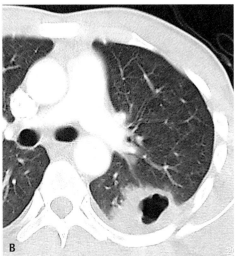

Fig. 50.5   **(A)** AP chest radiograph of a 35-year-old man with fever, cough, chest pain, and staphylococcal lung abscess shows an ill-defined focus of consolidation with associated cavitation in the left perihilar distribution. **(B)** Chest CT (lung window) demonstrates a corresponding focus of consolidation and cavitation in the lower lobe superior segment with adjacent pleural thickening.

Clinical Findings

Patients may present with fever, cough, and purulent sputum production. Those with complicating pulmonary infarcts may complain of chest pain and experience hemoptysis. Leukocytosis is common. Panton-Valentine leukocidin (PVL)–positive strains of *S. aureus* infections are often characterized by a temperature greater than 39°C, tachycardia (>140 beats per min), hemoptysis, pleural effusion, and leukopenia. PVL-positive strains are also associated with extensive necrotic ulcerations of the tracheal and bronchial mucosa and massive hemorrhagic necrosis of interalveolar septa. Abscesses develop in 15–20% of patients with staphylococcal pneumonia (**Figs. 50.1, 50.3, 50.4, 50.5, 50.6**). Pneumatoceles are uncommon in adults but occur in up to 40% of children with staphylococcal pneumonia (**Fig. 50.7**). These thin-walled cysts usually resolve over weeks to months but may rupture into the pleural space, causing spontaneous pneumothoraces. Empyema complicates staphylococcal pneumonia in 20% of affected adults (**Fig. 50.8**) and 75% of affected children.

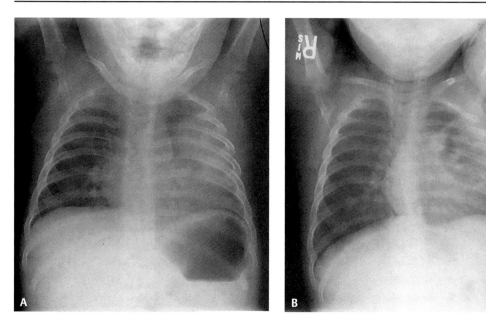

Figure 50.6 **(A)** AP chest radiograph of a 9-month-old child with staphylococcal pneumonia who remains toxic with high fever following a two-week course of antibiotics for otitis media shows focal, ill-defined consolidation in the left upper lobe with volume loss. **(B)** AP chest exam six days later shows irregular cavitation in the consolidated upper lobe consistent with lung abscess. (*Images courtesy of Lakshmana Das Narla, MD, VCU Medical Center, Richmond, Virginia.*)

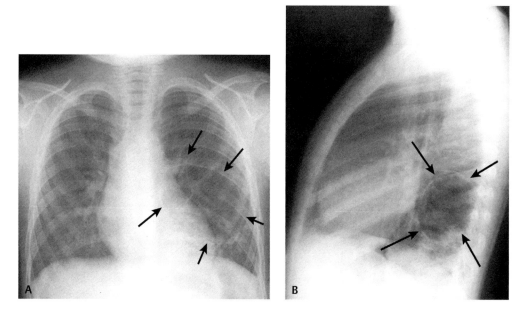

Figure 50.7 **(A)** AP and **(B)** lateral chest radiographs of a 5-year-old, six months after treatment for staphylococcal pneumonia, shows a well-defined, thin-walled 6.0 cm pneumatocele (*arrows*) at the site of previous consolidation (not shown).

Imaging Findings

Chest Radiography

- Lobular pattern of bilateral, multifocal, patchy, heterogeneous, segmental air space consolidations, usually affecting lower lobes (**Figs. 50.1A, 50.2, 50.5A, 50.6A**)
- Absent air bronchograms (**Figs. 50.1A, 50.2, 50.5A, 50.6A**)
- May progress to homogeneous air space consolidation

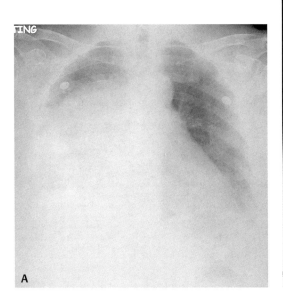

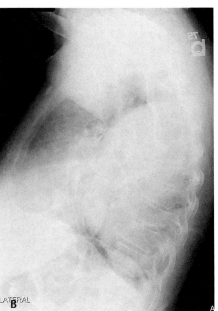

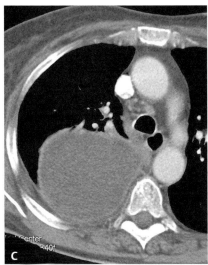

Fig. 50.8 **(A)** PA and **(B)** lateral chest radiographs of a 91-year-old woman with staphylococcal pneumonia complicated by empyema shows a large, lentiform opacity occupying most of the right thorax. Note the *positive spine sign* on the lateral exam **(B)**. **(C)** Contrast-enhanced chest CT (mediastinal window) reveals the large loculated pleural fluid collection. Note the mass effect on neighboring anatomic structures and the pleural enhancement.

- Volume loss may be present (**Fig. 50.6A**)
- May develop abscess(es) with cavitation; irregular, shaggy, internal walls; and air-fluid levels (**Figs. 50.1A, 50.1B, 50.5A, 50.6B**)
- Pleural effusion is common (30–50%); progression to empyema in 50% of cases (**Figs. 50.8A, 50.8B**)

MDCT

- Lobular pattern of bilateral, multifocal, patchy, heterogeneous, segmental air space consolidations, usually affecting lower lobes (**Figs. 50.1C, 50.1D, 50.9A**)
- Absent air bronchograms (**Figs. 50.1C, 50.1D, 50.9A**)
- May progress to homogeneous air space consolidation
- Focal or multi-focal nodule(s) or mass(es); may undergo cavitation, air-fluid levels (**Figs. 50.5B, 50.9A, 50.9B**)
- Centrilobular nodules and tree-in-bud opacities may be present (**Fig. 50.9A**)
- Peripheral and/or juxtapleural wedge-shaped opacities with associated feeding vessels; hematogenous dissemination (**Figs. 50.3, 50.4A, 50.4B**)
- Complicating parapneumonic effusion and/or empyema (**Fig. 50.8C**)

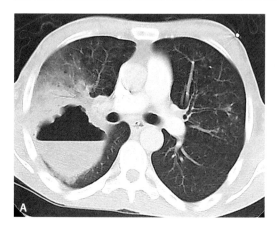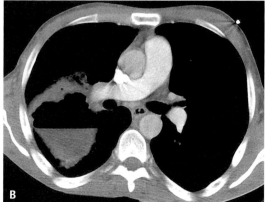

Fig. 50.9 Contrast-enhanced chest CT (**A**, lung window; **B**, mediastinal window) of a 35-year-old man with staphylococcal pneumonia shows a 6.0 cm lung abscess posterior segment right upper lobe. The abscess cavity demonstrates a lobular, shaggy internal wall from 9:00 to 12:00 and a large air-fluid level. Adjacent lobular bronchopneumonia pattern of air space disease extends further anteriorly into the right upper lobe **(A)**. Note the centrilobular nodules and tree-in-bud opacities in the left upper lobe resulting from endobronchial spread **(A)**.

Management

- Intravenous β-lactam agents (e.g., nafcillin, oxacillin) or first-generation cephalosporins (e.g., cefazolin)
- Vancomycin in cases of methicillin-resistant strains of *S. aureus* (MRSA)

Prognosis

- Mortality rate 25–30%; increases to over 80% with bacteremia
- PVL(+) *S. aureus* strains cause rapidly progressive, hemorrhagic, necrotizing pneumonia; higher morbidity and mortality than PVL(−) strains

PEARLS

- If air bronchograms are present, bronchopneumonia is less likely.
- Septic emboli manifest as poorly defined juxtapleural opacities; two-thirds of such lesions have associated feeding vessels appreciated on CT.
- Juxtapleural wedge-shaped consolidations represent septic emboli complicated by pulmonary infarction.
- PVL(+) methicillin-resistant *S. aureus* (MRSA) is an emerging pathogen worldwide causing rapidly progressive, hemorrhagic, often fatal necrotizing pneumonia, mainly in otherwise healthy children and young adults. This strain is often preceded by influenza-like symptoms.

Suggested Reading

1. Fraser RS, Müller NL, Colman N, Paré PD. Pulmonary infection. In: Fraser and Paré's Diagnosis of Diseases of the Chest, 4th ed. Philadelphia: Saunders; 1999:702–703, 743–748

2. Elizur A, Orscheln RC, Ferkol TW, et al. Panton-Valentine Leukocidin-positive methicillin-resistant *Staphylococcus aureus* lung infection in patients with cystic fibrosis. Chest 2007;131(6):1718–1725

3. Gillet Y, Issartel B, Vanhems P, et al. Association between *Staphylococcus aureus* strains carrying gene for Panton-Valentine leukocidin and highly lethal necrotising pneumonia in young immunocompetent patients. Lancet 2002;359(9308):753–759

4. Macfarlane J, Rose D. Radiographic features of staphylococcal pneumonia in adults and children. Thorax 1996;51(5): 539–540

5. Travis WD, Colby TV, Koss MN, Rosado-de-Christenson ML, Müller NL, King TE Jr. Lung infections. In: King DW, ed. Atlas of Nontumor Pathology: Non-Neoplastic Disorders of the Lower Respiratory Tract. First Series. Fascicle 2. Washington, DC: The American Registry of Pathology; 2002:541–544

CASE 51

■ Clinical Presentation

42-year-old woman with long-standing history of poorly controlled diabetes presented to the Emergency Department with purulent productive cough, shortness of breath, and fever

■ Radiologic Findings

PA (**Fig. 51.1A**) and lateral (**Fig. 51.1B**) chest X-rays demonstrate poorly defined nodular opacities and patchy areas of consolidation and a small right pleural effusion. Sputum and blood cultures confirmed the diagnosis.

■ Diagnosis

Haemophilus influenzae Pneumonia

■ Differential Diagnosis

• Other Community-Acquired Bronchopneumonias

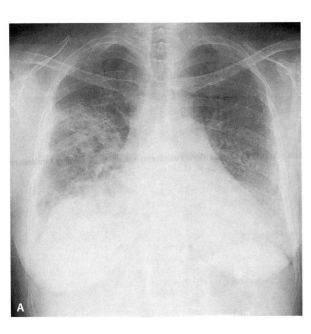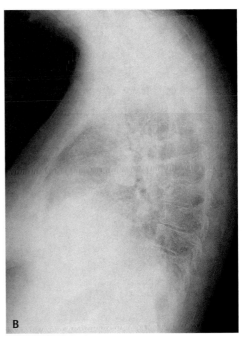

Fig. 51.1

■ Discussion

Background

H. influenzae pulmonary infection is acquired through person-to-person transmission via aerosolized droplets deposited in the nasopharynx. The nasopharynx is colonized in up to 90% of children by 5 years of age. Many patients with COPD are also colonized.

Etiology

The pleomorphic, Gram-negative bacterium *Haemophilus influenzae* causes *Haemophilus* pneumonia. Most organisms that colonize the nasopharynx are unencapsulated and non-typeable. Most strains that infect the lung are encapsulated and typeable. Type b is the most common strain responsible for *Haemophilus* pneumonia (Hib).

Clinical Findings

H. influenzae is a major cause of pneumonia in both children and adults. Despite reductions in frequency due to vaccination for *H. influenzae* type b, it remains one of the major pneumonias resulting in hospital admissions and is responsible for 5–20% of community-acquired pneumonia. Risk factors for infection include: children 2 months to 3 years of age, adults over 50 years of age, and patients with COPD, chronic alcoholism, diabetes mellitus, HIV-AIDS, sickle cell anemia, multiple myeloma, intravenous drug abuse, or hypogammaglobulinemia. *H. influenzae* is also an important cause of nosocomial pneumonia in patients without particular risk factors. Bronchopneumonia is often preceded by upper respiratory tract infection. Presenting symptoms include fever, purulent productive cough, and dyspnea. Leukocytosis is mild or absent. The clinical course may be complicated by bacteremia, meningitis, and pericarditis.

Imaging Findings

Chest Radiography

- Patchy air space opacities (i.e., bronchopneumonia pattern) (50–60%) (**Figs. 51.1A, 51.1B**)
- Lobar consolidation; more common in immunocompromised/immunosuppressed patients; unilateral or bilateral; usually lower lobe
- Combination of the two above patterns
- Acute non-segmental air space consolidation (30–50%)
- Volume expansion uncommon
- Reticular/nodular opacities associated with consolidation (15–30%) (**Figs. 51.1A, 51.1B**)
- Cavitation (<15%)
- Pleural effusion (40–50%) (**Figs. 51.1A, 51.1B**); empyema rare
- Slow resolution of disease

MDCT

- Any of the above patterns
- Ill-defined centrilobular nodules reflecting peribronchiolar inflammation (**Fig. 51.2**)
- Lobular consolidation
- Patchy distribution (i.e., bronchopneumonia pattern) typical (**Fig. 51.2**)

Management

- Resistant to penicillin family of antibiotics
- Intravenous third-generation cephalosporins until antibiotic sensitivities are available
- Vaccination with Hib conjugate vaccine is effective in preventing Hib infection; recommended for all children and high-risk patients

Prognosis

- Uncomplicated Hib pneumonia and non-encapsulated *H. influenzae* infections; usually good prognosis
- Overall mortality rate may approach 28% in adults (depending on co-morbidity); 5% in children

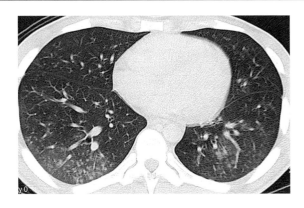

Fig. 51.2 Unenhanced CT (lung window) of bronchopneumonia due to *H. influenza* shows ill-defined centrilobular nodules and patchy ground glass. Areas of tree-in-bud are present due to infectious bronchiolitis.

PEARLS

- *H. influenzae* is one of the most common bacterial causes of acute COPD exacerbation.

Suggested Reading

1. Fact Sheet of the Centers for Disease Control and Prevention (CDC) Web Site at http://en.wikipedia.org/wiki/Haemophilus_influenzae accessed 17 July 2010

2. Lee KS, Kim TS, Han J, et al. Diffuse micronodular lung disease: HRCT and pathologic findings. J Comput Assist Tomogr 1999;23(1):99–106

3. Travis WD, Colby TV, Koss MN, Rosado-de-Christenson ML, Müller NL, King TE Jr. Lung infections. In: King DW, ed. Atlas of Nontumor Pathology: Non-Neoplastic Disorders of the Lower Respiratory Tract. First Series. Fascicle 2. Washington, DC: The American Registry of Pathology; 2002:541-544.

4. World Health Organization (WHO). *Haemophilus Influenzae* type b (Hib) Web Site at http://www.who.int/immunization/topics/hib/en/index.html accessesed 17 July 2010

CASE 52

■ Clinical Presentation

61-year-old woman with long-standing history of alcohol abuse presented with sudden onset of cough, pleuritic chest pain, dyspnea, fever, and rigors

■ Radiologic Findings

PA (**Fig. 52.1A**) and lateral (**Fig. 52.1B**) chest radiographs reveal a homogeneous, nonsegmental air space consolidation localized to the superior segment left lower lobe. No air bronchograms are seen. The affected lobe is overexpanded, and the oblique fissure bulges anteriorly and superiorly (*bulging fissure sign*) (**Fig. 52.1B**). Contrast-enhanced axial (**Fig. 52.1C**, mediastinal window; **Fig. 52.1D**, lung window) and accompanying sagittal (**Fig. 52.1E**, mediastinal window; **Fig. 52.1F**, lung window) chest CT shows the relationship between air space consolidation and the oblique fissure. Note the outward displacement of the cephalad aspect of the fissure (compare **Fig. 52.1B** and **Fig. 52.1F**). The superior segment is densely consolidated. The low-attenuation areas represent foci of necrosis. Enhancing blood vessels can be seen in the areas of low-attenuation consolidated lung parenchyma (*CT angiogram sign*). Also note the background of extensive centrilobular emphysema.

■ Diagnosis

Klebsiella Pneumonia (aka Friedländer's pneumonia)

■ Differential Diagnosis

- Pneumococcal Pneumonia
- Mixed Anaerobic Infection
- *Haemophilus influenza* Pneumonia
- Staphylococcal Pneumonia

■ Discussion

Background

Klebsiellae are ubiquitous in nature. In humans, they may colonize the skin, pharynx, gastrointestinal tract, sterile wounds, and urine and are regarded as normal flora in many parts of the gastrointestinal and biliary tracts. Oropharyngeal carriage is associated with endotracheal intubation, impaired host defenses, and antimicrobial use. The primary pathogenic reservoirs are the gastrointestinal tract of patients and hands of hospital personnel, the latter often responsible for nosocomial outbreaks. *Klebsiella* pneumonia usually results from aspiration of colonizing oropharyngeal microbes into the lower respiratory tract. *Risk factors* for *Klebsiella* pneumonia include alcoholism, diabetes mellitus, and COPD.

Etiology

Klebsiella pneumonia is caused by the Gram-negative bacterium *Klebsiella pneumoniae. K. pneumoniae* causes approximately 5% of community-acquired pneumonia and up to 30% of nosocomial pneumonia. The extensive clinical use of broad-spectrum antibiotics in hospitalized patients has led to increased carriage of *Klebsi-*

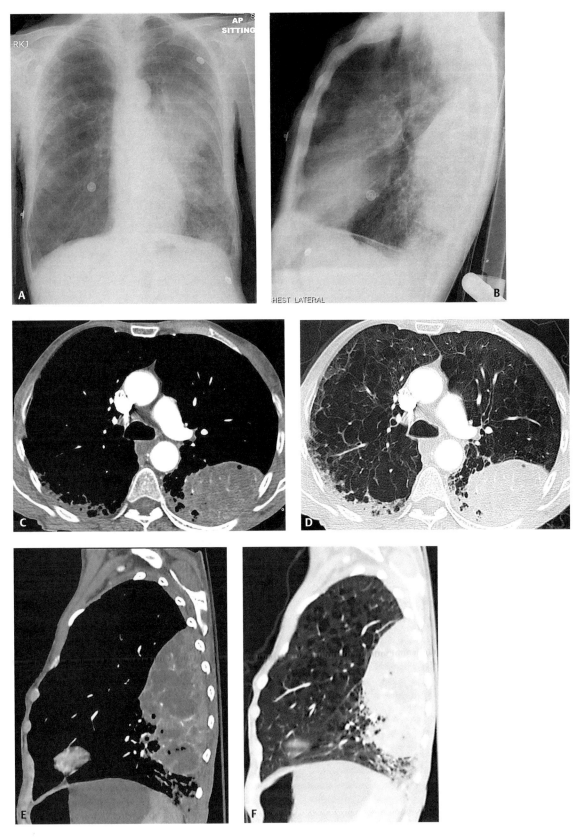

Fig. 52.1

ella as well as the evolution of multi-drug-resistant strains (MDRS). Lung infection by *K. pneumoniae* is often associated with production of large volumes of inflammatory exudate. The exudate may infiltrate the entire affected lobe, which enlarges, over-expands, and causes the abutting fissure to bulge toward the unaffected lobe (*bulging fissure sign*). Lung infection may also be associated with necrosis, tissue destruction, and hemorrhage, sometimes producing thick, bloody, mucoid sputum described as currant jelly.

Clinical Findings

Klebsiella pneumonia primarily affects persons with alcoholism (66%) and the debilitated (ICU and nursing home patients). Additional *risk factors* include indwelling central venous catheters and feeding tubes. Affected patients present with sudden onset of fever, rigors, dyspnea, pleuritic chest pain, and productive cough with the consistency of currant jelly. Prostration and hypotension may occur. White blood cell count may be elevated, diminished, or normal. *Klebsiella* pneumonia may be complicated by multicentric abscesses, cavitation, pulmonary gangrene, bronchiectasis, and empyema. Chronic pneumonia may be associated with interstitial fibrosis, organizing pneumonia, bronchiolitis, and necrotizing bronchitis.

Imaging Findings

Chest Radiography

- Usually involves upper lobes; lower lobe involvement is not uncommon (**Fig. 52.2**)
- Homogeneous, nonsegmental, lobar consolidation (**Figs. 52.1A, 52.1B**)
- Lobar expansion; *bulging fissure sign* (**Figs. 52.1B, 52.2**)
- Lung abscess(es) occur in up to 50% cases (**Fig. 52.2**)
- Pulmonary gangrene
  - Begins as lobar consolidation; usually in upper lobes
  - Coalescence of intrinsic lucencies to form large cavity
  - "Mass within a mass" or "air crescent" signs secondary to sloughed lung
  - Pleural effusion (70%) and/or empyema

MDCT

- Necrotizing pneumonia
  - Enhancing consolidations and poorly marginated low-attenuation areas with or without small air-containing cavities (**Figs. 52.1C, 52.1D, 52.1E, 52.1F**)
  - Scattered enhancing linear branching structures representing pulmonary vessels in atelectatic or consolidated lung (*CT angiogram sign*) (**Figs. 52.1C, 52.1D, 52.1E, 52.1F**)
  - Centripetal resolution from periphery to center with residual fibrosis

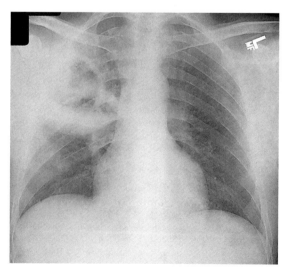

Fig. 52.2 AP chest radiograph of a 35-year-old woman with alcoholism and necrotizing *Klebsiella* pneumonia. Note the large irregular right upper lobe lung abscess and the inferiorly convex "bulging" horizontal fissure.

- Pulmonary gangrene
  - Multiple small abscesses coalesce into cavity containing sloughed necrotic lung
  - Narrowed or obliterated feeding bronchus impeding drainage of necrotic lung
  - Large-vessel thrombosis
  - Pleural effusion and/or empyema

Management

Community-Acquired Pneumonia

- Third-generation cephalosporins or quinolones and/or combination therapy with aminoglycosides
- Antibiotic therapy should be continued for at least 14 days
- Clinical and radiologic surveillance for surgically treatable complications
  - Pulmonary gangrene
  - Lung abscess(es)
  - Empyema

Nosocomial Pneumonia

- Imipenem, third-generation cephalosporins, quinolones, or aminoglycosides used alone or in combination
- Always confirm organism susceptibility
- Antibiotics should be continued for at least 14 days

Prognosis

- *Klebsiella* pneumonia: severe illness with rapid onset; mortality approaches 50% even with antimicrobial therapy
- Mortality may approach 100% for persons with alcoholism and bacteremia

PEARLS

- *Klebsiella* is among the top eight nosocomial pathogens in hospitals. Any organ system may be affected, but respiratory and urinary tract infections predominate.
- Because of the high prevalence of pneumococcal pneumonia in most communities, most patients with pneumonia manifesting with a *bulging fissure sign* are infected with *S. pneumoniae* rather than with *K. pneumoniae.*
- Cavitation, especially within a unilateral necrotizing pneumonia, strongly supports *Klebsiella* as the possible etiology.

Suggested Readings

1. Parker MS, Rosado-de-Christenson ML, Abbott GF. Pulmonary infections and aspiration pneumonia. common bacterial pneumonias. In: Teaching Atlas of Chest Imaging. New York: Thieme; 2006:223–226

2. Schmidt AJ, Stark P. Radiographic findings in *Klebsiella* (Friedlander's) pneumonia: the bulging fissure sign. Semin Respir Infect 1998;13(1):80–82

3. Travis WD, Colby TV, Koss MN, Rosado-de-Christenson ML, Müller NL, King TE Jr. Lung infections. In: King DW, ed. Atlas of Nontumor Pathology: Non-Neoplastic Disorders of the Lower Respiratory Tract. First series, fascicle 2. Washington, DC: American Registry of Pathology; 2002:549–550

CASE 53

■ Clinical Presentation

28-year-old quadriplegic ventilator-dependent man with fever, chills, and purulent sputum production

■ Radiologic Findings

PA (**Fig. 53.1A**) and lateral (**Fig. 53.1B**) chest X-rays demonstrate non-segmental right lower lobe consolidation without associated volume loss and an ipsilateral pleural effusion. Note the tracheostomy device. Sputum and blood cultures confirmed the diagnosis.

■ Diagnosis

Pseudomonas Pneumonia

■ Differential Diagnosis

Community-Acquired Pneumonia

*   *Staphylococcus aureus*
*   Group A *Streptococci*
*   *Klebsiella pneumoniae*

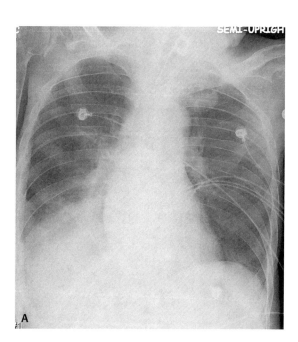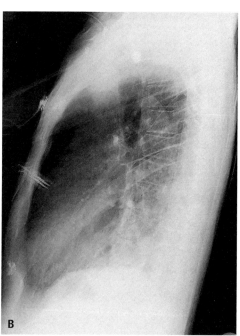

Fig. 53.1

Opportunistic Pneumonia

- *Escherichia coli*
- *Proteus* sp.
- *Enterobacter*
- *Serratia marcescens*

■ Discussion

Background

Pseudomonas may cause either *bacteremic* or *non-bacteremic* pneumonia. *Bacteremic* infection is acquired through breaks in the skin, the gastrointestinal mucosa, or respiratory tract, and most often occurs in patients with underlying hematologic or lymphoreticular malignancies, HIV-AIDS, immunosuppression, neutropenia, debilitation, or severe burns. *Non-bacteremic* infection is usually acquired through aspiration of infected oropharyngeal secretions. Risk factors for *non-bacteremic Pseudomonas* infection include advanced age, debilitation, chronic cardiopulmonary disease, COPD patients receiving steroids, cystic fibrosis, diffuse panbronchiolitis, and contaminated respiratory therapy equipment.

Etiology

Pseudomonas sp. is ubiquitous and survives in water, vegetation, and soil. Infection may result from exposure to contaminated hot tubs, whirlpools, vegetables, flowers, nails, and splinters. Because of resistance to many disinfectants, it is a common cause of nosocomial infection. In fact, *P. aeruginosa* is the most common pathogen isolated from patients who have been hospitalized longer than one week and a frequent cause of nosocomial infection of the lung and urinary tract. The overall prevalence of *P. aeruginosa* infections in U.S. hospitals is approximately 4 per 1,000 discharges (0.4%). *Pseudomonas* sp. also colonizes the gastrointestinal tracts of 5% of adults and of 50% of hospitalized patients with underlying neoplasia. *Pseudomonas* pneumonia is caused by infection from the Gram-negative aerobic bacteria *Pseudomonas* sp., most commonly *P. aeruginosa*.

Clinical Findings

Patients with *bacteremic Pseudomonas pneumonia* typically present with high fever, dyspnea, systemic toxicity, altered mental status, cough productive of scant non-purulent sputum, and skin lesions. Symptoms are often worse than expected based on radiographic findings. Alternatively, patients with *non-bacteremic Pseudomonas pneumonia* present with systemic toxicity, fever, chills, cough, and significant purulent sputum production. Pneumonia may be complicated by abscess formation and empyema.

Imaging Findings

Chest Radiography

Bacteremic Pneumonia

- Early pulmonary vascular congestion; rapidly progresses to pulmonary edema and necrotizing bronchopneumonia
- Within 48–72 hours: mixed alveolar and interstitial opacities; cavitation may occur
- Multifocal nodules or nodular opacities (>2.0 cm diameter)
- Nodules often coalesce into regions of frank consolidation

Non-Bacteremic Pneumonia

- Bronchopneumonia pattern of consolidation
- Multifocal, bilateral, non-segmental consolidation; lower lobe predilection although all lobes may be affected (**Figs. 53.1A, 53.1B**)
- Nodular and reticular opacities often present
- Abscess formation within foci of consolidation
- Small pleural effusions are common (**Figs. 53.1A, 53.1B**); empyema is rare

MDCT/HRCT

Bacteremic Pneumonia

- Multilobar air space consolidation (**Figs. 53.2A, 53.2B**); upper lobe predilection (82%)
- Nodular opacities (50%)
  - Centrilobular and tree-in-bud opacities (64%)
  - Larger, randomly distributed nodules (36%)
- Ground-glass opacities (31%)
- Bronchial wall thickening (57%)
- Necrosis (29%) (**Fig. 53.2B**)
- Pleural effusions
  - Unilateral (18%)
  - Bilateral (46%)

Management

- Antimicrobials are the mainstay of therapy; two-drug combination therapy (e.g., anti-pseudomonal β-lactam with aminoglycosides) is effective

Prognosis

- Infections caused by *P. aeruginosa* are treatable and potentially curable
- Acute fulminant *P. aeruginosa* infections (e.g., bacteremia, pneumonia, sepsis, meningitis): associated with extremely high mortality rates (36–81%)

PEARLS

- *P. aeruginosa* is the most common organism to cause pneumonia in ventilator-dependent patients; multifocal opacities and cavitation are not uncommon imaging features.
- Bacteremic pneumonia occurs in patients with neutropenia following chemotherapy and in HIV-AIDS patients.
- Chronic infection of the lower respiratory tract with *P. aeruginosa* is prevalent among patients with cystic fibrosis.

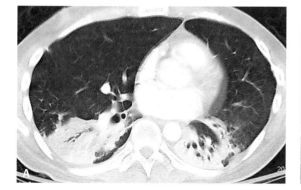 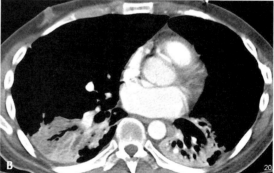

Fig. 53.2   Contrast-enhanced chest CT (**A**, lung window; **B**, mediastinal window) of a young man with AIDS and *P. aeruginosa* pneumonia manifest as multifocal bibasilar air space consolidations. Areas of decreased attenuation in the right lower lobe represent early necrosis that progressed to frank cavitation on follow-up study four days later (not illustrated).

Suggested Reading

1. Shah RM, Wechsler R, Salazar AM, Spirn PW. Spectrum of CT findings in nosocomial *Pseudomonas aeruginosa* pneumonia. J Thorac Imaging 2002;17(1):53–57

2. Travis WD, Colby TV, Koss MN, Rosado-de-Christenson ML, Müller NL, King TE Jr. Lung infections. In: King DW, ed. Atlas of Nontumor Pathology: Non-Neoplastic Disorders of the Lower Respiratory Tract. First series, fascicle 2. Washington, DC: American Registry of Pathology; 2002:550–553

3. Vikram HR, Shore ET, Venkatesh PR. Community acquired *Pseudomonas aeruginosa* pneumonia. Conn Med 1999; 63(5):271–273

4. Winer-Muram HT, Jennings SG, Wunderink RG, Jones CB, Leeper KV Jr. Ventilator-associated *Pseudomonas aeruginosa* pneumonia: radiographic findings. Radiology 1995;195(1):247–252

CASE 54

■ Clinical Presentation

53-year-old man with past CABG on chronic corticosteroids for remote kidney transplant presents with fever, non-productive cough, altered mental status, and diarrhea

■ Radiologic Findings

Baseline AP chest X-ray (**Fig. 54.1A**) shows patchy, non-segmental heterogeneous right upper lobe and bilateral perihilar opacities. AP chest X-ray two days later (**Fig. 54.1B**) demonstrates progression of disease, although confined to the same regions of lung. Follow-up chest X-ray two days later (**Fig. 54.1C**) reveals rapid progression of disease. Air space consolidation now replaces most of the right upper and left lower lobes. The left perihilar disease has progressed and extends into the upper lobe. Hypoxia necessitated intubation.

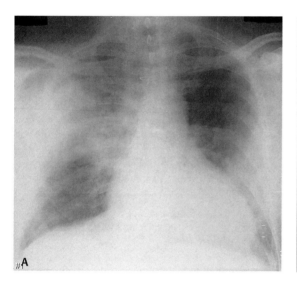

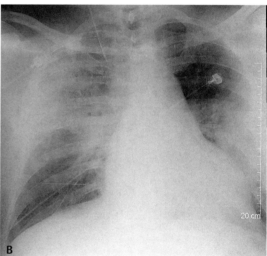

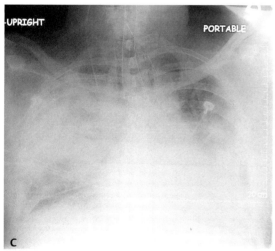

Fig. 54.1

■ Diagnosis

Legionella Pneumonia

■ Differential Diagnosis

• Other Community-Acquired Bronchopneumonias

■ Discussion

Background

Legionella was so named after a July 1976 outbreak of an unknown illness in Philadelphia at the American Legion Convention, during which 221 persons became ill and 34 died. On January 18, 1977, the unknown bacterium was identified and subsequently named *Legionella*. Since then, at least 50 species of *Legionella* have been identified. Pulmonary infection with *Legionella* is acquired through airborne spread of contaminated aerosolized water droplets that can travel up to 6 km (3.7 miles) from their source. No cases of person-to-person transmission have been reported. Most cases of *Legionella* pneumonia are traced to water, the natural habitat of *Legionella* sp. Typical sources include cooling towers, swimming pools, domestic hot water storage tanks, large central air conditioning units, shower heads, fountains, hot tubs, and freshwater ponds, rivers, lakes, and creeks.

Etiology

Legionella pneumonia is caused by the Gram-negative bacteria *Legionella* sp., most commonly *Legionella pneumophila*. It is responsible for 2–25% of community-acquired pneumonias requiring hospitalization and 1–40% of nosocomial pneumonias. The source of hospital-acquired *Legionella* pneumonia is typically the water distribution system. *Legionella* sp. is also the causative agent of Legionnaires' disease and Pontiac fever.

Clinical Findings

Legionella infects 8,000 to 18,000 individuals a year (USA). Most healthy individuals are not at risk of disease. *Risk factors* for infection include advanced age, diabetes, alcohol or tobacco abuse, immunocompromised or immunosuppressed states, male gender (2–3M:1F), malignancy (e.g., hairy cell leukemia), COPD, renal failure, transplantation, and corticosteroid therapy. Affected patients usually present after a 2–10-day incubation period with flu-like symptoms including fever, chills, lethargy, dry cough, and headache. Respiratory symptoms include non-productive cough or cough productive of watery or purulent sputum, dyspnea (50%), pleuritic chest pain (33%), and hemoptysis (33%). Symptoms tend to get worse during the first 4–6 days. Other signs and symptoms include diarrhea (50%), nausea and vomiting (25%), confusion, hallucinations, seizures, hyponatremia and hypophosphatemia (50%), and leukocytosis. One-third of patients require ventilatory support and 10% develop acute renal failure

Imaging Findings

Chest Radiography

• Patchy, peripheral, non-segmental consolidation (**Fig. 54.1A**); initially confined to one lobe
• Common, rapid contiguous and non-contiguous lobar progression and bilateral lung involvement (**Figs. 54.1A, 54.1B, 54.1C**)
• Nodular and mass-like consolidations
• Cavitation and lymphadenopathy; unusual
• Pleural effusion (50–66%)

MDCT

- Multilobar or multi-segmental pulmonary consolidation or ground glass opacities
- Cavitary lobar consolidation; more common in patients on high-dose steroids
- Sharply demarcated peribronchovascular foci of consolidation intermingled with ground glass opacity

Management

- Antibiotics; begun as soon as Legionnaires' disease is suspected, without waiting for laboratory confirmation
- Quinolones (ciprofloxacin, levofloxicin, moxifloxacin)
- Macrolides (azithromycin, clarithromycin, erythromycin)

Prognosis

- Radiographic improvement lags far behind clinical improvement; mean time for radiographic improvement is five weeks; may be complicated by pulmonary fibrosis
- Mortality rate: 5–25%
- Hospital-acquired *Legionella* pneumonia: 28% mortality rate

Suggested Reading

1. Stout JE, Muder RR, Mietzner S, et al. Role of environmental surveillance in determining the risk of hospital-acquired Legionellosis: a national surveillance study with clinical correlations. Infect Control Hosp Epidemiol 2007;28(7):818–824

2. Kim KW, Goo JM, Lee HJ, et al. Chest computed tomographic findings and clinical features of *Legionella* pneumonia. J Comput Assist Tomogr 2007;31(6):950–955

3. Nguyen TM, Ilef D, Jarraud S, et al. A community-wide outbreak of Legionnaires disease linked to industrial cooling towers—how far can contaminated aerosols spread? J Infect Dis 2006;193(1):102–111

4. Sakai F, Tokuda H, Goto H, et al. Computed tomographic features of *Legionella pneumophila* pneumonia in 38 cases. J Comput Assist Tomogr 2007;31(1):125–131

5. Travis WD, Colby TV, Koss MN, Rosado-de-Christenson ML, Müller NL, King TE. Lung infections. In: King DW, ed. Atlas of Nontumor Pathology: Non-Neoplastic Disorders of the Lower Respiratory Tract. First Series, Fascicle 2. Washington, DC: The American Registry of Pathology; 2002:553–556

CASE 55

■ Clinical Presentation

46-year-old man with chest pain, cough, and night sweats for several weeks

■ Radiologic Findings

PA chest radiograph (**Fig. 55.1A**) demonstrates patchy non-segmental right mid-lung air space disease, bilateral hilar lymphadenopathy, and poor visualization of the right posterolateral fifth rib. Unenhanced chest CT (lung window) (**Figs. 55.1B, 55.1C**) demonstrates a peripheral right upper lobe mass-like consolidation with a surrounding halo of ground glass opacity.

■ Diagnosis

Pulmonary Nocardiosis

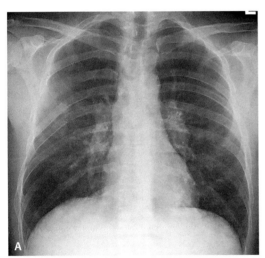
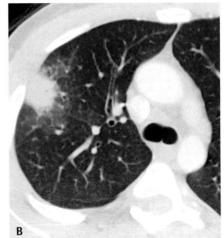
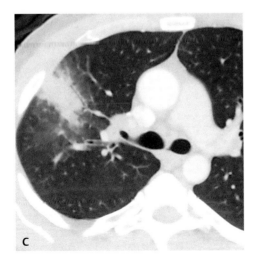

Fig. 55.1

■ Differential Diagnosis

- Other Atypical Pulmonary Infection (including tuberculosis and fungal infection)
- Septic Embolus
- Primary Lung Cancer
- Pulmonary Vasculitis

■ Discussion

Background

Pulmonary nocardiosis is usually acquired through inhalation of saprophytic organisms. Person-to-person transmission and blood-borne infection from infected catheters are rare. The primary risk factor for nocardiosis is immunodeficiency (e.g., lymphoreticular malignancy, solid organ transplantation). Other risk factors include chronic obstructive pulmonary disease (COPD), Cushing disease, acquired immunodeficiency syndrome (AIDS), systemic lupus erythematosus, treatment with methotrexate or corticosteroids, and pulmonary alveolar proteinosis.

Etiology

Nocardiosis is caused by the aerobic, Gram-positive, weakly acid-fast bacillus *Nocardia* sp. *Nocardia asteroides* accounts for 80–90% of pulmonary and disseminated infections. The bacterium is ubiquitous, found worldwide in soil and decaying vegetable matter.

Clinical Findings

Nocardiosis affects men more frequently than women, with a male-female ratio of 2:1 to 3:1. Immunocompetent patients may have a subacute presentation lasting several days to weeks. Symptoms may wax and wane, resulting in delayed diagnosis. Common symptoms include fatigue, low-grade fever, weight loss, and productive cough. Less often, patients experience dyspnea, pleuritic chest pain, and hemoptysis. Most patients have a moderate leukocytosis with neutrophilia. Immunocompromised patients may have a more acute presentation. Fifty percent of patients with pulmonary nocardiosis have disseminated infection to the brain, kidneys, skin, and bone. Pulmonary infection may be complicated by empyema and chest wall involvement.

Imaging Findings

Radiography

- Heterogenous, non-segmental parenchymal consolidation, often peripheral (**Fig. 55.1A**), multilobar, and abutting pleural surfaces (**Fig. 55.1A**)
- Less often, multifocal peripheral nodules or masses with irregular borders
- Cavitation in approximately one-third of nodules, masses, or consolidations
- Interstitial opacities
- Pleural effusion in approximately 50% of cases
- Chest wall involvement rare (**Fig. 55.1A**)

MDCT

- Focal (**Figs. 55.1B, 55.1C**) or multifocal consolidations
- Areas of low attenuation and peripheral enhancement
- Variable-sized pulmonary nodules
- Pleural effusion, empyema, pleural thickening
- Lymphadenopathy uncommon

Management

- Trimethoprim-sulfamethoxazole
- Empyema drainage

Prognosis

- Normal host: less than 5% mortality rate
- Immunocompromised host: 40% fatality rate
- Worse prognosis in patients with COPD, human immunodeficiency virus (HIV) infection, and disseminated disease (e.g., brain abscess)

PEARLS

- Although nocardiosis resembles actinomycosis, it is more likely to occur in immunocompromised hosts and to disseminate hematogeneously.

Suggested Reading

1. Mari B, Montón C, Mariscal D, Luján M, Sala M, Domingo C. Pulmonary nocardiosis: clinical experience in ten cases. Respiration 2001;68(4):382–388
2. Müller NL, Silva CIS. Bacterial pneumonia. In: Müller NL, Silva CIS, Hansell DM, Lee KS, Remy-Jardin M, eds. *Imaging of the Chest*. Philadelphia: Saunders Elsevier; 2008:240–321
3. Oszoyoglu AA, Kirsch J, Mohammed TL. Pulmonary nocardiosis after lung transplantation: CT findings in 7 patients and review of the literature. J Thorac Imaging 2007;22(2):143–148
4. Travis WD, Colby TV, Koss MN, Rosado-de-Christenson ML, Müller NL, King TE Jr. Lung infections. In: King DW, ed. Atlas of Nontumor Pathology: Non-Neoplastic Disorders of the Lower Respiratory Tract. First Series. Fascicle 2. Washington, DC: American Registry of Pathology; 2002:557–560

CASE 56

■ Clinical Presentation

39-year-old man presents with fever, cough, sputum production, and left-sided chest pain

■ Radiologic Findings

PA chest radiograph (**Fig. 56.1A**) shows an ill-defined left upper lobe perihilar mass-like opacity without air bronchograms. Contrast-enhanced chest CT (mediastinal window) (**Fig. 56.1B**) reveals a mass-like region of consolidation in the medial anterior segment of the left upper lobe that invades the adjacent anterior mediastinum and left anterior chest wall. Note the heterogeneous attenuation infiltrative process producing asymmetric thickening of the left pectoralis muscles.

■ Diagnosis

Pulmonary Actinomycosis with Chest Wall Invasion

■ Differential Diagnosis

- Atypical Infections (including nocardiosis, tuberculosis, and fungal infections)
- Primary Lung Cancer

■ Discussion

Background

Pulmonary actinomycosis results from aspiration of oropharyngeal secretions or by direct extension from a cervical or facial infection. Suppuration, sulfur granules, abscesses, and sinus tracts characterize actinomycosis. The diagnosis is established by the gross detection and microscopic assessment of yellow sulfur granules or grains (aggregates of mycelial fragments).

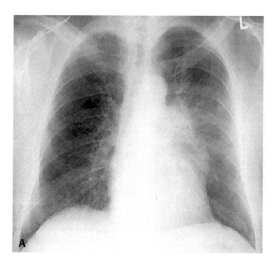 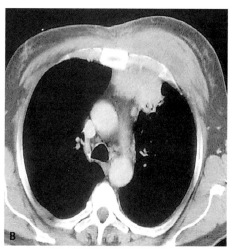

Fig. 56.1

294

Etiology

Actinomycosis is caused by the anaerobic saprophytic branching filamentous bacteria *Actinomyces* sp., and the usual pulmonary pathogen is *Actinomyces israelii*. *Actinomyces* sp. normally inhabit the oropharynx.

Clinical Findings

Actinomycosis most often manifests with cervicofacial infection following dental extraction. The incidence of pulmonary disease has markedly declined in most developed countries following the introduction of antibiotics. Most infections occur in immuno-competent individuals. Patients may present with productive cough, fever, weight loss, occasional hemoptysis, and pleuritic chest pain. Leukocytosis and anemia are common. Complications include rupture of abscesses into the pleura with subsequent empyema or bronchopleural fistula. Chronic lung involvement may result in pulmonary fibrosis. Infection may extend into the adjacent mediastinum or chest wall.

Imaging Findings

Radiography

- Peripheral small pulmonary nodules or segmental consolidations (**Fig. 56.1A**)
- Focal mass with or without associated cavitation; may mimic primary lung cancer (**Fig. 56.1A**)
- Less frequently, atelectasis, segmental opacities, multiple nodules (including miliary), biapical opacities
- Pleural effusion, empyema

MDCT

- Consolidation; may cross interlobar fissures and anatomic boundaries (**Fig. 56.1B**)
- Mass or nodule with intrinsic low attenuation and peripheral enhancement (**Fig. 56.1B**), frequent cavitation
- Pleural thickening; pleural effusion; empyema
- Chest wall involvement, soft-tissue mass or thickening (**Fig. 56.1B**), "wavy" periosteal reaction involving one or more contiguous ribs, skeletal involvement
- Endobronchial disease; may be associated with foreign bodies or broncholiths
- Hilar or mediastinal lymphadenopathy
- Mediastinal (**Fig. 56.1B**) or pericardial involvement (uncommon)

Management

- Penicillin; antibiotic of choice

Prognosis

- 90% cure with appropriate antibiotic therapy

PEARLS

- Actinomycosis manifests in a variety of forms; may mimic other infections or pulmonary neoplasms.
- A clinical pattern of remission and exacerbation of symptoms occurring in parallel with initiation and cessation of antibiotic therapy is a helpful diagnostic clue.

Suggested Reading

1. Kim TS, Han J, Koh W-J, et al. Thoracic actinomycosis: CT features with histopathologic correlation. AJR Am J Roentgenol 2006;186(1):225–231

2. Travis WD, Colby TV, Koss MN, Rosado-de-Christenson ML, Müller NL, King TE. Lung infections. In: King DW, ed. Atlas of Nontumor Pathology: Non-Neoplastic Disorders of the Lower Respiratory Tract. First Series, Fascicle 2. Washington, DC: The American Registry of Pathology; 2002:560–563

CASE 57

■ Clinical Presentation

Morbidly obese woman hospitalized for management of her diabetes who developed fever, productive cough, and dyspnea during her hospitalization

■ Radiologic Findings

AP (**Fig. 57.1**) chest radiograph reveals diffuse right perihilar nonsegmental air space disease without cavitation, pleural effusion, or lymphadenopathy. Subsequent bronchoscopy confirmed the diagnosis.

■ Diagnosis

Acinetobacter Hospital-Acquired Pneumonia

■ Differential Diagnosis

- Nosocomial Hospital-Acquired Pneumonia of Other Etiologies
- Aspiration Pneumonia
- Community-Acquired Pneumonias

■ Discussion

Background

Acinetobacter species are Gram-negative, nonmotile, aerobic coccobacillary organisms. However, they can be Gram-variable and occasionally Gram-positive on initial stains. The morphologic appearance is dependent on the growth phase with a rod-shaped appearance during rapid growth but a coccobacillary appearance during the stationary phase. *Acinetobacter* species are oxidase-negative, which differentiates this species from other Gram-negative organisms, such as *Pseudomonas*, *Neisseria*, and *Moraxella*.

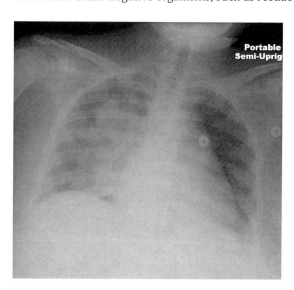

Fig. 57.1 *(Image courtesy of Kristin Miller, MD, VCU Medical Center, Richmond, Virginia.)*

296

Etiology

Acinetobacter grow easily in nature and are most commonly found in the soil and water. However, *Acinetobacter* has also been isolated from food, ventilator and suctioning equipment, infusion pumps, sinks, pillows, bed mattresses and railings, tap water, humidifiers, soap dispensers, etc. Such colonization is extremely problematic, as *Acinetobacter* survives an average of 20 days and can survive for as long as four months on hospital surfaces. Furthermore, up to 40% of healthy adults have skin colonization, with even higher rates among hospital employees and patients. The respiratory tract is frequently colonized in humans and is the most common site of infection.

Clinical Findings

Acinetobacter is primarily a colonizer of the hospital environment and of the ICU in particular and is an important cause of hospital-acquired (HAP) and ventilator-acquired (VAP) pneumonia. *Acinetobacter* is an uncommon but important cause of community-acquired pneumonia (CAP), with a high mortality rate. Hospital colonization most often occurs in intubated patients and those with multiple intravenous lines or monitoring devices, indwelling urinary or peritoneal catheters, and surgical drains. *Acinetobacter* isolates in respiratory secretions in intubated patients nearly always represent colonization as opposed to infection. *Acinetobacter* pneumonias occur in outbreaks and are usually associated with colonized respiratory support equipment or fluids. Patients with *Acinetobacter*-HAP or *Acinetobacter*-VAP present similarly to patients with HAP or VAP caused by other nosocomial pathogens. *Risk factors* for *Acinetobacter*-CAP include tobacco abuse, diabetes, and COPD. Most patients with *Acinetobacter*-CAP present with acute onset of fever, cough, severe respiratory distress, and pleuritic chest pain. However, cases have been reported in healthy individuals.

Imaging Findings

Community-Acquired

- Lobar consolidation pattern (one or more lobes); more common (68%) than bronchopneumonia pattern; often with rapid progression
- Pleural effusion/empyema; less common
- ARDS complicates up to 84% cases
- CT may reveal hilar and/or mediastinal lymphadenopathy

Hospital-Acquired

- Bronchopneumonia; non-segmental pattern; more common and often shows rapid progression (**Figs. 57.1, 57.3**)
- Parenchymal cavitation or abscess formation; more common
- Pleural effusion/empyema; up to 50% of cases (**Fig. 57.2**)

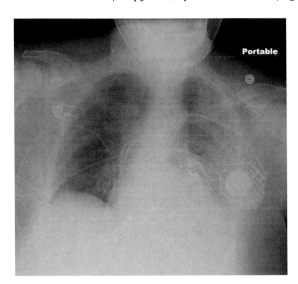

Fig. 57.2 AP chest radiograph of a woman with prolonged hospitalization for diabetes and renal failure shows patchy left perihilar non-segmental air space disease, and left lower lobe volume loss with pleural effusion. Bronchoscopy confirmed *Acinetobacter* pneumonia. *(Image courtesy of Kristin Miller, MD, VCU Medical Center, Richmond, Virginia.)*

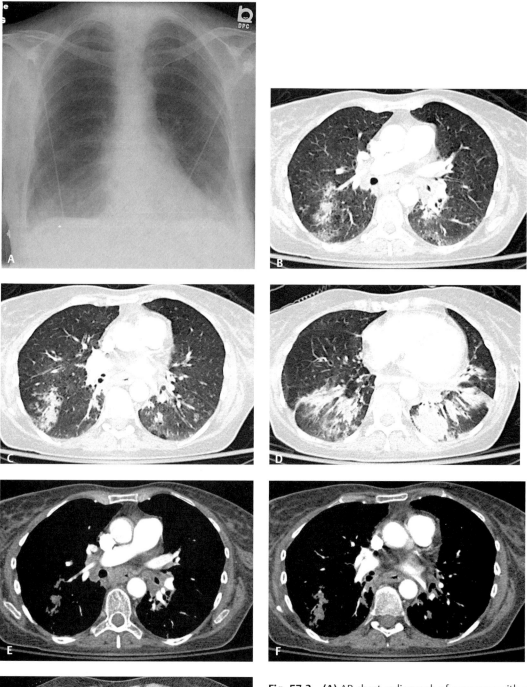

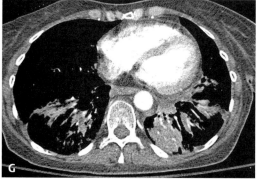

Fig. 57.3 **(A)** AP chest radiograph of a woman with prolonged hospitalization for diabetes shows bilateral perihilar and infrahilar non-segmental ground glass opacities and more coalescent disease in the left lower lobe. **(B–D)** Contrast-enhanced chest CT (lung window) reveals nonsegmental peribronchiolar ground glass and consolidation with scattered centrilobular and air space nodules in both lower lobes and more frank consolidation in the lung bases. **(E–G)** Accompanying mediastinal windows demonstrate extensive peribronchial, subcarinal, and paraesophageal lymphadenopathy. Bronchoscopy confirmed *Acinetobacter* pneumonia. *(Images courtesy of Kristin Miller, MD, VCU Medical Center, Richmond, Virginia.)*

- ARDS complicates up to 18% of cases
- CT may reveal hilar and/or mediastinal lymphadenopathy (**Figs. 57.3E, 57.3F, 57.3G**)

Management

- Multidrug-resistant *Acinetobacter*-HAP or *Acinetobacter*-VAP has become a formidable health care challenge
  - Polymyxins B and E (colistin) current antibiotics of choice; emerging resistance has been reported
- Most *Acinetobacter*-CAP remain sensitive to:
  - Amikacin, ticarcillin/clavulanate, and ampicillin/sulbactam

Prognosis

- *Acinetobacter*-CAP: higher incidence of bacteremia, ARDS, and death compared with *Acinetobacter*-HAP or *Acinetobacter*-VAP
- *Acinetobacter* infections
  - In-hospital mortality: 8–23%
  - ICU mortality: 10–43%

PEARLS

- Prevalence of *Acinetobacter* infections is increasing.
- *Acinetobacter* species are becoming a major cause of serious nosocomial infections, including HAP and VAP.
- *Acinetobacter* species have become increasingly resistant to antibiotics over the past several years and now present a significant challenge to physicians.
- Rates of bacteremia associated with *Acinetobacter*-CAP are higher than those associated with *Acinetobacter*-HAP or *Acinetobacter*-VAP.

Suggested Reading

1. Chen MZ, Hsueh PR, Lee LN, Yu CJ, Yang PC, Luh KT. Severe community-acquired pneumonia due to *Acinetobacter baumannii*. Chest 2001;120(4):1072–1077

2. Dijkshoorn L, van Dalen R, van Ooyen A, et al. Endemic *Acinetobacter* in intensive care units: epidemiology and clinical impact. J Clin Pathol 1993;46(6):533–536

3. Fournier PE, Richet H. The epidemiology and control of *Acinetobacter baumannii* in health care facilities. Clin Infect Dis 2006;42(5):692–699

4. Hartzell JD, Kim AS, Kortepeter MG, Moran KA. *Acinetobacter* pneumonia: a review. MedGenMed 2007;9(3):4

5. Leung WS, Chu CM, Tsang KY, Lo FH, Lo KF, Ho PL. Fulminant community-acquired *Acinetobacter baumannii* pneumonia as a distinct clinical syndrome. Chest 2006;129(1):102–109

CASE 58

■ Clinical Presentation

19-year-old woman with AIDS, employed as an equestrian trainer, with a CD4 count of 140 cells/µL presenting with fever, cough, increasing fatigue, and chest pain

■ Radiologic Findings

PA (**Fig. 58.1A**) and lateral (**Fig. 58.1B**) chest radiographs show focal region of lobar consolidation in the right middle lobe. Note the absence of appreciable volume loss, air bronchograms, and pleural effusion.

■ Diagnosis

Rhodococcus equi Pneumonia

■ Differential Diagnosis

*   Other Community-Acquired and Opportunistic Infections
*   *M. tuberculosis*
*   Various Fungal Infections
*   Primary and Secondary Lung Neoplasia

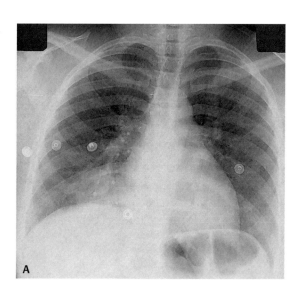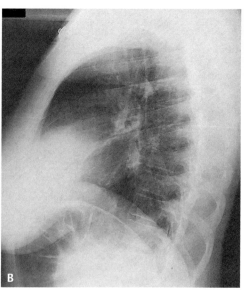

Fig. 58.1

■ Discussion

Background

Rhodococcus equi primarily causes zoonotic infections in grazing animals, namely horses and foals. Although *R. equi* rarely infects immunocompetent humans, it is emerging as an important pathogen in immunocompromised persons, especially those with AIDS and a CD4 count <200 cells/mm^3. Human infection results from inhalation of contaminated aerosols.

Etiology

R. equi is an aerobic, Gram-positive or Gram-variable, weakly acid-fast coccobacillus. It is found worldwide in the soil and in feces of some animals, especially horses. Thirty percent of infected persons have a history of animal exposure, particularly to horses.

Clinical Findings

Eighty to 90% of patients with *R. equi* infection are immunocompromised. Approximately 50–60% of these patients are HIV-positive, 15–20% have lymphoma, leukemia, or other underlying malignancies, and 10% are transplant recipients. Symptoms in immunocompetent patients are similar to those in immunocompromised patients. Necrotizing pneumonia is the most common pulmonary manifestation of infection. Affected patients have fever and cough (>80%). Fatigue, chest pain, dyspnea, hemoptysis, and weight loss may also occur. Extrapulmonary manifestations of *R. equi* infection include abscesses (e.g., soft tissues, brain, retroperitoneum), meningitis, pericarditis, endophthalmitis, lymphadenitis, osteomyelitis, septic arthritis, etc. *R. equi* infections occur in all age groups, with a mean age of 34–38 years. *Risk factors* for infection in immunocompetent patients include chronic renal insufficiency, alcoholism, and diabetes. Approximately 50% of *R. equi* infections in immunocompetent patients are due to trauma. Although the diagnosis of *R. equi* infection may be established from analysis of sputum, blood cultures, bronchial lavage fluid, or other infected tissue, the organism may be inadvertently dismissed as a contaminant.

Imaging Findings

Chest Radiography

- Multiple nodular air space opacities progressing to cavitation-abscess (54–77%)
- Dense parenchymal consolidation (**Figs. 58.1A, 58.1B**)
- Interstitial pneumonia
- Multifocal pulmonary opacities involving the bronchi consistent with tracheobronchial dissemination
- Pleural effusion; up to 20% of cases
- Mediastinal lymphadenopathy; not uncommon
- HIV-AIDS
  - Upper lobes preferentially involved; 55% of cases
  - Lower lobes; 35% of cases
  - Cavitation-abscess formation more common (67–77%)
- Immunocompetent patients
  - No definite lobar predilection

MDCT

- More sensitive; reveals more nodules and cavitation than conventional radiography
- Cavitation; single or multiple; thick-walled and may demonstrate air-fluid levels, indicating progression to abscess (**Figs. 58.2A, 58.2B**)
- Mediastinal lymphadenopathy; not uncommon

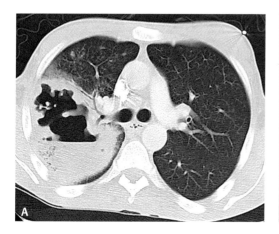 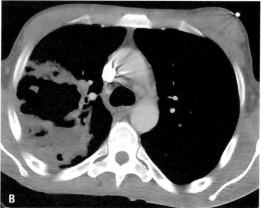

Fig. 58.2   Contrast-enhanced chest CT (**A**, lung window; **B**, mediastinal window) demonstrate thick-walled irregular cavity with an air-fluid level in the right upper lobe in this 35-year-old man with AIDS and *R. equi* lung abscess. Subtle centrilobular and air space nodules are seen in the upper lobe more anteriorly.

Management

- Mainstay is treatment of underlying infection with antibiotics and surgical therapy
- *R. equi* is usually *susceptible* to:
  - Erythromycin and azithromycin
  - Clarithromycin and ciprofloxacin
  - Vancomycin and aminoglycosides
  - Rifampin and imipenem
  - Meropenem and linezolid
- *R. equi* is usually *resistant* to:
  - Penicillin G and ampicillin
  - Carbenicillin and cefazolin
- *R. equi* pneumonia
  - Surgical treatment alone: no obvious benefit
  - Lobectomy or partial lung resection reserved for cases in which infection has evolved into large abscess or when infection is overwhelming
- Extrapulmonary *R. equi* infection
  - Local surgical resection or debridement recommended:
  - Endophthalmitis
  - Osteomyelitis
  - Subcutaneous abscess/paravertebral abscess
  - Pericardial effusion

Prognosis

- Extrapulmonary relapse: 13% of patients with *R. equi* pneumonia
- Complications include: pulmonary malakoplakia (i.e., unusual inflammatory disorder with accumulation of characteristic histiocytes with calcified lamellar Michaelis-Gutman bodies) and abscess formation
- Immunocompetent patients: 11% mortality
- Immunocompromised patients without HIV-infection: 20–25% mortality
- Immunocompromised patients with HIV-infection: 50–55% mortality

PEARLS

- Acid-fast nature/presence of aerial hyphae leads to misdiagnosis of *Nocardia* infection.
- Necrotizing pneumonia is the most common pulmonary manifestation of *R. equi* infection.

- *R. equi* can initially cause interstitial pneumonia mimicking *Pneumocystis jiroveci* pneumonia in HIV-positive patients.
- *R. equi* cavitary pneumonia in HIV-positive or neutropenic patients is often mistaken for fungal pneumonia.
- Immunocompromised/immunosuppressed patients should avoid contact with horses and foals, pastures, stalls, and barns.

Suggested Reading

1. Cornish N, Washington JA. *Rhodococcus equi* infections: clinical features and laboratory diagnosis. Curr Clin Top Infect Dis 1999;19:198–215

2. Haramati LB, Jenny-Avital ER. Approach to the diagnosis of pulmonary disease in patients infected with the human immunodeficiency virus. J Thorac Imaging 1998;13(4):247–260

3. Mayor B, Jolidon RM, Wicky S, Giron J, Schnyder P. Radiologic findings in two AIDS patients with *Rhodococcus equi* pneumonia. J Thorac Imaging 1995;10(2):121–125

4. Travis WD, Colby TV, Koss MN, Rosado-de-Christenson ML, Muller NL, King TE Jr. Lung infections. In: King DW, ed. Atlas of Nontumor Pathology: Non-Neoplastic Disorders of the Lower Respiratory Tract. First series, fascicle 2. Washington, DC: American Registry of Pathology; 2002:569–571

5. Wicky S, Cartei F, Mayor B, et al. Radiological findings in nine AIDS patients with *Rhodococcus equi* pneumonia. Eur Radiol 1996;6(6):826–830

CASE 59

■ Clinical Presentation

55-year-old man with history of alcohol and drug abuse presents with chronic cough, low-grade fever, and weight loss

■ Radiologic Findings

Posteroanterior (PA) (**Fig. 59.1A**) and lateral (**Fig. 59.1B**) chest radiographs demonstrate a large left upper lobe cavity with irregular nodular borders and adjacent pleural thickening. Note right lower lobe, lingular, and left lower lobe consolidations. Coned-down unenhanced chest CT (lung window) (**Figs. 59.1C, 59.1D**) demonstrates the irregular left upper lobe cavity (**Fig. 59.1C**) and tree-in-bud and centrilobular nodules in the lingula, left lower, and right lower lobes (**Fig. 59.1D**) consistent with endobronchial spread of pulmonary infection.

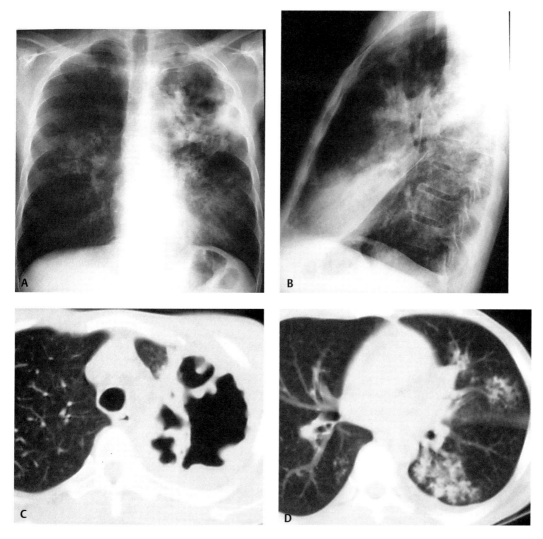

Fig. 59.1

304

■ Diagnosis

Mycobacterium tuberculosis

■ Differential Diagnosis

- Non-Tuberculous Mycobacterial Infection
- Other Necrotizing Pulmonary Infections (fungi, atypical organisms)
- Lung Abscess with Multifocal Bronchiolitis

■ Discussion

Background

Tuberculosis is the leading cause of death from infectious disease worldwide. More than two billion people (one-third of the world population) are infected, with approximately nine million new cases and nearly two million deaths reported annually and most of these occurring in developing countries. Tuberculosis is a worldwide pandemic, but over half of all new cases are reported in Asia and Africa. Approximately 1.4 million affected patients were infected with HIV in 2007, most of these in the African region. In the United States, approximately 13,000 new cases were reported in 2008, with a case rate per 100,000 population of approximately 4.2. Individuals at risk in the United States include those in ethnically diverse populations, immigrants, minorities, the homeless, the immunocompromised (particularly HIV-infected patients), and the elderly.

Etiology

Tuberculosis is caused by *M. tuberculosis,* an aerobic rod transmitted from person to person through inhalation of droplets containing tubercle bacilli. The organisms are initially deposited in the mid and lower lung zone alveoli, multiply within macrophages, and disseminate via lymphatic and hematogenous routes. Cell-mediated immunity develops up to 10 weeks after initial infection. Most patients contain their disease, but approximately 5% develop active tuberculosis within the first or second year after initial infection and approximately 10% develop active disease in their lifetime. Progression to active infection is more common in HIV-infected individuals, with a risk of up to 10% per year. Infection may also occur through re-activation of organisms that survive in areas of high oxygen tension or via exogenous exposure.

Clinical Findings

Patients with latent tuberculosis infection are asymptomatic and have a positive tuberculin skin test, but do not have active tuberculosis infection and are not infectious. These patients may be diagnosed via whole blood interferon-γ assay, which provides higher diagnostic accuracy than the traditional skin tests. Patients with tuberculosis disease have clinical, radiologic, and/or laboratory evidence of infection. The old concepts of primary and post-primary tuberculosis have been challenged, as tuberculosis infection worldwide is not likely to represent a single infectious event and re-infection is likely frequent. However, the nomenclature remains useful in categorizing the imaging manifestations of the disease. The radiologic features associated with primary and post-primary (or reactivation) tuberculosis correlate better with the host immune status than with the time elapsed since initial infection. Thus, severely immunocompromised patients typically exhibit the "primary pattern" of tuberculosis whereas immunocompetent individuals often exhibit the "post-primary pattern" of infection. The majority of patients with tuberculosis have pulmonary involvement. Extrapulmonary tuberculosis is more common in children and immunosuppressed patients. Affected patients may remain asymptomatic or present with a severe symptomatic pneumonia after initial infection. Patients with pulmonary tuberculosis may have an indolent clinical course and often present with cough, chest pain, and hemoptysis. Systemic complaints may include fever, chills, night sweats, anorexia, weight loss, weakness, and malaise. The diagnosis of tuberculosis is based on the identification of *M. tuberculosis* in body fluids or tissue.

Imaging Findings

Radiography

- Primary pattern of tuberculosis
  - Consolidation: usually unilateral (**Fig. 59.2**), dense, homogeneous; segmental, lobar, or multifocal; may be associated with ipsilateral lymphadenopathy (**Fig. 59.2**); rapidly progressive cavitary consolidation
  - Lymphadenopathy: typically unilateral, usually right hilar or right paratracheal; most common in children (**Fig. 59.2**)
  - Atelectasis: usually lobar and right-sided (30% of affected children)
  - Unilateral (typically self-limited) pleural effusion
  - Visualization of Ghon focus or Ranke complex (lung lesion and ipsilateral lymph nodes)
  - Miliary nodules
- Post-primary pattern of tuberculosis
  - Consolidation (**Figs. 59.1A, 59.1B**): patchy, heterogeneous, involving apical and posterior segments of upper lobes (85%) and superior segments of lower lobes (14%), ill-defined borders, satellite nodules
  - Cavitation (20–45%), thin or thick walls (**Figs. 59.1A, 59.1B**), focal or multifocal, air-fluid levels (while cavitation is traditionally considered a manifestation of the post-primary pattern disease, it also occurs in patients with the primary pattern of disease, particularly adolescents and young adults)
  - Nodular and linear opacities
  - Multifocal ill-defined 5–10 mm air space nodular opacities (**Figs. 59.1A, 59.1B**)
  - Tuberculoma; solitary (or multiple) pulmonary nodule, variable size, well-defined or ill-defined margins, may exhibit calcification
  - Pleural involvement; unilateral loculated pleural effusion, pleural calcification, may remain stable for years
  - Miliary nodules
- Normal chest radiographs, particularly in immunocompromised patients

MDCT/HRCT

- Central low attenuation; peripheral enhancement of affected lymph nodes
- Visualization of cavitation (**Figs. 59.1C, 59.3A, 59.3B, 59.4**)
- Linear branching opacities and centrilobular nodules (2–4 mm) (tree-in-bud) from endobronchial spread of infection (**Figs. 59.1D, 59.3A, 59.3B**); associated with cavitary disease
- Ill-defined nodules (4–8 mm), lobular consolidations, thick interlobular septa (**Figs. 59.3A, 59.3B, 59.5**)
- Miliary nodules (1–3 mm) with random distribution, thick nodular interlobular septa (**Fig. 59.5**)
- Tuberculoma: rim enhancement, calcification in 30%, satellite lesions in 80%
- Bronchial narrowing with mural thickening (**Fig. 59.3A**); upper lobe predominant bronchiectasis, may be severe
- Empyema; pleural calcification, bronchopleural fistula, empyema necessitatis

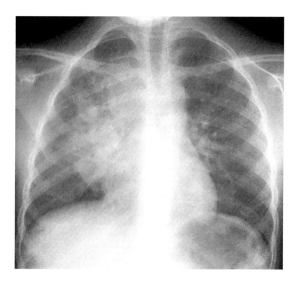

Fig. 59.2 PA chest radiograph of a 9-year-old boy with tuberculosis demonstrates a coalescent right perihilar consolidation with ipsilateral hilar and mediastinal lymphadenopathy.

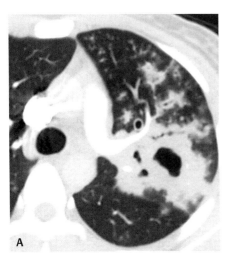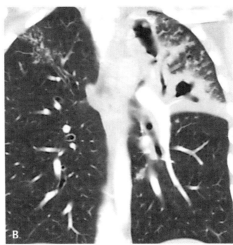

Fig. 59.3   Coned-down axial and coronal contrast-enhanced chest CT (lung windows) of a young woman with tuberculosis demonstrates a dominant left upper lobe cavitary mass with thick nodular walls surrounded by centrilobular nodules and tree-in-bud opacities. Note nodular bronchostenosis of left upper lobe bronchi **(A)** and focal cellular bronchiolitis in the right upper lobe **(B)** consistent with endobronchial dissemination of infection.

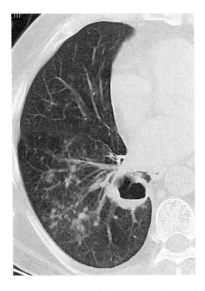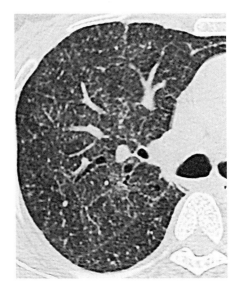

Fig. 59.4   Coned-down unenhanced chest CT (lung window) of an asymptomatic 45-year-old man with active tuberculosis demonstrates a right lower lobe thin-walled cavity with an air-fluid level and surrounding tree-in-bud centrilobular nodular opacities consistent with endobronchial spread of infection.

Fig. 59.5   Coned-down unenhanced chest CT (lung window) of a 50-year-old woman with miliary tuberculosis shows multifocal well-defined tiny pulmonary nodules randomly distributed throughout the lung.

- End-stage lung disease
- Mycetoma formation in chronic cavities
- Rarely fibrosing mediastinitis; pericardial calcification
- Evidence of old healed tuberculosis; dense or calcified lung nodules, upper lobe focal fibrosis, volume loss, bronchiectasis (may contain slowly multiplying *M. tuberculosis* organisms)
- Chest wall involvement; tuberculous spondylitis

Angiography

- Evaluation and treatment of significant hemoptysis
  - Identification of hypertrophied bronchial arteries and embolization
  - Identification of Rasmussen (pulmonary artery) aneurysm and embolization

Nuclear Scintigraphy

- Uptake of ^{18}F-FDG on PET imaging; false-positive findings for malignancy
- ^{11}C-choline PET imaging for differentiation between lung cancer and tuberculosis, low standard uptake values in tuberculomas

Management

- First-line drugs: isoniazid, rifampin, ethambutol, and pyrazinamide
- Treatment with a combination of first-line drugs with initial phase of 2 months and continuation phase of 4–7 months
- Latent tuberculosis infection: 6–12 months of isoniazid (occasionally rifampin and pyrazinamide) in selected patients in the United States
- Directly observed therapy (DOT): improved compliance and prevention of drug resistance in endemic areas and selected U.S. populations

Prognosis

- Adequate therapy; excellent prognosis, prevention of disease transmission
- Guarded prognosis in infections with drug-resistant strains

PEARLS

- Tuberculosis must be included in the differential diagnosis of patients with HIV-AIDS who exhibit intrathoracic lymphadenopathy. These patients are also more likely to manifest endobronchial spread of disease, miliary disease, extrapulmonary involvement, and a normal chest radiograph.
- Imaging findings in cases with delayed diagnosis of tuberculosis include normal radiograph, nodule or mass, parenchymal abnormalities attributed to inactive disease, isolated pleural effusion, isolated lymphadenopathy, and parenchymal abnormalities in unusual locations.
- Nodules, large cavities, consolidation, and ground glass opacity are associated with smear positivity.
- Healing may result in cicatricial atelectasis and lung destruction, typically affecting the upper lobe with hilar retraction and compensatory lower lobe hyperinflation. Linear opacities, nodules, traction bronchiectasis and pleural thickening can be encountered.
- Multidrug-resistant tuberculosis (MDR-TB) is resistant to isoniazid and rifampicin, and affected patients more commonly exhibit multifocal cavitary disease and imaging findings of chronicity, such as bronchiectasis and calcification. Extensively drug-resistant tuberculosis (XDR-TB) is resistant to isoniazid and rifampin, any fluoroquinolone, and at least one of three injectable second-line drugs (amikacin, kanamycin, or capreomycin).

Suggested Reading

1. Burrill J, Williams CJ, Bain G, Conder G, Hine AL, Misra RR. Tuberculosis: a radiologic review. Radiographics 2007;27(5):1255–1273

2. Jeong YJ, Lee KS. Pulmonary tuberculosis: up-to-date imaging and management. AJR Am J Roentgenol 2008;191(3): 834–844

3. Kim HY, Song K-S, Goo JM, Lee JS, Lee KS, Lim TH. Thoracic sequelae and complications of tuberculosis. Radiographics 2001;21(4):839–858, discussion 859–860

4. Ors F, Deniz O, Bozlar U, et al. High-resolution CT findings in patients with pulmonary tuberculosis: correlation with the degree of smear positivity. J Thorac Imaging 2007;22(2):154–159

5. Saurborn DP, Fishman JE, Boiselle PM. The imaging spectrum of pulmonary tuberculosis in AIDS. J Thorac Imaging 2002;17(1):28–33

CASE 60

■ Clinical Presentation

40-year-old woman with cough and weight loss

■ Radiologic Findings

PA chest radiograph (**Fig. 60.1A**) demonstrates middle lobe air space disease, a right apical thin-walled cavity, and multifocal bilateral lung nodules. Unenhanced thin-section chest CT (lung window) (**Figs. 60.1B, 60.1C, 60.1D**) demonstrates a thin-walled right apical lung cavity with surrounding architectural distortion (**Fig. 60.1B**), middle lobe atelectasis with intrinsic bronchiectasis (**Fig. 60.1D**), and scattered lung nodules with irregular borders (**Fig. 60.1C**).

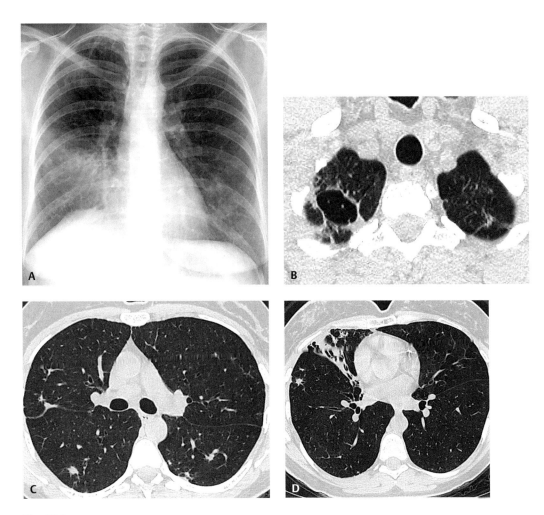

Fig. 60.1

309

■ Diagnosis

Mycobacterium avium-intracellulare Pulmonary Infection

■ Differential Diagnosis

- Other Pulmonary Infections (including tuberculosis, other non-tuberculous mycobacteria, and aspergillus)

■ Discussion

Background

Mycobacteria other than *M. tuberculosis* cause pulmonary and systemic infection in immunocompetent and immunocompromised individuals. These organisms occur ubiquitously in the environment (soil, water, plants, and animals).

Etiology

Non-tuberculous mycobacterial infections are produced by a variety of mycobacteria, including *M. avium-intracellulare* (MAI), *M. avium* complex (MAC), *M. kansasii, M. fortuitum, M. cheloneae, M. abscessus,* and *M. xenopi.* It is thought that infection occurs from environmental exposures as there are no documented cases of person-to-person transmission. Infection may occur through inhalation or via the gastrointestinal tract.

Clinical Findings

Nontuberculous mycobacterial pulmonary infection may exhibit various imaging manifestations depending on the patient population affected. The *classic form* of infection typically affects elderly Caucasian men with underlying chronic lung disease and is indistinguishable from pulmonary tuberculosis. The bronchiectatic form of infection (*non-classic*) typically affects elderly Caucasian non-smoking women. The so-called Lady Windermere syndrome is attributed to inspissated secretions resulting from voluntary cough suppression. Immunocompromised patients (typically those with the AIDS) and patients with deglutition problems may also be affected. In addition, hypersensitivity pneumonitis has been described in patients exposed to indoor hot tubs. Symptoms are often insidious and include cough, dyspnea, hemoptysis, and weight loss. Diagnostic criteria are based on clinical symptoms in the setting of nodular and cavitary lesions on radiography and multifocal bronchiectasis and small nodules on thin-section CT, supported by bacteriologic findings after exclusion of other diagnoses. Microbiologic criteria include positive cultures from at least two separate sputum samples or from at least one bronchial washing or lavage, or a transbronchial or lung biopsy positive for mycobacteria or showing typical histologic features (in addition to one or more positive culture (s) from sputum or bronchial washings).

Imaging Findings

Radiography

*Classic form (*Fig. 60.1A*)*

- Upper lobe (apical and posterior segment) cavitary disease
- Linear and nodular opacities
- Upper lobe volume loss
- Pleural thickening

*Non-classic form (*Fig. 60.1A*)*

- Multifocal small nodules
- Bronchiectasis and subsegmental/segmental atelectasis with preferential middle lobe and lingular involvement

Immunocompromised Patients (HIV-AIDS)

- Mediastinal/hilar lymphadenopathy
- Normal chest radiograph
- Consolidation, miliary nodules, pleural effusion

Hypersensitivity Pneumonitis

- Fine nodular, reticular-nodular opacities
- Consolidation

MDCT/HRCT

Classic form (Fig. 60.1B)

- Upper lobe (apical and posterior segment) cavitary disease
- Multifocal centrilobular nodules adjacent to cavities
- Cicatricial atelectasis
- Bronchiectasis
- Pleural thickening

Non-classic form (Figs. 60.1C, 60.1D, 60.2A, 60.2B)

- Multifocal centrilobular nodules, tree-in-bud opacities
- Bronchiectasis, bronchiolectasis with or without mucus plugging
- Middle lobe and lingular involvement and volume loss

Immunocompromised Patients (HIV-AIDS)

- Mediastinal/hilar lymphadenopathy; may exhibit low-attenuation centers
- Normal chest radiograph
- Consolidation, miliary nodules, pleural effusion

Hypersensitivity pneumonitis (Fig. 60.3)

- Diffuse bilateral ill-defined ground glass centrilobular nodules
- Diffuse ground glass opacities
- Expiratory air trapping

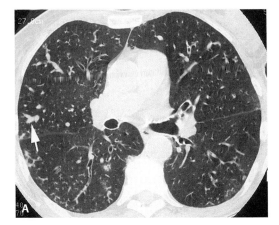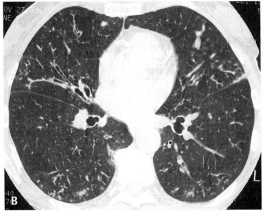

Fig. 60.2   Unenhanced chest CT (lung window) of an elderly woman with *M. avium* complex pulmonary infection demonstrates bronchiectasis and multifocal small pulmonary nodules. Note the mucus-filled dilated bronchi (*arrow*). *(Images courtesy of Diane C. Strollo, MD, University of Pittsburgh Medical Center, Pittsburgh, Pennsylvania.)*

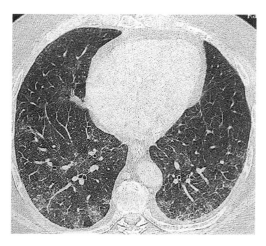

Fig. 60.3 Unenhanced HRCT (lung window) of an elderly man who developed dyspnea after consistent use of an indoor hot tub demonstrates patchy ground glass opacities and mosaic attenuation found to be secondary to hypersensitivity to *M. avium* complex recovered from the hot tub water.

Management

- Antimycobacterial drug therapy
- Pulmonary resection in selected cases

Prognosis

- Progression of untreated disease
- Colonized patients with repeated positive cultures may remain clinically stable
- Poor prognosis with severe underlying lung disease and disseminated infection in immunocompromised patients

Suggested Reading

1. Martinez S, McAdams HP, Batchu CS. The many faces of pulmonary nontuberculous mycobacterial infection. AJR Am J Roentgenol 2007;189(1):177–186

2. Jeong YJ, Lee KS, Koh W-J, Han J, Kim TS, Kwon OJ. Nontuberculous mycobacterial pulmonary infection in immunocompetent patients: comparison of thin-section CT and histopathologic findings. Radiology 2004;231(3):880–886

3. Koh W-J, Lee KS, Kwon OJ, Jeong YJ, Kwak SH, Kim TS. Bilateral bronchiectasis and bronchiolitis at thin-section CT: diagnostic implications in nontuberculous mycobacterial pulmonary infection. Radiology 2005;235(1):282–288

4. Travis WD, Colby TV, Koss MN, Rosado-de-Christenson ML, Müller NL, King TE Jr. Lung infections. In: King DW, ed. Atlas of Nontumor Pathology: Non-Neoplastic Disorders of the Lower Respiratory Tract, fasc 2, ser 1. Washington, DC: American Registry of Pathology and Armed Forces Institute of Pathology, 2001:539–727

OVERVIEW OF FUNGAL PNEUMONIAS

Fungal pneumonia is a lung infection caused either by *endemic* or *opportunistic fungi*. *Endemic fungi* occur in specific geographic locations around the world. In the United States, *endemic fungi* are prevalent in the Mississippi River Valley, the Ohio River Valley, and the southwest, and include pathogens such as *Histoplasma capsulatum, Coccidioides immitis, Blastomyces dermatitidis,* and *Paracoccidioides brasiliensis.* Such pathogens may cause lung infections in both immunocompetent and immunosuppressed persons. *Opportunistic fungi* are ubiquitous and tend to cause pneumonia in immunosuppressed and immunocompromised individuals (e.g., HIV-AIDS, chronic pulmonary disease, underlying neutropenia and or neoplasia, patients receiving chemotherapy or on chronic corticosteroid therapy, etc). *Opportunistic pathogens* include but are not limited to *Aspergillus* sp., *Pneumocystis jiroveci, Candida* sp., *Cryptococcus neoformans,* and *Mucor* sp. Pulmonary fungal infection occurs through four mechanisms: (1) inhalation of spores, (2) inhalation of conidia, (3) reactivation of latent infection, and (4) hematogenous dissemination. *Endemic fungal pneumonias* tend to be self-limited in immunocompetent persons but may be complicated by cavities, empyema, and bronchopleural fistula. *Opportunistic fungal pneumonia* has greater morbidity, and case fatality rates may approach 90%. This section will focus on some of the more common fungal pneumonias encountered in both healthy individuals and those with altered immune systems and defenses.

CASE 61

■ Clinical Presentation

Asymptomatic 30-year-old woman evaluated for an enlarging lung lesion

■ Radiologic Findings

PA chest radiograph (**Fig. 61.1A**) demonstrates a multi-lobulated left lower lobe nodule and ipsilateral calcified hilar lymph nodes. Contrast-enhanced chest CT (mediastinal and lung windows) (**Figs. 61.1B, 61.1C, 61.1D**) demonstrates clustered non-enhancing left lower lobe nodules with intrinsic round calcifications. The clustered nature of the lesions is best visualized on the coronal reformatted CT image (**Fig. 61.1D**).

■ Diagnosis

Histoplasmosis

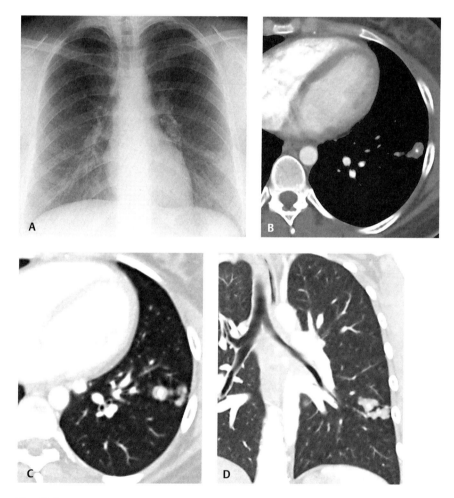

Fig. 61.1

314

■ Differential Diagnosis

- Granulomas; Other Fungal Infections
- Granulomas; Tuberculosis

■ Discussion

Background

Histoplasmosis is a fungal infection endemic to the south-central United States, especially the Mississippi and Ohio River valleys.

Etiology

Histoplasmosis is caused by *Histoplasma capsulatum*, a dimorphic fungus transmitted through inhalation of airborne spores typically released from infected soil enriched by bird droppings or guano. Inhaled organisms multiply within macrophages and undergo lymphatic and hematogenous dissemination. Cellular immunity develops within two weeks, with subsequent healing.

Clinical Findings

The vast majority of histoplasmosis infections are self-limited and do not produce symptoms. A small percentage of individuals experience an intense point-source exposure and present with fever, headache, myalgia, chest pain, and cough. Severe illness resembling acute respiratory distress syndrome may also occur. Chronic histoplasmosis typically affects middle-aged Caucasian men with a history of cigarette smoking and emphysema who present with cough, dyspnea, night sweats, and/or hemoptysis. Broncholithiasis may result in chronic cough, hemoptysis, and post-obstructive pneumonia. Disseminated histoplasmosis affects immunocompromised patients, who develop fever, weight loss, anorexia, malaise, cough, and organomegaly.

Imaging Findings

Radiography

Acute Histoplasmosis

- Focal or multifocal ill-defined consolidations; focal or multifocal lung nodules
- Lymphadenopathy
- Diffuse bilateral opacities with heavy exposures; may heal with calcification

Histoplasmoma (Fig. 61.1A)

- Single or multiple well-defined pulmonary nodules (0.5–3 cm)
- Central, diffuse, or concentric calcification
- Ipsilateral calcified hilar/mediastinal lymph nodes

Chronic Histoplasmosis (Fig. 61.2)

- Segmental or subsegmental apical consolidations
- Nodular or linear opacities
- Thick-walled apical bullae
- Upper lobe volume loss

Disseminated Histoplasmosis

- Miliary nodules
- Irregular linear opacities
- Air space opacities; may progress to diffuse consolidation

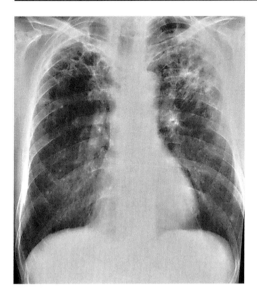

Fig. 61.2 PA chest radiograph of a 42-year-old man with chronic histoplasmosis and hemoptysis demonstrates bilateral asymmetric upper lobe predominant consolidations with intrinsic cavitation and architectural distortion and multiple bilateral scattered calcified pulmonary granulomas.

MDCT

Histoplasmoma (Figs. 61.1B, 61.1C, 61.1D)

- Nodule with central, diffuse, or laminated calcification; frequent satellite nodules
- Peripheral subpleural location, typically in posterior lower lobes

Lymphadenopathy

- Identification of calcification
- Broncholithiasis: endobronchial calcified or ossified material; typically from erosion of adjacent calcified lymph nodes with resultant atelectasis or consolidation

Disseminated Disease (Fig. 61.3)

- Random miliary micronodules (1–3 mm)

Scintigraphy

- Increased uptake of ^{18}F-FDG on PET imaging

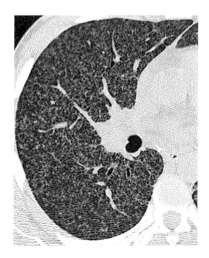

Fig. 61.3 Coned-down unenhanced chest CT of a 28-year-old man with AIDS, chills, fever, and disseminated histoplasmosis demonstrates profuse bilateral miliary pulmonary micronodules.

Management

- Antifungal therapy for chronic and disseminated histoplasmosis
- Lobectomy or segmentectomy for symptomatic broncholithiasis

Prognosis

- Good prognosis in self-limited infections
- Guarded prognosis in disseminated and progressive chronic disease

Suggested Reading

1. Gurney JW, Conces DJ Jr. Pulmonary histoplasmosis. Radiology 1996;199(2):297–306
2. Lindell RM, Hartman TE. Fungal infections. In: Müller NL, Silva CIS, Hansell DM, Lee KS, Remy-Jardin M, eds. Imaging of the Chest. Philadelphia: Saunders Elsevier; 2008:356–380
3. Seo JB, Song K-S, Lee JS, et al. Broncholithiasis: review of the causes with radiologic-pathologic correlation. Radiographics 2002;22(Spec No):S199–S213
4. Travis WD, Colby TV, Koss MN, Rosado-de-Christenson ML, Müller NL, King TE Jr. Lung infections. In: King DW, ed. Atlas of Nontumor Pathology: Non-Neoplastic Disorders of the Lower Respiratory Tract, fasc 2, ser 1. Washington, DC: American Registry of Pathology and Armed Forces Institute of Pathology, 2001:539–727

CASE 62

■ Clinical Presentation

78-year-old man from Arizona with cough, myalgias, and headache

■ Radiologic Findings

PA chest radiograph (**Fig. 62.1A**) demonstrates ill-defined nodular opacities in the right middle and lower lung zones. Unenhanced chest CT (lung window) (**Fig. 62.1B**) demonstrates a wedge-shaped right lower lobe consolidation and bilateral small pulmonary nodules. Unenhanced chest CT (lung window) (**Fig. 62.1C**) obtained six months after presentation demonstrates improvement of the right lower lobe consolidation with a residual pulmonary nodule as well as multiple right middle lobe centrilobular nodules. HRCT (**Fig. 62.1D**) obtained one year after presentation demonstrates a well-defined right lower lobe solitary pulmonary nodule in the region of the former right lower lobe consolidation.

■ Diagnosis

Coccidioidomycosis

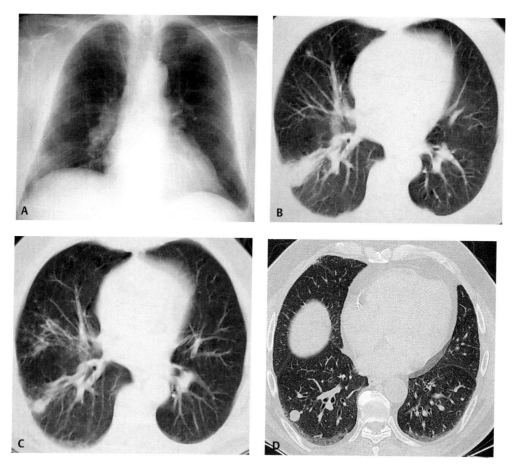

Fig. 62.1

318

■ Differential Diagnosis

- Other Fungal Infection
- Tuberculosis

■ Discussion

Background

Coccidioidomycosis is a highly infectious fungal disease endemic to the southwestern United States, northern and central Mexico, and Central and South America. It is estimated that there are 100,000 new cases of infection each year in the United States.

Etiology

Coccidioidomycosis is caused by *Coccidioides immitis*, a multimorphic fungus transmitted through inhalation of infected soil, typically in dry, hot climates.

Clinical Findings

Most patients (80%) with *primary coccidioidomycosis* are asymptomatic. Symptomatic patients with primary infection present with non-specific symptoms, including fever, cough, chest pain, and headache. *Valley fever* occurs in up to 20% of patients with symptomatic coccidioidomycosis and manifests with erythema nodosum, erythema multiforme, arthralgia, and occasional eosinophilia. Patients with *chronic coccidioidomycosis* have a prolonged symptomatic course with cough, weight loss, fever, and hemoptysis. *Disseminated disease* preferentially affects African Americans, Filipinos, pregnant women, and immunosuppressed patients, particularly those with AIDS. These patients may develop a severe pulmonary illness as well as skin, osseous, renal, and/or central nervous system involvement.

Imaging Findings

Primary Coccidioidomycosis

- Focal or multifocal, unilateral lower lobe consolidation (**Figs. 62.1A, 62.1B, 62.1C**)
- Lymphadenopathy in 20%
- Healing with pulmonary nodule (granuloma) (**Fig. 62.1D**) or chronic thin-walled ("grape skin") cavity (may change size over time) (**Figs. 62.2A, 62.2B**)
- Pleural effusion, typically small

Chronic Coccidioidomycosis (Figs. 62.2A, 62.2B)

- Upper lobe involvement
- Small nodular or linear opacities
- Single or multiple thin-walled cavities
- Volume loss

Disseminated Coccidioidomycosis (Fig. 62.3)

- Multifocal nodules and/or reticular opacities
- Miliary nodules

Scintigraphy

- Increased uptake of ^{18}F-FDG on PET imaging

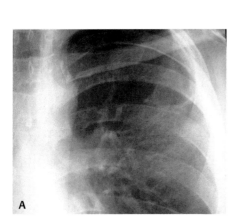
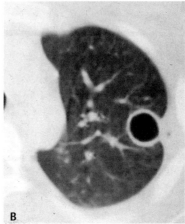

Fig. 62.2 Coned-down PA chest radiograph **(A)** of a 22-year-old man with chronic coccidioidomycosis demonstrates a thin-walled left upper lobe cavity. Coned-down unenhanced chest CT (lung window) **(B)** demonstrates the thin-walled cavity and adjacent pleural thickening.

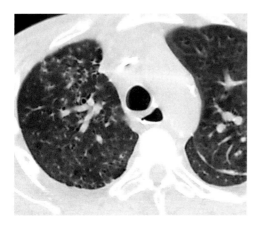

Fig. 62.3 Coned-down chest CT (lung window) of an immunocompromised patient with disseminated coccidioidomycosis demonstrates right upper lobe pulmonary micronodules and nodular pleural thickening of the left oblique fissure.

Management

- Fluconazole for acute uncomplicated disease
- Amphotericin B for disseminated disease and immunocompromised patients
- Surgical excision of chronic cavitary lesions, particularly in cases of hemoptysis or pleuropulmonary involvement

Prognosis

- Favorable prognosis with self-limited infection
- Poor prognosis with disseminated disease and impaired immunity

Suggested Reading

1. Lindell RM, Hartman TE. Fungal infections. In: Müller NL, Silva CIS, Hansell DM, Lee KS, Remy-Jardin M, eds. Imaging of the Chest. Philadelphia: Saunders Elsevier; 2008:356–380

2. Travis WD, Colby TV, Koss MN, Rosado-de-Christenson ML, Müller NL, King TE Jr. Lung infections. In: King DW, ed. Atlas of Nontumor Pathology: Non-Neoplastic Disorders of the Lower Respiratory Tract, fasc 2, ser 1. Washington, DC: American Registry of Pathology and Armed Forces Institute of Pathology; 2001:539–727

3. Wilde GE, Emery C, Lally JF. Radiological reasoning: miliary disease, vertebral osteomyelitis, and soft-tissue abscesses. AJR Am J Roentgenol 2008;190(3, Suppl):S11–S17

CASE 63

■ Clinical Presentation

39-year-old man with cough, fever, chills, and skin lesions

■ Radiologic Findings

PA chest radiograph (**Fig. 63.1A**) demonstrates a large mass-like consolidation in the right perihilar region affecting the right upper and lower lobes. Coned-down contrast-enhanced chest CT (lung window) (**Figs. 63.1B, 63.1C**) demonstrates a mass-like consolidation in the right lower lobe with central air bronchograms (**Fig. 63.1B**) and multifocal pulmonary nodules in the right lower and middle lobes (**Fig. 63.1C**). Note trace bilateral pleural effusions.

■ Diagnosis

Blastomycosis

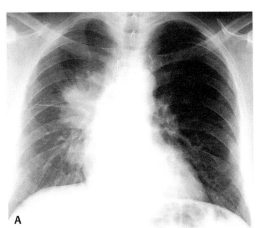

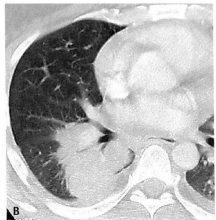

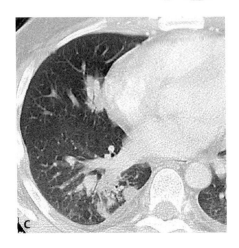

Fig. 63.1

321

■ Differential Diagnosis

- Primary Lung Cancer
- Lung Abscess
- Round Pneumonia

■ Discussion

Background

North American blastomycosis is a fungal infection endemic to the Mississippi and Ohio River valleys, the midwestern United States, the Canadian provinces near the Great Lakes, and the Saint Lawrence River valley, as well as other regions of the Americas, Europe, and Asia. The fungus grows in nitrogen-rich soil in wooded areas near streams, rivers, and lakes.

Etiology

Blastomycosis is caused by *Blastomyces dermatitidis*, a fungus acquired by inhalation of infected soil. Many outbreaks occur near recreational water.

Clinical Findings

Sporadic cases of blastomycosis are most common in adult men who engage in outdoor activities, but patients of all ages may become infected in highly endemic areas. Most symptomatic patients present with a subacute or chronic illness with low-grade fever, cough, hemoptysis, chest pain, night sweats, and/or weight loss. Affected patients may also present acutely with signs and symptoms resembling bacterial pneumonia: fever, cough, and pleuritic pain. Less frequently, patients may present with a self-limited flu-like illness or with a fulminant infection resulting in acute respiratory distress syndrome with high fever and hypoxemia. Infected individuals may be entirely asymptomatic. Late reactivation of disease may result in skin and osseous involvement.

Imaging Findings

Radiography

- Consolidation (**Fig. 63.1A**): focal, multifocal, patchy, or confluent; may be diffuse and slowly progressing with air bronchograms and satellite lesions
- Mass or nodule: focal, multifocal; when solitary may mimic lung cancer (**Fig. 63.1A**)
- Cavitation (15%)
- Interstitial nodular or micronodular opacities, miliary nodules
- Pleural thickening common, pleural effusion (10–15%)
- Rarely calcification or lymphadenopathy

MDCT

- Focal or multifocal mass(es) (**Fig. 63.1C**)
- Focal or multifocal consolidation(s) (**Figs. 63.1B, 63.1C**)
- Perihilar distribution (**Fig. 63.1B**)
- Air bronchograms (88%) (**Figs. 63.1B, 63.1C**)
- Nodules (**Figs. 63.1C, 63.2A**), centrilobular nodules with tree-in-bud opacities, satellite lesions (**Figs. 63.2A, 63.2B**)
- May demonstrate calcification in lymph nodes and pulmonary lesions
- Uncommon cavitation (**Fig. 63.2A**) and hilar/mediastinal lymphadenopathy
- Pleural effusion (**Figs. 63.1B, 63.1C**)

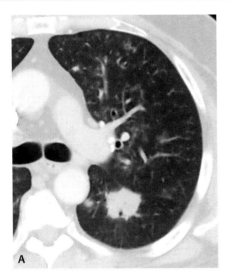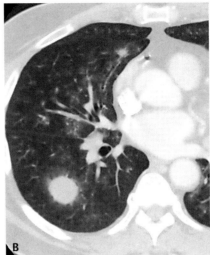

Fig.63.2 Contrast-enhanced chest CT (lung window) of a 58-year-old man with blastomycosis demonstrates multifocal pulmonary nodules and masses with ground glass opacity surrounding the right lower lobe mass (*CT halo sign*) **(B)** and a focus of cavitation in the left lower lobe mass **(A)**. Note multifocal middle and left upper lobe ground glass centrilobular nodules.

Scintigraphy

- Increased uptake of ¹⁸F-FDG on PET imaging; may mimic lung cancer

Management

- Oral itraconazole in most patients
- Severe acute presentation; amphotericin B

Prognosis

- Favorable prognosis in mild or self-limited infection even without therapy
- 90% cure rates in treated patients
- Poor prognosis with overwhelming infection, systemic dissemination, and/or immunocompromised patients

PITFALLS

- Slow radiographic and clinical improvement, absence of change, and/or progression should prompt exclusion of infectious granulomatous disease in patients undergoing treatment for presumed typical bacterial pneumonia.

Suggested Reading

1. Fang W, Washington L, Kumar N. Imaging manifestations of blastomycosis: a pulmonary infection with potential dissemination. Radiographics 2007;27(3):641–655

2. Lindell RM, Hartman TE. Fungal infections. In: Müller NL, Silva CIS, Hansell DM, Lee KS, Remy-Jardin M, eds. Imaging of the Chest. Philadelphia: Saunders Elsevier; 2008:356–380

3. Travis WD, Colby TV, Koss MN, Rosado-de-Christenson MI, Müller NL, King TE Jr. Lung infections. In: King DW, ed. Atlas of Nontumor Pathology: Non-Neoplastic Disorders of the Lower Respiratory Tract, fasc 2, ser 1. Washington, DC: American Registry of Pathology and Armed Forces Institute of Pathology; 2001:539–727

CASE 64

■ Clinical Presentation

67-year-old man with hemoptysis and prior tuberculosis

■ Radiologic Findings

Coned-down PA chest radiograph (**Fig. 64.1A**) demonstrates a cavitary left apical lesion with an intrinsic soft-tissue nodule and an air-fluid level. Coned-down unenhanced chest CT (lung window) (**Figs. 64.1B, 64.1C**) demonstrates a left apical thick-walled cavitary lesion with an intrinsic dependent soft-tissue nodule and small cavitary satellite nodules. Note adjacent pleural thickening as well as left apical centrilobular and paraseptal emphysema.

■ Diagnosis

Aspergillosis; Mycetoma

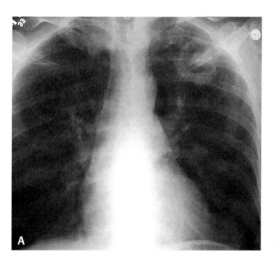
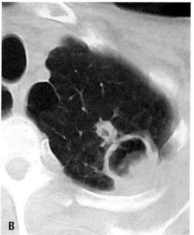
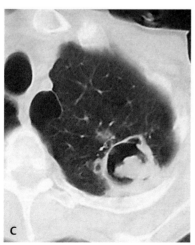

Fig. 64.1

■ Differential Diagnosis

- Mycetoma; Secondary to Other Fungi
- Chronic Necrotizing Aspergillosis
- Cavitary Lung Cancer with Necrotic Lung or Mycetoma Formation

■ Discussion

Background

The fungi classified as *Aspergillus* species occur worldwide and may produce disease through colonization of abnormal lung tissue or through vascular and tissue invasion in immunocompromised individuals.

Etiology

Aspergillosis is typically caused by three major species of fungi: *Aspergillus fumigatus, A. flavus,* and *A. niger.*

Clinical Findings

The clinical spectrum of *Aspergillus* infection is dependent upon the integrity of the host's immune system (**Table 64.1**). Patients with *saprophytic aspergilloma* (mycetoma, fungus ball) usually have a normal immunity and abnormal lung parenchyma, typically cavitary lung disease often secondary to tuberculosis or sarcoidosis. These patients may be entirely asymptomatic or may present with hemoptysis, which may be massive. *Angioinvasive aspergillosis* typically occurs in patients with severe neutropenia (absolute neutrophil count $<500 \times 10^3$/mL) who present with fever, dyspnea, cough, and chest pain. *Chronic necrotizing (semi-invasive) aspergillosis* affects patients with severe underlying lung disease who present with fever, productive cough, and dyspnea. *Allergic bronchopulmonary aspergillosis* is a hypersensitivity reaction (types I and III) to *Aspergillus* organisms in the tracheobronchial tree. Affected patients may have cystic fibrosis or chronic asthma and may present with wheezing, fever, productive cough, and chest pain. *Aspergillus* may produce necrotizing pseudomembranous tracheobronchitis (airway-invasive aspergillosis) in a small percentage of immunocompromised patients (neutropenia, AIDS) who present with dyspnea, wheezing, and cough.

Imaging Findings

Radiography

*Mycetoma (***Fig. 64.1A***)*

- Gravity-dependent soft-tissue nodule or mass within preexisting cavity
- *Air crescent sign*: crescent of air along non-dependent aspect of cavity surrounding the mycetoma
- Thin-walled cavities with focal mural thickening or air-fluid levels
- Adjacent pleural thickening

Angioinvasive Aspergillosis

- Normal radiographs in early disease
- Focal or multifocal pulmonary nodules or masses with ill-defined borders; may progress and coalesce
- Segmental or lobar consolidation

Table 64.1 Spectrum of Pulmonary *Aspergillus* Infection

Immune Status	Condition
Normal	Aspergilloma (mycetoma)
Hypersensitive	Allergic bronchopulmonary aspergillosis (ABPA)
Immunosuppressed (mild)	Chronic necrotizing aspergillosis
Immunosuppressed (severe)	Invasive pulmonary aspergillosis

- Cavitation during recovery from chemotherapy-induced neutropenia, intracavitary soft-tissue mass (necrotic lung) surrounded by a crescent of air

Chronic Necrotizing Aspergillosis

- Upper lobe consolidation with slowly progressive cavitation
- Intracavitary soft-tissue mass, adjacent pleural thickening

Allergic Bronchopulmonary Aspergillosis (ABPA)

- Upper lobe–predominant central tubular or branching opacities
- Intracavitary soft-tissue mass, adjacent pleural thickening

MDCT/HRCT

Mycetoma (Figs. 64.1B, 64.1C)

- Early lesions; focal or multifocal thickening of cavity wall
- Mobility of mycetoma within lung cavity or adherence to cavity wall
- Heterogeneous attenuation from calcification or air trapped within interstices in mycetoma
- Complete obliteration of cavity by intracavitary fungal mass
- Adjacent pleural thickening

Angioinvasive Aspergillosis

- Focal or multifocal nodules, masses, or consolidations with ill-defined borders
- *Halo sign*; ground glass attenuation surrounding nodules/consolidations (**Fig. 64.2**)
- Direct visualization of vascular occlusion with multidetector CT angiography
- Cavitation with air crescent around homogeneous intracavitary soft-tissue mass (necrotic lung); occurs during recovery from neutropenia (**Fig. 64.3**)
- Pleural effusion
- Chest wall, mediastinal invasion

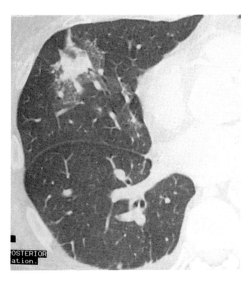

Fig. 64.2 HRCT targeted at the right lung of a neutropenic man with invasive aspergillosis demonstrates an irregular pulmonary nodule surrounded by ground glass opacity (*CT halo sign*).

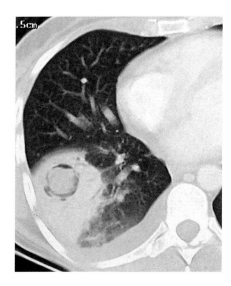

Fig. 64.3 Coned-down contrast-enhanced chest CT (lung window) of a 43-year-old woman with leukemia and invasive aspergillosis demonstrates a wedge-shaped consolidation in the right lower lobe with peripheral air bronchograms, central cavitation, an intracavitary soft-tissue nodule, and an ipsilateral pleural effusion.

Chronic Necrotizing Aspergillosis

- Lobar/segmental consolidation, ground glass opacity
- Bronchial wall thickening
- Multifocal pulmonary nodules with peripheral ground glass opacity
- Multiple cavities

Allergic Bronchopulmonary Aspergillosis (ABPA)

- Bronchiectasis
- Endobronchial non-enhancing soft-tissue or mucus plug; may exhibit high attenuation and/or cavitation (Case 25, Case 27)

Management

- Mycetoma: surgical excision, bronchial artery embolization to control hemoptysis, intracavitary instillation of antifungal agents
- Angioinvasive aspergillosis: first-line treatment—voriconazole (or other antifungal) with discontinuation of immunosuppressive if possible

Prognosis

- Mycetoma: good prognosis in symptomatic and treated patients; rarely death from massive hemoptysis
- Chronic necrotizing aspergillosis: indolent course
- Angioinvasive aspergillosis: generally poor prognosis, but recovery reported with early diagnosis, reversal of immunosuppression, and antifungal therapy

PEARLS

- Angioinvasive aspergillosis should be considered in the setting of severe neutropenia, signs and symptoms of infection, and new pulmonary abnormalities.
- Lesions of angioinvasive aspergillosis may show progression in size and number for up to nine days in spite of adequate treatment. Lesion cavitation is a marker of bone marrow recovery and correlates with improved prognosis. However, cavitary disease characteristically demonstrates slow resolution.

PITFALLS

- CT *halo sign* is *not* pathognomonic for angioinvasive fungal infection and has been described in other infections, vasculitides, neoplasms, and lymphoproliferative disorders.

Suggested Reading

1. Brodocfel H, Vogel M, Hebart H, et al. Long-term CT follow-up in 40 non-HIV immunocompromised patients with invasive pulmonary aspergillosis: kinetics of CT morphology and correlation with clinical findings and outcome. AJR Am J Roentgenol 2006;187(2):404–413

2. Franquet T, Müller NL, Giménez A, Guembe P, de La Torre J, Bagué S. Spectrum of pulmonary aspergillosis: histologic, clinical, and radiologic findings. Radiographics 2001;21(4):825–837

3. Martinez S, Heyneman LE, McAdams HP, Rossi SE, Restrepo CS, Eraso A. Mucoid impactions: finger-in-glove sign and other CT and radiographic features. Radiographics 2008;28(5):1369–1382

4. Sonnet S, Buitrago-Téllez CH, Tamm M, Christen S, Steinbrich W. Direct detection of angioinvasive pulmonary aspergillosis in immunosuppressed patients: preliminary results with high-resolution 16-MDCT angiography. AJR Am J Roentgenol 2005;184(3):746–751

5. Travis WD, Colby TV, Koss MN, Rosado-de-Christenson ML, Müller NL, King TE Jr. Lung infections. In: King DW, ed. Atlas of Nontumor Pathology: Non-Neoplastic Disorders of the Lower Respiratory Tract, fasc 2, ser 1. Washington, DC: American Registry of Pathology and Armed Forces Institute of Pathology; 2001:539–727

CASE 65

■ Clinical Presentation

42-year-old debilitated woman with advanced AIDS, cryptococcal meningitis, minimally productive cough, and fever.

■ Radiologic Findings

PA (**Fig. 65.1A**) and lateral (**Fig. 65.1B**) chest radiographs demonstrate subtle areas of air space disease in the left upper, right middle, and left lower lobes. No pleural effusion or lymphadenopathy is present. Chest CT (lung window) (**Figs. 65.1C, 65.1D, 65.1E**) confirms the presence of ground glass and nodular opacities in the left upper lobe, lingula, right middle and lower lobes, and frank left lower lobe consolidation with associated bronchial dilatation.

■ Diagnosis

Cryptococcal Pneumonia

■ Differential Diagnosis

- *Pneumocystis jiroveci* Pneumonia
- *Mycobacterium tuberculosis*
- *Histoplasma capsulatum*
- *Blastomyces dermatitidis*
- Other Fungal and Atypical Bacterial Pneumonias

■ Discussion

Background

The genus *Cryptococcus* contains more than 50 species; however, only *C. neoformans* and *Cryptococcus gattii* are considered human pathogens. Each species has five serotypes. *C. neoformans* is an encapsulated yeast found worldwide and is the most common species in the United States and other temperate climates. *C. neoformans* is found in soil, and soil contaminated with pigeon droppings in particular. *C. gattii* is found primarily in tropical and subtropical climates and can be isolated from certain species of eucalyptus trees. The virulence of cryptococcal infection depends on the immune system of the infected individual. *C. neoformans* serotype A causes most cryptococcal infections in immunocompromised patients, including patients with HIV-AIDS. Alternatively, *C. gattii* usually infects immunocompetent individuals.

Etiology

Cryptococcal infection is most often acquired by inhalation of airborne spores of *Cryptococcus neoformans*. Person-to-person transmission has not been documented.

Clinical Findings

Cryptococcal infection takes two major clinical forms: pulmonary infection and cerebromeningeal infection due to hematogenous spread from the lungs. Most patients with cryptococcal disease have meningitis. The

328

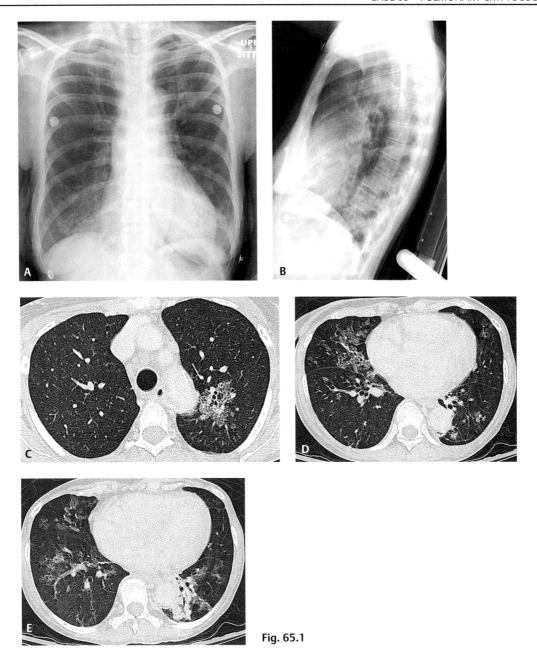

Fig. 65.1

most serious infections occur in patients with defective cell-mediated immunity. Those individuals with HIV-AIDS, organ transplantation, reticuloendothelial neoplasia, diabetes, or sarcoidosis or who are undergoing chronic corticosteroid therapy tend to develop the most serious cryptococcal infections. *Cryptococcosis* is a life-threatening fungal infection in HIV-AIDS patients. Approximately 7–15% of patients with HIV-AIDS develop cryptococcal infections, and patients with AIDS-associated cryptococcal infection account for 80–90% of all patients with cryptococcosis. Immunocompetent patients with pulmonary cryptococcosis may present with mild-to-moderate symptoms, including low-grade fever, malaise, cough (54%), cough with scant sputum production (30%), and pleuritic chest pain (46%). HIV-AIDS patients with cryptococcal lung infection more often have fever (80%), cough (60%), dyspnea (50%), headache, and weight loss.

Imaging Findings

Variable Presentations

- Focal nodule or mass with ill-defined or well-defined borders
- Multi-focal peripheral nodules or masses
- Unilateral or bilateral consolidation with or without air bronchograms; upper lobe predilection (**Figs. 65.1A, 65.1B, 65.1C, 65.1D, 65.1E**)
- Bronchial obstruction with distal atelectasis
- Reticular/reticulonodular opacities, miliary nodules, cavitation, calcification, pleural effusion, intrathoracic lymphadenopathy; more common in the immunocompromised

Management

- Intravenous amphotericin B combined with 5-fluorocytosine
- Surgical excision of lung nodules; select cases

Prognosis

- 14% mortality rate in patients with cryptococcal disease treated with amphotericin B and 5-fluorocytosine
- 28% mortality rate in patients treated with other regimens
- *C. gatti* strain infection in immunocompetent patients; greater mortality

PEARLS

- Patients with pulmonary cryptococcosis who develop focal mass-like pulmonary lesions and concomitant cerebromeningitis may have radiologic features misinterpreted as primary lung cancer with brain metastases.

Suggested Readings

1. Colen RR, Singer AE, McLoud TC. Cryptococcal pneumonia in an immunocompetent patient. AJR Am J Roentgenol 2007;188(3):W281–W282

2. Himmel JE, Stark P. Cryptococcal pneumonia in an immunocompetent host: radiographic findings. Semin Respir Infect 2003;18(2):129–131

3. Travis WD, Colby TV, Koss MN, Rosado-de-Christenson ML, Muller NL, King TE Jr. Lung infections. In: King DW, ed. Atlas of Nontumor Pathology: Non-Neoplastic Disorders of the Lower Respiratory Tract, first series, fascicle 2. Washington, DC: American Registry of Pathology; 2002:600–605

CASE 66

■ Clinical Presentation

26-year-old man with HIV-AIDS, CD4 count of 14 cells/μL, fever, non-productive cough, and dyspnea

■ Radiologic Findings

PA (**Fig. 66.1A**) and lateral (**Fig. 66.1B**) chest radiographs demonstrate patchy, bilateral, perihilar ground glass and reticular-nodular opacities without lymphadenopathy or pleural effusions.

■ Diagnosis

Pneumocystis jiroveci Pneumonia

■ Differential Diagnosis

- Mycoplasma Pneumonia
- Various Viral Pneumonias
- *Mycobacterium avium* Complex Pneumonia
- *Histoplasmosis* Pulmonary Infection
- *Cryptococcus* Pulmonary Infection
- Lymphocytic Interstitial Pneumonia (LIP)

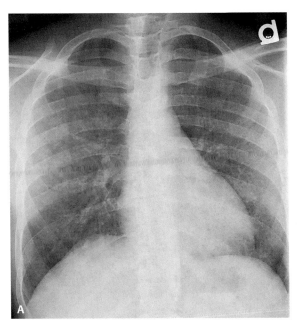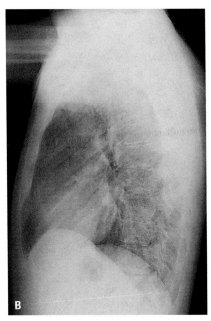

Fig. 66.1

■ Discussion

Background

Pneumocystis pneumonia (PCP) is caused by the yeast-like fungus *Pneumocystis jiroveci* (yee-row-vet-zee), named after the Czech parasitologist Otto Jirovec. The organism was previously misclassified as a proto-zoan and called *Pneumocystis carinii*. However, use of that nomenclature is now considered incorrect, as *Pneumocystis carinii* infection only occurs in animals, not humans. *Pneumocystis* infection has a worldwide distribution. *Pneumocystis* is commonly found in the lungs of immunocompetent individuals but usually causes infections only in those with altered immune systems. *Risk factors* for pulmonary infection include congenital or acquired disorders of cell-mediated immunity, organ transplantation, chemotherapy for hema-tologic or lymphoreticular neoplasia, and AIDS. *Pneumocystis jiroveci* is the second most common cause of pneumonia in AIDS patients and infects up to 80% of patients at some time during the course of their illness. *Pneumocystis* pneumonia is an AIDS-defining diagnosis.

Etiology

Pneumocystis pneumonia is likely acquired through inhalation of airborne respiratory secretions. *Pneumo-cystis jiroveci* causes subclinical infection in most persons during childhood. Latent infection develops into opportunistic pneumonia when an individual becomes immunosuppressed. The possibility of person-to-person transmission has been suggested but not yet definitively proven.

Clinical Findings

The clinical presentation of infected patients is variable. Signs and symptoms may be mild, but disease may be fulminant and may rapidly progress to respiratory failure. Patients with AIDS and *Pneumocystis* pneumo-nia tend to have a more indolent course. Non-productive cough (95%), dyspnea (95%), and fever (80%) are common symptoms and signs. Hypoxemia occurs in 80–95% of infected patients, and the DLCO is invariably diminished. Ninety percent (90%) of HIV-infected patients have an elevated lactate dehydrogenase (LDH) level, with a mean value of 375 ± 23 IU/L. Complications of *Pneumocystis* pneumonia include secondary spon-taneous pneumothorax, which complicates approximately 12% of infections and is a poor prognostic sign. Cytomegalovirus (CMV) pneumonia is the most common associated concomitant infection. The presump-tive diagnosis of *Pneumocystis* pneumonia can made by a combination of hypoxemia and its characteristic appearance on chest radiography in a patient with appropriate risk factors. Definitive diagnosis is made by histologic identification of the organism in the sputum or on BAL, by immunofluorescent staining of the specimen, and more recently by polymerase chain reaction (PCR) product molecular analysis. In addition to pulmonary infection, *Pneumocystis* may infect almost any other organ system.

Imaging Findings

Chest Radiography

Earliest Radiographic Manifestations

- Bilateral, symmetric, hazy or reticular opacities emanate from perihilar regions (**Figs. 66.1A, 66.1B**)
- Abnormalities can be diffuse
- Often there is perihilar, lower lung predominance (**Figs. 66.1A, 66.1B**)
- Less commonly, an upper lung predominance
- Pleural effusions and lymphadenopathy are characteristically absent (**Figs. 66.1A, 66.1B**)

More Advanced Cases

- Diffuse hazy and reticular opacities
- Slightly asymmetric but overall typical distribution
- Left untreated or if patient has been ill for some time, ground glass pattern of opacities may progress into multifocal air space consolidation

Other Unusual Patterns

- Upper lobe predominant disease
- Focal consolidation (**Fig. 66.2**)
- Nodules

MDCT/HRCT

- Multifocal ground glass opacities; most common manifestation (**Figs. 66.3, 66.4A, 66.4B, 66.4C**)
- Involvement tends to be bilateral (**Figs. 66.3, 66.4A, 66.4B, 66.4C**)
- Can be diffuse and homogeneous or patchy and asymmetric (**Figs. 66.3, 66.4A, 66.4B, 66.4C**)
- Superimposed patchy air space consolidation
- Often intervening areas of normal lung parenchyma; sharply marginated by interlobular septa (**Fig. 66.3**)
- "Crazy paving" pattern (**Fig. 66.3**)
- Nodules in bilateral upper lobes
- Pneumatoceles or thin-walled cysts (**Figs. 66.4A, 66.4B, 66.4C**)
  - Develop in 5–35% of patients
  - Range from 1 to 10 cm in diameter; walls ≤1 mm in thickness
  - Usually in upper lobes
  - Most cysts resolve over five days to one year (average five months); some might not change
  - Predispose to spontaneous pneumothoraces (5–10%); pneumomediastinum
- With healing, *P. jiroveci* may rarely lead to interstitial pulmonary fibrosis
- Pleural effusions (<17%) (**Figs. 66.4A, 66.4B, 66.4C**)
- Hilar and or mediastinal lymphadenopathy (<25%)

Management

- Preferred prophylaxis: trimethoprin-sulfamethoxazole
- Trimethoprin-sulfamethoxazole and intravenous pentamidine for acute infection
- Early administration of glucocorticoids within hours of beginning pharmacotherapy reduces risk of respiratory failure and death by more than 50% in hypoxic patients
- Other medications used, alone or in combination, include pentamidine, trimetrexate, and dapsone

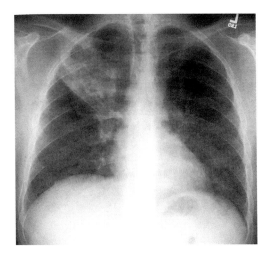

Fig. 66.2 PA chest radiograph of a 39-year-old man with AIDS, endobronchial *Pneumocystis jiroveci* infection, and post-obstructive pneumonia demonstrates focal right upper lobe consolidation and diffuse bilateral reticular opacities. Bronchoscopy revealed a right upper lobe endobronchial mass secondary to *Pneumocystis jiroveci*.

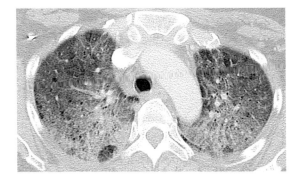

Fig. 66.3 Chest CT (lung window) in a patient with *Pneumocystis jiroveci* infection shows diffuse "crazy paving" pattern throughout both lungs with some intervening regions of minimally spared lung. Subtle subcentimeter cystic lesions are also present.

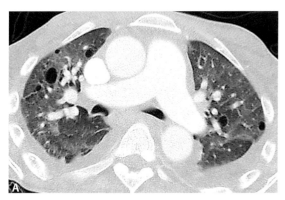
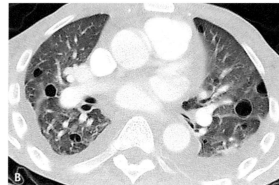
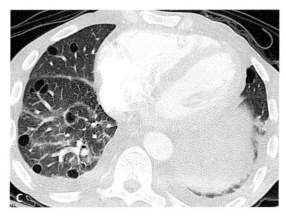

Fig. 66.4 Chest CT (lung windows) of a 44-year-old man with AIDS, CD4 count of 210 cells/μL, and *Pneumocystis* pneumonia reveals a background of bilateral, symmetric ground glass opacities and numerous variable-size thin-walled cystic lesions throughout both lungs. Note the uncommon bilateral pleural effusions.

Prognosis

- Usually favorable, with 50–90% survival rate if appropriately treated
- Incidence of *Pneumocystis* pneumonia has diminished with standard prophylaxis
- Poor prognosis in patients with rising LDH levels despite appropriate therapy
- Relapses in 50–75% of patients with AIDS and 10–20% of immunosuppressed patients without additional pharmacotherapy

PEARLS

- HIV-infected patients with CD4 counts <200 cells/μL are five times (5X) more likely to develop *Pneumocystis* pneumonia than patients with CD4 counts >200 cells/μL.

Suggested Readings

1. Hardak E, Brook O, Yigla M. Radiological features of *Pneumocystis jirovecii* pneumonia in immunocompromised patients with and without AIDS. Lung 2010;188(2):159–163
2. Demirkazik FB, Akin A, Uzun O, Akpinar MG, Ariyürek MO. CT findings in immunocompromised patients with pulmonary infections. Diagn Interv Radiol 2008;14(2):75–82
3. Luks AM, Neff MJ. *Pneumocystis jiroveci* pneumonia. Respir Care 2007;52(1):59–63
4. Tasaka S, Tokuda H, Sakai F, et al. Comparison of clinical and radiological features of *Pneumocystis* pneumonia between malignancy cases and acquired immunodeficiency syndrome cases: a multicenter study. Intern Med 2010;49(4): 273–281

OVERVIEW OF VIRAL PNEUMONIAS

Viral infections are the *most common* cause of symptomatic disease in children and adults. They cause a wide spectrum of illness, ranging from the common cold to pneumonia, and are associated with significant morbidity and mortality. The *most frequent* causes of viral pneumonia, in order of frequency, in adults are (1) the influenza virus, (2) respiratory syncytial virus (RSV), (3) adenovirus, and (4) the parainfluenza virus (PIV). Influenza virus types A (including the H1N1 subtype) and B are responsible for cases during influenza outbreaks. Less common causes of viral pneumonia include SARS *coronavirus, herpes simplex* virus (HSV), *herpes zoster* virus (HZV), cytomegalovirus (CMV), and hantavirus. Viruses are the *most common* cause of pneumonia in children, whereas in adults bacteria are a more common cause (see Cases 49–56). Viral pathogens cause 13–50% of virus-related community-acquired pneumonias and 8–27% of combined bacterial-viral infectious pneumonias. Immunocompromised patients are more susceptible to infection with CMV, HSV, HZV, influenza, RSV, and parainfluenza virus. Viruses enter the body through inhalation of aerosolized droplets in the nose and mouth. The virus must then invade the cells to replicate. The subsequent effects on the lung and immune system can extend to other systems, leading to constitutional symptoms and predisposing individuals to secondary bacterial infections. In the past, the diagnosis of viral pneumonia was made primarily on clinical findings. Today, diagnostic tests exist establishing the clinical diagnosis of viral pneumonias with a high level of confidence. Improved prevention and management strategies have also become available. This section will focus on some of the more common viral pneumonias encountered in both immunocompetent and immunosuppressed individuals.

Suggested Reading

1. Jennings LC, Anderson TP, Beynon KA, et al. Incidence and characteristics of viral community-acquired pneumonia in adults. Thorax 2008;63(1):42–48
2. Johnstone J, Majumdar SR, Fox JD, Marrie TJ. Viral infection in adults hospitalized with community-acquired pneumonia: prevalence, pathogens, and presentation. Chest 2008;134(6):1141–1148

CASE 67

■ Clinical Presentation

46-year-old woman admitted to the hospital with three-day history of progressive dyspnea, cough productive of whitish-yellow sputum, pleuritic chest pain, fever, and chills

■ Radiologic Findings

Baseline admission PA (**Fig. 67.1A**) and lateral (**Fig. 67.1B**) chest X-rays demonstrate subtle bilateral perihilar reticular opacities, right more so than left, and patchy, ill-defined consolidation in the right base paralleling the right heart border. Follow-up PA (**Fig. 67.1C**) and lateral (**Fig. 67.1D**) chest radiographs two days later reveal rapid progression of disease. Extensive ill-defined patchy and confluent consolidations are now present bilaterally. Note the absence of pleural effusion.

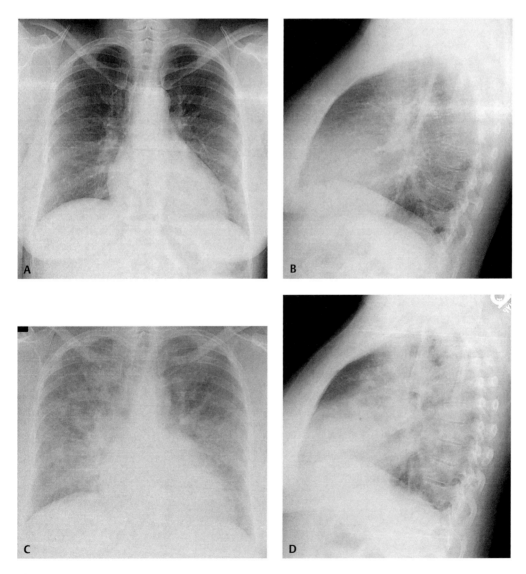

Fig. 67.1

336

■ Diagnosis

Influenza Pneumonia

■ Differential Diagnosis

• Other Viral Pneumonias
• Various Atypical Pneumonias

■ Discussion

Background

Influenza Virus

The influenza virus is a leading respiratory pathogen that affects persons of all ages and is responsible for annual epidemics worldwide.

Etiology

Seasonal influenza is an acute respiratory illness that occurs primarily during winter months. *Influenza pneumonia* is caused by the influenza virus, an RNA virus. Three types (A, B, and C) are identified based on antigenic differences in internal proteins. Most human infections are caused by types A and B. Type A is the most virulent and can be divided into various antigenic subtypes based on the presence of two structurally, functionally, and genetically distinct surface glycoproteins: hemagglutinin (H) and neuraminidase (N). Variations of these surface glycoproteins result in evasion of pre-existing host immunity (*antigenic drift*) and in the emergence of viruses to which there is no pre-existing immunity (*antigenic shift*). *Antigenic drift* is responsible for annual winter outbreaks. *Antigenic shift* is responsible for influenza pandemics. The influenza epidemic of 1918 killed 20–40 million people and accounted for 80% of the deaths in the U.S. Army in World War I. The virus is highly contagious and transmitted from person to person via inhalation of infected airborne secretions or contact with infected secretions. The incubation period is only 24–48 hours, allowing for rapid spread of the disease.

H1N1 Virus

The novel swine-origin influenza type A (H1N1) virus (S-OIV), also referred to as "swine flu" by the lay press and media, and was first reported in Mexico in April 2009. Infection rapidly spread to many other countries around the world prompting the World Health Organization (WHO) to declare the emergence of a global pandemic by June 2009. As of the May 30, 2010 WHO update, more than 214 countries and overseas territories or communities reported laboratory confirmed cases of pandemic influenza H1N1 2009, including over 18,138 deaths. H1N1 is a highly contagious acute respiratory disease, spread similarly to that of seasonal influenza viruses, which includes person-to-person large-particle respiratory droplet transmission produced by coughing or sneezing or touching contaminated surfaces. The incubation period is 1–7 days.

Clinical Findings

Influenza Pneumonia

Affected patients have an acute presentation with fever, chills, prostration, myalgias, arthralgias, malaise and headache. By the end of the first week, rhinorrhea, sore throat, and dry cough develop. During the second week of illness, patients develop non-productive cough, and easy fatigability. Infection in immunocompetent patients typically follows a self-limited course. Adults with underlying chronic diseases, women in the third trimester of pregnancy and immunosuppressed patients may develop severe life-threatening pneumonia often complicated by secondary bacterial infection. Systemic complications, including Guillain-Barre syndrome, toxic shock syndrome and Reyes' syndrome, may also occur.

H1N1

In contrast to seasonal influenza, which typically affects persons of extreme ages (i.e., young children and the elderly), H1N1 commonly affects the young to middle-aged. Affected patients are considered infectious one day before and seven days after the onset of symptoms. Clinical features vary and include flu-like symptoms such as fever and chills, cough, sore throat, myalgias, headache, and fatigue. Some patients also experience nausea, vomiting, and diarrhea. Most patients have mild illness. Infection in high-risk patients more often follows a severe and complicated course that can result in respiratory failure and death. The time course between hospital admission and the need for mechanical ventilatory support can be less than 24 hours in some case. High-risk groups include children under 5 years of age, adults 65 years of age and older, patients with underlying chronic disease (e.g., asthma, COPD, diabetes, heart disease, and renal disease), the immunosuppressed, and obese patients with a body mass index (BMI) ≥30. Laboratory findings include lymphopenia, elevated serum LDH and creatinine kinase levels, and sometimes thrombocytopenia. Although sepsis and ARDS represent hypercoagulable states, acute PTE disease is not a common complication of seasonal influenza but has a reported increased prevalence in severely ill patients with H1N1.

Imaging Findings

Chest Radiography

Influenza Pneumonia

- Perihilar reticular (**Figs. 67.1A, 67.1B**) or reticular nodular opacities
- Poorly defined lower lobe segmental consolidation
- Ill-defined patchy consolidation; may rapidly progress to confluent lung disease (**Figs. 67.1A, 67.1B, 67.1C, 67.1D**)
- Patchy areas of air space consolidation; 1–2 cm diameter; rapidly become confluent
- Lung involvement may be unilateral or bilateral (**Figs. 67.1A, 67.1B, 67.1C, 67.1D**)
- Pleural effusion rare

H1N1

- Normal in more than 50% of patients
- Abnormal: bilateral disease (71%); unilateral disease (29%) (**Figs. 67.2A, 67.2B, 67.2C, 67.2D, 67.2E**)
- Patchy consolidation (50%) (**Figs. 67.2A, 67.2B, 67.2C, 67.2D, 67.2E**)
- Ground glass alone (25%); mixture of ground glass and consolidation (25%) (**Figs. 67.2A, 67.2B, 67.2C, 67.2D, 67.2E**)
- Ill-defined nodular opacities, 1–2 cm in diameter; rapidly become confluent (**Figs. 67.2C, 67.2D**)
- Lower lung zone predilection (71%); diffuse (25%)
- Central lung zones (71%)
- More extensive disease (≥3 lung zones) in patients requiring mechanical ventilation (**Figs. 67.2A, 67.2B, 67.2C, 67.2D, 67.2E**)
- No significant lymph node enlargement
- Pleural effusion (8%)

MDCT/HRCT

Influenza Pneumonia

- Bilateral areas of ground glass attenuation with a lobular distribution
- Multi-focal peribronchovascular or juxtapleural consolidation
- Air space nodules
- Small centrilobular nodules representing alveolar hemorrhage
- Diffuse ground glass opacities with irregular linear areas of increased attenuation

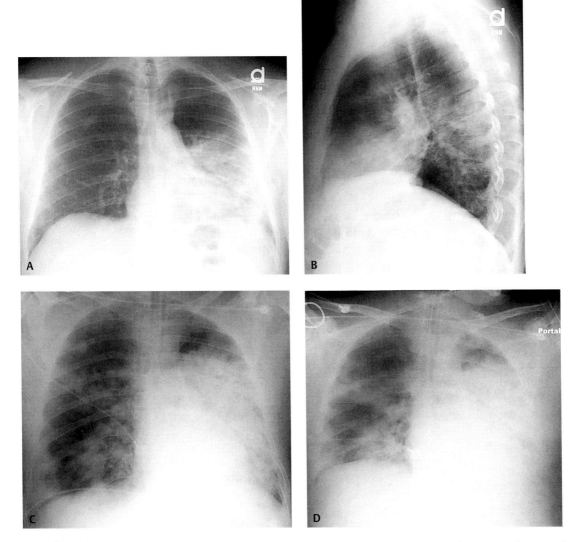

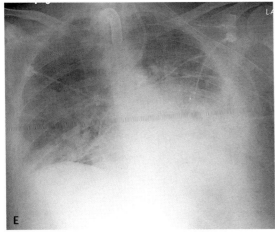

Fig. 67.2   42-year-old man with acute myelogenous leukemia and laboratory confirmed S-OIV (H1N1). **(A)** PA and **(B)** lateral chest X-rays demonstrate a mixture of patchy ground glass and air space consolidations involving primarily the left lower lobe and lingula. Left upper lobe involved to a lesser extent. Note the absence of pleural effusion and lymphadenopathy. By hospital day 2 the patient required intubation and mechanical ventilatory support. **(C)** AP chest exam shows progression to confluent disease in the left lung and evolution of patchy nodular opacities and consolidations throughout the right lung but more concentrated in the lower lobe. **(D)** Chest exam on hospital day 4 reveals more confluent progression of disease in the right lung. By hospital day 10, the patient required tracheostomy. There was no clinical or radiographic **(E)** improvement and progressive respiratory failure followed. The patient did not survive.

H1N1

- Pattern resembles that seen with severe acute respiratory syndrome (SARS) (**Figs. 67.3A, 67.3B, 67.3C**)
- Unilateral or bilateral ground glass opacities with or without associated focal or multi-focal consolidations (**Figs. 67.3A, 67.3B, 67.3C**)
  - Peribronchovascular and juxtapleural distribution resembling organizing pneumonia; most common (**Figs. 67.3A, 67.3B, 67.3C**)
  - Other patterns
    - Diffuse without zonal predominance
    - Basal or axial predominance
- No centrilobular nodules or tree-in-bud opacities
- No mediastinal or hilar lymph node enlargement
- Pleural effusion uncommon

Management

Influenza Pneumonia

- Prevention through annual vaccination with inactivated influenza virus, particularly elderly patients and those with chronic disease
- Supportive therapy with bed rest, antipyretics, hydration, and antitussives
- Antiviral drugs in high-risk individuals

H1N1

- CDC recommends influenza vaccination as the first and most important step in protecting against flu
- Nasal spray vaccine (live attenuated H1N1 virus) released early October 2009: approved for healthy individuals aged 2–49 years; should not be used in pregnant or immunocompromised individuals

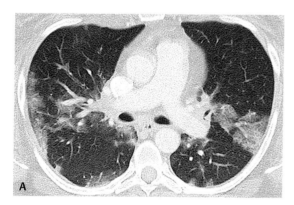
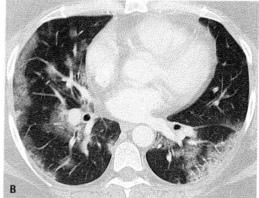
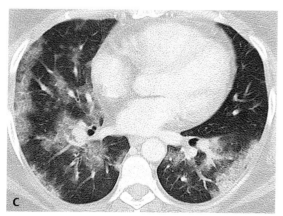

Fig. 67.3 Chest CT (lung window) of a 39-year-old woman with laboratory confirmed S-OIV (H1N1) shows bilateral ground glass opacities with a predominant peribronchovascular and juxtapleural distribution resembling organizing pneumonia.

- Injectable vaccine (killed H1N1) released second week of October 2009; approved for use in ages 6 months to the elderly; pregnant women; high-risk patients (e.g., asthma, COPD, diabetes, heart disease, neurocognitive disorders)
- Zanamivir (Relenza [GlaxoSmithKline, Research Triangle Park, NC]): initial choice for antiviral prophylaxis or treatment when influenza A infection or exposure is suspected; high prevalence of influenza A (H1N1) virus strains resistant to oseltamivir (Tamiflu [Genentech, San Francisco, CA])

Prognosis

Influenza

- Generally favorable
- Increased likelihood of bacterial superinfection and fatal course in immunocompromised patients and patients in developing countries

H1N1

- Most patients have mild illness
- High-risk patients have severe illness complicated by respiratory failure and death
- Case fatality rate (CFR) 0.5%

PEARLS

- Most frequent imaging pattern seen with H1N1 is bilateral lower lobe and central lung predominant air space disease. In hospitalized patients, disease is rapidly progressive and confluent.
- H1N1 is associated with an increased prevalence of acute PTE disease in severely ill patients and has been postulated as one of the leading causes of death during pandemics.

Suggested Reading

1. Agarwal PP, Cinti S, Kazerooni EA. Chest radiographic and CT findings in novel swine-origin influenza A (H1N1) virus (S-OIV) infection. AJR Am J Roentgenol 2009;193(6):1488–1493

2. Ajlan AM, Quiney B, Nicolaou S, Müller NL. Swine-origin influenza A (H1N1) viral infection: radiographic and CT findings. AJR Am J Roentgenol 2009;193(6):1494–1499

3. Kim EA, Lee KS, Primack SL, et al. Viral pneumonias in adults: radiologic and pathologic findings. Radiographics 2002; 22(Spec No, suppl):S137–S149

4. Tanaka N, Matsumoto T, Kuramitsu T, et al. High resolution CT findings in community-acquired pneumonia. J Comput Assist Tomogr 1996;20(4):600–608

5. Travis WD, Colby TV, Koss MN, Rosado-de-Christenson ML, Müller NL, King TE Jr. Lung infections. In: King DW, ed. Atlas of Nontumor Pathology: Non-Neoplastic Disorders of the Lower Respiratory Tract, fasc 2, ser 1. Washington, DC: American Registry of Pathology and Armed Forces Institute of Pathology; 2001:657–660

CASE 68

■ Clinical Presentation

28-year-old man with acute myelogenous leukemia (AML) and neutropenia and recent non-productive cough, fever, and headache following bone marrow transplantation

■ Radiologic Findings

Unenhanced HRCT (lung window) (**Figs. 68.1A, 68.1B**) demonstrates profuse bilateral patchy nodular centrilobular ground glass opacities and scattered reticular opacities

■ Diagnosis

Cytomegalovirus Pneumonia

■ Differential Diagnosis

- Other Opportunistic Infections (fungal, viral)
- Other Causes of Bronchiolitis

■ Discussion

Background

Based on antibody titers, the prevalence of infection by cytomegalovirus (CMV) ranges from 40% to 100% in adults worldwide and approximates 100% for HIV-infected homosexual men and 80% for intravenous drug users. Disease is very rarely documented in immunocompetent individuals.

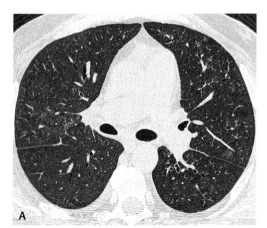 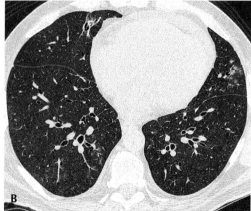

Fig. 68.1   *(Images courtesy of Santiago Rossi, MD, Buenos Aires, Argentina.)*

Etiology

Cytomegalovirus pneumonia is caused by CMV, a herpes virus with a double-stranded DNA. The virus may remain dormant within host cells for years but can be reactivated when host immunity is compromised.

Clinical Findings

CMV produces opportunistic infections that typically affect allogeneic hematopoietic stem cell and organ transplant recipients. CMV pneumonia usually occurs between 60 days and six months after transplantation. CMV infections may also occur after treatment with immunosuppressive drugs and in patients with HIV-AIDS and other immunodeficiency states. While the virus is commonly isolated from the lungs of patients with AIDS, recovery of CMV does not always correlate with clinical disease. Presenting symptoms include fever, cough, dyspnea, tachypnea, and hypoxemia. Extrapulmonary manifestations include retinitis and gastrointestinal involvement.

Imaging Findings

Radiography

- Bilateral reticular opacities
- Bilateral small and large nodular opacities
- Bilateral diffuse air space consolidation/ground glass opacity

MDCT/HRCT

- Ground glass opacities
- Nodular opacities; centrilobular nodules (<10 mm) (**Figs. 68.1A, 68.1B**)
- Large nodules, consolidations
- Linear opacities, interlobular septal thickening
- Rarely pleural effusion, mediastinal lymphadenopathy

Management

- Antiviral therapy with ganciclovir; also used for prophylaxis

Prognosis

- High mortality; approximately 80% over a 10-year period

Suggested Reading

1. Horger MS, Pfannenberg C, Einsele H, et al. Cytomegalovirus pneumonia after stem cell transplantation: correlation of CT findings with clinical outcome in 30 patients. AJR Am J Roentgenol 2006;187(6):W636-43

2. Miller WT Jr, Shah RM. Isolated diffuse ground-glass opacity in thoracic CT: causes and clinical presentations. AJR Am J Roentgenol 2005;184(?):613 G22

3. Travis WD, Colby TV, Koss MN, Rosado-de-Christenson ML, Müller NL, King TE Jr. Pulmonary infections. In: King DW, ed. Atlas of Nontumor Pathology: Non-Neoplastic Disorders of the Lower Respiratory Tract, fasc 2, ser 1. Washington, DC: American Registry of Pathology and Armed Forces Institute of Pathology; 2001:539–727

CASE 69

■ Clinical Presentation

53-year-old woman status post kidney transplant eight months earlier with five-day history of vesicular skin rash followed by progressive dyspnea, cough, tachypnea, and chest pain

■ Radiologic Findings

PA (**Fig. 69.1A**) and lateral (**Fig. 69.1B**) chest radiographs show multiple subcentimeter nodules of varying size distributed throughout both lungs. Chest CT (lung window) (**Figs. 69.1C, 69.1D, 69.1E, 69.1F**) reveals 1–10 mm well-defined and ill-defined nodules randomly disseminated bilaterally. At least one nodule in the left lower lobe has surrounding ground glass (**Fig. 69.1E**). Note the absence of pleural effusion and lymphadenopathy.

■ Diagnosis

Varicella-Zoster Pneumonia

■ Differential Diagnosis

- Cytomegalovirus (CMV)
- Adenovirus
- Measles
- Respiratory Syncytial Virus (RSV)
- Disseminated Fungal Pulmonary Infection
- *Mycobacterium tuberculosis*
- Metastatic Pulmonary Disease

■ Discussion

Background

Varicella-zoster virus (VZV) is a contagious herpes virus that can cause two distinct clinical syndromes. The first, *varicella* (*chickenpox*), is most commonly a self-limited mucocutaneous process that occurs primarily in children, and less often in adults. The second, *herpes zoster* (*shingles*), occurs primarily in adults from reactivation of latent infection residing in the posterior dorsal root ganglia. The latter spreads along sensory nerves, causing severe, unilateral, painful cutaneous lesions in a specific dermatome. In immunocompetent individuals, *herpes zoster* is usually limited to a post-herpetic neuralgia. However, *herpes zoster* is more likely to occur in immunosuppressed persons. Up to 50% of these latter patients develop disseminated disease that may be complicated by hepatitis, meningoencephalitis, uveitis, and pneumonia. VZV pneumonia is the most serious complication of disseminated VZV infection.

Etiology

Varicella-zoster pneumonia is caused by infection of the lung by the herpes varicella-zoster virus.

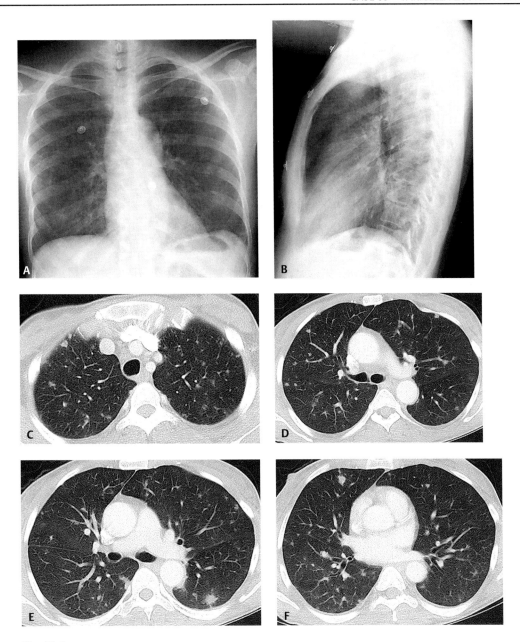

Fig. 69.1

Clinical Findings

Clinical manifestations of VZV pneumonia range from asymptomatic disease to mild illness, to respiratory failure and death. When present, symptoms typically evolve within one to six days after the skin rash appears. In patients in whom pneumonia develops, the skin rash tends to be severe and often involves the mucosa of the mouth and pharynx. Signs and symptoms of pulmonary infection include fever, cough, dyspnea, pleuritic chest pain, tachypnea, cyanosis, and rarely hemoptysis. Most cases occur in young adults. Pregnant and bone marrow transplant patients and those with lymphoma and leukemia are at risk.

Imaging Findings

Chest Radiography

- Differs from that of other viral pneumonias
- Multiple 5–10 mm well-defined to ill-defined nodules (**Figs. 69.1A, 69.1B**)
- Nodules may become confluent; may appear migratory
- Hilar lymphadenopathy/pleural effusion may occur in acute phase; otherwise unusual
- Small round consolidations usually resolve within one week after skin lesions disappear; alternatively may persist for months
- Lesions may calcify and persist indefinitely as innumerable randomly distributed 2–3 mm calcified nodules throughout both lungs (<2% of patients)

MDCT/HRCT

- Variable patterns
- Multiple, soft-tissue attenuation, often ill-defined, 5–10 mm nodules randomly distributed throughout both lungs; may mimic metastatic disease (**Figs. 69.1C, 69.1D, 69.1E, 69.1F**)
- Nodules regress as skin lesions and other symptoms improve clinically
- Nodules with surrounding ground glass attenuation (**Fig. 69.1E**)
- Patchy foci of ground glass attenuation
- Coalescence of lesions

Management

- Intravenous acyclovir
- Possible steroids
- Isolation precautions to control spread of disease

Prognosis

- Complications of *varicella pneumonia* include respiratory failure and pulmonary infarction
- Disseminated *zoster* infection may be complicated by hepatitis, meningoencephalitis, and uveitis
- Mortality rate: 9–50%

PEARLS

- Ten percent of pregnant women with varicella infection develop pneumonia, which can be severe and is often life-threatening.
- Clinical improvement precedes radiologic clearing by several weeks or longer.

Suggested Reading

1. Kim JS, Ryu CW, Lee SI, Sung DW, Park CK. High-resolution CT findings of varicella-zoster pneumonia. AJR Am J Roentgenol 1999;172(1):113–116

2. Picken G, Booth AJ, Williams MV. Case report: the pulmonary lesions of chickenpox pneumonia—revisited. Br J Radiol 1994;67(799):659–660

3. Travis WD, Colby TV, Koss MN, Rosado-de-Christenson ML, Muller NL, King TE Jr. Lung infections. In: King DW, ed. Atlas of Nontumor Pathology: Non-Neoplastic Disorders of the Lower Respiratory Tract, first series, fascicle 2. Washington, DC: American Registry of Pathology; 2002:646–648

OVERVIEW OF ATYPICAL PNEUMONIAS

Typical pneumonia is a term that describes disease characterized by an abrupt onset with associated fever, chills, productive cough, pleurisy, and clinical or radiologic signs of lung consolidation. In contradistinction, *atypical pneumonia* more often describes the insidious onset of pneumonia associated with non-productive cough, minimal pulmonary signs, and a host of extrapulmonary symptoms (e.g., malaise, nausea and vomiting, diarrhea, and sore throat). However, there is a significant degree of both clinical and radiologic overlap. Whereas most *typical pneumonias* are caused by various bacterial pathogens (see Cases 49–56), *atypical pneumonias* result from non-bacterial pathogens, most commonly *M. pneumoniae and C. pneumoniae.* Some authorities also place *Legionella* sp. (see Case 54) in this category. The case that follows in this section will focus on *M. pneumoniae* infection.

Suggested Reading

1. Burillo A, Bouza E. *Chlamydophila pneumoniae.* Infect Dis Clin North Am 2010;24(1):61–71 Review

2. Cunha CB. The first atypical pneumonia: the history of the discovery of *Mycoplasma pneumoniae.* Infect Dis Clin North Am 2010;24(1):1–5 Review

3. Cunha BA. Atypical pneumonias: current clinical concepts focusing on Legionnaires' disease. Curr Opin Pulm Med 2008;14(3):183–194 Review

CASE 70

■ Clinical Presentation

33-year-old man with three- to four-day history of dyspnea, non-productive cough, fevers, and chills admitted to the hospital with presumptive diagnosis of community-acquired pneumonia. Antibiotic therapy was initiated without improvement. He developed progressive hypoxia. CTPA for pulmonary embolism on hospital day 4 revealed no embolism. Two days later, ARDS ensued.

■ Radiologic Findings

Admission PA (**Fig. 70.1A**) chest X-ray shows bilateral, perihilar, segmental ground glass and air space consolidations. Follow-up AP portable chest exam three days later (**Fig. 70.1B**) reveals significant progression of disease. Chest CT (lung window) (**Figs. 70.1C, 70.1D, 70.1E, 70.1F**) acquired on hospital day 4 demonstrates a patchy pattern of variable attenuation characterized by foci of ground glass, consolidation, hypoattenuated lung with reduced perfusion, and intervening areas of normal lung. The combination of "mixed densities" throughout the lung gives it a geographic appearance similar to a preserved meat product called *head cheese* or *hog's head cheese* (**Fig. 70.2**) and it is therefore referred to as the *head cheese sign*.

■ Diagnosis

Mycoplasma Pneumonia

■ Differential Diagnosis

- Typical Bacterial Pneumonias
- Other Atypical Pneumonias
- Viral Pulmonary Infection
- Hypersensitivity Pneumonitis
- Acute Interstitial Pneumonia (AIP)

■ Discussion

Background

Mycoplasma is considered an "atypical" bacterium; it lacks a cell wall and produces pulmonary infection through extracellular growth and interference with ciliary function. It is a common cause of community-acquired pneumonia and is probably responsible for approximately 20–30% of the pneumonias that affect the general population. Infections occur year-round, but typically in the fall and winter months. The incidence of *M. pneumoniae* infection in the United States is approximately 1/1,000 persons. Epidemics of *Mycoplasma* pneumonia occur every 4–8 years in the general population and are more frequent within closed populations (e.g., college dorms, military barracks, and prisons).

Etiology

Mycoplasma pneumonia is caused by the organism *Mycoplasma pneumoniae*. The disease is transmitted through close contact with infected individuals and inhalation of infected respiratory droplets. The incubation period averages three weeks, in contrast to that of influenza and other viral pneumonias, which is generally a few days.

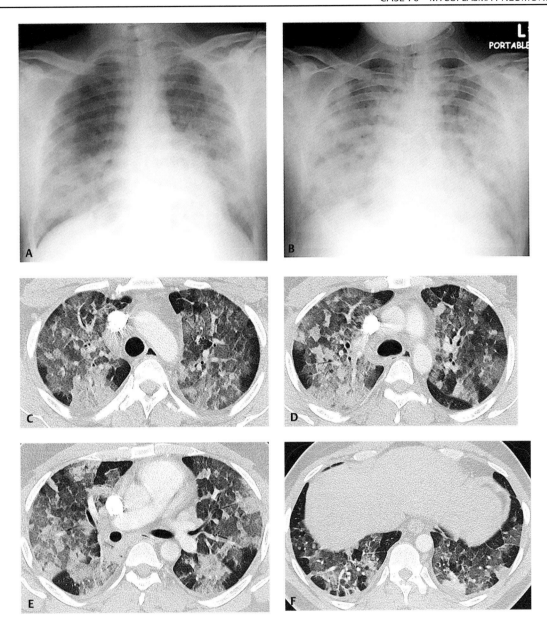

Fig. 70.1

Clinical Findings

Mycoplasma pneumonia typically occurs in children, adolescents, and young adults, although approximately 15% of affected patients are over the age of 40 years. The earliest symptoms include fever, chills, malaise, anorexia, and headache. Subsequently, sore throat and non-productive cough develop. One-third of patients complain of earache. Dyspnea and pleuritic chest pain are rare. As the disease progresses, up to 100% of patients develop a persistent low-grade fever and an intractable, hacking cough. Extrapulmonary manifestations include cervical lymphadenopathy, arthralgias, pharyngitis, skin rash, and conjunctivitis. Infected patients may also have gastrointestinal (nausea, vomiting, diarrhea), central nervous system (aseptic meningitis, cranial nerve palsies, transverse myelitis), and cardiac (conduction abnormalities, heart failure) involvement. Rarely, affected patients may develop ARDS. The diagnosis is usually based on clinical presentation, normal white blood cell count or mild leukocytosis, and elevated titers of serum cold agglutinins (>1:32).

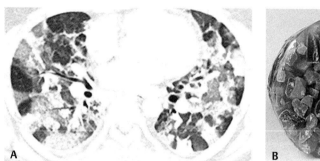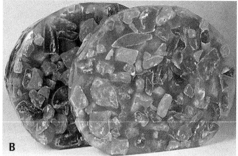

Fig. 70.2 Whereas the CT "geographic" pattern of disease is created by a combination of ground glass opacities, consolidation, mosaic perfusion, and intervening normal lung **(A)**, that of actual "head cheese" is created by the mixture of boiled pork scraps and pigs' feet in a gelatinous background **(B)**.

Imaging Findings

Chest Radiography

- Bilateral ground glass or air space segmental or lobar consolidations (**Figs. 70.1A, 70.1B, 70.3**)
- Lower lobe predilection
- Reticular or nodular opacities
- Bronchial wall thickening
- Pleural effusions (30%)

MDCT/HRCT

- Poorly defined centrilobular nodules consistent with bronchiolitis (**Figs. 70.4A, 70.4B**)
- Lobular patchy air space consolidation and ground glass attenuation consistent with bronchopneumonia (**Fig. 70.4B**)
- Geographic pattern of disease created by combination of ground glass opacities, consolidation, mosaic perfusion, and intervening normal lung (*head cheese sign*) (**Figs. 70.1C. 70.1D, 70.1E, 70.1F, 70.2A, 70.2B**)
- Peribronchovascular and interlobular septal thickening
- ± Mediastinal lymphadenopathy

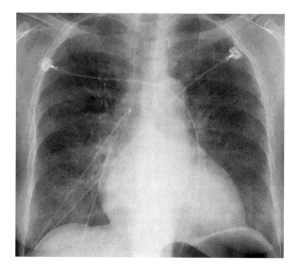

Fig. 70.3 AP chest-ray of a 60-year-old woman presenting with malaise and dyspnea and subsequently diagnosed with *M. pneumoniae* shows bilateral ground glass opacities. *(Image courtesy of Rosita M. Shah, MD, University of Pennsylvania Abramson Cancer Center, Philadelphia, Pennsylvania.)*

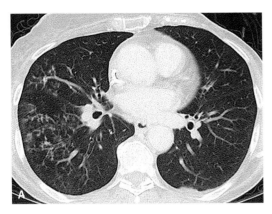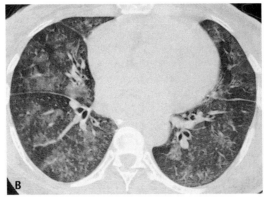

Fig. 70.4 CT features of *M. pneumoniae* in two different patients. A pattern of ill-defined centrilobular nodules and tree-in-bud opacities most heavily concentrated in the right middle and lower lobe **(A)**. Bilateral widespread ill-defined centri-lobular nodules and ground glass lobular opacities **(B)**. *(Images courtesy of Rosita M. Shah, MD, University of Pennsylvania Abramson Cancer Center, Philadelphia, Pennsylvania.)*

Management

- Antimicrobials against *M. pneumoniae* are bacteriostatic
- Tetracycline; erythromycin; second-generation tetracyclines (doxycycline) and macrolides: drugs of choice
- Penicillins and cephalosporins: ineffective because organism lacks a cell wall

Prognosis

- Infection may exacerbate underlying bronchial asthma
- Most patients recover completely; those patients that develop ARDS have increased mortality
- Resolution of radiographic abnormalities is relatively rapid and occurs within four to eight weeks in most patients; delayed resolution in appropriately treated patients suggests superimposed bacterial infection
- Following infection with *M. pneumoniae*, patients may develop interstitial fibrosis, Swyer-James syndrome with a unilateral hyperlucent lung, bronchial wall thickening, bronchiectasis, mosaic perfusion, and air trapping

Suggested Reading

1. Drugs of choice for community-acquired bacterial pneumonia. Med Lett Drugs Ther 2007;49(1266):62–64
2. Reittner P, Müller NL, Heyneman L, et al. *Mycoplasma pneumoniae* pneumonia: radiographic and high-resolution CT features in 28 patients. AJR Am J Roentgenol 2000;174(1):37–41
3. Smith LG. Mycoplasma pneumonia and its complications. Infect Dis Clin North Am 2010;24(1):57–60
4. Travis WD, Colby TV, Koss MN, Rosado-de-Christenson ML, Müller NL, King TE Jr. Pulmonary infections. In: King DW, ed. Atlas of Nontumor Pathology: Non-Neoplastic Disorders of the Lower Respiratory Tract, fasc 2, ser 1. Washington, DC: American Registry of Pathology and Armed Forces Institute of Pathology; 2001:539–727

OVERVIEW OF PARASITIC PNEUMONIAS

Parasitic pneumonia is a rare cause of pneumonia attributable to an infection of the lung by parasites. Although parasitic diseases are most prevalent in tropical and subtropical climates, such infections are being increasingly reported worldwide because of globalization and transcontinental travel. Most parasites enter the body via the skin or after being swallowed. Parasitic pneumonia occurs as the larvae of some of these parasites pass through the lungs via the bloodstream. Most parasitic pneumonias occur in immunosuppressed or immunocompromised patients. The clinical manifestations of parasitic pneumonia range from asymptomatic disease to life-threatening. The most important parasites responsible for parasitic pneumonia include:

Pulmonary amoebiasis. Causative agent is the protozoan *Entamoeba histolytica*. Pulmonary amoebiasis occurs primarily by extension from an amoebic liver abscess. Signs and symptoms include fever, right upper quadrant abdominal pain, chest pain, cough, and expectoration of an "anchovy-like" paste. Pulmonary involvement in the absence of liver disease may cause SVC syndrome. Imaging may reveal hemidiaphragm elevation, pleural effusion, and basilar air space disease. Active trophozoites may be found in sputum or pleural fluid.

Pulmonary leishmaniasis. Caused by the protozoan *Leishmania donovani*; infection is transmitted by the sand fly (*Phlebotomus* species). Pneumonia, pleural effusion, and mediastinal lymphadenopathy have been reported in patients with HIV-AIDS.

Pulmonary malaria. Caused by the obligate intraerythrocytic protozoan *Plasmodium*; primarily transmitted by the bite of an infected female mosquito (*Anopheles* species). Four types of malarial parasites infect humans: *P. falciparum, P. malaria, P. ovale, and P. vivax*, of which *P. falciparum* is the most deadly. Clinical manifestations range from cough to rapidly fatal ARDS and respiratory failure. Imaging findings include lobar consolidation, diffuse interstitial pulmonary edema, pleural effusion, and ARDS.

Pulmonary hydatid disease. Caused by the cestodes *Echinococcus granulosus* and *Echinococcus multilocularis*. Hydatid cysts most often form in the liver and lungs. Pulmonary echinococcosis results from hematogenous dissemination from infected liver lesions. Signs and symptoms can occur from compression of adjacent structures by cysts. Infected patients may also experience cough, fever, dyspnea, chest pain, hemoptysis, asthma-like symptoms, non-resolving pneumonia, pleural effusions, empyema and pneumothorax from cyst rupture into the pleural space, sepsis, and respiratory failure. Imaging studies may demonstrate isolated or multiple variable-size rounded opacities, an air-fluid level, and the *water lily sign*. Pulmonary hydatid disease is discussed in further detail in Case 71.

Pulmonary schistosomiasis. Caused by infection with the trematode *Schistosoma haematobium, S. mansoni*, or *S. japonicum*. Pulmonary schistosomiasis can manifest as an acute or chronic form of disease. *Acute pulmonary schistosomiasis* presents with fever and chills, dyspnea, dry cough and wheezing, weight loss, abdominal pain, diarrhea, hives, and myalgias. Imaging studies may reveal small pulmonary nodules. *Chronic pulmonary schistosomiasis* may be characterized by pulmonary artery hypertension, cor pulmonale, lobar collapse and consolidation, and hemoptysis.

Paragonimiasis pneumonia. Caused by the food-borne zoonosis *Paragonimus westermani* and is most prevalent in Asia. Infected patients experience fever, chest pain, cough, and hemoptysis. Imaging studies may demonstrate ground glass and air space opacities, one or more variable-size nodules with or without cavitation, pleural effusion, and pneumothorax.

***Ascaris* pneumonia.** Caused by infection with the nematode *Ascaris lumbricoides*. The larvae cause bronchial inflammation, increased sputum production, and bronchospasm. Infected patients may present with dyspnea, dry cough, fever, and blood eosinophilia. Imaging studies often reveal migratory peripheral air space opacities and consolidations.

***Strongyloides* pneumonia.** Caused by the nematode *Strongyloides stercoralis*. Filariform larvae migrate through the lungs, causing hemorrhage and bronchopneumonia. Larvae that penetrate the intestinal mucosa cause disseminated and usually fatal disease. Patients with pulmonary *Strongyloides* are often misdiagnosed with new-onset asthma or asthma exacerbation or present in acute respiratory distress. *Strongyloides* dissemination may manifest as an immune reconstitution inflammatory syndrome in HIV-AIDS patients receiving highly active antiretroviral therapy (HAART).

Pulmonary dirofilariasis. Caused by zoonotic nematode infection with *Dirofilaria immitis* or *Dirofilaria repens*. Humans are accidental hosts infected by mosquito bite. The parasites often lodge in the pulmonary arterial circuit, causing pulmonary embolism and apparent arteriovenous malformation on imaging studies. Many infected patients are asymptomatic. Others complain of chest pain, cough, fever, dyspnea, and hemoptysis.

Suggested Reading

1. Kuzucu A. Parasitic diseases of the respiratory tract. Curr Opin Pulm Med 2006;12(3):212–221 Review
2. Santivanez S, Garcia HH. Pulmonary cystic echinococcosis. Curr Opin Pulm Med 2010;16(3):257–261 Review
3. Vijayan VK. How to diagnose and manage common parasitic pneumonias. Curr Opin Pulm Med 2007;13(3):218–224
4. Vijayan VK. Parasitic lung infections. Curr Opin Pulm Med 2009;15(3):274–282

CASE 71

■ Clinical Presentation

Asymptomatic 35-year-old man

■ Radiologic Findings

PA chest radiograph (**Fig. 71.1A**) demonstrates a well-marginated polylobular mass in the right lower lobe. Coned-down contrast-enhanced chest CT (lung and mediastinal windows) (**Figs. 71.1B, 71.1C**) demonstrates a polylobular right lower lobe mass with well-defined borders and intrinsic homogeneous fluid attenuation contents. Note linear peripheral enhancement of the wall of the cystic lesion (**Fig. 71.1C**).

■ Diagnosis

Pulmonary Cystic Hydatid Disease (Echinococcosis)

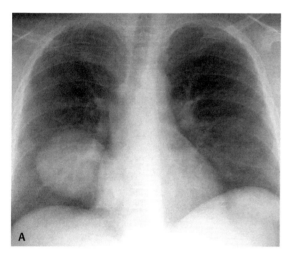

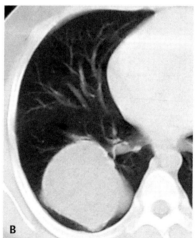

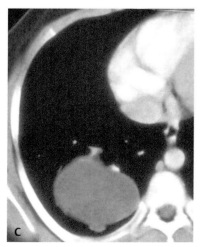

Fig. 71.1

■ Differential Diagnosis

- Pulmonary Bronchogenic Cyst
- Primary or Solitary Secondary Malignant Neoplasm

■ Discussion

Background

The misuse of the term *echinococcosis* to denote human infection is prevalent, although, by strict definition, *echinococcosis* refers to infection of non-human carnivores by the adult parasite, while *hydatidosis* refers to human infection by metacestodes. Pulmonary hydatidosis is a parasitic infectious disease endemic to many parts of the world, particularly underdeveloped sheep- and cattle-raising areas of South America, the Mediterranean region, the Middle East, Africa, and Australia. It is estimated that 65 million individuals are infected worldwide. The life cycle of these organisms requires two hosts: the *definitive host,* which is a carnivorous dog (or other member of the Canidae or Felidae family) infected with adult egg-producing intestinal tapeworms, and the *intermediate host,* which is typically a sheep or a pig (or other mammal) that develops infective metacestodes after ingesting viable eggs. The cycle is completed when the carnivore mammal ingests infected intermediate hosts. Humans are accidental or aberrant intermediate hosts who typically present a dead end to the parasite's life cycle. Human infection results from ingestion of food or water contaminated by fecal material containing the parasite's eggs. Most affected patients have hepatic involvement, and the lung is the second most frequently affected organ. *Echinococcus granulosus* grows in tissue by forming well-defined fluid-filled cysts. The inner lining of the cyst, the *endocyst,* consists of a germinal layer that contains brood capsules and *protoscolices* and may form daughter cysts. The *endocyst* is surrounded by the *exocyst,* a tough outer laminated membrane. The *pericyst* is the host reaction that surrounds the *exocyst,* composed of fibrous tissue with giant cell formation and eosinophilic infiltration. The macroscopic features of the parasitic cyst and the surrounding tissue reaction are the basis for its characteristic imaging features.

Etiology

Most cases of hydatidosis are caused by *Echinococcus granulosus*, endemic to Mediterranean countries, Eastern Europe, the Middle East, Africa, South America, Australia, and New Zealand. *E. multilocularis* is found in the Arctic, portions of Asia, and Northern Europe. *E. vogeli* is found in tropical South America. *E. oligarthrus* is characteristically found in Central and South America.

Clinical Findings

Patients with cystic pulmonary hydatidosis infected with *E. granulosus* may remain asymptomatic for years. Symptoms are usually the result of cyst rupture, which may produce cough, hemoptysis, chest pain, or anaphylactic reaction.

Radiography

- Well-defined spherical nodule or mass (**Fig. 71.1A**); solitary or multiple; variable size (up to 20 cm or larger)
- Mediastinal or pleural mass (with mediastinal or pleural involvement)
- Complicated hydatidosis (cyst rupture)
  - Crescent of air surrounding soft-tissue nodule or mass; air between *pericyst* and *exocyst*
  - Air-fluid level related to *exocyst* rupture
  - *Water lily sign* related to *exocyst* rupture and visualization of undulating contour of collapsed *exocyst* floating in cyst fluid contained by *pericyst*
  - Surrounding air space disease; adjacent pleural effusion or pneumothorax

MDCT

- Spherical unilocular cystic lesion with fluid attenuation contents, well-defined borders (**Figs. 71.1B, 71.1C**)
- Enhancement of cyst wall (**Fig. 71.1C**); no enhancement of cyst contents
- Mediastinal or pleural cystic lesions (with mediastinal or pleural involvement)
- Linear/reticular opacities
- Rarely, pleural effusion, mediastinal lymphadenopathy

Management

- Disease prevention: strict personal hygiene, careful washing of food, avoidance of contaminated water, treatment or euthanasia of infected domestic dogs and cats
- Diagnosis inferred from characteristic imaging findings in patients at risk; immunodiagnosis based on antibody and/or circulating antigen detection
- Surgical excision of cysts in patients with limited disease with or without prior chemotherapy with benzimidazoles (albendazone, mebendazole)
- PAIR—Puncture-Aspiration-Injection-Reaspiration—technique with peri-interventional chemotherapy

Prognosis

- Asymptomatic patients (intact hydatid cysts); may be followed for decades
- Spontaneous healing of pulmonary cysts in some cases
- Superinfection, anaphylaxis, and death from cyst rupture

Suggested Reading

1. Eckert J, Gemmell MA, Meslin F-X, et al. WHO/OIE Manual on Echinococcosis in Humans and Animals: A Public Health Problem of Global Concern. Paris: WHO; 2001. http://www.who.int/zoonoses/resources/echinococcosis/en/

2. Martínez S, Restrepo CS, Carrillo JA, et al. Thoracic manifestations of tropical parasitic infections: a pictorial review. Radiographics 2005;25(1):135–155

3. Marty AM, Johnson LK, Neafie RC. Hydatidosis (Echinococcosis). In: Meyers WM, Neafie RC, Marty AM, Wear DJ, eds. Pathology of Infectious Diseases. Volume 1. Washington, DC: American Registry of Pathology and Armed Forces Institute of Pathology; 2000:145–164

4. Polat P, Kantarci M, Alper F, Suma S, Koruyucu MB, Okur A. Hydatid disease from head to toe. Radiographics 2003; 23(2):475–494, quiz 536–537

CASE 72

■ Clinical Presentation

35-year-old woman with mental retardation and pre-existing gastric bezoar with a witnessed aspiration and respiratory distress necessitating emergent intubation

■ Radiologic Findings

Baseline AP portable chest X-ray (**Fig. 72.1A**) demonstrates clear lungs and a heterogeneous gastric mass consistent with her known bezoar. AP portable chest exam (**Fig. 72.1B**) following the witnessed aspiration and subsequent intubation shows acute onset of air space consolidation in the right lower lobe with hilar extension. Patchy ground glass foci are also seen in the right upper lobe and in the left apex to a lesser degree.

■ Diagnosis

Aspiration Pneumonia

■ Differential Diagnosis

None

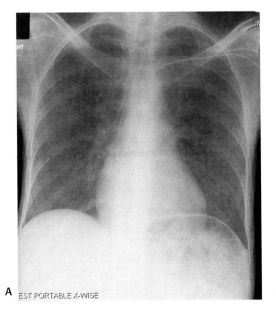 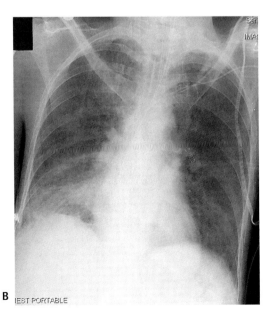

A EST PORTABLE X-WISE

B IEST PORTABLE

Fig. 72.1

357

■ Discussion

Background

Aspiration is the presence of foreign material in the airways of the lung, the sequelae of which depends on the volume and nature of the aspirated material and the frequency of aspiration. Small volumes of aspirate are common and are readily handled by normal defense mechanisms (e.g., glottic closure, cough reflex) without complication. Predisposing risk factors for aspiration are summarized in **Table 72.1**.

Etiology

Aspiration or inhalation of particulate matter, fluids, or secretions from the stomach and/or oropharynx into the lungs may result in any of four different clinical syndromes: (1) *chemical pneumonia (CP)*, aspiration of gastric acid and contents incites a chemical pneumonitis (Mendelson syndrome); (2) *bacterial pneumonia (BP)*, aspiration of bacteria from the oropharynx; (3) *exogenous lipoid pneumonia*, aspiration of animal, mineral, or vegetable oil (see Case 113); and (4) *foreign body aspiration*, which may be complicated by lobar atelectasis, respiratory distress, and bacterial pneumonia. The incidence of *CP* is not known. *BP* sequelae of aspiration accounts for 5–15% of cases of community-acquired pneumonia. *Aspiration-related nosocomial BP* is the second most common cause of nosocomial infection, and the leading cause of death from health care–related infections.

Clinical Findings

CP (Mendelson syndrome) is typically caused by aspiration of a large volume of non-infected gastric acid. The lower the pH (<2.5) and the greater the volume of aspirate (>20 mL), the greater the likelihood of chemical pneumonitis. Affected patients typically present acutely within minutes to a few hours of the inciting event. Signs and symptoms often include respiratory distress, tachypnea, tachycardia, wheezing and rales, cough, frothy pink sputum production, and fever. *BP* caused by aspiration may be community-acquired or nosocomial. Anaerobic organisms and or various aerobes are usually responsible. *Anaerobic BP* is usually related to a large volume of aspirate in alcoholics or persons with poor dentition. *Nosocomial aspiration BP* is usually related to colonization of hospital devices and the oropharynx by Gram-negative bacteria. *BP* is typically characterized by an insidious onset over a period of days (aerobic infections) or weeks (anaerobic infection). Signs and symptoms may include purulent productive cough with a putrid odor (anaerobic infection), halitosis, and fever.

Table 72.1 Predisposing Risk Factors for Aspiration

Altered Levels of Consciousness	Neurologic Disorders	Mechanical Conditions	Esophageal Disorders	Miscellaneous
Drug overdose or over-sedation	Dementia	Nasogastric tube	GERD	Critical or chronic illness
Alcohol	Parkinson disease	Various enteric feeding tubes	UGI bleed	Generalized deconditioning
Anesthesia	Multiple sclerosis	Endotracheal or tracheostomy tube	Achalasia	Debilitation
Post-ictal	Amyotrophic lateral sclerosis	Bronchoscopy	Strictures	Protracted vomiting
Head trauma	Myasthenia gravis	Esophagoscopy	Diverticula	Recumbent positioning
Cerebral vascular accident			Neoplasia	
			Tracheoesophageal fistula	

Imaging Findings

- Influenced by type and severity of aspiration
- CT useful in assessing for complications

Chemical Pneumonia

Sterile Secretions at Low pH

- Patchy areas of air space consolidation; involves mainly dependent lung (**Figs. 72.1A, 72.1B, 72.2A, 72.2B, 72.3A, 72.3B**)
- Predilection for posterior segment upper lobes and superior segment lower lobes; supine patients (**Figs. 72.1A, 72.1B, 72.2A, 72.2B, 72.3A, 72.3B**)
- Extensive bilateral consolidation simulates ARDS; large volume aspirate (**Fig. 72.2A**)
- Bronchopneumonia or abscess formation as a complication
- Resolution 7–10 days in survivors

Bacterial Pneumonia

- Focal or multi-focal air space consolidation with or without cavitation
- Predilection for dependent lung zones
- Abscess formation, parapneumonic effusion, empyema, bronchopleural fistula as complications

Management

Chemical Pneumonia

- Tracheal suctioning to remove particulate matter in cases of witnessed aspiration
- Supportive care with intubation and mechanical ventilation
- Antibiotics indicated only if secondary infection develops

Bacterial Pneumonia

- Supportive therapy and antibiotics are the mainstays of therapy

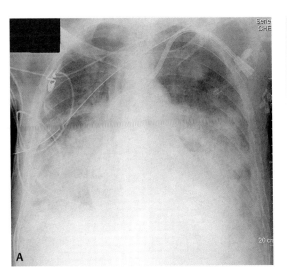 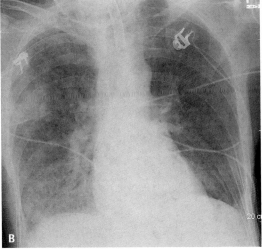

Fig. 72.2 Radiographic depiction of aspiration pneumonia in two separate patients. **(A)** AP chest X-ray of a patient with witnessed aspiration during a pulseless electrical activity arrest (PEA) shows extensive bilateral consolidation from the large volume aspirate that simulates ARDS. **(B)** AP chest exam of a quadriplegic ventilator-dependent man with witnessed aspiration of tube feedings reveals patchy air space consolidations in the dependent right upper and lower lobe.

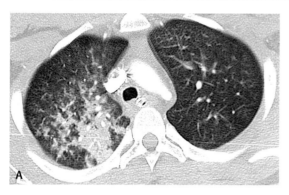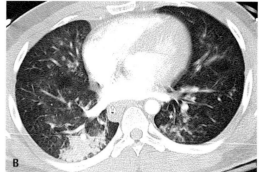

Fig. 72.3 Chest CT (lung window) of a young patient with heroin overdose found lying down in a large pool of vomit demonstrates foci of consolidation in the dependent right upper and lower lobes. There are also scattered ground glass, centrilobular nodules, and tree-in-bud opacities from the aspirate.

Prognosis

Chemical Pneumonia

- Dependent upon underlying disease and ensuing complications
- Two-thirds patients: rapid radiographic clearing
- 25% of patients: initial rapid clinical improvement followed by new or expanding radiographic opacities from complicating bacterial pneumonia, ARDS, acute PTE
- May be complicated by ARDS, or bacterial or nosocomial pneumonia
- Mortality rate: 30–50%

Bacterial Pneumonia

- Dependent upon underlying disease and ensuing complications
- May be complicated by lung abscess, empyema, bronchopleural fistula
- Nosocomial infection associated with prolonged hospital course, more complications, higher mortality rates

PEARLS

- Particulate matter aspiration usually follows a segmental distribution, affecting one or more posterior segments of upper or lower lobes; may resemble bronchopneumonia.
- Repeated bouts of aspiration may be complicated by bronchiectasis and pulmonary fibrosis.

Suggested Reading

1. Franquet T, Giménez A, Rosón N, Torrubia S, Sabaté JM, Pérez C. Aspiration diseases: findings, pitfalls, and differential diagnosis. Radiographics 2000;20(3):673–685

2. Marik PE. Aspiration pneumonitis and aspiration pneumonia. N Engl J Med 2001;344(9):665–671

3. Mendelson CL. The aspiration of stomach contents into the lungs during obstetric anesthesia. Am J Obstet Gynecol 1946;52:191–205

4. Travis WD, Colby TV, Koss MN, Rosado-de-Christenson ML, Müller NL, King TE Jr. Lung infections. In: King DW, ed. Atlas of Nontumor Pathology: Non-Neoplastic Disorders of the Lower Respiratory Tract, first series, fascicle 2. Washington, DC: American Registry of Pathology; 2002:187–196

Section VI

Neoplastic Disease

OVERVIEW OF NEOPLASTIC DISEASE

Pulmonary neoplasms produce extensive morbidity and mortality among the United States (U.S.) population and worldwide. Most pulmonary neoplasms are malignant. Both primary and secondary pulmonary neoplasms affect the lung. Lung cancer accounts for approximately 95% of all primary neoplasms of the lung. It has a strong association with cigarette smoking, but other environmental and occupational carcinogens are also implicated. It is estimated that approximately 222,520 malignant neoplasms of the lung and bronchus will be diagnosed in U.S. men and women in 2010. While death rates from lung cancer have recently decreased in men, they have increased in women, and lung cancer remains the most common cause of cancer death for both men and women in the United States. Other malignant neoplasms of the lung and airways, such as bronchial carcinoid and pulmonary lymphoma, are relatively rare. The lung is a common site for secondary malignant neoplasia, and pulmonary metastases represent the most common pulmonary neoplasms.

Most patients with primary lung cancer present with symptoms that may be related to obstructive effects by central lesions, extrapulmonary involvement by advanced tumors, metastatic disease, and less frequently paraneoplastic syndromes or systemic effects of the primary neoplasm not related to metastatic disease. Approximately 10% of lung cancers occur in asymptomatic individuals and are discovered incidentally on imaging studies obtained for other reasons.

The most common cell type of lung cancer is adenocarcinoma, followed by squamous cell carcinoma and small cell carcinoma. The histologic classification of lung cancer continues to evolve. The most recent classification addresses the complexities related to the histologic diagnosis of adenocarcinoma, introduces new terminology for pre-malignant conditions and minimally invasive cancers, no longer includes the term *bronchioloalveolar carcinoma,* and discourages the use of the term *non–small cell lung cancer* (not otherwise specified). The new classification of adenocarcinoma promotes a multidisciplinary approach to the diagnosis and provides guidelines for diagnosing adenocarcinoma on biopsy specimens.

All cell types of lung cancer may initially manifest as solitary pulmonary nodules, and pulmonary nodules are frequent findings on chest CT. A pulmonary nodule is defined as a round or irregular lung opacity with well- or poorly defined borders that measures up to 3 cm in diameter in any imaging plane on CT. Nodules may be solid or subsolid. A *solid nodule* typically exhibits homogeneous attenuation and obscures the underlying pulmonary anatomy. In general, size stability of a solid pulmonary nodule for a period of two years is a reliable criterion for benignity. Likewise, absence of contrast enhancement or enhancement of less than 15 Hounsfield units on CT of a homogeneous pulmonary nodule measuring less than 3 cm in diameter virtually excludes lung cancer.

Subsolid nodules include part-solid and non-solid nodules. *Non-solid nodules* exhibit pure ground glass attenuation and allow visualization of the underlying pulmonary architecture. A *part-solid nodule* is composed of both solid and ground glass components. Up to 50% of part-solid solitary nodules <1.5 cm are malignant, and risk increases with increasing nodule size. Unfortunately, benign conditions may also manifest as solitary pulmonary nodules, and various imaging follow-up recommendations have been proposed to distinguish between benign and malignant entities. The Fleischner Society published management recommendations for *solid pulmonary nodules,* summarized in **Table VI.1**. These recommendations take into account risk factors for lung cancer, including exposure to carcinogens and history of lung cancer in a first-degree relative. Management recommendations for *subsolid nodules* are not as clear, but interim recommendations have been proposed by Godoy et al. and are summarized in **Table VI.2**.

Table VI.1   Fleischner Society Management Guidelines for Solid Nodules

Size	Low-Risk Patient	High-Risk Patient
≤4 mm	No follow-up	Follow-up at 12 months; if unchanged no follow-up
>4–6 mm	Follow-up at 12 months; if unchanged no follow-up	Follow-up at 6–12 months; if unchanged follow-up at 12–24 months
>6–8mm	Follow-up 6–12 months; if unchanged follow-up at 18–24 months	Follow-up at 3–6 months; if unchanged follow-up at 9–12 months and 24 months
>8 mm	Follow-up at 3, 9, and 24 months; or dynamic contrast-enhanced CT, PET, and/or biopsy	Same

In August 2009 a new staging system for lung cancer was introduced by the International Association for the Study of Lung Cancer (IASLC). Unlike prior staging systems, the new system is based on a study of over 81,000 lung cancer cases collected at multiple institutions in 20 countries and four continents. T, N, and M descriptors are still used for the primary tumor (T), lymph node metastases (N), and metastatic disease (M). The system addresses distinctions between clinical (prior to any treatment) and pathologic (at resection) staging. Although pathologic staging is preferable, clinical staging guides management decisions for individual patients. Imaging findings are considered part of the clinical staging of lung cancer. The system introduces changes in the categorization of the extent of the primary tumor (T descriptor), mostly related to tumor size, and the largest lesion dimension is used (**Table VI.3**). Satellite nodules in the primary tumor lobe are now categorized as T3 disease, and the T4 descriptor now includes separate tumor nodules in a different but ipsilateral lobe. The N descriptor has undergone little change, but there are new anatomic definitions of the different nodal stations (**Table VI.4**). The M1 descriptor now includes M1a and M1b categories (**Table VI.5**). Stages I, II, and III are stratified into A and B categories. **Table VI.6** shows the distribution of the T, N, and M components of each different stage. The new classification of adenocarcinoma will potentially impact the T descriptor, which may have to be adjusted to take into account the solid (or invasive) component of lung cancers manifesting as part-solid nodules.

Table VI.2 Godoy and Naidich Interim Guidelines for Assessment and Management of Subsolid Nodules

Morphology	Management
Non-solid/ground glass nodules	
<5 mm	No follow-up
5 to <10 mm	Follow-up CT in 3–6 months; if unchanged, annual follow-up for up to 5 years
10 mm or larger	Follow-up CT in 3–6 months; if unchanged, resection
Part-solid nodules	
Solitary regardless of size	Consider resection
Multifocal subsolid nodules	
<5 mm	Follow-up at 1 year
5 to <10 mm	Follow-up CT surveillance
>10 mm	Consider resection of dominant lesions

Table VI.3 T-N-M System for Lung Cancer: T Descriptor—Primary Tumor

T0	No primary tumor
T1	Tumor ≤3 cm surrounded by lung or visceral pleura Tumor at or distal to lobar bronchus Superficial tumor confined to tracheal or mainstem bronchial wall
T1a T1b	Tumor ≤2 cm >2 cm but ≤3 cm
T2	>3 cm but ≤7 cm Visceral pleural invasion Involvement of main bronchus ≥2 cm distal to carina Atelectasis/obstructive pneumonia extending to hilum but involving less than one lung
T2a T2b	>3 cm but ≤5 cm >5 cm but ≤7 cm
T3	Tumor >7 cm Direct chest wall, diaphragm, phrenic nerve, mediastinal, pleural, or parietal pericardium invasion Tumor in main bronchus <2 cm from carina Atelectasis/pneumonitis of entire lung Separate tumor nodules in same lobe
T4	Invasion of heart, great vessels, trachea, recurrent laryngeal nerve, esophagus, vertebral body, carina Separate tumor nodules in separate ipsilateral lobe

Table VI.4   T-N-M System for Lung Cancer: N Descriptor—Regional Lymph Nodes

N0	No lymph node metastases
N1	Metastases to ipsilateral peribronchial and/or perihilar lymph nodes and intrapulmonary lymph nodes
N2	Metastases to ipsilateral mediastinal and/or subcarinal lymph nodes
N3	Metastases to contralateral mediastinal, contralateral hilar, ipsilateral or contralateral scalene, or supraclavicular lymph nodes

Table VI.5   T-N-M System for Lung Cancer: M Descriptor—Distant Metastases

M0	No distant metastases
M1a	Separate tumor nodules in contralateral lobe Pleural nodules or malignant pleural effusion
M1b	Distant metastases

Table VI.6   Lung Cancer Staging

	N0	N1	N2	N3
T1a	IA	IIA	IIIA	IIIB
T1b	IA	IIA	IIIA	IIIB
T2a	IB	IIA	IIIA	IIIB
T2b	IIA	IIB	IIIA	IIIB
T3	IIB	IIIA	IIIA	IIIB
T4	IIIA	IIIA	IIIB	IIIB
M1 = IV				

Suggested Reading

1. Detterbeck FC, Boffa DJ, Tanoue LT. The new lung cancer staging system. Chest 2009;136(1):260–271

2. Girvin F, Ko JP. Pulmonary nodules: detection, assessment, and CAD. AJR Am J Roentgenol 2008;191(4):1057–1069

3. Godoy MCB, Naidich DP. Subsolid pulmonary nodules and the spectrum of peripheral adenocarcinomas of the lung: recommended interim guidelines for assessment and management. Radiology 2009;253(3):606–622

4. MacMahon H, Austin JHM, Gamsu G, et al; Fleischner Society. Guidelines for management of small pulmonary nodules detected on CT scans: a statement from the Fleischner Society. Radiology 2005;237(2):395–400

5. Travis WD, Brambilla E, Noguchi M, et al. IASLC/ATS/ERS International Multidisciplinary Classification of Lung Adenocarcinoma. J Thorac Oncol 2010; In press

6. Winer-Muram HT. The solitary pulmonary nodule. Radiology 2006;239(1):34–49

CASE 73

■ Clinical Presentation

65-year-old man with cough and chest pain

■ Radiologic Findings

PA (**Fig. 73.1**) and lateral (**Fig. 73.2**) chest radiographs demonstrate a roughly spherical mass of lobular contours in the left lung. Contrast-enhanced chest CT (mediastinal window) (**Figs. 73.3, 73.4**) demonstrates a heterogeneously enhancing mass with irregular central low attenuation, representing necrosis. The mass abuts central bronchi medially (**Fig. 73.4**) and the adjacent pleura laterally.

■ Diagnosis

Lung Cancer; Invasive Adenocarcinoma

■ Differential Diagnosis

- Lung Cancer; Other Cell Types
- Other Primary Malignant Neoplasm
- Lung Abscess
- Solitary Metastasis (rare)

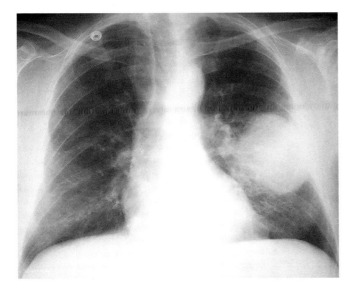

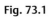
Fig. 73.1

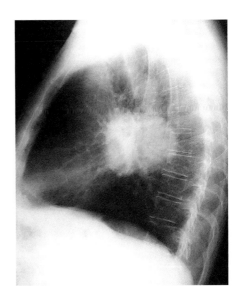
Fig. 73.2

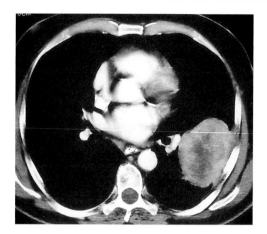

Fig. 73.3

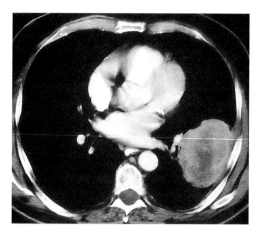

Fig. 73.4

■ Discussion

Background

Lung cancer is the most frequent primary malignancy of the lung and the most common fatal malignancy of men and women in the United States. Four principal cell types (adenocarcinoma, squamous cell carcinoma, small cell carcinoma, and large cell carcinoma) are recognized, but multi-differentiated tumors also occur. Adenocarcinoma is the most frequently diagnosed cell type of lung cancer. It typically manifests as a peripheral mass in the lung parenchyma, but central neoplasms also occur.

Etiology

Lung cancer is strongly associated with exposure to inhaled carcinogens, particularly cigarette smoke. While all cell types are related to cigarette smoking, adenocarcinoma exhibits a weak association and is the most common cell type diagnosed in non-smokers and in women. Lung cancer is also associated with exposure to occupational and environmental agents such as asbestos and radon. Conditions characterized by pulmonary fibrosis (such as usual interstitial pneumonia and progressive systemic sclerosis) are associated with an increased incidence of lung cancer, particularly adenocarcinoma. *Atypical adenomatous hyperplasia* (*AAH*) and *mucinous* and *non-mucinous adenocarcinomas in situ* (*AIS*) are pre-invasive or precursor lesions of adenocarcinoma. AAH is most common in women and is found most frequently in cancer-bearing lungs, particularly in association with adenocarcinoma. Epidermal growth factor receptor (EGFR) is a cell surface receptor that may be overexpressed in adenocarcinoma of the lung. Cell types of *invasive adenocarcinoma* include lepidic predominant, acinar predominant, papillary predominant, micropapillary predominant, and solid predominant adenocarcinomas.

Clinical Findings

Over 90% of patients with lung cancer are symptomatic at presentation. Large masses may produce cough, dyspnea, and/or chest discomfort. Pleural and chest wall invasion results in pleuritic and/or localized chest pain. Central adenocarcinomas may produce symptoms of bronchial obstruction. Paraneoplastic syndromes such as thrombophlebitis and non-bacterial thrombotic endocarditis may occur in association with adenocarcinoma. A minority of affected patients are asymptomatic and diagnosed incidentally because of abnormal chest radiography or an incidentally found lesion on CT. Adenocarcinomas should be tested for EGFR mutations since tumors that exhibit such mutations are more responsive to treatment with EGFR tyrosine kinase inhibitors. Patients with adenocarcinoma may exhibit improved outcomes when treated with pemetrexed.

Imaging Findings

Chest Radiography

- Solitary pulmonary nodule or mass of variable border characteristics; ill-defined, spiculated, or well-defined lobular contours (**Figs. 73.1, 73.2**)
- Associated hilar and/or mediastinal lymphadenopathy

MDCT

- Peripheral solid pulmonary nodule or mass with lobular or spiculated borders (**Figs. 73.3, 73.4, 73.5A, 73.5B, 73.6**); may exhibit pleural retraction (**Fig. 73.5A**)
- Subsolid pulmonary nodule; increased likelihood of invasive adenocarcinoma with increasing size of solid component and with solid components larger than 50% of the lesion; occasionally a ground glass nodule
- Nodule or mass with bubble-like or cystic lucencies, air bronchograms
- *CT angiogram sign* (vessels traversing the tumor) described in mucinous adenocarcinomas
- Cavitation (in up to 15% of lung cancers) (**Fig. 73.6**) and calcification (usually eccentric, in up to 10% of lung cancers); more common in large tumors
- Contrast enhancement (**Figs. 73.3, 73.4**)
- Pleural effusion, pleural masses, or both suggest pleural metastases (**Fig. 73.7**) and advanced malignancy
- Osseous destruction indicates chest wall involvement
- Lesion characterization, staging, and biopsy/resection planning; evaluation of adjacent structures (pleura, chest wall, mediastinum) to exclude invasion

MRI

- More sensitive than CT for demonstration of chest wall involvement
- Demonstration of hilar/mediastinal lymphadenopathy, particularly if contraindication for intravenous administration of iodinated contrast media

PET-CT

- Non-invasive evaluation of patients with lung cancer; imaging after intravenous administration of 2-(fluorine-18)-fluoro-2-deoxy-D-glucose (^{18}FDG); FDG accumulation from increased glucose utilization by malignant cells

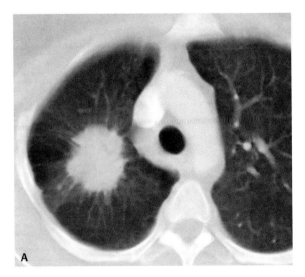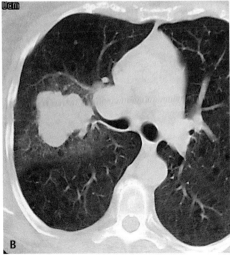

Fig. 73.5 **(A)** Coned-down chest CT (lung window) of a middle-aged woman with adenocarcinoma shows a spiculated right upper lobe mass. Note that some tumor spicules extend to the pleural surface, producing "pleural tags" or "tails" and focal retraction. **(B)** Coned-down unenhanced chest CT (lung window) of a 59-year-old woman with adenocarcinoma shows a polylobular right upper lobe mass that obstructs the lumen of the right upper lobe posterior segmental bronchus and is surrounded by ground glass attenuation. Note surrounding centrilobular emphysema.

- High sensitivity and negative predictive value in nodules over 7 mm in diameter
- Elevated standard uptake values (SUV); but SUV lower for adenocarcinoma than for other cell types of lung cancer; inverse correlation of SUV and survival

Management

- Lobectomy and lymph node dissection based on resectable stage at presentation
- EGFR mutations as predictors of response to erlotinib (Tarceva; Genentech) and gefitinib (Iressa; Astrazeneca); EGFR mutations most frequent in East Asian patients and those without a history of cigarette smoking

Prognosis

- Based on tumor stage at presentation
- Main independent prognostic factors: stage, performance status, age, and gender; smoking history may be an independent prognostic factor

PEARLS

- All cell types of lung cancer exhibit a predilection for the upper lobes.
- Doubling time (time required for doubling of tumor volume) of adenocarcinomas ranges between 7 and 465 days.
- Tumor size does not allow distinction between benign and malignant pulmonary nodules, but large masses (over 3 cm) are more likely to be malignant (**Figs. 73.1, 73.2, 73.3, 73.4**).
- While irregular spiculated lesion borders are suggestive of malignancy (**Figs. 73.5A, 73.6**), they are also described in benign conditions. However, lung cancer may also manifest as a well-defined non-lobular pulmonary nodule.
- *Tail sign* refers to a linear opacity that extends from a peripheral mass to the adjacent pleura with associated focal retraction (**Fig. 73.5A**). It is seen in up to 80% of peripheral lung cancers imaged with HRCT and is most commonly associated with adenocarcinoma.
- Patients with pulmonary fibrosis have a higher incidence of lung cancer, typically adenocarcinoma. These tumors exhibit a predilection for the lower lobes and the lung periphery (**Fig. 73.6**).
- Malignant pleural mesothelioma typically manifests with circumferential nodular pleural thickening. However, peripheral adenocarcinoma may diffusely involve the pleura and may manifest with similar imaging findings (**Fig. 73.7**).

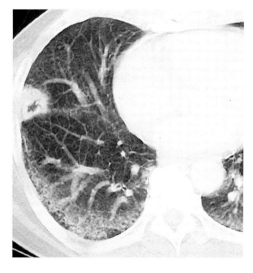

Fig. 73.6 Coned-down unenhanced chest CT (lung window) of a 66-year-old man with idiopathic pulmonary fibrosis shows a peripheral right middle lobe cavitary nodule, which represents an adenocarcinoma. Note the spiculated lesion borders and the thick nodular cavity wall.

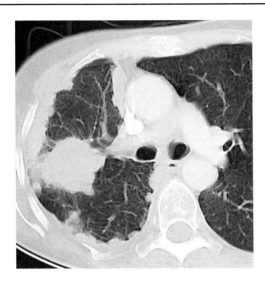

Fig. 73.7 Unenhanced chest CT (lung window) of a 43-year-old woman with adenocarcinoma demonstrates a lobular right upper lobe mass and ipsilateral circumferential nodular pleural thickening with encasement and volume loss of the right lung. The imaging findings mimic those of malignant pleural mesothelioma.

Suggested Reading

1. Beckles MA, Spiro SG, Colice GL, Rudd RM. Initial evaluation of the patient with lung cancer: symptoms, signs, laboratory tests, and paraneoplastic syndromes. Chest 2003;123(1, Suppl):97S–104S

2. Colby TV, Noguchi M, Henschke C, et al. Adenocarcinoma. In: Travis WD, Brambilla E, Müller-Hermelink HK, Harris CC, eds. World Health Organization Classification of Tumours. Pathology & Genetics. Tumours of the Lung, Pleura, Thymus and Heart. Lyon: IARC Press; 2004:35–44

3. Travis WD, Brambilla E, Noguchi M, et al. IASLC/ATS/ERS International Multidisciplinary Classification of Lung Adenocarcinoma. J Thorac Oncol 2010; In press

4. Travis WD. Lung cancer: overview and classification. In: Müller NL, Silva CIS, Hansell DM, Lee KS, Remy-Jardin M, eds. Imaging of the Chest. Philadelphia: Saunders Elsevier; 2008:471–486

CASE 74

■ Clinical Presentation

Asymptomatic 77-year-old woman

■ Radiologic Findings

Coned-down unenhanced axial and coronal chest CT (lung window) (**Figs. 74.1, 74.2**) demonstrates a right upper lobe peripheral subpleural part-solid pulmonary nodule that represents a minimally invasive adenocarcinoma. Coned-down unenhanced chest CT (lung window) of the left lung (**Fig. 74.3**) shows a 5 mm ground glass left upper lobe nodule presumed to represent a focus of atypical adenomatous hyperplasia based on imaging stability.

■ Diagnosis

Lung Cancer; Minimally Invasive Adenocarcinoma

■ Differential Diagnosis

- Pulmonary Infection
- Adenocarcinoma In Situ; Invasive Adenocarcinoma
- Lymphoma

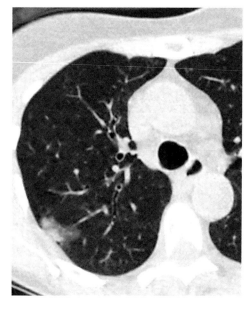

Fig. 74.1

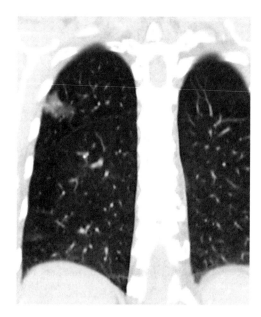

Fig. 74.2

■ Discussion

Background

The new histologic classification of adenocarcinoma does not include the former bronchioloalveolar carcinoma subtype, which was previously applied to a broad spectrum of neoplasms with widely varied mortality rates and prognostic characteristics. Instead, the new classification introduces the subtypes *adenocarcinoma in situ* (*AIS*) and *minimally invasive adenocarcinoma* (*MIA*). AIS and atypical adenomatous hyperplasia (AAH) are recognized as precursor or preinvasive lesions for invasive adenocarcinoma of the lung. AIS refers to small lesions (≤3 cm) with pure lepidic growth and no stromal, vascular, or pleural invasion. MIA refers to small lesions (≤3 cm) that exhibit a predominantly lepidic growth and ≤5 mm of locally invasive tumor in any one focus. The term *lepidic* means "related to scales" or "scaly covering layer" and is used to describe tumors that grow with a replacement pattern or along pre-existing alveolar structures.

Etiology

The etiology of AIS and MIA is poorly understood. However, AAH is recognized as the precursor lesion for both cell types and for invasive adenocarcinoma.

Clinical Findings

AIS and MIA are typically found incidentally in asymptomatic patients who undergo chest CT. Subclinical pulmonary infections may mimic these lesions. For this reason, patients with such incidentally discovered lesions may be given a course of antibiotics to document resolution of these abnormalities. Persistent lesions are characteristically managed based on findings at serial chest CT according to the criteria proposed by Godoy and Naidich.

Imaging Findings

Chest Radiography

- Normal chest radiograph
- Subtle, ill-defined, small pulmonary nodule(s) or ground glass nodular opacity(ies)

MDCT

AAH

- Focal or multi-focal, small (≤5 mm) pure ground glass nodule(s) (**Figs. 74.3, 74.4A, 74.4B**)
- May be seen in association with invasive adenocarcinoma

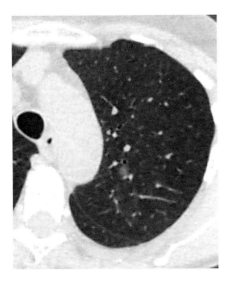

Fig. 74.3

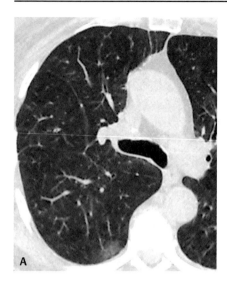 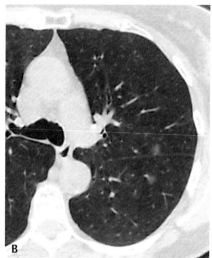

Fig.74.4 **(A)** Coned-down unenhanced chest CT (lung window) of the right lung of an asymptomatic woman with multifocal ground glass nodules demonstrates a dominant ground glass nodule in the right lower lobe. **(B)** Coned-down unenhanced chest CT (lung window) of the left lung shows smaller ground glass nodules in the left upper and lower lobes. These lesions were stable and are thought to represent AAH or AIS. The lesions are being followed, as the patient is not a surgical candidate.

AIS

- Focal or multifocal
- Ground glass, part-solid or solid lung nodule(s) (**Fig. 74.5**)

MIA

- Part-solid nodule with predominant ground glass opacity; solid component typically measures 5 mm or less (**Fig. 74.6**)
- AAH, AIS, and MIA may exhibit overlapping imaging features (**Fig. 74.7**)

Management

- Lobectomy and lymph node dissection for solid nodules
- Use of sublobar resection for AIS and MIA; awaits results of randomized clinical trials currently underway in North America and Japan

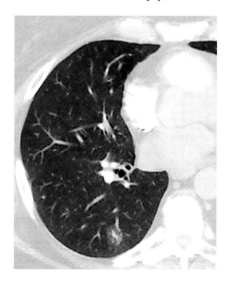

Fig. 74.5 Coned-down chest CT (lung window) of an asymptomatic 55-year-old woman demonstrates a part-solid right lower lobe ground glass nodule that represents an AIS.

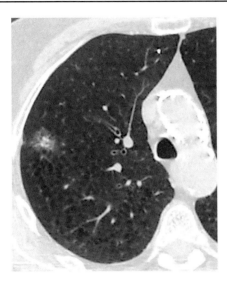

Fig. 74.6 Coned-down chest CT (lung window) of an asymptomatic 78-year-old woman with a part-solid nodule in the right upper lobe. The solid component occupies more than 50% of the lesion, making it suspicious for MIA or invasive adenocarcinoma.

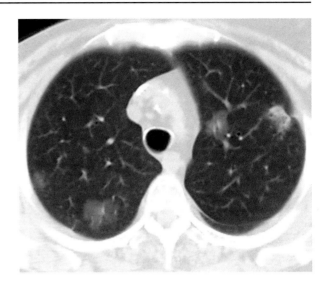

Fig. 74.7 Unenhanced chest CT (lung window) of an asymptomatic 73-year-old woman demonstrates multifocal bilateral nodules in the upper lobes. The peripheral nodule in the left upper lobe is mostly solid, exhibits intrinsic cystic changes, and was thought to represent an invasive adenocarcinoma. The rest of the lesions are non-solid or part-solid and may represent AAH, AIS, and/or MIA. The patient is not a surgical candidate and is being observed. Had the patient been a surgical candidate, excision of the dominant, mostly solid left upper lobe lesion would have been strongly considered.

Prognosis

• Nearly 100% disease-specific survival for surgically resected AIS and MIA

PEARLS

• Thin-section CT is used to follow small non-solid and part-solid nodules as these are rarely visible on radiography.
• Multiplanar reformatted images may be of value, as some neoplasms may only demonstrate growth in the craniocaudad dimension.
• AIS and MIA are not felt to be FDG avid when compared with other cell types of lung cancer and are expected to result in false negative PET-CT.

Suggested Reading

1. Godoy MCB, Naidich DP. Subsolid pulmonary nodules and the spectrum of peripheral adenocarcinomas of the lung: recommended interim guidelines for assessment and management. Radiology 2009;253(3):606–622

2. Marom EM, Sarvis S, Herndon JE II, Patz EF Jr. T1 lung cancers: sensitivity of diagnosis with fluorodeoxyglucose PET. Radiology 2002;223(2):453–459

3. Travis WD, Brambilla E, Noguchi M, et al. IASLC/ATS/ERS International Multidisciplinary Classification of Lung Adenocarcinoma. J Thorac Oncol 2010; In press

4. Colby TV, Noguchi M, Henschke C, et al. Adenocarcinoma. In: Travis WD, Brambilla E, Müller-Hermelink HK, Harris CC, eds. World Health Organization Classification of Tumours. Pathology & Genetics. Tumours of the Lung, Pleura, Thymus and Heart. Lyon: IARC Press; 2004:35–44

CASE 75

■ Clinical Presentation

56-year-old woman evaluated because of left upper extremity pain

■ Radiologic Findings

Coned-down PA chest radiograph (**Fig. 75.1**) shows a left apical lung mass with spiculated borders, associated pleural thickening, and destruction of the left posterior second rib (*arrow*). Contrast-enhanced chest CT (mediastinal window) (**Figs. 75.2, 75.3**) demonstrates the locally invasive left apical soft-tissue mass which partially encases the left subclavian artery. Contrast-enhanced coronal T1-weighted MR with fat saturation (**Fig. 75.4**) reveals to better advantage the extent of the soft-tissue mass, which completely encases the left subclavian artery and surrounds portions of the left brachial plexus

■ Diagnosis

Pancoast Tumor; Adenocarcinoma

■ Differential Diagnosis

* Pancoast Tumor; Other Cell Type
* Pulmonary Lymphoma

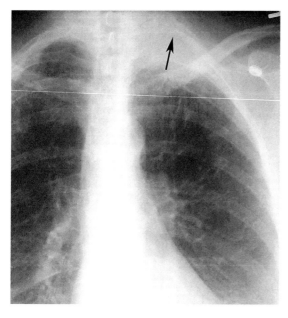

Fig. 75.1

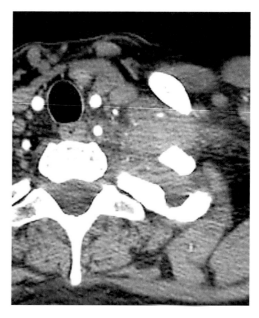

Fig. 75.2

376

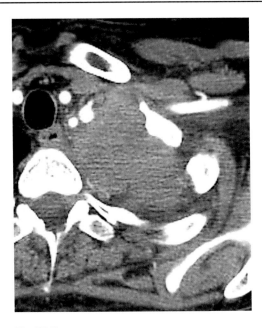

Fig. 75.3

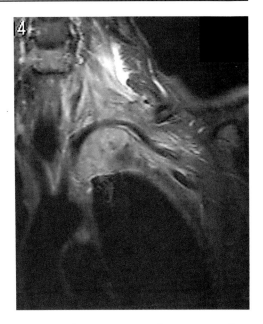

Fig. 75.4   *(Images courtesy of Santiago Martínez-Jiménez, MD, Duke University Medical Center, Durham, North Carolina.)*

■ Discussion

Background

Pancoast tumor or superior pulmonary sulcus tumor refers to lung carcinomas arising in the apical lung parenchyma and represents approximately 3% of primary non–small cell lung cancers. These lesions may involve the chest wall soft tissues of the adjacent thoracic inlet and may produce a characteristic clinical syndrome known as the Pancoast syndrome. The superior sulcus is anatomically divided into anterior, middle, and posterior compartments by the scalene muscles. Evaluation of patients with Pancoast tumor is directed at evaluation of the structures of the superior sulcus, including the subclavian vein, the subclavian artery, the brachial plexus, and the stellate ganglion. While Pancoast tumors were previously thought to primarily represent peripheral squamous cell carcinomas, recent series report that most are adenocarcinomas.

Etiology

The etiology of Pancoast tumors is poorly understood. These peripheral lung cancers produce local invasion of the adjacent chest wall rather than extending inferiorly into the adjacent lung parenchyma.

Clinical Findings

Patients with Pancoast tumor may present with characteristic symptoms and signs of the Pancoast syndrome, namely shoulder and arm pain and Horner syndrome, characterized by ipsilateral ptosis, anhydrosis, myosis, and enophthalmos. These tumors were originally described by Henry Pancoast in four patients who presented with shoulder and upper extremity pain, atrophy of the ipsilateral hand muscles, and Horner syndrome.

Imaging Findings

Chest Radiography

- Apical mass; may mimic apical pleural thickening (**Fig. 75.1**)
- Associated skeletal involvement, including rib (usually first or second posterior rib) or vertebral body destruction (**Fig. 75.1**)

MDCT

- Right apical soft-tissue mass arising in the lung parenchyma (**Figs. 75.2, 75.3**)
- Evidence of chest wall involvement; skeletal or soft-tissue invasion; modality of choice for evaluation of skeletal structures (**Figs. 75.2, 75.3**)

MRI

- Optimal modality for evaluating superior sulcus soft tissues and determining tumor resectability (**Fig. 75.4**)
- Superior for differentiating tumor from adjacent soft tissues and for detecting involvement of the spinal canal, neuroforamina, vascular structures, and brachial plexus (**Fig. 75.4**)

PET-CT

- Detection of lymph node and distant metastasis; baseline staging

Management

- Multimodality therapy consisting of surgery and pre- or postoperative radiation therapy with or without chemotherapy
- Absolute contraindications to surgical resection: brachial plexus invasion above T1, invasion of >50% of a vertebral body, invasion of esophagus or trachea, distant metastases, N2 or contralateral N3 nodal metastases
- Relative contraindications to surgical resection: invasion of the subclavian artery, invasion of <50% of a vertebral body, neuroforaminal extension, invasion of common carotid or vertebral arteries, ipsilateral N1 or N3 nodal metastases

Prognosis

- Up to 47% five-year survival in patients undergoing multimodality treatment (surgery and radiation therapy)

PEARLS

- Patients with Pancoast tumor do not typically present with characteristic symptoms of lung cancer, such as cough, dyspnea, or hemoptysis. In fact, many present with shoulder pain that is often thought to be related to musculoskeletal disease.

Suggested Readings

1. Bruzzi JF, Komaki R, Walsh GL, et al. Imaging of non-small cell lung cancer of the superior sulcus: part 1: anatomy, clinical manifestations, and management. Radiographics 2008;28(2):551–560, quiz 620
2. Bruzzi JF, Komaki R, Walsh GL, et al. Imaging of non-small cell lung cancer of the superior sulcus: part 2: initial staging and assessment of resectability and therapeutic response. Radiographics 2008;28(2):561–572

CASE 76

■ Clinical Presentation

57-year-old woman with cough, hemoptysis and weight loss

■ Radiologic Findings

PA (**Fig. 76.1**) and lateral (**Fig. 76.2**) chest radiographs demonstrate a large right hilar mass with associated upper lobe volume loss. Note the reverse "S" shape produced by the concave outline of the lateral aspect of the minor fissure and the convex outline of the central mass (**Fig. 76.1**), the so-called reverse "S" sign of Golden. Contrast-enhanced chest CT (lung and mediastinal windows) (**Figs. 76.3, 76.4**) reveals a large central mass that produces severe irregular narrowing of the right mainstem bronchus (**Fig. 76.3**), atelectasis of the right upper lobe (**Fig. 76.4**), and deformity of the superior vena cava consistent with local invasion (**Fig. 76.4**).

■ Diagnosis

Lung Cancer; Squamous Cell Carcinoma

■ Differential Diagnosis

* Lung Cancer, Other Cell Type
* Other Primary Malignant Neoplasm
* Lymphoma
* Metastatic Disease

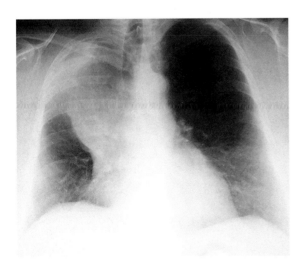

Fig. 76.1

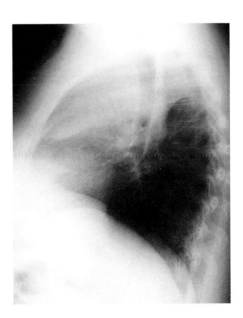

Fig. 76.2

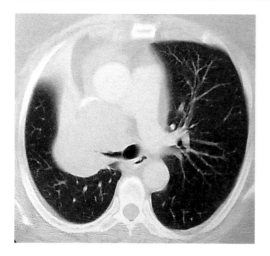

Fig. 76.3

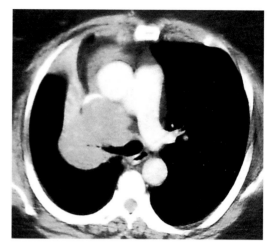

Fig. 76.4

■ Discussion

Background

Squamous cell carcinoma accounts for approximately 30% of all lung carcinomas. It is a malignant epithelial neoplasm characterized by microscopic keratinization and/or intercellular bridges. It exhibits rapid local growth and relatively late distant metastases.

Etiology

Squamous cell carcinoma has a strong association with cigarette smoking (over 90% affect smokers) and exposure to inhaled carcinogens, particularly arsenic. Squamous dysplasia and squamous carcinoma in situ are precursor lesions.

Clinical Findings

Squamous cell carcinomas are rapidly growing neoplasms with a predilection for the central airways. Affected patients usually exhibit early signs and symptoms of airway obstruction, including cough, hemoptysis, wheezing, and obstructive pneumonia. Some patients present with paraneoplastic syndromes, such as hypercalcemia, resulting from a parathyroid hormone–related peptide produced by the tumor. Digital clubbing and hypertrophic pulmonary osteoarthropathy (HPOA) are most frequently associated with squamous cell lung carcinoma and adenocarcinoma. HPOA manifests as a painful bilateral arthropathy of the ankles, knees, and wrists and periosteal new bone formation of the distal long bones of the extremities. Squamous cell carcinoma is the cell type of lung cancer most likely to cavitate, and cavitary lesions may exhibit epidermal growth factor receptor (EGFR) over-expression, which is taken into consideration for targeted therapy.

Imaging Findings

Chest Radiography

- Frequent secondary atelectasis (absent air bronchograms) (**Figs. 76.1, 76.2**), obstructive pneumonia, or mucoid impaction; may be dominant radiologic abnormalities
- Central mass (**Figs. 76.1, 76.2, 76.5A**)
- Bronchial wall thickening; thickened (>3 mm) intermediate stem line (i.e., posterior wall of the bronchus intermedius) (lateral radiography) (**Fig. 76.5A**)
- Peripheral lung nodule or mass
- Cavitation
- Lymphadenopathy (**Figs. 76.1, 76.2, 76.5A**)

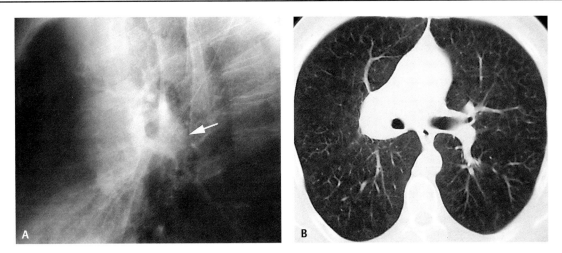

Fig. 76.5   **(A)** Coned-down lateral chest radiograph of a 41-year-old man with a central squamous cell carcinoma demonstrates thickening of the posterior wall of the bronchus intermedius (intermediate stem line) with a nodular posterior contour (*arrow*) suggestive of malignancy and lymphadenopathy. **(B)** Unenhanced chest CT (lung window) reveals the right central mass/lymphadenopathy and associated bronchial wall thickening.

MDCT

- Irregular central mass with abrupt obstruction of bronchial lumen (**Figs. 76.3, 76.4, 76.6**)
- Post-obstructive consolidation (**Figs. 76.6, 76.7**), atelectasis (**Figs. 76.3, 76.4**); contrast administration may help differentiate tumor from adjacent consolidation and atelectasis (**Fig. 76.4**), as tumor typically enhances less than atelectatic lung
- Bronchial wall thickening (**Figs. 76.3, 76.5B**)
- Peripheral mass or nodule (**Figs. 76.7B, 76.8**)
- Cavitation; central or eccentric, irregular inner surface (**Figs. 76.7B, 76.8**)
- Mediastinal (**Figs. 76.3, 76.4**), osseous or soft-tissue invasion
- Lymphadenopathy (**Figs. 76.3, 76.4, 76.5B**)

MRI

- More sensitive than CT for demonstration of chest wall involvement
- Distinction of tumor from surrounding atelectasis/consolidation
- Demonstration of hilar/mediastinal lymphadenopathy, particularly when intravenous contrast is contraindicated

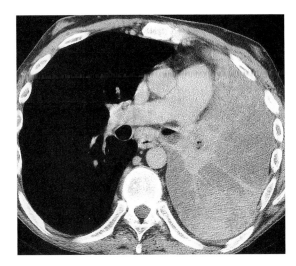

Fig. 76.6 Unenhanced chest CT (mediastinal window) demonstrates a central spiculated soft-tissue mass encasing the left mainstem bronchus surrounded by low-attenuation "drowned" lung. Note the absence of air bronchograms.

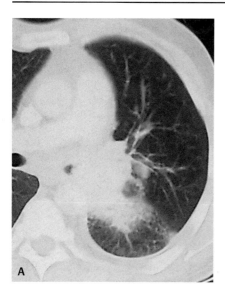
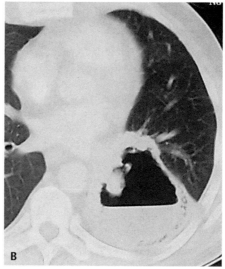

Fig. 76.7 Coned-down chest CT (lung window) of a 58-year-old man with a central squamous cell carcinoma demonstrates an irregular soft-tissue mass obstructing the left lower lobe bronchus **(A)** with distal lower lobe consolidation and cavitation **(B)**.

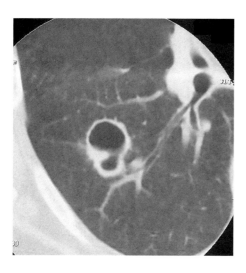

Fig. 76.8 HRCT (lung window) targeted at the right lung of an asymptomatic 50-year-old man with squamous cell carcinoma demonstrates a 2.8 cm right lower lobe cavitary nodule. Note the irregular nodular cavity wall.

PET-CT

- Non-invasive evaluation of patients with lung cancer; imaging after intravenous administration of 2-(fluorine-18)-fluoro-2-deoxy-D-glucose (^{18}FDG); FDG accumulation from increased glucose utilization by malignant cells
- High sensitivity and negative predictive value in tumors over 1 cm in diameter

Management

- Based on tumor stage at presentation; surgical excision of resectable lesions
- Targeted therapy with anti-EGFR agents in tumors with EGFR over-expression

Prognosis

- Main independent prognostic factors: stage, performance status, age, and gender; smoking history
- Cavitation with EGFR over-expression identified as a predictor of poor outcome in Stage I lung cancers

PEARLS

- *Reverse "S" sign of Golden* refers to lobar collapse associated with a central obstructing mass, which produces a convex contour medial to the concave contour of atelectatic right upper lobe on frontal radiography (**Fig. 76.1**) (see Case 38). Similar contour abnormalities are seen on other lobes, on lateral radiography (**Fig. 76.2**) and on chest CT (**Fig. 76.3**). This finding is highly suggestive of malignancy.
- Squamous cell carcinoma is the most frequent cell type of lung cancer to exhibit cavitation. Most cavitary cancers exhibit irregular nodular inner cavity walls measuring 0.5–3.0 cm in thickness (**Figs. 76.7B, 76.8**), but thin, smooth cavity walls (that may mimic benign conditions) are also described.
- Airway obstruction from a central lung carcinoma is often complete. Resultant consolidations do not typically exhibit air bronchograms and are characterized by volume loss (**Figs. 76.1, 76.2**). However, obstructive pneumonitis with consolidation may limit loss of volume, and air spaces may fill with fluid, a finding known as *drowned lung* (**Fig. 76.6**). However, long-standing obstruction may also result in infection and abscess formation (**Fig. 76.7B**).

Suggested Reading

1. Felson B. The lobes. In: Felson B, ed. Chest Roentgenology. Philadelphia: WB Saunders; 1973:71–142

2. Onn A, Choe DH, Herbst RS, et al. Tumor cavitation in stage I non-small cell lung cancer: epidermal growth factor receptor expression and prediction of poor outcome. Radiology 2005;237(1):342–347

3. Hammar SP, Brambilla C, Pugatch B, et al. Squamous cell carcinoma. In: Travis WD, Brambilla E, Müller-Hermelink HK, Harris CC, eds. World Health Organization Classification of Tumours. Pathology & Genetics. Tumours of the Lung, Pleura, Thymus and Heart. Lyon: IARC Press; 2004:26–30

4. Travis WD. Lung cancer: overview and classification. In: Müller NL, Silva CIS, Hansell DM, Lee KS, Remy-Jardin M, eds. Imaging of the Chest. Philadelphia: Saunders Elsevier; 2008:471–486

CASE 77

■ Clinical Presentation

60-year-old woman with facial swelling and weight loss

■ Radiologic Findings

PA (**Fig. 77.1**) and lateral (**Fig. 77.2**) chest radiographs demonstrate a mediastinal mass of lobular contours that extends to both sides of midline and is predominantly located in the anterior mediastinum (**Fig. 77.2**). Note the small right pleural effusion. Contrast-enhanced chest CT (mediastinal window) (**Figs. 77.3, 77.4**) demonstrates extensive mediastinal lymphadenopathy encasing the great vessels and the central tracheo-bronchial tree as well as a small right pleural effusion. Note the almost complete obliteration of the lumen of the superior vena cava (**Fig. 77.4**), enhancing chest wall collateral vessels (*arrow*) (**Fig. 77.3**), and intense enhancement of the azygos vein (**Fig. 77.4**), consistent with superior vena cava obstruction.

■ Diagnosis

Lung Cancer; Small Cell Carcinoma

■ Differential Diagnosis

- Lung Cancer, Other Cell Type
- Lymphoma
- Mediastinal Metastases

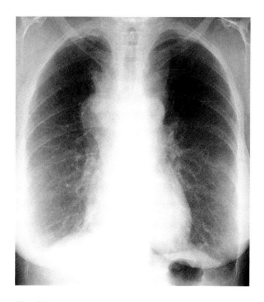

Fig. 77.1

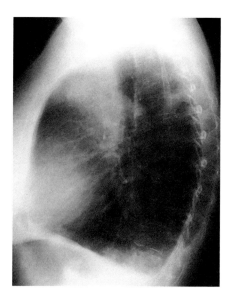

Fig. 77.2

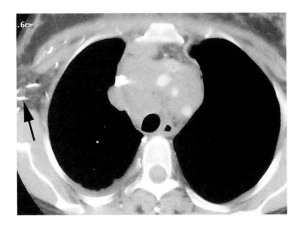

Fig. 77.3

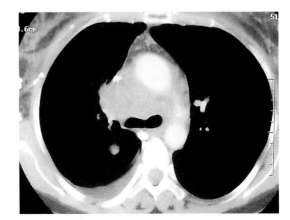

Fig. 77.4

■ Discussion

Background

Small cell carcinoma is a malignant epithelial neoplasm characterized by small cells with scant cytoplasm and poorly defined cell borders. It is a highly aggressive neoplasm that accounts for approximately 13.8–20% of all lung cancers. It is characterized by rapid local tumor growth and frequent metastases at presentation.

Etiology

All cell types of lung cancer are associated with cigarette smoking, but small cell carcinoma demonstrates the strongest association. This cell type is also strongly associated with occupational exposure to chloromethyl ether and radon gas.

Clinical Findings

Patients with small cell carcinoma are typically elderly males with a significant history of cigarette smoking. Symptoms such as cough and dyspnea often relate to central airway obstruction. Locally invasive tumors may grow into the mediastinum, with resultant retrosternal pain, hoarseness, and vocal cord paralysis. Small cell carcinoma is the most common neoplasm to produce superior vena cava syndrome, characterized by facial and upper extremity swelling, headache, and dizziness. Patients with small cell carcinoma may also present with signs and symptoms related to metastatic disease, such as anorexia, malaise, fever, and weight loss. Secretion of peptide hormones may result in paraneoplastic syndromes related to excessive production of adrenocorticotropic (ACTH) or antidiuretic (ADH) hormones. Small cell carcinoma may also be associated with paraneoplastic autoimmune neurologic syndromes, such as Lambert-Eaton myasthenic syndrome, peripheral neuropathy, and cortical cerebellar degeneration.

Imaging Findings

Chest Radiography

- Large central mass with hilar and/or mediastinal lymphadenopathy
- Hilar and/or mediastinal lymphadenopathy as dominant finding without visualization of primary tumor (**Figs. 77.1, 77.2**)
- Rarely peripheral nodule/mass with or without lymphadenopathy

MDCT

- Primary tumor assessment, demonstration of local invasion (**Figs. 77.3, 77.4**)
- Identification of lymphadenopathy (**Figs. 77.3, 77.4**)
- Demonstration of superior vena cava obstruction on contrast-enhanced CT; non-visualization of superior vena cava lumen, enhancement of chest wall/mediastinal collateral vessels (**Fig. 77.4**)
- Identification of liver, adrenal gland, and/or chest wall metastases

MRI

- May be superior to CT in demonstrating mediastinal invasion; multiplanar imaging assessment of vascular/pericardial invasion without need for intravenous contrast

Management

- Chemotherapy
- Limited-stage small cell lung cancer: consideration of concurrent radiotherapy
- Very limited-stage disease (rare) (T1/T2, N0): surgical excision with combination chemotherapy
- Endovascular stenting for patients with superior vena cava syndrome, with prompt relief of symptoms and return to normal hemodynamics

Prognosis

- Poor prognosis; five-year survival of 1–5%
- Poor prognosis, particularly with extensive disease, poor performance status, elevated LDH or alkaline phosphatase, low plasma albumin, and low plasma sodium levels
- Median survival without treatment: 2–4 months
- Response to chemotherapy frequent but of short duration (4 months for patients with extensive-stage disease; 12 months for patients with limited-stage disease)

Suggested Reading

1. Lanciego C, Chacón JL, Julián A, et al. Stenting as first option for endovascular treatment of malignant superior vena cava syndrome. AJR Am J Roentgenol 2001;177(3):585–593

2. Simon GR, Wagner H; American College of Chest Physicians. Small cell lung cancer. Chest 2003;123(1, Suppl):259S–271S

3. Travis W, Nicholson S, Hirsch FR, et al. Small cell carcinoma. In: Travis WD, Brambilla E, Müller-Hermelink HK, Harris CC, eds. World Health Organization Classification of Tumours. Pathology & Genetics. Tumours of the Lung, Pleura, Thymus and Heart. Lyon: IARC Press; 2004:31–34

4. Travis WD. Lung cancer: overview and classification. In: Müller NL, Silva CIS, Hansell DM, Lee KS, Remy-Jardin M, eds. Imaging of the Chest. Philadelphia: Saunders Elsevier; 2008:471–486

5. Zakowski MF. Pathology of small cell carcinoma of the lung. Semin Oncol 2003;30(1):3–8

CASE 78

■ Clinical Presentation

70-year-old woman with right chest wall pain

■ Radiologic Findings

PA (**Fig. 78.1**) and lateral (**Fig. 78.2**) chest radiographs demonstrate a large ovoid right upper lobe mass of lobular contours with adjacent right apical pleural thickening and suggestion of destruction of the anterolateral portions of the second and third right ribs.

■ Diagnosis

Lung Cancer: Large Cell Carcinoma

■ Differential Diagnosis

- Lung Cancer; Other Cell Type
- Lymphoma
- Lung Abscess

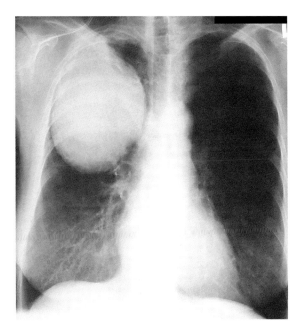

Fig. 78.1

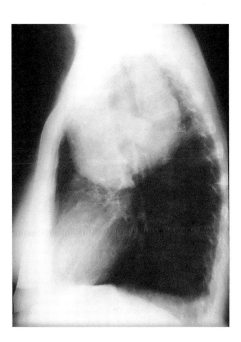

Fig. 78.2

387

■ Discussion

Background

Large cell carcinoma is an undifferentiated lung cancer that lacks features of adenocarcinoma, squamous cell carcinoma or small cell carcinoma and is considered a diagnosis of exclusion. It is an aggressive cell type of lung cancer that accounts for approximately 9% of all lung carcinomas. These neoplasms are characterized by rapid growth and frequent metastases at presentation.

Etiology

Large cell carcinomas are strongly associated with cigarette smoking.

Clinical Findings

Patients with large cell carcinoma may present with cough, dyspnea, and/or chest pain related to tumor size, obstruction, and/or local invasion.

Imaging Findings

Chest Radiography

- Large peripheral lung mass (**Figs. 78.1, 78.2**)
- Large central mass
- Mass with associated hilar and/or mediastinal lymphadenopathy

MDCT

- Large mass
- Frequent heterogeneous attenuation, particularly after intravenous contrast
- Frequent lymphadenopathy
- Assessment of local invasion

MRI

- Superior to CT for visualization of chest wall/mediastinal invasion

Management

- Based on tumor stage at presentation; surgical excision of resectable lesions

Prognosis

- Generally poor prognosis
- Prognostic criteria include performance status and tumor stage at presentation

Suggested Reading

1. Brambilla E, Pugatch B, Geisinger K, et al. Large cell carcinoma. In: Travis WD, Brambilla E, Müller-Hermelink HK, Harris CC, eds. World Health Organization Classification of Tumours. Pathology & Genetics. Tumours of the Lung, Pleura, Thymus and Heart. Lyon: IARC Press; 2004:45–50
2. Travis WD. Lung cancer: overview and classification. In: Müller NL, Silva CIS, Hansell DM, Lee KS, Remy-Jardin M, eds. Imaging of the Chest. Philadelphia: Saunders Elsevier; 2008:471–486

CASE 79

■ Clinical Presentation

76-year-old woman with chest discomfort and weight loss

■ Radiologic Findings

PA chest radiograph (**Fig. 79.1**) demonstrates a dominant polylobular mass in the left upper lobe and a poly-lobular nodule in the right upper lobe. Unenhanced chest CT (lung window) (**Figs. 79.2, 79.3**) shows the dominant polylobular mass in the left upper lobe (**Fig. 79.2**) and the right upper lobe polylobular nodule, which exhibits slightly spiculated borders and a pleural tag (**Fig. 79.3**). Coronal reformatted unenhanced chest CT (lung window) (**Fig. 79.4**) illustrates the bilateral upper lobe lung cancers.

■ Diagnosis

Multicentric Synchronous Lung Cancers

■ Differential Diagnosis

- Multifocal Infection
- Pulmonary Vasculitis
- Pulmonary Metastases; Atypical Manifestation because of Upper Lobe Involvement

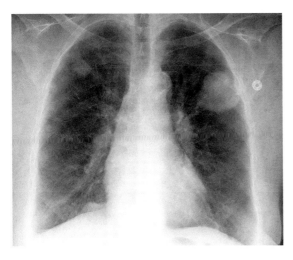

Fig. 79.1

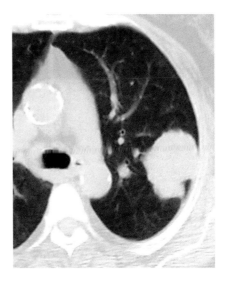

Fig. 79.2

389

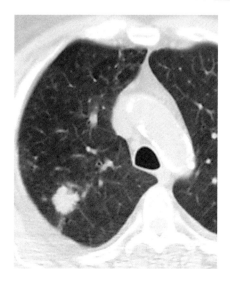

Fig. 79.3

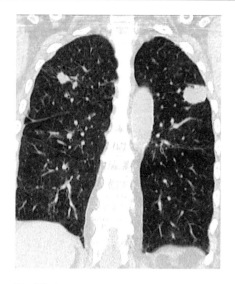

Fig. 79.4

■ Discussion

Background

Multicentric primary lung cancers can be classified as synchronous or metachronous types. *Synchronous lung cancers* are detected or resected simultaneously, whereas in the case of *metachronous lung cancers*, there is a time interval between the detection of the first lesion and the detection of a subsequent lesion. In these cases, the additional pulmonary lesion may represent a second primary neoplasm, a recurrence of the original primary neoplasm, or a pulmonary metastasis. *Metachronous lung cancers* are more common and occur in up to 70% of cases. Some primary lung cancers, particularly adenocarcinomas, may manifest as multicentric neoplasms. The incidence of *synchronous* multiple primary lung cancers is estimated to range from 0.2% to 20% and is increasing, likely due to widespread early detection with chest CT and PET imaging.

Etiology

The etiology of synchronous lung cancers is poorly understood.

Clinical Findings

Patients with synchronous lung cancers may be entirely asymptomatic. Large and advanced lesions may result in local symptoms, including dyspnea, cough, chest pain, and respiratory failure. Advanced metastatic lung cancers may produce systemic complaints.

Imaging Findings

Chest Radiography

- Multifocal nodules and/or masses; may be unilateral or bilateral (**Fig. 79.1**)
- Variable size (**Fig. 79.1**)
- Variable morphologic features; well- or poorly defined borders, lobulated contours (**Fig. 79.1**), spiculated borders, cavitation
- May exhibit associated hilar/mediastinal lymphadenopathy
- May exhibit associated pleural effusion

MDCT

- Multifocal nodules and/or masses (**Figs. 79.4–79.6**)
- Variable morphologic features (**Figs. 79.2–79.6**); may exhibit well- or poorly-defined borders, lobulated contours, spiculated borders and/or cavitation (**Fig. 79.5**)
- May exhibit associated lymphadenopathy and/or pleural effusion

Management

- Complete anatomic tumor resection with radical lymphadenectomy when feasible
- In the case of a dominant lung cancer with associated multi-focal stable non-solid nodules, resection of the dominant lesion and observation of the ground glass nodules may be considered

Prognosis

- Influenced by cell type and tumor stage
- Influenced by size of largest neoplasm
- Reported two- and five-year overall survivals of 61.6% and 34%, respectively, in surgically treated patients
- Survival adversely affected by smoking status, low FEV_1, postoperative complications, and necessity of pneumonectomy
- Consideration of adjuvant treatment

PEARLS

- Synchronous lung cancers may present difficulties in tumor staging. It may not always be possible to prospectively determine if lesions are truly synchronous lung cancers; bilateral tumors may be designated as M1a lesions, placing affected patients in the unresectable Stage IV category.

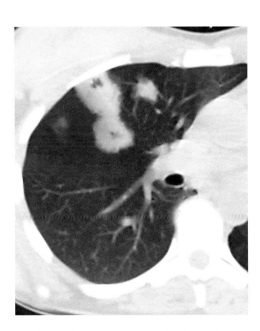

Fig. 79.5 Coned-down chest CT (lung window) of an asymptomatic 40-year-old woman demonstrates three of several multicentric synchronous right upper lobe lung cancers. The lesions exhibit polylobular borders and small intrinsic cavitation.

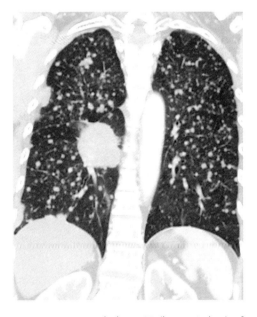

Fig. 79.6 Coronal chest CT (lung window) of a 60-year-old woman who presented with chest pain and weight loss shows a dominant polylobular, slightly spiculated mass in the right lower lobe and synchronous multifocal bilateral pulmonary nodules consistent with metastatic disease. Peripheral elongated right pleural lesions likely represent pleural metastases.

Suggested Reading

1. Asamura H. Multiple primary cancers or multiple metastases, that is the question. J Thorac Oncol 2010;5(7):930–931

2. De Leyn P, Moons J, Vansteenkiste J, et al. Survival after resection of synchronous bilateral lung cancer. Eur J Cardiothorac Surg 2008;34(6):1215–1222

3. Trousse D, Barlesi F, Loundou A, et al. Synchronous multiple primary lung cancer: an increasing clinical occurrence requiring multidisciplinary management. J Thorac Cardiovasc Surg 2007;133(5):1193–1200

4. Tsutsui S, Ashizawa K, Minami K, et al. Multiple focal pure ground-glass opacities on high-resolution CT images: Clinical significance in patients with lung cancer. AJR Am J Roentgenol 2010;195(2):W131–W138

CASE 80

■ Clinical Presentation

50-year-old woman status post hysterectomy for uterine cancer

■ Radiologic Findings

PA (**Fig. 80.1**) and lateral (**Fig. 80.2**) chest radiographs demonstrate multiple bilateral well-defined spherical pulmonary nodules and masses, which are most numerous in the lung bases.

■ Diagnosis

Pulmonary Metastases

■ Differential Diagnosis

- Primary Pulmonary Lymphoma
- Multicentric Lung Cancer
- Hematogenous Infection
- Vasculitis

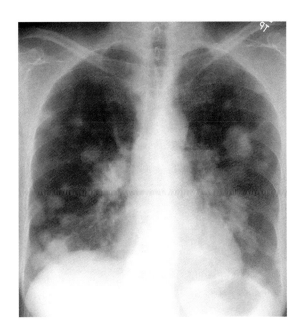

Fig. 80.1

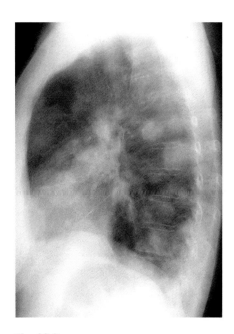

Fig. 80.2

■ Discussion

Background

The term *metastasis* is generally defined as the transfer of disease from one organ to another that is not in direct contiguity. In the setting of neoplasia, metastases are characteristic of malignancy. Pulmonary metastases represent the most frequent pulmonary neoplasm. Depending on the location of the primary tumor, lung metastases may represent early or late neoplastic dissemination. Secondary lung neoplasia may occur via hematogenous, lymphatic, and tracheobronchial routes.

Etiology

Pulmonary metastases typically result from hematogenous dissemination of malignancy. The neoplastic cells are transported to the lung and "arrest" in its capillary bed. Thus, most primary neoplasms that produce lung metastases have a rich vascular supply and a venous drainage into the systemic circulation, with the lung as the filtering organ. Pulmonary metastases may in turn metastasize and produce disseminated malignancy.

Clinical Findings

Patients with pulmonary metastases may be entirely asymptomatic. When metastases are numerous, large, and/or involve the airways and pleura, affected patients may experience dyspnea, cough, chest pain, and respiratory failure. Patients with lymphangitic carcinomatosis typically present with dyspnea. Patients with sarcoma metastatic to the lung may present with acute chest pain because of secondary spontaneous pneumothorax. Most patients with pulmonary metastases have a known history of malignancy. Rarely, patients present with pulmonary metastases from an unknown primary neoplasm.

Imaging Findings

Chest Radiography

- Bilateral multifocal well-defined nodules/masses; spherical morphology (**Figs. 80.1, 80.2**)
- Variable size (miliary nodules to large *cannon ball* masses)
- Multi-focal opacities with ill-defined borders; may mimic air space disease
- Most numerous in the lower lobes (**Figs. 80.1, 80.2**)
- May exhibit associated hilar/mediastinal lymphadenopathy
- May exhibit associated pleural effusion
- Rarely
  - Cavitation, most frequent in metastases from squamous cell carcinomas, but also described in adenocarcinomas and sarcomas
  - Calcification
  - Solitary nodule/mass
  - Endobronchial lesion; may exhibit atelectasis/consolidation
  - Lymphangitic carcinomatosis

MDCT

- Multi-focal well-defined spherical pulmonary nodules/masses (**Figs. 80.3, 80.4**)
- Variable shape; larger nodules may be lobular or exhibit irregular margins
- Most numerous in lung bases and subpleural lung periphery (outer one-third of lung) (**Fig. 80.3**)
- May exhibit associated lymphadenopathy and/or pleural effusion
- May exhibit a vascular relationship (angiocentric), a pulmonary vessel coursing into the metastasis (*feeding vessel sign*) (**Fig. 80.3**)
- Rarely
  - Cavitation (**Fig. 80.4**)
  - Calcification (e.g., osteogenic sarcoma, synovial cell sarcoma, or chondrosarcoma metastases)
  - Solitary nodule/mass

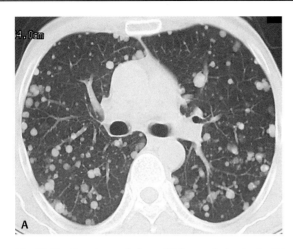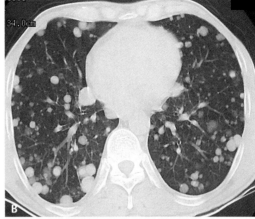

Fig. 80.3   Unenhanced chest CT (lung window) of a 58-year-old man with metastatic salivary gland carcinoma demonstrates multiple bilateral, well-defined pulmonary nodules. Note the spherical morphology of the lesions, their angiocentric distribution, and the preferential involvement of the lung periphery and the lower lobes.

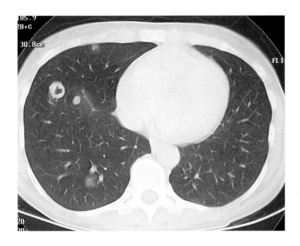

Fig. 80.4   Chest CT (lung window) of a middle-aged woman with metastatic ovarian carcinoma reveals several right lung metastases, one of which exhibits cavitation. Note the nodular morphology and irregular thickness of the cavity wall.

- ○ Lymphangitic carcinomatosis
- ○ Endobronchial metastases
- ○ Intravascular tumor emboli (most commonly hepatocellular carcinoma; adenocarcinoma of breast and stomach)

Management

- Systemic therapy based on cell type
- Radiation therapy in selected cases
- Surgical excision of solitary or limited pulmonary metastases (when the lung is the only affected site) with continued surveillance and possible additional metastasectomies
- Radiofrequency ablation

Prognosis

- Poor
- Better in patients with limited metastases who are candidates for metastasectomy

PEARLS

- CT is more sensitive than radiography in detecting pulmonary metastases, particularly for nodules over 3 mm in size. However, it is also less specific as it detects unrelated benign, previously unsuspected pulmonary nodules. The likelihood of benign disease increases when pulmonary nodules are detected only on CT.
- Solitary pulmonary metastases are rare. Thus, lung cancer must always be included in the differential diagnosis of a patient with known malignancy who presents with a new solitary pulmonary nodule or mass. Solitary metastases typically result from sarcomas, melanoma, or colon, breast, and genitourinary cancers. A new solitary nodule in a patient with known invasive melanoma or skeletal sarcoma is more likely to represent a metastasis. A new solitary nodule in a patient with known squamous cell carcinoma or lymphoma is more likely to represent a new primary lung cancer.
- Patients with endobronchial metastases may exhibit findings of bronchial obstruction (pneumonia, atelectasis) mimicking the presentation of central lung cancer.
- Differential diagnosis for Cannonball metastases includes colorectal, renal cell, and breast carcinomas; sarcoma; seminomatous and non-seminomatous germ cell tumors; melanoma; follicular thyroid cancer.

Suggested Reading

1. Aquino SL. Imaging of metastatic disease to the thorax. Radiol Clin North Am 2005;43(3):481–495, vii

2. Gillams AR, Lees WR. Radiofrequency ablation of lung metastases: factors influencing success. Eur Radiol 2008; 18(4):672–677

3. Seo JB, Im JG, Goo JM, Chung MJ, Kim MY. Atypical pulmonary metastases: spectrum of radiologic findings. Radiographics 2001;21(2):403–417

CASE 81

■ Clinical Presentation

18-year-old woman with cough and hemoptysis

■ Radiologic Findings

PA (**Fig. 81.1**) and lateral (**Fig. 81.2**) chest radiographs demonstrate left lower lobe atelectasis. Contrast-enhanced chest CT (mediastinal window) (**Figs. 81.3, 81.4**) reveals a small, lobular, enhancing, partially endobronchial lesion obstructing the left lower lobe bronchus, with resultant volume loss, consolidation, and bronchiectasis (**Fig. 81.4**).

■ Diagnosis

Bronchial Carcinoid

■ Differential Diagnosis

- Mucoepidermoid Carcinoma
- Adenoid Cystic Carcinoma
- Central Lung Cancer (rare in adolescents and young adults)

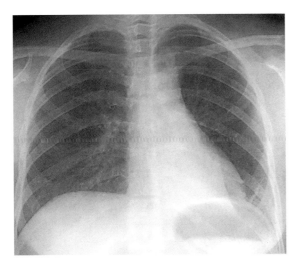

Fig. 81.1

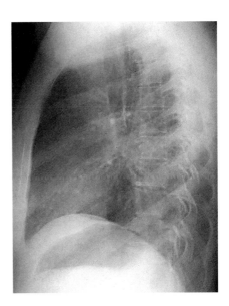

Fig. 81.2

397

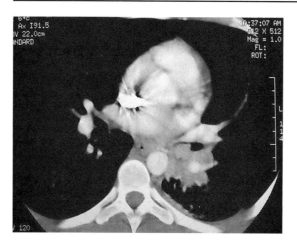

Fig. 81.3

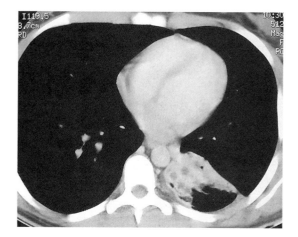

Fig. 81.4

■ Discussion

Background

Carcinoid is a rare malignant primary pulmonary neoplasm of neuroendocrine origin and accounts for approximately 2% of all lung neoplasms. Eighty to 90% of bronchial and pulmonary carcinoids are *typical* (<2 mitoses per 10 high-power fields and absent necrosis) and 10–20% are *atypical* (2–10 mitoses per 10 high-power fields and necrosis) carcinoids.

Etiology

Bronchial carcinoids are thought to derive from the neuroendocrine cells of the bronchial epithelium. Atypical carcinoids are more common in men and are associated with cigarette smoking.

Clinical Findings

Carcinoid characteristically affects adult men and women, with an average age of 45 years and a wide age range, and is the most common primary lung neoplasm of young persons, typically adolescents. Affected patients are often symptomatic and present with cough and recurrent pulmonary infection. Hemoptysis, chest pain, wheezing, and dyspnea may also occur. Up to half of patients with carcinoid are asymptomatic and are diagnosed incidentally. Rarely, patients with bronchial carcinoid present with symptoms related to ectopic ACTH production by the lesion. Most *typical carcinoids* exhibit no evidence of metastatic disease, whereas approximately 50% of *atypical carcinoids* have metastases at presentation.

Imaging Findings

Chest Radiography

- Well-defined hilar or perihilar mass
- Well-defined endobronchial nodule or mass
- Nodule or mass in the lung periphery
- Atelectasis, consolidation, mucoid impaction (may be dominant findings and may obscure central mass) (**Figs. 81.1, 81.2**); rare identification of mucus plugging on radiography
- Size ranges from 2 to 5 cm; atypical carcinoids usually larger
- Peripheral well-defined solitary pulmonary nodule/mass

MDCT

- Spherical/ovoid, well-defined smooth or lobular nodule/mass within or near central bronchi (**Fig. 81.3**)
- Intralesional calcification (diffuse or punctate) in approximately 30% (**Fig. 81.5**)
- Marked contrast enhancement (**Figs. 81.3, 81.5**)
- Visualization of endoluminal tumor or bronchial relationship (**Figs. 81.3, 81.5, 81.6**)
- Evaluation of distal lung parenchyma; volume loss, air trapping, consolidation, bronchiectasis (**Figs. 81.4, 81.5**)
- Lymphadenopathy; up to 50% of patients with atypical carcinoid

Scintigraphy

- No increased FDG uptake on PET-CT in most cases of *typical carcinoid*
- Increased FDG uptake reported in *atypical carcinoid*
- Octreotide uptake in hormonally active and/or occult carcinoids; correlation with cross-sectional imaging for localization of abnormal activity

Management

- Surgical excision; typically lobectomy or pneumonectomy
- Tracheobronchial sleeve resection for central carcinoids with normal distal lung parenchyma

Prognosis

- Typical carcinoid: 87% five-year survival
- Atypical carcinoid: 56% five-year survival; increased risk of local recurrence, particularly with lymph node metastases

---

PEARLS

- Positron emission tomography (PET) imaging is not typically useful in the diagnosis of carcinoid tumors, as many exhibit low metabolic activity.

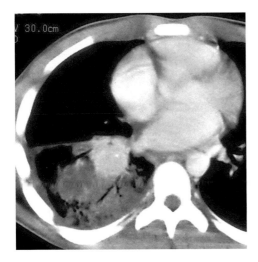

Fig. 81.5 Contrast-enhanced chest CT (mediastinal window) of a young man with recurrent right lower lobe pneumonia and hemoptysis secondary to a typical bronchial carcinoid demonstrates a lobular enhancing central mass with a small focus of punctuate calcification. Note distal right lower lobe consolidation and bronchiectasis.

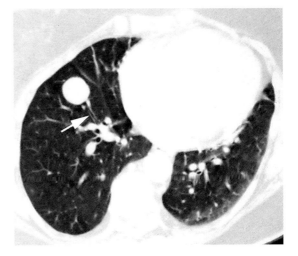

Fig. 81.6 Chest CT (lung window) of an asymptomatic 61-year-old woman status post bilateral lumpectomies for breast carcinoma with an incidental bronchial carcinoid demonstrates a well-defined spherical lobular right lower lobe soft-tissue mass. Note the bronchus (*arrow*) that courses to the lesion.

Suggested Reading

1. Beasley MB, Thunnissen FB. Hasleton PhS, et al. Carcinoid tumour. In: Travis WD, Brambilla E, Müller-Hermelink HK, Harris CC, eds. World Health Organization Classification of Tumours. Pathology & Genetics. Tumours of the Lung, Pleura, Thymus and Heart. Lyon: IARC Press; 2004:59–62

2. Chong S, Lee KS, Chung MJ, Han J, Kwon OJ, Kim TS. Neuroendocrine tumors of the lung: clinical, pathologic, and imaging findings. Radiographics 2006;26(1):41–57, discussion 57–58

3. Park CM, Goo JM, Lee HJ, Kim MA, Lee CH, Kang MJ. Tumors in the tracheobronchial tree: CT and FDG PET features. Radiographics 2009;29(1):55–71

CASE 82

■ Clinical Presentation

Asymptomatic 71-year-old man evaluated because of an abnormal chest radiograph

■ Radiologic Findings

PA chest radiograph (**Fig. 82.1**) demonstrates multi-focal bilateral nodular opacities without associated lymphadenopathy or pleural effusion. Unenhanced chest CT (lung window) (**Fig. 82.2**) shows multi-focal subpleural nodular opacities of heterogeneous attenuation. Biopsy confirmed the diagnosis of primary pulmonary lymphoma of mucosa-associated lymphoid tissue (MALT). PA chest radiograph (**Fig. 82.3**) obtained three years later demonstrates interval growth and coalescence of multi-focal nodular opacities. Unenhanced chest CT (lung window) (**Fig. 82.4**) confirms interval growth of pulmonary lesions, which exhibit internal air bronchograms.

■ Diagnosis

Primary Pulmonary Lymphoma; Marginal Zone B-Cell Lymphoma of MALT

■ Differential Diagnosis

- Multicentric Lung Cancer
- Pulmonary Metastases
- Multi-focal Pneumonia
- Cryptogenic Organizing Pneumonia

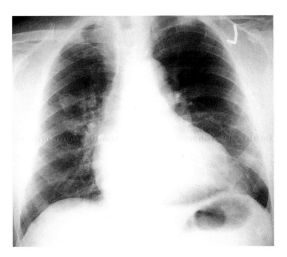

Fig. 82.1

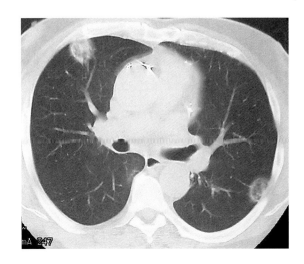

Fig. 82.2

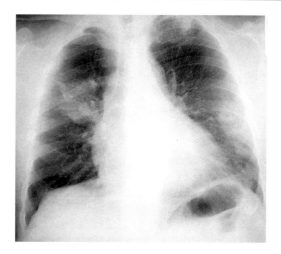

Fig. 82.3

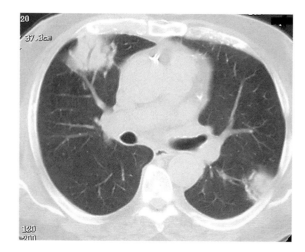

Fig. 82.4

■ Discussion

Background

Pulmonary lymphomas are subdivided into those lymphomas limited to the lung (primary) and those in which the lung is affected secondarily. A *primary pulmonary lymphoma* is defined as an *extranodal pulmonary lymphoma* without evidence of extrapulmonary involvement at diagnosis and during the subsequent three months. It is a rare lung malignancy and comprises approximately 0.5% of all primary lung neoplasms. Most (70–90%) primary pulmonary lymphomas are marginal zone lymphomas of MALT. Primary pulmonary diffuse large B-cell lymphomas account for approximately 5–20% of all primary pulmonary lymphomas. A *secondary pulmonary lymphoma* is much more frequent, occurs in approximately 50% of patients with lymphoma, and is more common in patients with Hodgkin lymphoma.

Etiology

Primary pulmonary lymphomas are typically non-Hodgkin lymphomas. Although their etiology is not known, MALT lymphomas are thought to arise in response to inflammatory or autoimmune disorders, and diffuse large B-cell lymphomas have been associated with pulmonary involvement by collagen vascular diseases with or without underlying pulmonary fibrosis as well as with AIDS and other immunodeficiencies. *Secondary pulmonary lymphoma* is thought to represent hematogenous and/or lymphatic dissemination of nodal lymphoma and in some cases direct pulmonary invasion by lymphoma involving adjacent lymph nodes.

Clinical Findings

Patients with *primary pulmonary lymphoma* are typically asymptomatic and often diagnosed incidentally because of an abnormal chest radiograph. Symptomatic patients may present with pulmonary complaints, including cough, dyspnea, chest pain, and hemoptysis, or systemic complaints. Patients with *secondary pulmonary lymphomas* characteristically have a known lymphoma. Patients with primary pulmonary lymphoma are typically in the sixth or seventh decade of life. Affected individuals may have immunologic disorders, including Sjögren syndrome, Hashimoto thyroiditis, systemic lupus erythematosus, and infection by the human immunodeficiency virus (HIV).

Imaging Findings

Chest Radiography

- Focal nodule, mass, or consolidation (**Fig. 82.5A**)
- Multi-focal nodules, masses, or consolidations (**Figs. 82.1, 82.3**)
- Frequent air bronchograms (**Fig. 82.3**); may exhibit cavitation
- Indolent course with slow growth over months to years (**Figs. 82.1, 82.3**); may exhibit rapid progression
- Diffuse interstitial opacities

MDCT

- Focal or multi-focal nodules, masses, or consolidations (**Figs. 82.2, 82.4, 82.5B, 82.6A**)
- Ground glass opacities, CT *halo sign*
- Air bronchograms (90%) (**Figs. 82.2, 82.4, 82.5B, 82.6A**); bronchial stretching, narrowing or dilatation; bubble-like lucencies; cavitation
- Reticular opacities
- Pleural effusion in up to 10% of cases
- Lymphadenopathy in 5–30% of cases

PET-CT

- Modality of choice for staging and assessment of patients with extranodal Hodgkin lymphoma and non-Hodgkin lymphoma; increased FDG activity of affected sites (**Fig. 82.6B**)
- Used as a guide for selection of biopsy sites for confirmation of the diagnosis

Management

- Surgical excision in patients with focal primary pulmonary lymphoma
- Surgical excision and/or adjuvant chemotherapy in patients with bulky or multi-focal lymphoma
- Consideration of follow-up without treatment of asymptomatic elderly patients

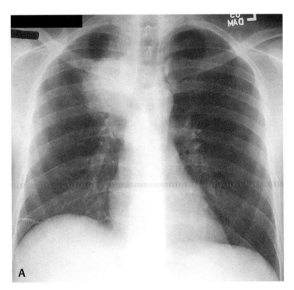
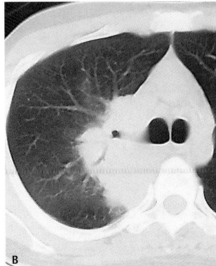

Fig. 82.5 **(A)** PA chest radiograph of a 37-year-old man with HIV infection, cough, and chest pain shows a large right upper lobe mass, which abuts the superior mediastinum. **(B)** Chest CT (lung window) demonstrates a large right upper lobe consolidation of irregular borders with internal air bronchograms. There was no lymphadenopathy. At surgery, primary pulmonary lymphoma was diagnosed.

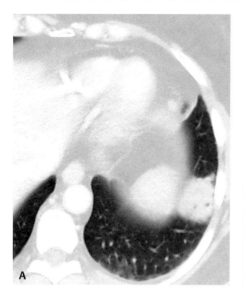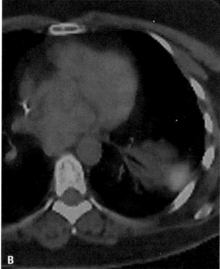

Fig. 82.6 **(A)** Coned-down chest CT (lung window) of a 54-year-old woman with primary pulmonary lymphoma of MALT demonstrates left lower lobe mass-like consolidation with intrinsic air bronchograms. **(B)** FDG PET-CT shows intense FDG uptake in the lesion. No other areas of involvement by lymphoma were identified. (*See color insert following page 108.*)

Prognosis

- 84–94% five-year survival reported in patients with marginal zone lymphoma of MALT origin
- 0–60% five-year survival reported in patients with diffuse large B-cell pulmonary lymphoma

PEARLS _____

- Mediastinal Hodgkin lymphoma is common and may progress to secondary pulmonary involvement manifesting with coarse perihilar reticular opacities, multi-focal nodular opacities, or subpleural nodules/masses (**Fig. 82.7**). Air bronchograms may be present (**Fig. 82.7**).
- Primary pulmonary Hodgkin lymphoma is rare.

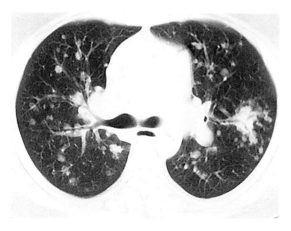

Fig. 82.7 Chest CT (lung window) of a young woman with secondary pulmonary involvement by Hodgkin lymphoma shows multi-focal pulmonary nodules, some of which cluster along the airways, exhibiting intrinsic air bronchograms.

Suggested Reading

1. Lee DK, Im JG, Lee KS, et al. B-cell lymphoma of bronchus-associated lymphoid tissue (BALT): CT features in 10 patients. J Comput Assist Tomogr 2000;24(1):30–34

2. Nicholson AG, Harris NL. Marginal B-cell lymphoma of the mucosa-associated lymphoid tissue (MALT) type. In: Travis WD, Brambilla E, Müller-Hermelink HK, Harris CC, eds. World Health Organization Classification of Tumours. Pathology & Genetics. Tumours of the Lung, Pleura, Thymus and Heart. Lyon: IARC Press; 2004:88–90

3. Nicholson AG, Harris NL. Primary pulmonary diffuse large B-cell lymphoma. In: Travis WD, Brambilla E, Müller-Hermelink HK, Harris CC, eds. World Health Organization Classification of Tumours. Pathology & Genetics. Tumours of the Lung, Pleura, Thymus and Heart. Lyon: IARC Press; 2004:88–90

4. Paes FM, Kalkanis DG, Sideras PA, Serafini AN. FDG PET/CT of extranodal involvement in non-Hodgkin lymphoma and Hodgkin disease. Radiographics 2010;30(1):269–291

5. Toma P, Granata C, Rossi A, Garaventa A. Multimodality imaging of Hodgkin disease and non-Hodgkin lymphomas in children. Radiographics 2007;27(5):1335–1354

CASE 83

■ Clinical Presentation

40-year-old man with hemoptysis

■ Radiologic Findings

PA (**Fig. 83.1**) chest radiograph demonstrates a 3 cm mass with well-defined lobular borders in the right mid-lung. Unenhanced chest CT (mediastinal window) (**Fig. 83.2**) shows a well-defined polylobular middle lobe mass with intrinsic fat and soft-tissue attenuation as well as a small focus of punctate calcification.

■ Diagnosis

Hamartoma

■ Differential Diagnosis

None

■ Discussion

Background

Pulmonary hamartoma is a benign pulmonary neoplasm composed of mesenchymal tissues, including cartilage, fat, connective tissue, and smooth muscle. These tissues are found in varying proportions. Entrapped respiratory epithelium may also be found within the lesion. Hamartomas account for approximately 8% of lung neoplasms, are considered the most common benign tumor of the lung, and represent approximately 77% of all benign lung neoplasms.

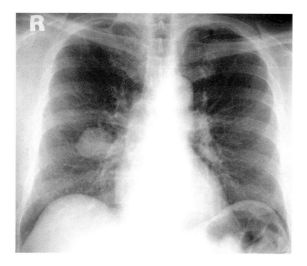

Fig. 83.1

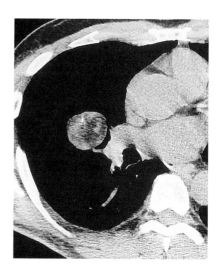

Fig. 83.2

Etiology

Pulmonary hamartoma is thought to arise from peribronchial mesenchymal tissues, but its etiology remains unknown.

Clinical Findings

Pulmonary hamartomas typically affect asymptomatic patients who are diagnosed incidentally because of an abnormal chest radiograph. Symptomatic patients may present with symptoms related to bronchial obstruction by an endobronchial hamartoma. Men are more commonly affected than women, with a male-to-female ratio of approximately 2:1. Most affected patients are older than 40 years, and the peak incidence is in the sixth decade of life. Most hamartomas occur as solitary lung nodules or masses. Rare cases of multi-focal hamartomas are reported.

Imaging Findings

Chest Radiography

- Well-defined solitary pulmonary nodule/mass (**Figs. 83.1, 83.3A**)
- Rare visualization of cartilaginous ("popcorn") calcification; increased frequency with increasing lesion size
- Obstructive pneumonia or atelectasis in cases of endobronchial hamartoma

MDCT

- CT diagnostic criteria:
  - Well-defined smooth or lobular borders (**Figs. 83.2, 83.3B**)
  - Diameter of 2.5 cm or less (**Fig. 83.3B**)
  - Internal fat attenuation or fat and calcification (**Figs. 83.2, 83.3B, 83.4**); fat attenuation in approximately 50%
- Thin-section CT, more sensitive in detecting small foci of fat or calcification (**Fig. 83.3B**)
- May manifest as a non-calcified lesion without fat attenuation

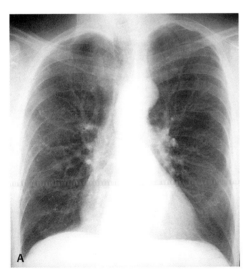
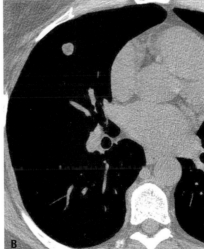

Fig. 83.3 **(A)** PA chest radiograph of an asymptomatic elderly man with a long history of cigarette smoking and an incidentally discovered pulmonary hamartoma demonstrates a well-defined soft-tissue nodule in the middle lobe. **(B)** Coned-down unenhanced chest CT (mediastinal window) shows a lobular well-defined solitary pulmonary nodule of heterogeneous attenuation with internal fat attenuation.

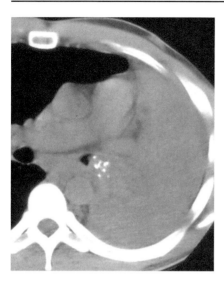

Fig. 83.4 Coned-down unenhanced chest CT (mediastinal window) of an elderly woman who presented with cough demonstrates left lung atelectasis secondary to an obstructive endoluminal hamartoma in the left mainstem bronchus. Note foci of punctate calcification within the lesion

- Internal enhancing septa on contrast-enhanced CT
- Endobronchial hamartoma (**Fig. 83.4**); foci of fat and/or calcification within endoluminal well-defined nodule/mass; bronchial obstruction

MRI

- Lobular nodule/mass of intermediate signal intensity on T1WI; increased SI on T2WI
- Demonstration of internal fat signal
- Enhancing intralesional tissue septa

PET-CT

- Characteristic low metabolic activity/FDG uptake
- Rare reports of increased FDG uptake in hamartomas

Management

- Surgical excision; wedge resection or enucleation, easily "shelled out" from surrounding lung
- Sleeve excision, lobectomy, pneumonectomy for central lesions
- Observation of asymptomatic patients with typical imaging findings

Prognosis

- Excellent
- Excision is curative; rare recurrences, no reports of malignant transformation

PEARLS

- Hamartomas exhibit slow growth over time, ranging from 1 to 10 mm per year.
- Transthoracic needle biopsy of pulmonary hamartoma exhibits 85% diagnostic accuracy.
- *Carney triad* describes the coexistence of (1) gastric epithelioid leiomyosarcoma (now considered to represent gastrointestinal stromal tumor [GIST]); (2) extra-adrenal paraganglioma, and (3) pulmonary chondroma. The latter is considered distinct from pulmonary hamartoma.

Suggested Readings

1. Gaerte SC, Meyer CA, Winer-Muram HT, Tarver RD, Conces DJ Jr. Fat-containing lesions of the chest. Radiographics 2002;22(Spec No):S61–S78

2. Girvin F, Ko JP. Pulmonary nodules: detection, assessment, and CAD. AJR Am J Roentgenol 2008;191(4):1057–1069

3. Nicholson AG, Tomashefski JF Jr, Popper H. Hamartoma. In: Travis WD, Brambilla E, Müller-Hermelink HK, Harris CC, eds. World Health Organization Classification of Tumours. Pathology & Genetics. Tumours of the Lung, Pleura, Thymus and Heart. Lyon: IARC Press; 2004:113–114

4. Winer-Muram HT. The solitary pulmonary nodule. Radiology 2006;239(1):34–49

Section VII

Thoracic Trauma

OVERVIEW OF THORACIC TRAUMA

Trauma is the third leading cause of death in the United States and the most frequent cause of death for individuals under 35 years of age. The rate of thoracic trauma in the United States alone is approximately 12 per million population per day, resulting in more than 300,000 hospitalizations each year. Thoracic injuries account for 25–35% of trauma-related deaths or approximately 16,000 deaths per year. Thoracic trauma is broadly categorized as *blunt* or *penetrating*. *Blunt thoracic trauma* accounts for 90% of chest trauma and is most often the result of deceleration forces associated with motor vehicle collisions (75–80%); automobile versus pedestrian collisions, falls, assaults, blast injuries, and compression injuries. Injuries of the thorax are a major cause of morbidity (36%) and mortality (16%) in cases of blunt trauma. The latter is usually due to aortic or great vessel injury. Most *penetrating injuries* to the chest are caused by knives or handgun bullets. Approximately 4–15% of admissions to major trauma centers today are attributable to penetrating thoracic injuries. For every firearm-related death it is estimated there are 3–5 other, nonfatal firearm injuries. Penetrating trauma can be further categorized as *low-* versus *high-energy injuries*. All stabbings are considered *low-energy injuries*. Hand-driven low-energy weapons damage tissue only with their sharp cutting edge or point. The interpretation of radiologic imaging studies to assess the extent of underlying injuries must take into consideration the length and width of the projectile, its depth of penetration and angle of entry, as well as the nature and mechanism of the force applied (e.g., single thrust, repetitive thrust, twisting and rotation with entry, etc.). Gunshot wounds can be divided into *low-energy* (e.g., handguns, air-powered pellet guns) and *high-energy* injuries (e.g., rifles and military weapons). *High-energy* gunshot wounds are associated with a muzzle velocity of 1,000–2,500 feet per second. Most civilian penetration trauma results from knives or handguns (i.e., low-energy injuries). The extent of tissue damage caused by a projectile is more severe for *high-energy* missiles. *High-energy* projectiles are associated with the formation of both temporary and permanent cavities that result in substantial tissue damage along the wound tract and surrounding tissues and organ systems. This latter concept is critical to the appropriate analysis of diagnostic imaging studies of such penetrating trauma victims.

Suggested Reading

1. Costantino M, Gosselin MV, Primack SL. The ABC's of thoracic trauma imaging. Semin Roentgenol 2006;41(3): 209–225

2. Primack SL, Collins J. Blunt nonaortic chest trauma: radiographic and CT findings. Emerg Radiol 2002;9(1):5–12

3. Shanmuganathan K, Matsumoto J. Imaging of penetrating chest trauma. Radiol Clin North Am 2006;44(2):225–238, viii

4. Tocino I, Miller MH. Computed tomography in blunt chest trauma. J Thorac Imaging 1987;2(3):45–59

CASE 84

■ Clinical Presentation

20-year-old man involved in a motorcycle collision with complicating head trauma and diminished breath sounds over the right thorax

■ Radiologic Findings

AP chest exam (**Fig. 84.1**) reveals right upper lobe consolidation and right lower lobe ground glass opacities consistent with pulmonary contusions. The right hemidiaphragm and ipsilateral costophrenic sulcus appear more pronounced, crisp, and hyperlucent than the left counterpart. Note the underlying backboard.

■ Diagnosis

Right Pneumothorax; *Deep Sulcus Sign*

■ Differential Diagnosis

None

■ Discussion

Background

Pneumothorax is a frequent complication after blunt or penetrating chest trauma. In blunt trauma, it is the *second most common injury* after rib fractures, occurring in 30–40% of patients. *Occult pneumothorax*, defined as a pneumothorax on chest or abdominal CT but not evident on chest radiography, is found in 2–12% of blunt trauma victims (**Figs. 84.2A, 84.2B**). Although many pneumothoraces are often initially small in volume, diagnosis is important, as an unsuspected pneumothorax may rapidly enlarge and become symptomatic in patients receiving mechanical ventilation. In the *supine* trauma patient, pleural air may preferentially accu-

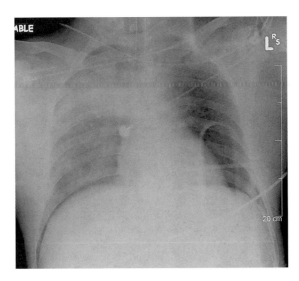

Fig. 84.1

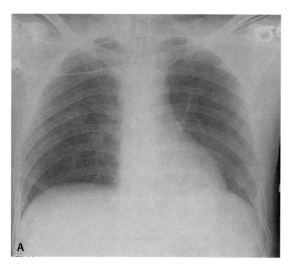 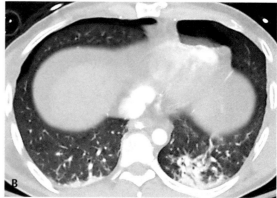

Fig. 84.2 Radiographically occult pneumothoraces detected on CT in a young man who sustained both head and abdominal trauma following a motor vehicle collision. **(A)** Supine chest radiography reveals no conspicuous pneumothorax. **(B)** Abdominal CT (lung window) at the thoraco-abdominal level shows clinically and radiographically unsuspected bilateral pneumothoraces.

mulate in several recesses (also see Case 174). The *anteromedial recess* accumulates air first and accounts for up to 30% of pneumothoraces, but the problem is unrecognized on frontal supine chest exams in 30–50% of trauma patients. Left unrecognized and untreated, such pneumothoraces progress to tension in one-third of patients. Radiographic features of an anterior medial pneumothorax include the *deep sulcus sign* (**Figs. 84.1, 84.3**), manifest by a deep lucent costophrenic sulcus. *Tension pneumothorax* is an emergent clinical and not a radiologic condition that should be diagnosed and treated *before* the acquisition of imaging studies. However, unexpected tension pneumothoraces are not infrequently encountered on imaging (**Fig. 84.4**). Once they are identified, prompt and emergent management is indicated.

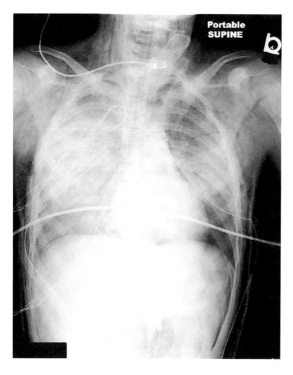

Fig. 84.3 AP supine chest X-ray of a 16-year-old involved in an ATV rollover shows bilateral ground glass opacities and consolidations, right more so than left, consistent with pulmonary contusions; pneumomediastinum; and subcutaneous air in the chest wall and deep cervical fascia of the neck bilaterally. Persistent left pneumothorax despite chest tube placement is manifest by a crisp left diaphragm and heart border and a deep lateral costophrenic sulcus (*deep sulcus sign*).

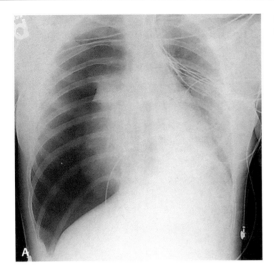
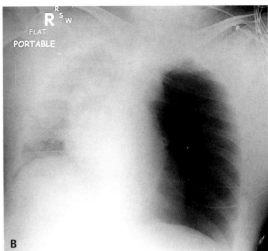
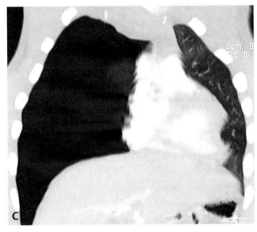

Fig. 84.4   Radiologic features of **(A)** right- and **(B)** left-sided tension pneumothorax in two different trauma patients. Both cases demonstrate ipsilateral parenchymal volume loss and diaphragmatic inversion as well as contralateral mediastinal shift. Note that the affected thorax appears hyperlucent and is over-expanded due to a "ball-valve" phenomenon with air trapping in the pleural space and that the intercostal spaces are widened. **(C)** Coronal CT (lung window) in another patient reveals a right-sided tension pneumothorax with contralateral mediastinal displacement. Compare the relative size of the right and left thoraces. The right is much larger secondary to the underlying ball-valve effect.

Etiology

Traumatic pneumothoraces may result from alveolar compression, parenchymal laceration, pleural tears, tracheobronchial disruption, and barotrauma.

Clinical Findings

Most patients with pneumothorax present with sudden onset of acute pleuritic chest pain and dyspnea. The former may be difficult to assess in the acute trauma setting. Additional clinical signs and symptoms may be present or may evolve depending on the size of the pneumothorax and the patient's underlying respiratory reserve. These may include tachypnea, tachycardia, hypoxia, hypotension, jugular venous distension, cyanosis, and tracheal deviation. The significance of a pneumothorax depends not on its absolute "size" but on its physiologic effect. All pneumothoraces in trauma victims are potentially "significant" regardless of size, because even seemingly inconsequential pneumothoraces may rapidly become life threatening under the influence of positive-pressure ventilation.

Imaging Findings

Supine Chest Radiography

Anteromedial Recess Pleural Air

- Deep lucent costophrenic sulcus (*deep sulcus sign*) (**Figs. 84.1, 84.3**) or cardiophrenic angle
- Relative increase in lucency over affected lung base
- Air outlines central dome and anterior insertion of diaphragm (*double diaphragm sign*)

Subpulmonic Recess

- Air accumulates between visceral pleura of lung base and parietal pleura of diaphragm (**Fig. 84.5**)

Posteromedial Recess

- Lucent line sharply delineating ipsilateral paraspinal line, descending thoracic aorta, and/or posterior costophrenic sulcus

Tension Pneumothorax

- Contralateral mediastinal shift (**Figs. 84.4A, 84.4B**)
- Collapse of ipsilateral lung (**Figs. 84.4A, 84.4B**)
- Flattening or inversion of ipsilateral diaphragm (**Figs. 84.4A, 84.4B**)
- Widening of ipsilateral intercostal spaces (**Figs. 84.4A, 84.4B**)
- Effacement of ipsilateral heart border

Ultrasound

- Now used more frequently to diagnose occult pneumothorax at bedside and in unstable patients
- Three signs may be observed along anterolateral chest wall in supine patients: *lung sliding*, the *A-line* sign, and the *lung point*
- Normal lung *glides* smoothly under pleura during respiratory cycle
  - Abolition of *lung sliding* alone (sensitivity 100%, specificity 78%) for diagnosis of occult pneumothorax
  - Absent *lung sliding* plus the *A-line sign* (sensitivity 95%, specificity 94%)
  - *Lung point* (sensitivity 79%, specificity 100%)
  - Either vertical (comet tail artifacts) or horizontal reverberation artifacts arise from lung-wall interface during respiration
    - *Positive* study for pneumothorax when only *horizontal artifacts* are visible
    - *Negative study* when artifacts arise from the pleural line and spread up to the edge of the screen (i.e., "comet tail artifacts")

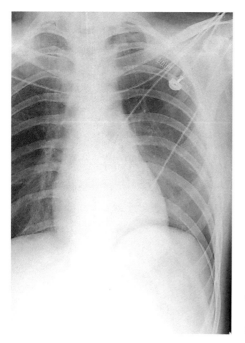

Fig. 84.5   Coned-down frontal chest X-ray shows a curvilinear collection of intrapleural air insinuated between the left lung base and diaphragm consistent with a subpulmonic pneumothorax following knife stabbing to the left chest wall.

MDCT

- Identifies twice as many pneumothoraces as supine chest radiography (**Fig. 84.2**)
- Air in nondependent aspect of pleural space and pleural recesses (**Figs. 84.2A, 84.2B, 84.6A, 84.6B**)

Management

- *Small* (minuscule, <10 mm) to *moderate* (anterior; fails to extend beyond mid-coronal line) radiographically occult pneumothoraces can be managed without chest tubes in patients not requiring positive-pressure ventilation
- Anterolateral pneumothoraces, especially those crossing the mid-coronal line, are likely best managed with pleural drainage
- Video thoracoscopy (VATS) and small wedge resections may be indicated for persistent post-traumatic pneumothoraces secondary to lung lacerations

Prognosis

- Good if recognized and managed appropriately

PEARLS

- Subcutaneous air on imaging studies should alert the radiologist to the presence of possible occult pneumothorax.
- Limited imaging through the lung bases in trauma patients undergoing head or abdominal CT can readily reveal the presence or absence of radiographically inconspicuous or unsuspected pneumothoraces.
- Air within the pulmonary ligament is infrequent and should not be misinterpreted as posteromedial pneumothorax. The former is characterized by a linear lucent band with a convex lateral border and a superior border that curves toward the upper hilum. The latter has a triangular morphology.

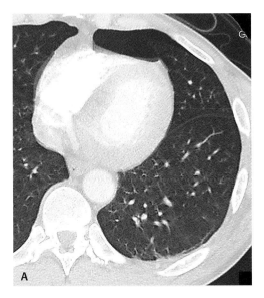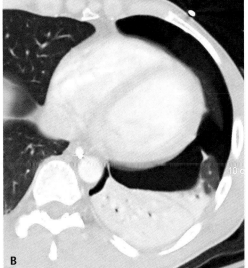

Fig. 84.6   Left-sided pneumothoraces on chest CT (lung window) in two different trauma patients. **(A)** shows a small anteromedial pneumothorax. **(B)** reveals a larger pneumothorax with anteromedial, lateral, posterior, and posteromedial components of pleural separation and left lower lobe collapse.

Suggested Reading

1. Gavelli G, Canini R, Bertaccini P, Battista G, Bnà C, Fattori R. Traumatic injuries: imaging of thoracic injuries. Eur Radiol 2002;12(6):1273–1294

2. Primack SL, Collins J. Blunt nonaortic chest trauma: radiographic and CT findings. Emerg Radiol 2002;9(1):5–12

3. Rivas LA, Fishman JE, Múnera F, Bajayo DE. Multislice CT in thoracic trauma. Radiol Clin North Am 2003;41(3): 599–616

4. Lomoschitz FM, Eisenhuber E, Linnau KF, Peloschek P, Schoder M, Bankier AA. Imaging of chest trauma: radiological patterns of injury and diagnostic algorithms. Eur J Radiol 2003;48(1):61–70

5. Koh DM, Burke S, Davies N, Padley SPG. Transthoracic US of the chest: clinical uses and applications. Radiographics 2002;22(1):e1

6. Wolfman NT, Gilpin JW, Bechtold RE, Meredith JW, Ditesheim JA. Occult pneumothorax in patients with abdominal trauma: CT studies. J Comput Assist Tomogr 1993;17(1):56–59

CASE 85

■ Clinical Presentation

Series of five different unrelated trauma patients who share in common placement of pleural thoracostomy tubes in anomalous clinically undesirable but unsuspected locations

■ Radiologic Findings

Malpositioned thoracostomy tubes (**Figs. 85.1, 85.2, 85.3, 85.4, 85.5**). Axial (**Fig. 85.1A**) and accompanying sagittal MIP (**Fig. 85.1B**) chest CTs (lung window) show intrafissural placement of the left pleural drain in the oblique fissure. Note the persistent, inadequately decompressed pneumothorax. Axial CT (**Fig. 85.2**) (lung window) reveals intraparenchymal placement of the right chest tube. The anterior-placed pleural drain pierces the right middle lobe. Note the intraparenchymal hemorrhage along the course of the pleural drain. AP chest X-ray (**Fig. 85.3A**) demonstrates a left inferomedial pleural drain overlying the left heart. There is a persistent left subpulmonic pneumothorax, pneumomediastinum, and extensive subcutaneous air in the chest wall bilaterally. Accompanying axial CT images (**Fig. 85.3B**, mediastinal window; and **Fig. 85.3C**, lung window) confirm mediastinal placement of the left pleural drain. Note the chest tube relationship to the left atrial appendage. Coned-down frontal chest X-ray (**Fig. 85.4**) shows three extrapleural thoracostomy tubes inappropriately positioned in the subcutaneous tissues of the chest wall. Note the persistent hydropneumothorax and air space disease. CT topogram (**Fig. 85.5A**) demonstrates a kinked right chest tube and a subdiaphragmatic left chest tube. Note its relationship to the ipsilateral diaphragm. Axial CT (mediastinal window) (**Fig. 85.5B**) confirms subdiaphragmatic placement of the chest tube insinuated between the stomach and the splenic hilum.

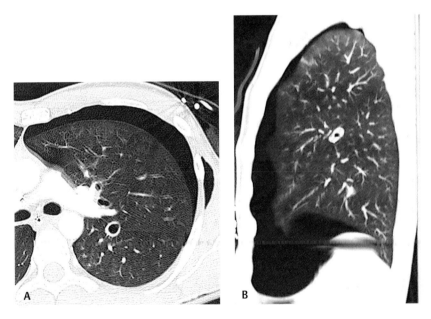

Fig. 85.1

421

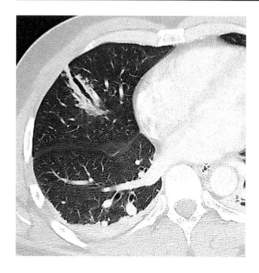

Fig. 85.2

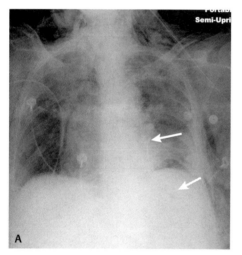

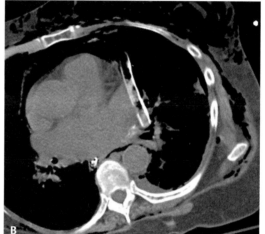

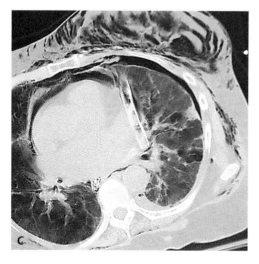

Fig. 85.3

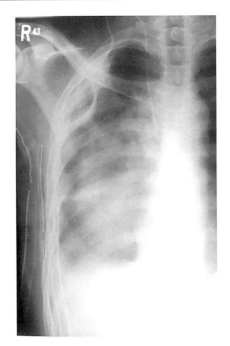

Fig. 85.4

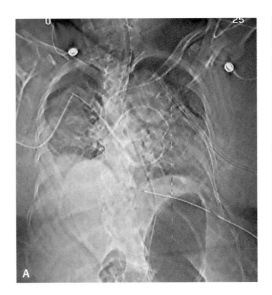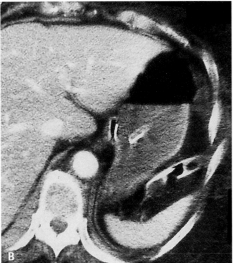

Fig. 85.5

■ Diagnosis

Malpositioned Thoracostomy Tubes

■ Differential Diagnosis

None

■ Background

Discussion

Malpositioning of thoracostomy tubes occurs in 26–58% of placements under emergent conditions. Failure of pneumothorax to decompress following thoracostomy tube placement may be the result of such chest tube malpositioning. Anomalous positioning may be difficult to appreciate on chest radiography. CT is an excellent tool for delineating thoracostomy tubes inadvertently positioned in aberrant locations: *intrafissural* (**Fig. 85.1**), *intraparenchymal* (**Fig. 85.2**), *mediastinal* (**Fig. 85.3**), *extrathoracic chest wall soft tissues* (**Fig. 85.4**), and *below the diaphragm* (**Fig. 85.5**).

Etiology

Inadvertent anomalous placement of thoracostomy tubes may be the result of operator inexperience but more often is related to loss of normal palpable landmarks used to guide placement. The latter may occur with morbidly obese patients or deformity of the chest wall (e.g., crush injuries, flail chest, burns, severe scoliosis).

Clinical Findings

An *intrafissural thoracostomy tube* (**Fig. 85.1**) may adequately decompress a pneumothorax but is often less effective in evacuating hemothorax and other pleural fluid collections. *Intraparenchymal thoracostomy tube* placement (**Fig. 85.2**) can be difficult to recognize clinically and radiographically. Landay et al. reported 26% of patients in their series experienced clinical and radiographic improvement after inadvertent misplacement of an intraparenchymal chest tube and 42% of such patients had no ill sequelae. The authors postulated such malpositioned tubes may evacuate pleural air or fluid collections as they penetrate the pleural space to or from the lung parenchyma. However, such tube thoracostomy lung penetration may produce air leaks or vascular injuries, the latter resulting in pseudoaneurysm or bleeding (i.e., hemothorax). *Mediastinal chest tube placements* (**Fig. 85.3**) may be complicated by injuries to the thoracic aorta, great vessels, coronary arteries, myocardium, and hemopericardium. *Extrathoracic subcutaneous pleural drains* (**Fig. 85.4**) will not evacuate either pleural air or fluid and may be complicated by chest wall hematoma and subsequent infection. *Subdiaphragmatic pleural drain placements* (**Fig. 85.5**) are rare but more problematic and may be complicated by injuries to various hollow and solid viscera and the diaphragm.

Imaging Findings

Radiographic clues to possible *intraparenchymal* thoracostomy tube placement:

- Sudden-onset extensive extra-alveolar air (e.g., marked increase in size of pre-existing pneumothorax or development of extensive subcutaneous air) following pleural tube placement
- Hemorrhage or hematoma manifest as ground glass opacity or consolidation surrounding the intraparenchymal thoracostomy tube; often difficult to appreciate with concomitant non-iatrogenic pulmonary contusion, laceration, or hemothorax
- Abrupt or gradual increase in either parenchymal or pleural opacity following pleural tube placement
- MDCT and multiplanar reconstructions in sagittal, sagittal oblique, and coronal planes more sensitive for delineating aberrant course and lung penetration (**Fig. 85.1A, 85.1B, 85.3C, 85.5B**)

Management

- All malpositioned subcutaneous, intraparenchymal, mediastinal, and subdiaphragmatic thoracostomy tubes need to be removed as soon as possible
- Many patients with *intraparenchymal* chest tube placements only require tube removal; others require additional pleural tube placements or surgical repair of parenchymal laceration(s)
- *Subdiaphragmatic* pleural drain placements may necessitate surgical repair of diaphragm and injured hollow or solid subdiaphragmatic viscera

Suggested Reading

1. Baldt MM, Bankier AA, Germann PS, Pöschl GP, Skrbensky GT, Herold CJ. Complications after emergency tube thoracostomy: assessment with CT. Radiology 1995;195(2):539–543

2. Landay M, Oliver Q, Estrera A, Friese R, Boonswang N, DiMaio JM. Lung penetration by thoracostomy tubes: imaging findings on CT. J Thorac Imaging 2006;21(3):197–204

3. Lim KE, Tai SC, Chan CY, et al. Diagnosis of malpositioned chest tubes after emergency tube thoracostomy: is computed tomography more accurate than chest radiograph? Clin Imaging 2005;29(6):401–405

CASE 86

■ Clinical Presentation

Young male victim of an assault and stabbing to the right chest with diminished breath sounds over the affected thorax.

■ Radiologic Findings

AP chest radiograph (**Fig. 86.1A**) shows asymmetric hazy ground glass opacification of the right hemithorax from dependent layering pleural fluid. Fluid also tracks along the right lateral chest wall toward the apex. Contrast-enhanced chest CT through the upper (**Fig. 86.1B**), mid (**Fig. 86.1C**), and lower (**Fig. 86.1D**) thorax reveals a large dependent layering, mixed-attenuation pleural fluid collection and relaxation atelectasis in the posterior segment right upper lobe and portions of the middle and lower lobe. Locules of air are present in the pleural space (**Figs. 86.1B, 86.1D**). Subcutaneous air is seen in the right chest wall (**Fig. 86.1D**).

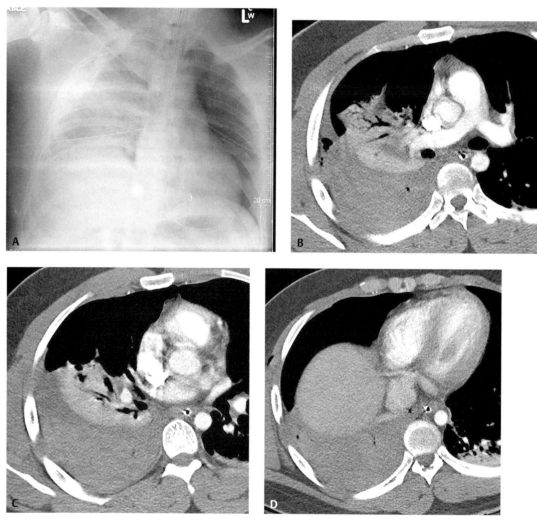

Fig. 86.1

■ Diagnosis

Hemothorax

■ Differential Diagnosis

None

■ Discussion

Background

Traumatic pleural fluid collections may result from bleeding of the chest wall, mediastinal, or diaphragmatic blood vessels; traumatic central venous catheter line insertions; and thoracic duct injury. Such fluid collections following chest trauma usually represent hemothorax. In fact, hemothorax occurs in approximately 50% of major trauma injuries, especially those caused by penetrating trauma. A small hemothorax also typically occurs in association with post-traumatic ipsilateral pneumothorax.

Etiology

Venous injuries or direct injuries to the lung parenchyma result in low-pressure bleeding with little mass effect and are usually self-limited. *Arterial injuries* (e.g., intercostals, subclavian, internal mammary) are under greater pressure, may continue to bleed and rapidly fill the affected hemithorax, and may be associated with lung compression and mediastinal displacement. Continued bleeding may require tube thoracostomy drainage.

Clinical Findings

Affected patients may demonstrate tachypnea, tachycardia, dyspnea, cyanosis, and hypotension. Breath sounds may be diminished or absent on the affected side and the thorax may sound dull on percussion. Large hemothoraces or tension hemothoraces may be associated with contralateral tracheal deviation.

Imaging Findings

Chest Radiography

Supine Exams

- Pleural effusions <200–300 mL; usually undetected
- Larger effusions first collect posteriorly in the dependent hemithorax (see Case 171)
- Relative increased opacity with preserved vascular markings compared with contralateral hemithorax (see Case 171)
- Still larger effusions extend laterally along chest wall, producing a band-like radio-opacity; eventually spill into ipsilateral apex, forming an apical cap (**Fig. 86.1A**)
- Further increases in volume; contralateral displacement of cardiomediastinal silhouette and physiologically may behave similar to tension pneumothorax

Ultrasonography

- Increasingly used to exclude pleural effusion, evaluate volume when present, assess potential composition, and guide thoracentesis and pleural drain placement
- During respiration, an effusion demonstrates *fluid color sign*
  - Color Doppler signal is returned from within the effusion
  - Sign is useful in distinguishing pleural effusion from pleural thickening

○ Sonographic appearances and patterns of pleural effusion subclassified as anechoic, complex nonseptated, complex septated, or homogeneously echogenic
○ Complicated effusions (e.g., exudative and hemorrhagic) more often demonstrate complex nonseptated, complex septated, and homogeneously echogenic patterns (see Case 171)

MDCT

- Superior to chest radiography in identifying traumatic pleural fluid collections
- Acute hemothorax attenuation coefficients: 35–75 HU (**Figs. 86.1B, 86.1C, 86.1D, 86.2A, 86.2B, 86.2C**).
- Focal areas of high attenuation within pleural fluid collection usually represent clot or fibrin; may occlude even properly positioned pleural drains precluding evacuation
- Hemothorax may be associated with atelectasis, pulmonary contusion, pulmonary or vascular lacerations with active extravasation (**Figs. 86.2A, 86.2B, 86.2C**), and pneumothorax

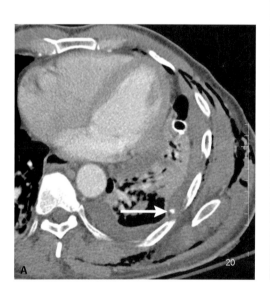
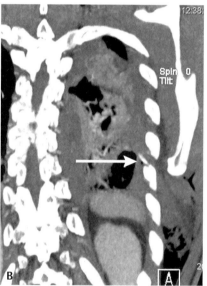
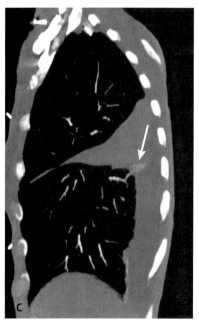

Fig. 86.2 Acute hemothorax with foci of active extravasation. **(A)** Contrast-enhanced axial and **(B)** coronal MIP CT of a young man repeatedly stabbed in the chest demonstrates a left hemothorax and active extravasation of contrast from a lacerated eighth intercostal artery (*arrow*). This lacerated intercostal artery was subsequently embolized angiographically. **(C)** Contrast-enhanced sagittal MIP CT in another blunt trauma victim reveals hemothorax related to pulmonary laceration in the superior segment right lower lobe with active blush of extravasation (*arrow*).

Management

- Low-pressure (venous) bleeding: usually self-limited
- High-pressure (arterial) bleeding: may require thoracostomy tube drainage
  - Closed drainage: may be used for hemothorax (500–1,500 mL) that stops bleeding after thoracostomy tube placement
  - Open thoracotomy: may be necessary in up to 10–15% of patients
    - Usually reserved for hemothorax >1,500–2,000 mL
    - Continued bleeding and pleural tube output >200–300 mL per hour
  - Massive bleeding from an intercostal artery or pulmonary artery laceration can also be managed by selective arteriography and transcatheter embolization

Prognosis

- Early evacuation of retained hemothorax (video thoracoscopy or thoracotomy) improves pulmonary function, prevents empyema and delayed fibrothorax
- Evacuation should ideally be performed within three days of injury

PEARLS

- Hemothorax often appears several hours *after* the traumatic insult. That is, the initial chest X-ray following blunt chest trauma may demonstrate no pleural effusion or only a small effusion that markedly enlarges over the next several hours and in some cases even progresses to tension physiology.

Suggested Reading

1. Bouhemad B, Zhang M, Lu Q, Rouby JJ. Clinical review: Bedside lung ultrasound in critical care practice. Crit Care 2007;11(1):205

2. Carrillo EH, Heniford BT, Senler SO, Dykes JR, Maniscalco SP, Richardson JD. Embolization therapy as an alternative to thoracotomy in vascular injuries of the chest wall. Am Surg 1998;64(12):1142–1148

3. Kessel B, Alfici R, Ashkenazi I, et al. Massive hemothorax caused by intercostal artery bleeding: selective embolization may be an alternative to thoracotomy in selected patients. Thorac Cardiovasc Surg 2004;52(4):234–236

4. Lomoschitz FM, Eisenhuber E, Linnau KF, Peloschek P, Schoder M, Bankier AA. Imaging of chest trauma: radiological patterns of injury and diagnostic algorithms. Eur J Radiol 2003;48(1):61–70

CASE 87

■ Clinical Presentation

59-year-old man stabbed in *Zone I* (demarcated by thoracic inlet inferiorly and cricoid cartilage superiorly) and *Zone II* (mid-portion of neck from cricoid cartilage to angle of mandible) of the left neck six days earlier. Emergent tracheostomy was required. A left pleural effusion evolved on chest radiography (not illustrated) over the past several days.

■ Radiologic Findings

Contrast-enhanced CT at the T1 level (**Fig. 87.1A**) reveals a mid-line tracheostomy device and a large, eccentric, left-sided retrotracheal fluid collection. Note the lateral displacement of the great vessels and residual foci of pneumomediastinum. CT images at the branch vessel (**Fig. 87.1B**) and aortic pulmonary window level (**Fig. 87.1C**) show a low-attenuation left pleural effusion (–10 to –23 HU). Subsequent pleural fluid analysis showed a high concentration of emulsified fats and triglycerides (>110 mg/dL).

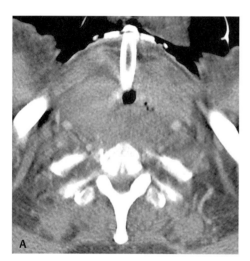
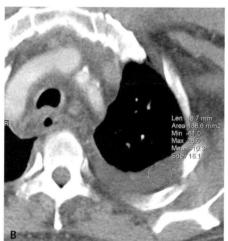
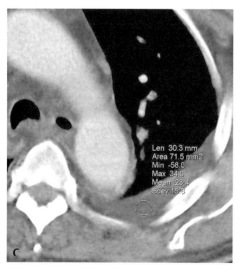

Fig. 87.1

430

■ Diagnosis

Chyloma with Chylothorax; Traumatic Thoracic Duct Injury

■ Differential Diagnosis

None

■ Discussion

Background

Chylothorax is the accumulation of chyle (i.e., lymphatic fluid) in the pleural space. Trauma is the *second* leading cause of chylothorax (25%). Thoracic duct disruption is complicated by accumulation of lymph in the extrapleural mediastinum, which forms a mass-like lesion called a *chyloma*. Subsequent rupture of the chyloma into the pleural space causes the chylothorax. The anatomic course of the thoracic duct and the site of injury determine the situs of the chylous effusion. The thoracic duct originates off the cisterna chyli at L2 and courses to the right of the spine ventral and medial to the azygos vein. Therefore, injury to the *lower half* of the duct results in a right-sided effusion. Between T5 and T8, the thoracic duct crosses the midline and then ascends to the left of the spine until it drains into the angle of the junction of the left subclavian and left internal jugular veins. Therefore, injuries to the upper half of the duct result in left-sided effusions. In normal adults, the thoracic duct transports up to 4 L of chyle per day; thus a large volume of chyle may accumulate quite rapidly in the pleural cavity in cases of duct injury. Although usually unilateral, chylous effusions can be bilateral.

Etiology

Although rare, iatrogenic injury to the thoracic duct has been reported with most invasive thoracic surgical procedures (e.g., central line and thoracostomy tube placements, coronary artery revascularization, thyroidectomy, lobectomy and pneumonectomy, esophagectomy, radical neck dissection, spinal surgery). Nonsurgical traumatic thoracic duct injury is rare and usually secondary to penetrating trauma but may also be associated with fracture-dislocation of the thoracic spine.

Clinical Findings

Initial signs and symptoms are usually related to the presence of a large hydrothorax compressing the lung and most often manifest as dyspnea. However, cyanosis and hypotension may also occur.

Imaging Findings

Chest Radiography

Unilateral or, less often, bilateral pleural effusion

MDCT

- Rarely provides much additional diagnostic information
- Chylous effusion appears similar to other pleural effusions (**Figs. 87.1A, 87.1B, 87.1C**)
- Attenuation may decrease below simple fluid following ingestion of fatty meals
- Prior to rupture, the chyloma may be identified as a low or fluid attenuation mediastinal mass-like lesion (**Fig. 87.1A**)

MRI

- Signal intensities equivalent to that of proteinaceous fluid
- Increased signal on T1WI
- Homogeneous increased signal intensity on T2WI

Lymphangiography

- Powerful and highly reliable imaging tool; best demonstrates site of injury (**Fig. 87.2**)
- May assist with occlusion of the postoperatively damaged lymphatic duct, thereby avoiding need for reoperation

Lymphoscintigraphy

- May localize thoracic duct injuries; can be performed by oral administration of I-123 β-methyl-iodophenyl pentadecanoic acid (BMIPP) as well as intravenous administration of technetium-99m human serum albumin or filtered sulfur colloid

Management

- Conservative management
    - Pleural fluid drainage
    - Supportive ventilation
    - Fluid replenishment, elemental diet supplementation, and total parenteral nutrition
- Conservative management failures
    - CT-guided percutaneous needle ablation
    - Video-assisted thoracoscopic duct ligation, laparoscopic duct ligation, or thoracotomy and/or laparotomy may be necessary

Prognosis

- Effusion often spontaneously resolves after several months
- 10% recurrence rate

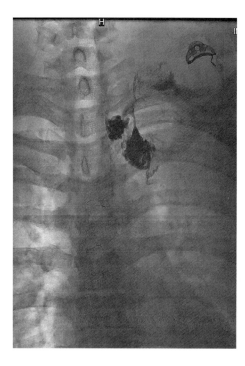

Fig. 87.2 Chylous leak depicted with lymphangiography. Pedal ascending lymphangiography was performed following the infusion of 10 mL of Ethiodol (Savage Laboratory, Melville, NY). Coned-down inverted AP chest X-ray centered over the left thorax of a 17-year-old man with a chylous effusion refractory to conservative management shows diffuse extravasation of contrast in the left supraclavicular region. *(Image courtesy of Jamie Tisnado, MD, and Sonya Bhole, BS, Department of Radiology, Division of Interventional Radiology, VCU Medical Center, Richmond, Virginia.)*

PEARLS

- *Zone I neck injuries.* Structures at greatest risk: aortic arch/great vessels, thoracic duct, trachea, esophagus, lung apex, cervical spine, spinal cord, cervical nerve roots
- *Zone II neck injuries.* Structures at greatest risk: carotid and vertebral arteries, jugular veins, pharynx, larynx, trachea, esophagus, cervical spine and cord
- *Zone III* (bound by angle of mandible and skull base). Structures at greatest risk of injury: salivary and parotid glands, esophagus, trachea, vertebral bodies, carotid arteries, jugular veins, and cranial nerves IX–XII

Suggested Reading

1. Gray H. The lymphatic system: the thoracic duct. In: Charles Mayo Goss, ed. Gray's Anatomy: Anatomy of the Human Body, 29th ed. Philadelphia: Lea & Febiger; 1973:738–739

2. Kos S, Haueisen H, Lachmund U, Roeren T. Lymphangiography: forgotten tool or rising star in the diagnosis and therapy of postoperative lymphatic vessel leakage. Cardiovasc Intervent Radiol 2007;30(5):968–973

3. Pandey R, Lee DF. Laparoscopic ligation of the thoracic duct for the treatment of traumatic chylothorax. J Laparoendosc Adv Surg Tech A 2008;18(4):614–615

4. Silen ML, Weber TR. Management of thoracic duct injury associated with fracture-dislocation of the spine following blunt trauma. J Trauma 1995;39(6):1185–1187

5. Sugiura K, Tanabe Y, Ogawa T, Tokushima T. Localization of chyle leakage site in postoperative chylothorax by oral administration of I-123 BMIPP. Ann Nucl Med 2005;19(7):597–601

CASE 88

■ Clinical Presentation

Young male victim of a gunshot wound to the right chest

■ Radiologic Findings

AP chest X-ray (**Fig. 88.1A**) demonstrates extensive right upper lobe air space disease. Metallic shrapnel fragments follow a path from the mid-clavicle to the first intercostal space and continue over the fractured third to fifth posterior ribs to a retained bullet over T4-T5. Foci of subcutaneous air overlie the right coracoid process. Axial (**Figs. 88.1B, 88.1C**) and coronal (**Fig. 88.1D**) chest CT (lung window) through the right upper lobe show the ground glass with acinar opacities and consolidation to better advantage. Note the comminuted rib fractures and subcutaneous air. A chest tube has been placed.

■ Diagnosis

Pulmonary Contusion

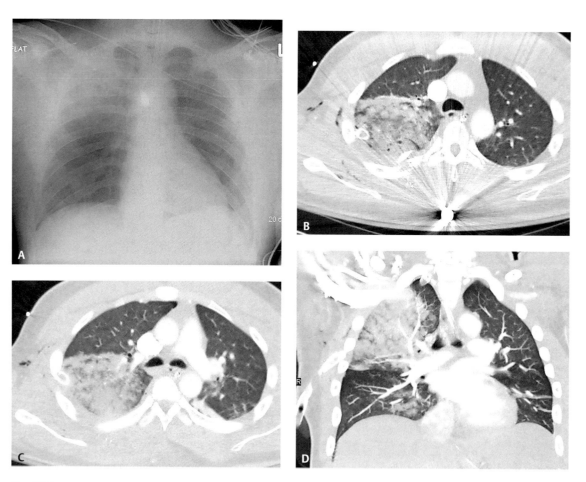

Fig. 88.1

434

◾ Differential Diagnosis

None

◾ Discussion

Background

Pulmonary contusion is equivalent to a bruise of the lung that leads to edema and blood accumulation in alveolar spaces and loss of normal lung function. Pulmonary contusions are the *most common* pulmonary injury after blunt thoracic trauma and are present in 17–70% of patients with severe chest trauma.

Etiology

Contusions result from either a direct blow immediately adjacent to normal lung parenchyma or from a contrecoup injury. Such force disrupts small blood vessels and capillary alveolar membranes, with subsequent extravasation of blood and edema into the interstitium and alveoli. Contusions generally occur in the lung parenchyma adjacent to rigid or solid structures (e.g., thoracic spine, ribs, heart, and liver) or at the lung base (i.e., increased basilar mobility) and are one of the principal factors affecting patient morbidity and mortality, the latter of which varies from 14% to 40% depending upon the severity of the contusion and presence of concomitant thoracic and non-thoracic injuries.

Clinical Findings

Severe pulmonary contusions may be complicated by intrapulmonary shunts, reduced lung compliance, ventilation-perfusion mismatch, hemoptysis, tachypnea, hypoxemia, hypoxia, bronchorrhea, and reduced cardiac output.

Imaging Findings

Chest Radiography

- Peripheral focal or multifocal (**Fig. 88.2**) non-segmental ground glass opacities or consolidations; do not respect fissural boundaries
- Severe contusions can affect an entire lobe, lung, or both lungs (**Fig. 88.1A**)
- Air bronchograms may be absent because of airway obstruction by retained secretions and/or blood (**Figs. 88.1A, 88.2**)

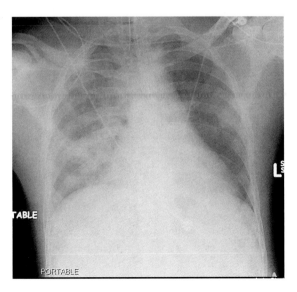

Fig. 88.2 AP chest radiograph of a young man involved in a motor vehicle collision with complicating roll-over demonstrates bilateral patchy areas of ground glass and non-segmental consolidations, right more so than left. Note the high-riding endotracheal tube that needs to be advanced and the right clavicular fracture.

MDCT

- More accurately reveals size and extent of lung injury as well as the presence of concomitant lung laceration(s) (see Case 89)
- Injury to the interstitium with partial alveolar compromise presents as diffuse, non-segmental, heterogeneous ground glass opacities (**Figs. 88.1B, 88.1C, 88.1D, 88.3A-88.3B**)
- Severe alveolar injury or concomitant pulmonary laceration; air spaces fill with blood (acinar opacities), forming parenchymal consolidations (**Figs. 88.1B, 88.1C, 88.1D**)

Management

- Supportive therapy directed at pain control (i.e., concomitant chest wall injuries) and use of pulmonary toilet and supplemental oxygen
- Severe contusions associated with significant pulmonary shunting may require mechanical ventilation

Prognosis

- Reported mortality ranges from 10% to 25%
- 40–60% of patients will require mechanical ventilation

Complications

- Main complications: ARDS and pneumonia
- Approximately 50% of patients with pulmonary contusion develop ARDS
- 80% of patients with pulmonary contusions involving over 20% of lung volume develop ARDS
- Blood in alveolar spaces provides an excellent culture medium for bacteria and subsequent pneumonia

PEARLS

- Severe contusions manifest early on chest X-rays, often within 3–4 hours; become most conspicuous within 24–72 hours; and then gradually clear over 3–10 days.
- Opacities which fail to clear in the above time frame or alternatively progress radiographically raise the suspicion of secondary infection or ARDS.
- *Non-segmental* distribution of *pulmonary contusion* is often helpful in differentiating contusion from *aspiration*, which is usually *segmental.*

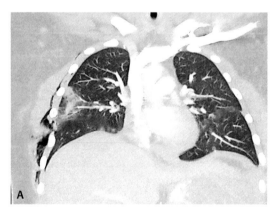 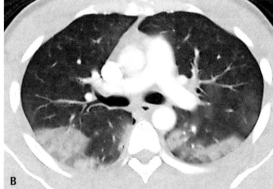

Fig. 88.3 Pulmonary contusions in two different trauma patients. **(A)** Coronal CT MIP (lung window) shows a peripheral, non-segmental, focal area of ground glass and consolidation in the right upper lobe. Note the adjacent chest wall injury and subcutaneous air. **(B)** Axial CT (lung window) reveals bilateral, multi-focal, non-segmental ground glass and acinar opacities and a minuscule right posteromedial pneumothorax.

Suggested Reading

1. Cohn SM. Pulmonary contusion: review of the clinical entity. J Trauma 1997;42(5):973–979

2. Miller PR, Croce MA, Bee TK, et al. ARDS after pulmonary contusion: accurate measurement of contusion volume identifies high-risk patients. J Trauma 2001;51(2):223–228, discussion 229–230

3. Sangster GP, González-Beicos A, Carbo AI, et al. Blunt traumatic injuries of the lung parenchyma, pleura, thoracic wall, and intrathoracic airways: multidetector computer tomography imaging findings. Emerg Radiol 2007;14(5):297–310

CASE 89

■ Clinical Presentation

Young construction worker who fell 25 feet from a platform.

■ Radiologic Findings

Type 1 laceration with *hematopneumocele,* anterior segment left upper lobe. More laterally a contusion parallels the chest tube. Contusions in the left lower lobe and a contusion with *Type 2 laceration,* superior segment right lower lobe (**Fig. 89.1A**). Pulmonary contusion with intraparenchymal *hematoma,* left upper lobe. Contusion with *Type 3* laceration, left upper lobe. and *Type 2* laceration, superior segment right lower lobe (**Fig. 89.1B**). Pulmonary contusions with *Type 1* lacerations with *hematopneumocele* in the lingula and left lower lobe. Contusion with an intraparenchymal *hematoma* also parallels the thoracic spine in the left lower lobe (**Fig. 89.1C**). *Type 2* lacerations in the posterobasal segment right lower lobe and contusions in the posterobasal segment left lower lobe and lingula (**Fig. 89.1D**). A residual left pneumothorax is present

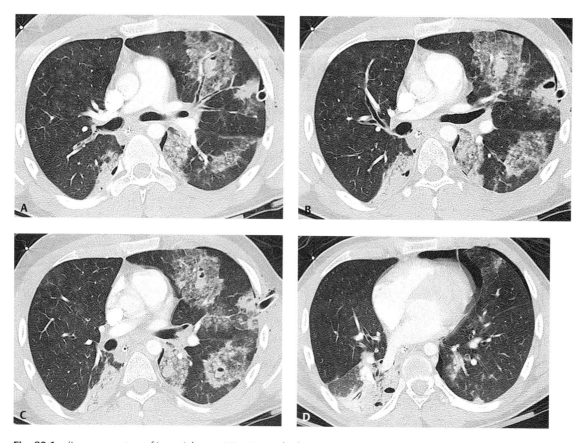

Fig. 89.1   *(Images courtesy of Janae Johnson, MD, VCU Medical Center, Richmond, Virginia.)*

438

■ Diagnosis

Multifocal Pulmonary Lacerations and Contusions

■ Differential Diagnosis

None

■ Discussion

Background

Pulmonary Lacerations

Pulmonary lacerations represent serious sequelae of chest trauma characterized by disruption of normal lung architecture, unlike pulmonary contusions, and are therefore a potentially more serious lung injury. Lacerations may be caused by perforation of the lung parenchyma or pleura (e.g., stab wounds, gunshot wounds, and rib fractures) or by inertial deceleration. As with contusions, pulmonary lacerations usually occur near solid structures in the chest such as the ribs or thoracic spine.

Etiology

Pulmonary lacerations are classified into four categories based upon the nature of the applied force and the CT appearance. *Type I* laceration (compression rupture) is the *most common*, results from chest wall compression causing lung parenchyma to rupture, and is located centrally (**Figs. 89.1A, 89.1C**). *Type II* laceration (compression shear) is the result of a lateral compression force between the lung and the thoracic spine and is most often seen as a paravertebral tubular lesion in the lung bases (**Figs. 89.1A, 89.1B, 89.1D**). *Type III* laceration (rib penetration tear) is usually small, rounded, peripherally located, and often associated with rib fractures and pneumothorax (**Fig. 89.1B**). *Type IV* laceration (adhesion tear) results from shearing of peripheral lung from previously formed pleuropulmonary adhesions and is diagnosed only at surgery or on pathologic specimens. Multiple laceration types may coexist in the same patient, lung or even lobe (**Figs. 89.1A, 89.1B, 89.1C, 89.1D**). A *pneumatocele* forms if the space created by the laceration fills with air from the tracheobronchial tree. An intraparenchymal *hematoma* forms if this space instead fills with blood originating from a disrupted lung vessel (**Figs. 89.1B, 89.1C**). Pneumatocele and hematoma may coexist (i.e., *hematopneumocele*), characterized by an air-fluid level (**Figs. 89.1A, 89.1C**). *Pulverized lung* may occur in severe blunt chest trauma, is best appreciated on CT, and is characterized by multiple small 5–10 mm lucencies in a region of dense air space consolidation.

Imaging Findings

Chest Radiography

- May be inconspicuous or difficult to appreciate on initial chest exams
- Often obscured by surrounding contusion, consolidation, and not infrequently, an ipsilateral hemothorax
- Faint linear opacity corresponding to the air-filled pneumatocele: *earliest* findings
- Usually round or oval; may take several days to develop classic morphology
- Isolated or multiple
- Average size: 2–5 cm in diameter
- May contain air-fluid levels
- Rapid enlargement of pneumatoceles in patients on positive-pressure ventilation

MDCT

- More readily demonstrates lacerations as localized air collections of varying shapes and morphologies within areas of parenchymal consolidation (**Figs. 89.1A, 89.1B, 89.1C, 89.1D**)

- Spherical or variable-shape air-fluid collection(s) surrounded by ground glass opacities or consolidation (**Figs. 89.1A, 89.1B, 89.1C, 89.1D**)
- Isolated or multiple (**Figs. 89.1A, 89.1B, 89.1C, 89.1D**)
- Average size: 2–5 cm in diameter (**Figs. 89.1A, 89.1B, 89.1C, 89.1D**); can exceed 10 cm

Management

- Supportive; supplemental oxygen, ventilation, and drainage of pleural fluid
- Thoracotomy indications (5% of cases)
  - Lung fails to re-expand; persistent pneumothorax, bleeding, or hemoptysis
  - Suturing, stapling, over-sewing, wedging out the laceration, and occasionally lobectomy

Prognosis

- Pulmonary lacerations usually resolve over three to five weeks
- Complicated lacerations may persist for as long as one year

Complications

- Bronchopleural fistula; further complicated by pneumothorax or tension pneumothorax
- Post-traumatic pneumatoceles; may progressively enlarge in patients on mechanical ventilation

PEARLS

- In the absence of complications or pulverized lung, *isolated* lacerations are an indicator of injury severity, but otherwise have little clinical significance.
- Organized hematomas may persist for months following an injury and may be misdiagnosed as lung abscess or neoplasia in the absence of clinical history. Evaluation of serial chest radiographs is necessary for the correct diagnosis.

Suggested Reading

1. Costantino M, Gosselin MV, Primack SL. The ABC's of thoracic trauma imaging. Semin Roentgenol 2006;41(3): 209–225
2. Gavelli G, Canini R, Bertaccini P, Battista G, Bnà C, Fattori R. Traumatic injuries: imaging of thoracic injuries. Eur Radiol 2002;12(6):1273–1294
3. Sangster GP, González-Beicos A, Carbo AI, et al. Blunt traumatic injuries of the lung parenchyma, pleura, thoracic wall, and intrathoracic airways: multidetector computer tomography imaging findings. Emerg Radiol 2007;14(5): 297–310

CASE 90

■ Clinical Presentation

39-year-old man involved in a high-speed motor vehicle collision

■ Radiologic Findings

Chest CT (**Fig. 90.1**) (lung window) demonstrates a focal intercostal herniation of the anterolateral right upper lobe (*arrow*). The hernia was subsequently reduced at surgery.

■ Diagnosis

Traumatic Lung Herniation

■ Differential Diagnosis

None

■ Discussion

Background

Lung herniation may be congenital, spontaneous, pathologic, or the result of thoracic wall trauma. Traumatic lung hernias may occur following various surgical procedures, falls, motor vehicle collisions (MVCs), and penetrating chest injuries. Focal lung herniation is a rare complication that may result from acquired defects in the chest wall (e.g., rib fractures, sternoclavicular or costochondral dislocations) following blunt chest

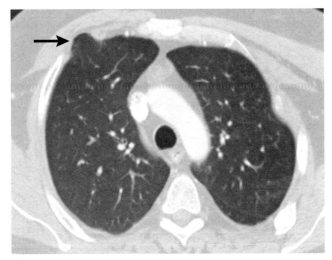

Fig. 90.1

441

trauma. Traumatic lung herniation most often occurs in the anterolateral chest wall, where there is minimal soft-tissue support (e.g., intercostal muscles) and may be complicated by pneumothorax, hemothorax, lung incarceration, and strangulation. The latter requires prompt recognition and surgical reduction.

Etiology

An important factor in the etiology of this traumatic entity is the relative lack of muscular support afforded by the anterior thorax. Motor vehicle collisions have replaced penetrating trauma as the most common etiologic agent of traumatic lung herniation.

Clinical Findings

The true incidence of traumatic lung herniation is unknown. Many such injuries remain occult because of a low index of suspicion, subtle physical exam findings, and lack of symptoms. Incarceration is unusual but when it occurs, it most often results from entrapment of the herniated lung on spicules of fractured ribs.

Imaging Findings

Chest Radiography

- Rarely occurs in isolation
- Concomitant signs of acute traumatic chest injuries common; pneumothorax, hemothorax, pulmonary contusion, rib fractures, costosternal or costal cartilage disruption
- Herniation itself may go unrecognized
- Well-circumscribed loculation of subcutaneous air; tangential or expiratory views may be necessary in some patients to demonstrate the herniation

MDCT

- More often demonstrated (**Figs. 90.1, 90.2**)
- Better defines dimensions of herniated lung (**Figs. 90.1, 90.2**)
- Concomitant chest wall deformity/injury (**Figs. 90.1, 90.2**)

Management

- Repair of lacerated lung with running sutures and reduction of herniated lung to the thoracic cavity; wedge resection or lobectomy in select cases
- Repair of thoracic wall defect

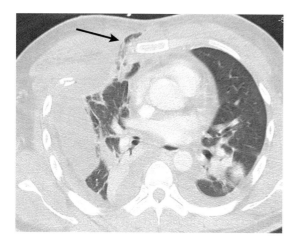

Fig. 90.2 Chest CT of a 25-year-old man involved in a MVC with vehicular ejection shows traumatic lung herniation of a portion of the medial segment right middle lobe along the disrupted costosternal articulation and anteromedial chest wall. Loculated hemothorax is present along the right lateral chest wall (*arrow*). An ipsilateral extrapleural hematoma and pleural effusion as well as atelectatic changes in the right lower lobe are also seen. Note the right chest wall deformity and acutely angulated rib fractures. The hernia was surgically reduced.

Prognosis

- Early surgical repair offers best results with low morbidity
- Long-term prognosis: excellent

Suggested Reading

1. Allen GS, Fischer RP. Traumatic lung herniation. Ann Thorac Surg 1997;63(5):1455–1456

2. May AK, Chan B, Daniel TM, Young JS. Anterior lung herniation: another aspect of the seatbelt syndrome. J Trauma 1995;38(4):587–589

CASE 91

■ Clinical Presentation

26-year-old man involved in a MVC with vehicular ejection

■ Radiologic Findings

Axial (**Fig. 91.1A**) and coronal MIP (**Fig. 91.1B**) chest CT (lung window) shows a right main bronchus injury and a *fallen lung sign*. Note the caliber change in the right main bronchus relative to the left, persistence of a large right pneumothorax despite chest tube placement, and lateral-inferior collapse of the detached right lung away from its hilum.

■ Diagnosis

Tracheobronchial Injury with *Fallen Lung Sign*

■ Differential Diagnosis

None

■ Discussion

Background

Injuries of the tracheobronchial tree are relatively rare, but may occur with blunt or penetrating trauma, and with iatrogenic injuries resulting from traumatic intubation or over-inflation of an ET tube balloon cuff or tracheostomy placement. The incidence is estimated at 2% in blunt chest and neck trauma and 1–2% in penetrating chest trauma. Laryngotracheal injuries occur in 8% of patients with penetrating neck injuries. Bronchial injuries are more common than tracheal injuries, and more than 80% occur within 2 cm of the carina.

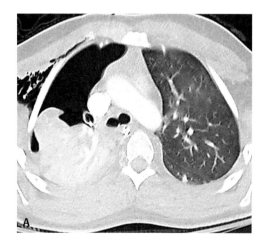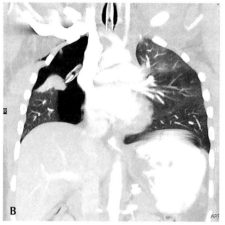

Fig. 91.1

Right-sided bronchial injuries are also more common than left-sided injuries. Those bronchial injuries within the pleural envelop (i.e., distal to insertion of the pulmonary ligament) more likely result in an ipsilateral *pneumothorax*, whereas those occurring outside the pleural envelop (i.e., medial to the pulmonary ligament) are associated with *pneumomediastinum*. Additionally, because the left main bronchus has a longer mediastinal course than the right main bronchus, injuries to the left main bronchus are more often associated with *pneumomediastinum* and right main bronchus injuries are more commonly associated with *pneumothorax.*

Etiology

Blunt trauma usually produces shear forces associated with vertical tears in the membranous trachea, axially oriented tears in the cartilaginous rings, or transections of the mainstem bronchi. *Penetrating trauma* most often involves the cervicothoracic trachea.

Clinical Findings

A clinical feature characteristic of bronchial injury is a persistent pneumothorax (also see Case 95) or a persistent air leak (e.g., pneumomediastinum; significant and increasing subcutaneous air) despite appropriate chest tube placement and functioning. Additional signs and symptoms include cough, hemoptysis, hypoxia, and respiratory distress.

Imaging Findings

Chest Radiography

- Atelectasis of affected lung, lobe, or segment
- Extra-alveolar air manifest as persistent pneumothorax, pneumomediastinum, and/or subcutaneous air (also see Cases 92 and 95)
- *Bayonet sign*—rare; thin, tapering air-filled structure at proximal end of ruptured bronchus
- *Double wall sign*—manifests as intramural air in proximal airways
- *Fallen lung sign*—caused by detachment of lung from mainstem bronchus; affected lung "falls" or collapses away from ipsilateral hilum and toward lateral chest wall into most dependent portion of thoracic cavity

MDCT

- Many of the same features seen on chest radiography including *fallen lung sign* (**Figs. 91.1A, 91.1B**)
- Acute angulation or change in caliber of affected airway (**Figs. 91.1A, 91.2**)
- Tract(s) of air extending from injured bronchus or trachea
- Frank discontinuity of affected airway (**Fig. 91.2**)

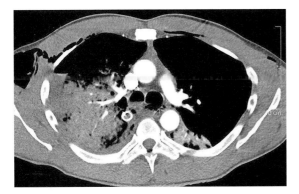

Fig. 91.2 Contrast-enhanced chest CT (mediastinal window) of a 30-year-old man involved in a MVC complicated by ejection demonstrates complete traumatic disruption of the posterior wall of the left main bronchus. Note the gross discrepancy in caliber of the right and left main bronchi. Foci of pneumomediastinum, extensive right upper lobe air space disease, right hemothorax, and partial left lower lobe collapse are also present.

- Findings often more readily appreciated on multiplanar reconstructions
- Virtual bronchoscopy complements CT; helpful adjunct to guiding conservative medical or surgical management

Management

- Early diagnosis is important to prevent complications, including airway stenosis, pneumonia, and bronchiectasis
- Short lacerations involving the upper one-third of the trachea may be treated with antibiotics and intubation beyond the level of the injury
- Some small or peripheral bronchial tears can also be treated conservatively but may be complicated by stenosis
- Surgical repair is indicated for transmural tears >1 cm and those associated with a persistent pneumothorax unrelieved by tube thoracostomy

Prognosis

- Tracheobronchial injury is potentially fatal; mortality rate may be as high as 30%
- Other injuries often accompany tracheobronchial injury (50% of cases)

PEARLS

- Rupture of the trachea or bronchus is the most common type of blunt airway injury.

Suggested Reading

1. Faure A, Floccard B, Pilleul F, et al. Multiplanar reconstruction: a new method for the diagnosis of tracheobronchial rupture? Intensive Care Med 2007;33(12):2173–2178
2. Johnson SB. Tracheobronchial injury. Semin Thorac Cardiovasc Surg 2008;20(1):52–57
3. Karmy-Jones R, Wood DE. Traumatic injury to the trachea and bronchus. Thorac Surg Clin 2007;17(1):35–46 Review
4. Savaş R, Alper H. Fallen lung sign: radiographic findings. Diagn Interv Radiol 2008;14(3):120–121
5. Wintermark M, Schnyder P, Wicky S. Blunt traumatic rupture of a mainstem bronchus: spiral CT demonstration of the "fallen lung" sign. Eur Radiol 2001;11(3):409–411

CASE 92

■ Clinical Presentation

Middle-aged female victim of domestic violence brought into the Emergency Department after being severely beaten

■ Radiologic Findings

PA (**Fig. 92.1A**) and lateral (**Fig. 92.1B**) chest X-rays demonstrate extensive streaky lucencies of air in the mediastinum at the thoracic inlet and paralleling the superior vena cava and great vessels (**Fig. 92.1A**) and in the retrosternal clear space (**Fig. 92.1B**). A radiolucent line parallels the descending thoracic aorta from the aortic pulmonary window to the diaphragm (**Fig. 92.1A**). Extensive subcutaneous air is present in the chest wall and deep cervical fascia of the neck bilaterally. Right rib fractures are seen as well as an incidental right upper lobe mass (later diagnosed as primary lung adenocarcinoma). Coronal CT MIP (lung window) through the anterior (**Fig. 92.1C**), mid- (**Fig. 92.1D**), and posterior (**Fig. 92.1E**) thorax reveals extensive mediastinal air dissecting along the mediastinal pleural reflections of the heart and great vessels (**Figs. 92.1C, 92.1D**), descending aorta, and left diaphragm (**Fig. 92.1E**). A large left pneumothorax is seen, inconspicuous on the chest X-ray because of the extensive extra-alveolar air (**Fig. 92.1E**). Free air is present below the left diaphragm (**Fig. 92.1E**). The spiculated right upper lobe mass is also seen to better advantage (**Fig. 92.1E**).

■ Diagnosis

Pneumomediastinum

■ Differential Diagnosis

None

■ Discussion

Background

Pneumomediastinum is the presence of air or gas in the mediastinal compartment. It occurs in approximately 10% of blunt chest trauma victims but may also be seen with penetrating chest injuries.

Etiology

In more than 95% of cases, pneumomediastinum results from alveolar rupture following an abrupt increase in intra-alveolar pressure. The extra-alveolar air then dissects along the pulmonary interstitium and peribronchovascular sheaths centrally to enter the mediastinum (i.e., Macklin effect). Such abrupt increases in intra-alveolar pressure may occur with simple straining against a closed glottis (e.g., weight-lifting, childbirth), mechanical ventilation with barotrauma, or deep inhalation of illicit recreational drugs (e.g., crack cocaine, marijuana). Air may also enter the mediastinum from injuries to the aerodigestive tract (e.g., tracheobronchial tree, larynx, retropharynx, esophagus) or via the retroperitoneum. When extensive, air from the mediastinum can rupture into the pleural space, creating a pneumothorax; extend inferiorly into the retroperitoneum and rupture into the peritoneal space, resulting in pneumoperitoneum; or impede venous return to the heart (i.e., tension pneumomediastinum with cardiac tamponade).

447

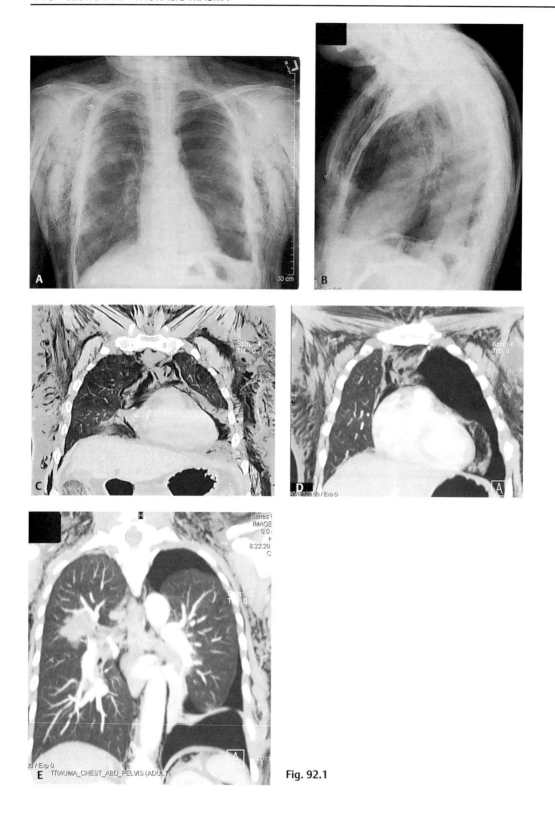

Fig. 92.1

Clinical Findings

Affected patients may or may not be symptomatic. The most common symptoms include chest pain (67%); persistent cough (42%); sore throat (25%); and dysphagia, dyspnea, or nausea and vomiting (8% each). The chest pain is usually substernal; often radiates to the neck, back, and shoulders; and is exacerbated with deep inspiration. Some patients exhibit no physical signs. Others may exhibit soft-tissue crepitus on palpation and *Hamman's sign* (i.e., precordial rasping noise synchronous with the heartbeat and accentuated during expiration).

Imaging Findings

Chest Radiography

- Streaky lucencies of mediastinal air in thoracic inlet (**Fig. 92.1A**) or retrosternal clear space (**Fig. 92.1B**)
- Air outlining great vessels, thoracic aorta, myocardium, thymus (**Figs. 92.1A, 92.1B, 92.2A**)
- Air outlining various mediastinal structures and contributing to the creation of numerous radiologic signs
  - *Double bronchial wall sign*—air accumulates adjacent to the bronchial walls, allowing visualization of both sides
  - *"Ring around the artery" sign*—air dissects around the pulmonary artery(ies) (**Fig. 92.2B**)
  - *Continuous diaphragm sign*—air becomes trapped posterior to the pericardium and the entire diaphragm becomes conspicuous (**Fig. 92.2C**)
  - *Tubular artery sign*—air outlines ascending aorta, aortic arch, and or major branches of aorta (**Figs. 92.2A, 92.2B**)
  - *Naclerio's V sign*—air outlines descending thoracic aorta and extends laterally between the parietal pleura and the medial left hemidiaphragm (**Fig. 92.2D**)
  - *Spinnaker sail sign*—pediatric cases; air elevates the thymus gland

MDCT

- Reveals the same imaging findings to better advantage (**Figs. 92.1C, 92.1D, 92.1E**)
- May reveal underlying cause of pneumomediastinum (e.g., aerodigestive tract injury)
- ± concomitant pneumoperitoneum, pneumoretroperiteoneum, pneumothorax (**Figs. 92.1C, 92.1D, 92.1E**)

Prognosis

- Generally benign, self-limited condition
- Mortality rate approaches 70% in patients with Boerhaave syndrome (**Fig. 92.2D**), even with surgical intervention

Management

- Most patients with pneumomediastinum should be admitted and observed for signs of serious complications (e.g., pneumothorax, tension pneumothorax, mediastinitis)
- Follow-up chest radiography should be obtained in 12–24 hours to detect any progression or complications
- Tension pneumomediastinum may require surgical decompression

PEARLS

- Pneumoretroperitoneum and pneumoperitoneum may dissect into the mediastinum and manifest as pneumomediastinum on chest radiography.
- Not infrequently, it may be difficult to differentiate *pneumomediastinum* from *pneumopericardium* or *medial pneumothorax*.
- *Pneumopericardium* allows direct visualization of the pericardium.
  - Intra-pericardial air respects normal pericardial borders.
  - As volume of air increases, it assumes a more ovoid as opposed to linear morphology.

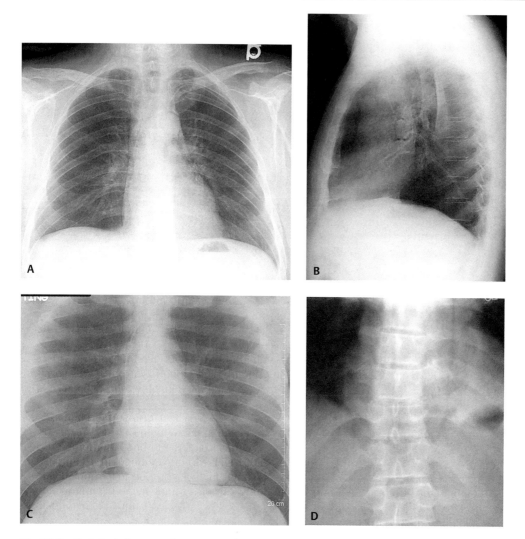

Fig. 92.2   Radiologic features of pneumomediastinum. **(A)** PA chest X-ray shows air outlining the contour of various mediastinal structures such as the right atrial border, ascending aorta, transverse aorta (*tubular artery sign*) and left heart border. **(B)** Lateral X-ray demonstrates a crescent of air outlining the right pulmonary artery ("*ring around the artery*" sign). **(C)** Coned-down frontal radiograph of another patient with pneumomediastinum reveals air dissecting along the transverse aorta and left heart border and continuity of the left and right diaphragm through the heart shadow (*continuous diaphragm sign*). **(D)** Coned-down frontal chest X-ray of a 25-year-old man with severe retching following heavy alcohol consumption at a bachelor party and esophageal rupture (Boerhaave syndrome) shows a longitudinal hyperlucent stripe outlining the descending aorta and a hyperlucent triangle between the medial aspect of the left diaphragm and descending aorta (*V sign of Naclerio*). *(Images A and B courtesy of Judson Frye, MD, VCU Medical Center, Richmond, Virginia.)*

- *Medial pneumothoraces* are often characterized by additional signs of pleural air elsewhere in the affected hemithorax (see Cases 84 and 174).
- Lateral decubitus exams may aid in differentiation in problematic cases.
  - In the setting of both pneumothorax and pneumopericardium, air moves to the non-dependent surface with patient manipulation.
  - Air within the mediastinum does not move with such manipulation.
- *Black mach band* may mimic pneumomediastinum and or pneumothorax. Mach band phenomenon is secondary to retinal inhibition with adjacent light and dark stimulation (e.g., soft-tissue density adjacent to air density [left heart and lung]) and will disappear if one edge is obscured (i.e., with a finger or hand).

Suggested Reading

1. Costantino M, Gosselin MV, Primack SL. The ABC's of thoracic trauma imaging. Semin Roentgenol 2006;41(3): 209–225

2. Gavelli G, Canini R, Bertaccini P, Battista G, Bnà C, Fattori R. Traumatic injuries: imaging of thoracic injuries. Eur Radiol 2002;12(6):1273–1294

3. Iyer VN, Joshi AY, Ryu JH. Spontaneous pneumomediastinum: analysis of 62 consecutive adult patients. Mayo Clin Proc 2009;84(5):417–421

4. Primack SL, Collins J. Blunt nonaortic chest trauma: radiographic and CT findings. Emerg Radiol 2002;9(1):5–12

CASE 93

■ Clinical Presentation

30-year-old man who sustained multiple stab wounds to his chest

■ Radiologic Findings

Contrast-enhanced chest CT (**Figs. 93.1A, 93.1B, 93.1C,** mediastinal window; **Fig. 93.1D,** lung window) demonstrates air in the pericardial sac and foci of pneumomediastinum. Note the concomitant left hemothorax, bibasilar volume loss, and subcutaneous air in the left chest wall.

■ Diagnosis

Pneumopericardium

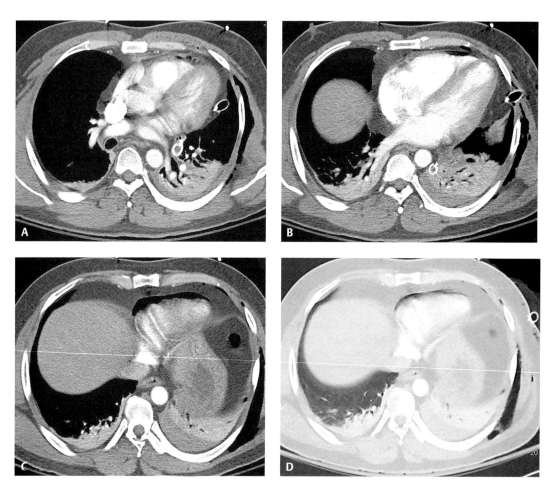

Fig. 93.1

452

■ Differential Diagnosis

None

■ Discussion

Background

Pneumopericardium is defined as air within the pericardial sac. Post-traumatic pneumopericardium is rare; however, its presence is likely associated with an underlying cardiac injury. Pericardial and cardiac injuries are more commonly associated with penetrating as opposed to blunt trauma and result from direct violation of the pericardium and/or myocardium. Although less common with blunt thoracic trauma, injuries may occur following severe blows to the anterior chest. Such injuries may be complicated by cardiac contusion, cardiac rupture, valvular injuries, coronary artery injuries, conducting system injuries, hemopericardium, and cardiac tamponade.

Etiology

Pneumopericardium may result from cardiac or mediastinal surgery, penetrating or blunt trauma, infectious pericarditis with gas-producing organisms, and a fistulous communication between the pericardium and an adjacent air-containing organ (i.e., stomach or esophagus). Pneumopericardium secondary to blunt chest trauma is generally due to one of three mechanisms: (1) air extension along pulmonary venous perivascular sheaths from ruptured alveoli to the pericardium, (2) pneumothorax associated with pleuropericardial tear. or (3) direct tracheobronchial-pericardial communication.

Clinical Findings

Cardiac contusion is the most common injury of the heart, occurring in up to 76% of blunt chest trauma victims. The anteriorly located right heart chambers are more commonly injured than the left heart chambers. *Cardiac laceration* and *rupture* are rare (0.21–2.0% incidence) but most often involve the right atrium, right ventricle, or both. Acute tamponade may be caused by as little as 250–300 mL of hemopericardium. Pneumopericardium may be associated with respiratory distress and/or hemodynamic compromise, the degree of which depends on the amount of trapped air and circulation blocked in the systemic and pulmonary veins. *Tension pneumopericardium* causing cardiac tamponade is extremely rare but carries a reported mortality of 56%; thus rapid diagnosis and definitive surgical treatment are necessary.

Imaging Findings

Chest Radiography

Pneumopericardium

- *Halo sign*—radiolucent band of air partially or completely surrounds the heart and does not extend above the upper limit of the pericardial reflections; confined below the aortic arch (**Fig. 93.2**)

Differentiating Pneumopericardium from Pneumomediastinum and/or Medial Pneumothorax

- Lateral decubitus exam shows shift of pericardial air; pneumomediastinum does not
- *"Transverse band of air"* sign—delineates air in transverse sinus of the pericardium
- *"Triangle of air"* sign—hyperlucency behind the sternum, anterior to the cardiac base and aortic root, differentiates pneumopericardium from pneumomediastinum
- In typical pneumopericardium, the cardiac silhouette is normal or large in size (**Fig. 93.2**), whereas in tension pneumopericardium, the cardiac silhouette appears small

Cardiac Laceration/Contusion

- Limited value

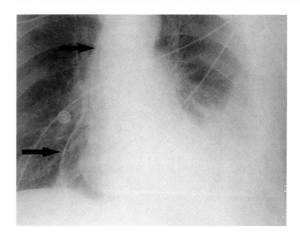

Fig. 93.2 Coned-down AP chest radiograph of a young man stabbed in the chest demonstrates pneumopericardium. The trapped pericardial air collection forms a double contour along the cardiac borders (*arrows*) that surrounds the myocardium (*halo sign*) but is limited superiorly by the attachment of the pericardial reflections differentiating it from pneumomediastinum. A left hemothorax is also present.

Non-specific Signs

- Cardiomegaly
- Heart failure
- Abnormal cardiac contours
- Pneumopericardium

MDCT

- Air within the pericardial sac and delimited by pericardial reflections (**Figs. 93.1A, 93.1B, 93.1C, 93.1D**)
- Associated findings may include hemopericardium, pneumothorax, pneumomediastinum (**Figs. 93.1B, 93.1C**)
- *Universal sign* of *cardiac injury* on CT is hemopericardium

Additional Findings

- Compression of right-sided cardiac chambers
- Pneumopericardium
- Active arterial extravasation

Transthoracic or Transesophageal Echocardiography

- Should be readily performed in any suspect cases without hesitation

MRI

- Demonstrates traumatic cardiac, valvular, and possible coronary vessel injuries
- Limited value in the acute setting

Management

- Small pneumopericardium in a hemodynamically stable patient without signs of tamponade usually requires no specific treatment; air reabsorbs over two weeks
- Symptomatic pneumopericardium
  - Immediate needle aspiration
  - Pericardial drain or creation of pericardial window for continuous drainage

Prognosis

- Tension pneumopericardium; mortality rate as high as 56%
- Right atrial rupture; mortality rate up to 54%
- Right ventricular rupture; mortality rates up to 29%

PEARLS

- Differentiating small traumatic pneumopericardium from left medial pneumothorax or pneumomediastinum may be difficult. *"Transverse band of air" sign* on frontal radiography, representing air in the transverse sinus of the pericardium, and the *"triangle of air" sign* noted on lateral radiography are features of pneumopericardium.
- When in doubt, left lateral decubitus radiography can establish the diagnosis.

Suggested Reading

1. Gavelli G, Canini R, Bertaccini P, Battista G, Bnà C, Fattori R. Traumatic injuries: imaging of thoracic injuries. Eur Radiol 2002;12(6):1273–1294

2. Lomoschitz FM, Eisenhuber E, Linnau KF, Peloschek P, Schoder M, Bankier AA. Imaging of chest trauma: radiological patterns of injury and diagnostic algorithms. Eur J Radiol 2003;48(1):61–70

3. Polhill JL, Sing RF. Traumatic tension pneumopericardium. J Trauma 2009;66(4):1261

4. Van Gelderen WFC. Stab wounds of the heart: two new signs of pneumopericardium. Br J Radiol 1993;66(789): 794–796

CASE 94

■ Clinical Presentation

Young man involved in a MVC with respiratory distress and dull breath sounds over the left thorax

■ Radiologic Findings

AP (**Fig. 94.1**) chest radiograph shows marked rightward displacement of the cardiomediastinal silhouette by herniated hollow viscera into the left thorax. A left-sided hemothorax extends into the apex. Note the large radiolucent focus at the left lung base.

■ Diagnosis

Acute Traumatic Rupture Left Diaphragm

■ Differential Diagnosis

- Eventration or Elevation of the Diaphragm
- Diaphragmatic Paralysis

■ Discussion

Background

Most diaphragmatic injuries are caused by *penetrating trauma*. Approximately 15% of stab wounds and 45% of gunshot wounds to the lower chest are complicated by diaphragmatic injuries. Diaphragmatic injuries should be suspected in any penetrating trauma victim with wounds below the fourth anterior, the sixth lateral, and

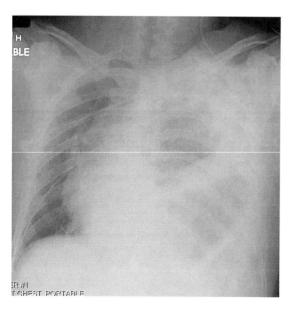

Fig. 94.1

456

eighth posterior intercostal spaces (*4-6-8 rule*). The incidence of diaphragmatic injury among *blunt trauma* victims varies from 0.8% to 8.0% and is more frequently observed with abdominal as opposed to thoracic trauma. Left-sided injuries are three times more common than right-sided injuries; however, as up to 4.5% of blunt trauma victims sustain bilateral diaphragmatic injuries. Most diaphragmatic tears are more than 10 cm in length and involve the muscular posterior or posterolateral diaphragm.

Etiology

A sudden increase in either intra-abdominal or intra-thoracic pressure against a fixed diaphragm accounts for most blunt diaphragmatic injuries. Other postulated mechanisms of injury include shearing stress on a stretched diaphragm and avulsion of the diaphragm from its points of attachment.

Clinical Findings

Acute diaphragmatic injury should be considered in patients who sustain significant abdominal or thoracoabdominal trauma and present with dyspnea or respiratory distress. The majority of affected trauma patients (<94%) have concomitant injuries. Associated injuries often include hepatic (16%) and/or splenic lacerations (48%), rib fractures (52%), pelvic fractures (52%), and closed head injuries (32%). Left-sided diaphragmatic injuries are associated with herniation of subdiaphragmatic viscera into the chest. The stomach and colon are the most commonly herniated organs. As many as three-quarters of affected patients have herniation of other intra-abdominal organs (e.g., omentum, spleen, kidney, pancreas). Diaphragmatic injuries may go unrecognized in patients on positive-pressure ventilation, only declaring their presence following extubation (**Fig. 94.2**). Delayed herniation may be complicated by bowel strangulation. Intrathoracic splenosis may manifest as a sequela of remote diaphragmatic and splenic injuries on imaging studies decades later and should not be confused with neoplastic disease.

Imaging Findings

Chest Radiography

Initial chest radiography is diagnostic in 27–60% of left-sided diaphragmatic injuries, but in only 17% of right-sided injuries.

- May initially appear normal
- Non-specific findings may include:
    ○ Elevated asymmetric, poorly visualized, or irregular-appearing diaphragm (**Figs. 94.1, 94.2, 94.3**)
    ○ Hemothorax, pneumothorax, and hemopneumothorax (**Figs. 94.1, 94.2, 94.3**)

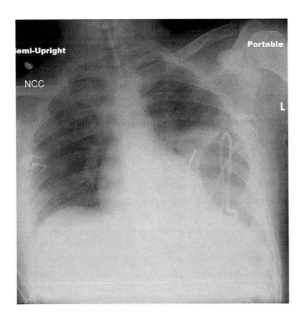

Fig. 94.2 AP chest radiograph of a young trauma victim with delayed presentation of a left diaphragmatic rupture following extubation. Feeding tube is redundantly coiled within the herniated intrathoracic stomach. The patient had been intubated for the past seven days. He was subsequently extubated and the feeding tube was placed in preparation for transfer to a skilled nursing facility because of a concomitant severe closed head injury.

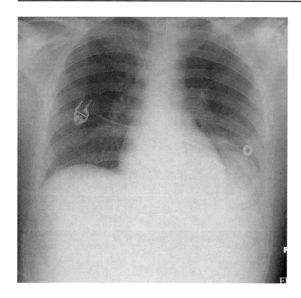

Fig. 94.3 AP chest radiograph of a 38-year-old man who sustained a rupture of the left diaphragm following a MVC. Non-specific radiographic signs include a poorly defined, asymmetrically elevated left diaphragm and lower lobe opacification by hemothorax. A 9.0 cm tear was seen intra-operatively and subsequently repaired.

- ○ Lower lobe opacification in the presence of an elevated diaphragm (**Fig. 94.3**)
- ○ Contralateral mediastinal shift in the absence of pneumothorax or large effusion (**Fig. 94.1**)
- ○ Persistent contralateral mediastinal shift despite the presence of a pleural drain
- ○ Lower rib fractures
- • More specific findings may include:
  - ○ An abnormal or U-shaped course of nasogastric or enteric tube (**Fig. 94.2**)
  - ○ Herniation of abdominal contents into the thorax (**Figs. 94.1, 94.2**)

Ultrasonography

Scanning is performed in the oblique transverse subxiphoid plane at the midline to obtain comparative images of both hemidiaphragms. A transducer is then positioned in each subcostal area, and each hemidiaphragm is scanned separately in the coronal plane.

- • Permits direct visualization of diaphragm
- • More useful in evaluation of right-sided injuries
- • Stomach/bowel gas limits evaluation of left-sided injuries
- • Normal diaphragm demonstrates continuous echogenic lines; injured diaphragm shows focal disruptions or interruptions of diaphragmatic echoes at site of injury
- • Diminishment or absence of expected respiratory excursion of the ruptured diaphragm

MDCT

Blunt Trauma

- • Sensitivity 50–100%; specificity 86–100%

Imaging Findings

- • Abrupt discontinuity of diaphragm (73–82%) with or without herniation of stomach or other viscera into thorax (**Fig. 94.4**)
- • *Absent diaphragm sign*
  - ○ Non-visualization of diaphragm in an area where it does not contact another organ and should otherwise be seen
- • *Dependent viscera sign*
  - ○ Loss of the superior support of the liver, stomach, and/or bowel, allowing them to fall dependently against the posterior ribs (**Fig. 94.5**)

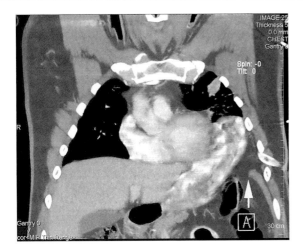

Fig. 94.4 Coronal chest CT (mediastinal window) of a 50-year-old man involved in a high-speed MVC reveals abrupt discontinuity of the left diaphragm (*arrow*) with intrathoracic herniation of the stomach.

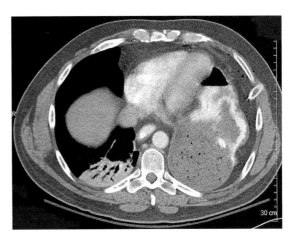

Fig. 94.5 Axial chest CT (mediastinal window) of man involved in an ATV accident demonstrates rupture of the left diaphragm. The herniated intrathoracic stomach is in contact with the left ventricle. Loss of superior support of the stomach by the ruptured diaphragm has allowed the stomach to fall dependently against the posterior ribs (*dependent viscera sign*).

- *CT collar sign*
  - Waist-like or focal constriction of herniated viscera, stomach or bowel through diaphragmatic defect (**Fig. 94.6**)
- Visualization of peritoneal fat, bowel, or viscera lateral to the lung or diaphragm or posterior to the diaphragmatic crus
- *Hump sign*
  - Variant of the *collar sign*
  - Rounded portion of herniated liver through the diaphragm forms a hump-shaped mass (**Fig. 94.7**)
  - May also manifest as a mushroom-like mass in the right hemithorax where the herniated liver is constricted by the tear
- *Band sign*
  - Linear lucency across the liver along the torn edges of the hemidiaphragm
- Irregularly thickened diaphragm
  - Highly suggestive of diaphragmatic rupture in the absence of retroperitoneal contusion; does not distinguish between injury requiring surgical repair and partial-thickness tears
- Concomitant proximity injuries of ribs, liver and/or spleen, adrenal gland

Penetrating Trauma

Sensitivity 88%; specificity 82%

- Most accurate sign is the presence of a contiguous injury on either side of the diaphragm in single-entry penetrating trauma (**Fig. 94.8**)

MRI

- Primary role is in nonacute or difficult cases (e.g., eventration/elevation versus injury)
- Both cardiac and respiratory gating should be used to minimize motion artifacts
- T1WI sagittal and coronal images: delineate left diaphragm as a low-signal-intensity curvilinear band of soft tissue outlined by higher-signal-intensity abdominal and mediastinal fat
- Evaluation of the right diaphragm more problematic

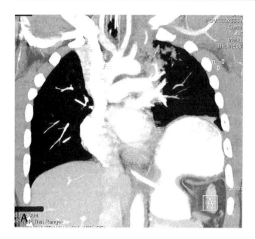
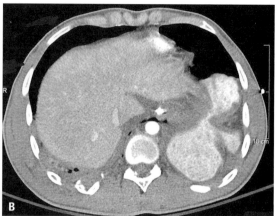

Fig. 94.6 **(A)** Coronal and **(B)** axial chest CT (mediastinal window) of a young man involved in a motorcycle collision reveals a focal waist-like constriction in the herniated stomach at the location of the diaphragmatic rent (*CT collar sign*). Most of the stomach has herniated into the left thorax.

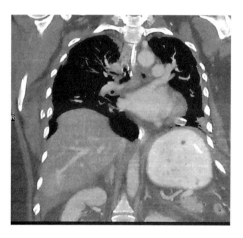

Fig. 94.7 Coronal chest CT (mediastinal window) of a young trauma victim with a ruptured right diaphragm shows the dome of the liver projecting into the lower right chest cavity. The herniated liver has a "hump-like" or "mushroom-like" morphology where it is constricted by the diaphragmatic rent.

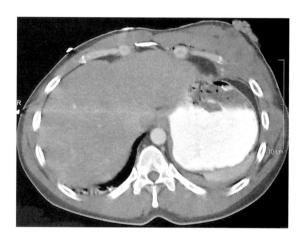

Fig. 94.8 Axial chest CT (mediastinal window) of a young patient stabbed in the left thoracoabdominal region shows an irregularly thickened left diaphragm. There is an associated hematoma on both sides of the injured diaphragm and foci of active contrast extravasation. Note the adjacent chest wall hematoma. A near full-thickness tear of the diaphragm was subsequently surgically repaired.

Management

- Small diaphragmatic lacerations
  - Laparoscopy; alternative to open repair
- Open laparotomy for large (>10 cm) tears adjacent to or near esophageal hiatus
  - Most injuries can be repaired primarily
  - Synthetic mesh (e.g., polypropylene, Dacron) occasionally required for large tears
- Centrally located injuries
  - Most easily repaired
- Posterolateral injury of right diaphragm
  - Best approached through the chest, as the liver obscures an abdominal approach
- Lateral injuries near chest wall
  - May require reattachment of the diaphragm to the chest wall by encirclement of the ribs with suture material

Prognosis

- Mortality approaches 30%
- May be adversely affected by
  - Associated abdominal and thoracic injuries
  - Delays in diagnosis and surgical repair; bowel strangulation

PEARLS

- Positive-pressure ventilation can prevent herniation of bowel into the thorax, delaying diagnosis of diaphragmatic injury in some cases until after patient has been extubated.
- Atelectasis and or hemothorax may obscure visualization of diaphragmatic tears.
- Normal focal areas of discontinuity in the posterior diaphragm are seen in 6–11% of nontrauma patients (e.g., congenital Bochdalek defects) and in up to 35% of elderly persons. The presence or absence of concomitant proximity trauma is helpful in appropriately directing the diagnosis.

Suggested Reading

1. Bagheri R, Tavasoli A, Sadrizadeh A, et al. The role of thoracoscopy for the diagnosis of hidden diaphragmatic injuries in penetrating thoracoabdominal trauma. Interact Cardiovasc Thorac Surg 2009; May 25 [Epub ahead of print]

2. Bodanapally UK, Shanmuganathan K, Mirvis SE, et al. MDCT diagnosis of penetrating diaphragm injury. Eur Radiol 2009; Mar 31

3. Costantino M, Gosselin MV, Primack SL. The ABC's of thoracic trauma imaging. Semin Roentgenol 2006;41(3): 209–225

4. Lomoschitz FM, Eisenhuber E, Linnau KF, Peloschek P, Schoder M, Bankier AA. Imaging of chest trauma: radiological patterns of injury and diagnostic algorithms. Eur J Radiol 2003;48(1):61–70

5. Primack SL, Collins J. Blunt nonaortic chest trauma: radiographic and CT findings. Emerg Radiol 2002;9(1):5–12

CASE 95

■ Clinical Presentation

45-year-old pedestrian struck by a bus traveling at approximately 35 mph

■ Radiologic Findings

AP (**Fig. 95.1A**) chest radiograph reveals a persistent large right pneumothorax despite the chest tube. Diffuse ground glass opacity throughout the right lung consistent with extensive pulmonary contusion. The left lower lobe is collapsed. Multiple contiguous, segmental anterior and posterior right-sided rib fractures are present, many of which are acutely angulated. Extensive subcutaneous air is present in the ipsilateral chest wall. 3-D CT reconstruction (**Fig. 95.1B**) illustrates the acutely fractured first through eighth anterior and more inferiorly displaced posterior rib fractures to better advantage.

■ Diagnosis

Flail Chest with Complicating Bronchial Fracture and Pneumothorax

■ Differential Diagnosis

None

■ Discussion

Background

Rib fractures are the *most common* injury in blunt chest trauma, occurring in at least 50% of patients. The location and number of involved ribs serve as clues to possible concomitant injuries and to the severity of the trauma. For example, *ribs 1–3* are very stable, protected by the shoulder girdle and adjacent musculature.

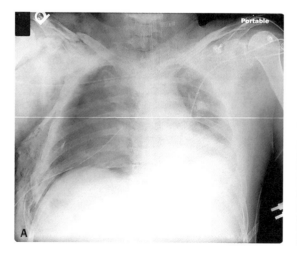 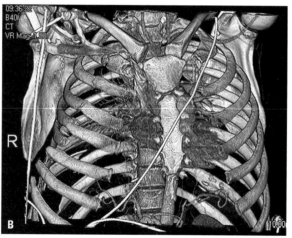

Fig. 95.1 (*See color insert following page 108.*)

Acute fractures of the *upper* first three ribs require a substantial force. There is a high correlation of such fractures or fractures of the first two ribs and clavicle with maxillofacial, cranial, brachial plexus, branch vessel, and tracheobronchial injuries. Fractures of *ribs 4–9* are common and most significant when associated with *flail chest*. Fractures of the *lower ribs 10–12* are less common but may be associated with traumatic injuries of the liver, spleen, kidneys, and diaphragm. *Flail chest* is the most severe traumatic injury of the chest wall in blunt trauma. It is characterized by anterior and posterior segmental fractures of more than three congruent ribs or single fractures of more than four contiguous ribs. These fractures create an abnormally mobile, free-floating, unstable chest wall segment that moves paradoxically during the respiratory cycle. The traumatic separation of ribs from their costochondral cartilages (**Figs. 95.2A, 95.2B, 95.2C, 95.2D, 95.2E**) may also result in a flail segment.

Etiology

Flail chest requires significant blunt force trauma to the torso, fracturing the ribs in multiple locations. Such trauma may be caused by motor vehicle collisions, falls, blast or crushing injuries, and assaults in younger, healthy patients. However, it may also occur with lesser trauma in persons with underlying osteoporosis, with neoplastic disease, including multiple myeloma, and with congenital absence of the sternum.

Clinical Findings

Clinically, flail chest is characterized by chest wall instability and focal paradoxical chest wall motion during spontaneous respiration that inhibits normal respiratory excursion and impairs ventilation. This clinical finding may disappear after intubation with positive-pressure ventilation, often delaying diagnosis. Associated intrathoracic injuries are common and include pulmonary contusion (46%) and pneumothorax, hemothorax, or hemopneumothorax (70%). The incidence of great vessel, tracheobronchial, and diaphragmatic injuries is not greater than that of trauma patients without flail chest. Most patients with flail chest complain of severe pain, experience dyspnea, and require prolonged ventilator support. Respiratory failure results primarily from underlying lung injury (e.g., contusion and/or laceration); however, pendelluft (i.e., contralateral movement of dead space gas from the flail to nonflail side) may contribute in some cases. Twenty-seven percent of patients with flail chest develop ARDS.

Imaging Findings

Chest Radiography

- Limited value, demonstrates only 40–50% of acute rib fractures and is even less sensitive in detecting costochondral fractures (**Fig. 95.2A**)
- Primary role—detection of otherwise unsuspected concomitant injuries (e.g., pneumothorax, hemothorax, mediastinal hematoma, diaphragmatic rupture) (**Fig. 95.1**)

MDCT

- Multiplanar and 3-D reconstruction are more sensitive and better delineate extent of chest wall injury; helpful in planning surgical stabilization (**Figs. 95.1B, 95.2B, 95.2C, 95.2D, 95.2E**)
- Concomitant injuries
  - Pneumothorax/hemothorax
  - Diaphragmatic and subdiaphragmatic solid and hollow visceral injuries

Management

- Pain control
  - Oral and/or parenteral analgesics
  - Epidural analgesics
  - Intercostal nerve blocks
- Surgical chest wall stabilization (e.g., external fixation devices; pins and/or plates for internal fixation) of affected ribs up to six days post-injury
  - Allows intercostal muscle healing, reducing or alleviating discoordinated paradoxical chest wall motion

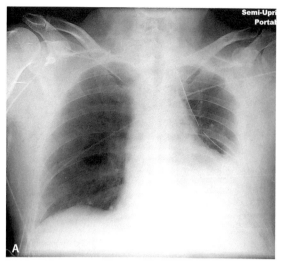
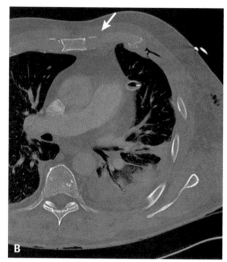
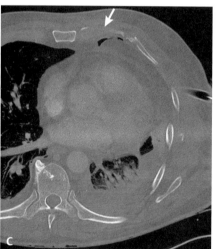
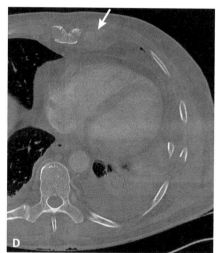
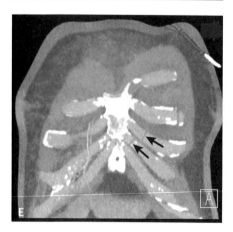

Fig. 95.2 **(A)** AP chest radiograph of a 35-year-old man involved in a high-speed MVC demonstrates a left hemothorax and lower lobe volume loss. Axial chest CT (bone window) **(B–D)** shows unsuspected and radiographically inconspicuous fractures with associated hematoma of the left third through fifth costochondral cartilages (*arrows*). These latter injuries are nicely depicted on the coronal MIP chest CT (mediastinal window) **(E,** *arrows*).

- o Improves gas exchange and expedites extubation in patients with respiratory insufficiency but without pulmonary contusion
- Supportive care for patients with pulmonary contusion; no benefit from surgical chest wall stabilization

Prognosis

- Morbidity and mortality range from 3% to 60%; dependent on extent of intrathoracic injury, concomitant nonthoracic injuries, and patient's age
- Number and location of rib fractures may be helpful in predicting the degree of underlying radiographically inconspicuous intercostal muscle injury in flail chest
- Intercostal muscular injury may be more important to patient morbidity and long-term disability than the actual osseous trauma itself

PEARLS

- Flail chest wall injuries may be clinically unrecognized if the affected segment is "fixed" in place by a large chest wall hematoma and may be responsible for otherwise unexplained respiratory failure.

Suggested Reading

1. Costantino M, Gosselin MV, Primack SL. The ABC's of thoracic trauma imaging. Semin Roentgenol 2006;41(3): 209–225

2. Lardinois D, Krueger T, Dusmet M, Ghisletta N, Gugger M, Ris HB. Pulmonary function testing after operative stabilisation of the chest wall for flail chest. Eur J Cardiothorac Surg 2001;20(3):496–501

3. Lomoschitz FM, Eisenhuber E, Linnau KF, Peloschek P, Schoder M, Bankier AA. Imaging of chest trauma: radiological patterns of injury and diagnostic algorithms. Eur J Radiol 2003;48(1):61–70

4. Primack SL, Collins J. Blunt nonaortic chest trauma: radiographic and CT findings. Emerg Radiol 2002;9(1): 5–12

5. Weyant MJ, Bleier JI, Naama H, et al. Severe crushed chest injury with large flail segment: computed tomographic three-dimensional reconstruction. J Trauma 2002;52(3):605

CASE 96

■ Clinical Presentation

59-year-old unrestrained driver involved in a high-speed MVC with complaints of chest pain. The vehicle's steering wheel was severely deformed in the collision.

■ Radiologic Findings

Contrast-enhanced sagittal MIP (bone window) (**Fig. 96.1A**) and axial (mediastinal window) (**Fig. 96.1B**) chest CT shows a markedly depressed mid-sternal body fracture; associated peri-sternal, para-sternal, and retrosternal hematoma; and soft-tissue stranding overlying the sternum. Note the preserved fat plane between the retrosternal hematoma and the aorta.

■ Diagnosis

Sternal Fracture

■ Differential Diagnosis

None

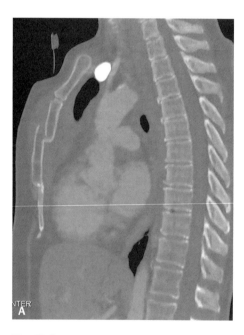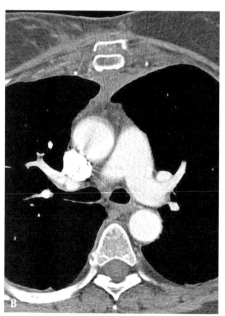

Fig. 96.1

466

■ DISCUSSION

Background

The incidence of sternal fracture as a result of motor vehicle collisions ranges between 3% and 10%, although the incidence may decrease with airbags. The *most common* location for sternal fractures is within 2 cm of the sternal-manubrial joint. Most fractures are associated with a retrosternal hematoma (**Fig. 96.1B**). *Simple sternal fractures* are usually benign. *Depressed, segmental sternal fractures* have an increased association with myocardial contusions, traumatic hemopericardium, coronary vessel lacerations, thoracic aorta lacerations, tracheobronchial tears, thoracic spine fractures (see Case 99), and head trauma.

Etiology

Motor vehicle collisions account for 60–90% of sternal fractures. Most of these occur in restrained occupants but in the absence of airbag deployment. It is postulated that the deceleration forces are concentrated into the non-elastic 2-inch seatbelt harness strap, which delivers this force directly to the sternum. Unrestrained occupants usually sustain injury during vehicular ejection or from direct impact with the steering wheel or dashboard. Direct impact from contact sports, falls from a height, pedestrians struck by motor vehicles, and assaults account for most of the remainder.

Clinical Findings

Signs and symptoms include crepitus, pain, edema, contusion, and ecchymosis (40–45% of patients) over the fracture site. The fracture may visibly move during respiration and a "step-off" deformity may be palpable. Whereas *simple isolated fractures* are usually benign and unassociated with myocardial contusion, patients with *complex sternal fractures* have a higher incidence of cardiac injuries, and further evaluation with ECG and cardiac enzymes is warranted.

Imaging Findings

Chest Radiography

- Usually not evident on frontal chest exams
- Mediastinal widening may or may not be present
- Can be difficult to appreciate on oblique sternal views
- Usually well delineated on lateral chest or dedicated lateral sternal views (**Fig. 96.2**)

Ultrasound

- More sensitive than lateral radiography in detecting sternal fractures but not as good in assessing degree of displacement
- Hematoma; hypoechoic area over sternum
- Disruption of cortical bone or a step in the bone outline
- Identification of fragment dislocation

MDCT

- Direct fracture visualization and assessment of degree of displacement (**Fig. 96.1B**); optimized with MPR and MIP sagittal reformations (**Fig. 96.1A**)
- Indirect evidence of fracture: soft-tissue, parasternal, or retrosternal hematoma (**Fig. 96.1B**)
- Concomitant associated injuries

Management

- Rest and pain control with analgesics for isolated sternal fracture
- Minimize activities involving use of pectoral and shoulder girdle muscles
- Surgical stabilization for displaced or unstable sternal fractures

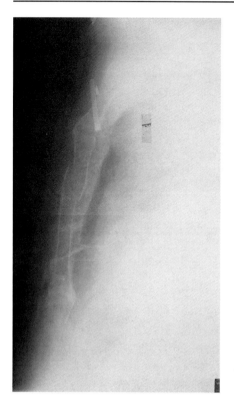

Fig. 96.2   Lateral sternal view reveals a displaced sternal fracture approximately 4.0 cm below the sternomanubrial joint. Retrosternal hematoma and fat create the opacity behind the sternum. AP chest radiograph (not illustrated) was grossly unremarkable.

- ○ Open reduction and internal fixation (ORIF)
- ○ Wire suturing and placement of plates and screws

Prognosis

- >50% of persons with sternal fractures have ECG and radionuclide abnormalities indicating some degree of blunt cardiac injury and dysfunction
- Good; *isolated sternal fractures* and normal ECG
- Mortality rate 25–45% with *complex sternal fractures*; related to associated injuries

PEARLS

- Traumatic aortic injury occurs in <2% of persons with sternal fractures; rate is similar to that of persons with blunt chest trauma without sternal fracture.
- Fat plane preservation between the hematoma and aorta suggests the hematoma is not related to aortic or great vessel injury.
- Manubrial fractures have a greater association with intrathoracic and upper mediastinal (e.g., great vessel) injuries.

Suggested Reading

1. Gavelli G, Canini R, Bertaccini P, Battista G, Bnà C, Fattori R. Traumatic injuries: imaging of thoracic injuries. Eur Radiol 2002;12(6):1273–1294

2. Lomoschitz FM, Eisenhuber E, Linnau KF, Peloschek P, Schoder M, Bankier AA. Imaging of chest trauma: radiological patterns of injury and diagnostic algorithms. Eur J Radiol 2003;48(1):61–70

3. Primack SL, Collins J. Blunt nonaortic chest trauma: radiographic and CT findings. Emerg Radiol 2002;9(1):5–12

4. Recinos G, Inaba K, Dubose J, et al. Epidemiology of sternal fractures. Am Surg 2009;75(5):401–404

CASE 97

■ Clinical Presentation

Young patient struck by a car

■ Radiologic Findings

Chest CT coronal MIP (bone window) (**Fig. 97.1A**) and 3-D reformatted image of the left scapula (bone window) (**Fig. 97.1B**) show a comminuted fracture of the scapula and bilateral upper lobe pulmonary contusions. 3-D reformation (**Fig. 97.1B**) reveals the articular surface of the glenoid is intact.

■ Diagnosis

Comminuted Left Scapular Fracture

■ Differential Diagnosis

None

■ Discussion

Background

Scapular fracture is present in approximately 1% of cases of blunt trauma. High-speed motor vehicle collisions are the *most common cause* of acute scapular fractures, but falls and direct blows to the area can also be responsible. A significant force is required to fracture the scapula. Therefore, the presence of such an injury should alert the radiologist and clinician to the possibility of additional thoracic injuries. Eighty to 90% of trauma patients with scapular fractures have associated rib fractures, pulmonary contusion (**Fig. 97.1A**), pneumotho-

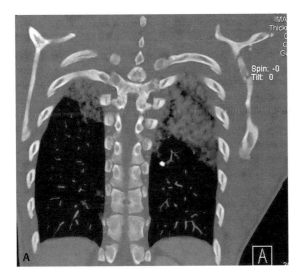
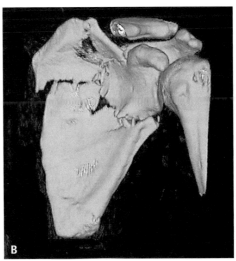

Fig. 97.1

rax, or hemothorax. There is also a relationship between scapular fractures and thoracic spine as well as head injuries. *Scapulothoracic dissociation* is a rare but serious devastating closed forequarter amputation of the upper extremity resulting from a direct blow to or severe traction on the shoulder girdle. Fifty to 60% of patients with scapulothoracic dissociation are motorcyclists. The postulated mechanism of injury involves attempting to hold onto the handlebars while being forcibly thrown. Injuries to ATV riders occur in a similar manner and are becoming more common. Clinically, there is near complete disruption of the forequarter from the torso.

Clinical Findings

Scapular Fractures

Signs and symptoms are similar to those of other acute fractures and include pain, tenderness, and reduced range of motion.

Scapulothoracic Dissociation

Massive soft-tissue swelling and partial or complete tears of the deltoid, pectoralis minor, rhomboids, levator scapulae, trapezius, and latissimus dorsi muscles are usually present. Concomitant injury to the ipsilateral brachial plexus, subclavian artery, and/or subclavian vein invariably occurs. The axillary artery is not infrequently injured. The neurologic deficit is most often the result of complete avulsion of the brachial plexus. There is also a high prevalence of other, often severe injuries.

Imaging Findings

Scapular Fractures

Chest Radiography

- May be inconspicuous or difficult to fully characterize on chest radiography (**Fig. 97.2**) and require dedicated AP and lateral views in the scapular plane (Grashey and "Y" views); axillary views help clarify degree of displacement and deformity
- Presence or absence of displacement, comminution, or articular extension should always be determined
- Apical-lateral extrapleural hematoma is a helpful radiologic clue
- Rib fractures and pneumothorax: frequently associated injuries
- Concomitant displaced acromial, glenoid, humeral head injuries may be apparent

MDCT

- Depicts scapular fractures not readily appreciated on chest radiography (**Fig. 97.1A**)

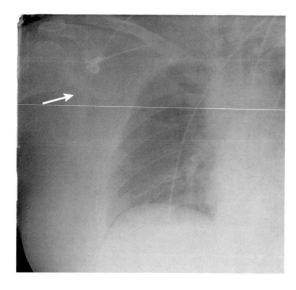

Fig. 97.2 Coned-down AP chest radiograph over the right thorax and axilla of a woman involved in a motorcycle collision shows a comminuted fracture of the right scapula extending into the base of the glenoid and diastasis of the acromial-clavicular joint (*arrow*).

- 3-D reformatted images delineate intra-articular extension of fractures and are very helpful in planning surgical reconstruction and stabilization (**Fig. 97.1B**)

Scapulothoracic Dissociation

Chest Radiography (Figs. 97.3A, 97.3B)

- Radiographic hallmark: lateral displacement of the scapula
  - Scapulothoracic ratio (i.e., thoracic spinous process to medial scapular border distance): ≥1.40 (abnormal:normal, on well-centered frontal exam)
- Concomitant fracture of ipsilateral clavicle with lateral displacement of distal fragment, acromioclavicular separation, and sternoclavicular fracture

MDCT/MRI (Figs. 97.3C, 97.3D, 97.3E)

- Depicts conventional radiographic findings to better advantage
- Separation of scapula from chest wall
- Excessively large hematoma may be suggestive of serious vascular injury
- Chest wall or paraspinous hematoma may be identified
- Pseudomeningocele; indicative of spinal root avulsion
  - Three or more pseudomeningoceles diagnostic of an irreparable neurologic injury
- MRI offers more detailed information regarding brachial plexus injury

Management

Scapular Fractures

- Pain control and immobilization
- Intra-articular extension: often deciding factor between surgical repair and conservative management

Scapulothoracic Dissociation

- Urgent surgical exploration mandatory for patients with active hemorrhage, expanding hematoma, or severe hand ischemia
- Complete disruption of brachial plexus; primary amputation should be considered
- Partial brachial plexus injury; some potential for functional recovery
  - Direct repair of nerve injuries may be considered if patient is stable
  - Urgent revascularization of ischemic upper extremity

Prognosis

Scapular Fracture

- Accompanying injuries have greater impact on patient's outcome than scapular fracture itself

Scapulothoracic Dissociation

- Early recognition and aggressive treatment are crucial; outcome is not dependent on management of the arterial injury, but rather on the severity of the neurologic deficit
- Severe long-term disability may result from ischemia and brachial plexus damage
- Complications may ultimately require shoulder arthrodesis and amputation

---

PEARLS

- Ninety percent of patients with both scapular and rib fractures have a pneumothorax.
- Vascular injuries associated with scapulothoracic dissociation are often limb- or life-threatening; upper extremity CTA or conventional arteriography is indicated to assess the nature and extent of arterial injuries in the limb of an affected patient.

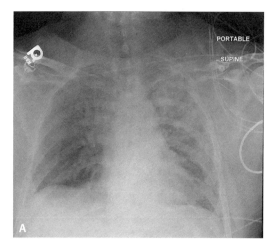
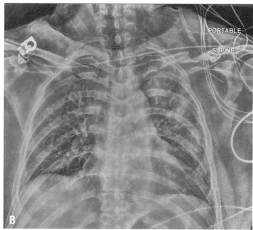
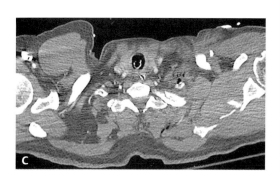
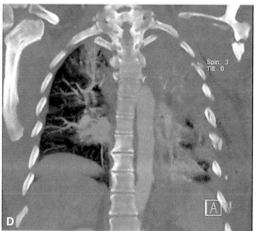
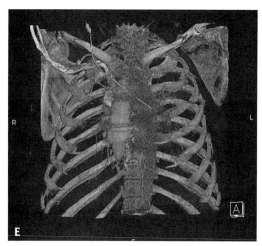

Fig. 97.3 AP portable trauma bay chest radiograph **(A)** with accompanying edge-enhanced image **(B)** of a young man involved in a high-speed motorcycle collision with diminished left upper extremity pulses demonstrate a widened mediastinum with poor definition of the transverse aorta, aorticopulmonary window, and right tracheo-broncial angle consistent with hemomediastinum in this setting. Left perihilar and upper lobe air space disease consistent with pulmonary contusion. The left diaphragm and left heart border is crisp, reflective of an ipsilateral pneumothorax. Note the significant left chest wall trauma characterized by acute fractures of the 1st through 8th ribs; comminuted scapular fracture; displaced left mid-shaft clavicular fracture; and the marked separation of the left scapula from the chest wall. The scapulothoracic ratio (i.e., thoracic spinous process-medial scapular border distance) is 1.8. Selected contrast-enhanced chest CT axial **(C)** (mediastinal window); coronal **(D)** (bone windows); and 3-D volume-rendered images **(E)** demonstrate these injuries to better advantage. Compare the relationship of the left and right scapula to the thoracic cage on the 3-D images **(E)**. (*See color insert following page 108.*)

Suggested Reading

1. Gavelli G, Canini R, Bertaccini P, Battista G, Bnà C, Fattori R. Traumatic injuries: imaging of thoracic injuries. Eur Radiol 2002;12(6):1273–1294

2. Lee GK, Suh KJ, Choi JA, Oh HY. A case of scapulothoracic dissociation with brachial plexus injury: magnetic resonance imaging findings. Acta Radiol 2007;48(9):1020–1023

3. Lomoschitz FM, Eisenhuber E, Linnau KF, Peloschek P, Schoder M, Bankier AA. Imaging of chest trauma: radiological patterns of injury and diagnostic algorithms. Eur J Radiol 2003;48(1):61–70

4. Witz M, Korzets Z, Lehmann J. Traumatic scapulothoracic dissociation. J Cardiovasc Surg (Torino) 2000;41(6): 927–929

CASE 98

■ Clinical Presentation

15-year-old male who fell off dirt bike while attempting to jump over an embankment

■ Radiologic Findings

AP CT scout (**Fig. 98.1A**) shows asymmetric alignment of the clavicles. The right clavicle lies lower than the left. A right paratracheal opacity is also present. Contrast-enhanced chest CT (mediastinal window) (**Fig. 98.1B**) reveals posterior displacement of the right sternoclavicular joint with the medial edge encroaching on the innominate artery and a right paratracheal hematoma.

■ Diagnosis

Posterior Dislocation of the Right Sternoclavicular Joint

■ Differential Diagnosis

None

■ Discussion

Background

Significant direct or indirect blunt force to the shoulder girdle can cause traumatic dislocation of the sterno-clavicular joint (SCJ). *Anterior sternoclavicular dislocations* are much more common (9:1) and usually result from an indirect mechanism such as a blow to the anterior shoulder that rotates the shoulder backward.

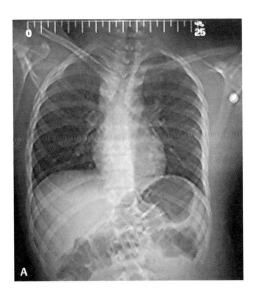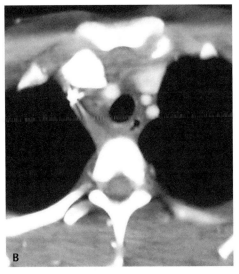

Fig. 98.1

473

Posterior sternoclavicular dislocations are relatively rare, accounting for <1% of all dislocations. Traumatic forces that drive the shoulder forward can cause such posterior dislocations. The proximity of the dislocated medial clavicular head to critical structures in the thoracic inlet (e.g., aerodigestive tract, great vessels, brachial plexus, and apical pleural reflections) can result in serious concomitant injuries the exclusion of which should be part of the radiologist's search pattern.

Clinical Findings

Affected patients commonly complain of chest and shoulder pain exacerbated by arm movement. Pain tends to be more severe with posterior SCJ dislocations. Additional signs and symptoms caused by associated injuries or by compression of adjacent structures by posterior SCJ dislocations may include paresthesias, dysphagia, stridor, tachypnea, venous congestion of the head and neck, and respiratory distress.

Imaging Findings

Chest Radiography

Anterior SCJ Dislocation

- Limited value
- Diagnosis usually made on physical exam

Posterior SCJ Dislocation

- Relatively inconspicuous; high false negative rate
- Subtle findings on a neutrally positioned frontal exam may include
  - Lateral displacement proximal end of clavicle
  - Apparent asymmetry in clavicular head height (**Fig. 98.1A**)

Specialized View

Serendipity View

- Central beam is tilted to 40° from the vertical and directed cephalad through the manubrium while patient is supine
- Normal clavicles appear in the same horizontal plane
- Anterior and posterior dislocations appear above and below the plane, respectively

MDCT

- Imaging modality of choice (**Figs. 98.2, 98.3**)
- Diagnosis readily established by comparing non-injured side with injured side (**Figs. 98.1A, 98.2, 98.3**)

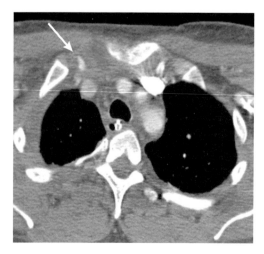

Fig. 98.2 Contrast-enhanced chest CT (mediastinal window) of a trauma patient involved in an ATV incident shows posterior and lateral disruption of the right sternoclavicular joint (*arrow*). Note the peri-joint space hematoma and the right lateral chest wall extrapleural hematoma.

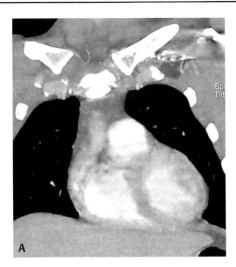 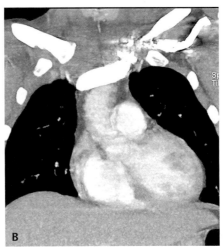

Fig. 98.3 Contrast-enhanced coronal MIP CT (mediastinal window) progressing from a more anterior **(A)** to posterior **(B)** location in the chest demonstrates anterior and superior displacement of the medial right clavicle from its normal articulation with the manubrium. Note the peri-joint space diastasis and hematoma. The left sternoclavicular joint is normal.

- Peri-joint space and/or mediastinal hematoma (**Figs. 98.2, 98.3**)
- Exclusion of associated injuries
- MPR/MIP images: delineate the injury and relationship to adjacent structures

Management

Acute Anterior SCJ Dislocations

- Usually managed non-operatively
- Manual reduction with local anesthesia and sedatives
    - Arm abducted and extended while lateral traction is applied to affected extremity
    - Direct pressure exerted over medial clavicle

Acute Posterior SCJ Dislocations

- More serious injury because of association with vascular, intrathoracic, and superior mediastinal injuries
- Pain control, possibly including general anesthesia
- Open reduction and surgical stabilization if closed reduction fails
- Treatment of associated injuries

Prognosis

- Posterior SCJ dislocation: estimated 25% complication rate related to pneumothorax, SVC laceration, subclavian artery or vein occlusion, and aerodigestive tract injury

Suggested Reading

1. Ernberg LA, Potter HG. Radiographic evaluation of the acromioclavicular and sternoclavicular joints. Clin Sports Med 2003;22(2):255–275
2. Garretson RB III, Williams GR Jr. Clinical evaluation of injuries to the acromioclavicular and sternoclavicular joints. Clin Sports Med 2003;22(2):239–254
3. McCulloch P, Henley BM, Linnau KF. Radiographic clues for high-energy trauma: three cases of sternoclavicular dislocation. AJR Am J Roentgenol 2001;176(6):1534
4. Torretti J, Lynch SA. Sternoclavicular joint injuries. Curr Opin Orthop 2004;15(4):242–247

CASE 99

■ Clinical Presentation

25-year-old man involved in a high-speed MVC with vehicular ejection

■ Radiologic Findings

AP chest radiograph (**Fig. 99.1A**) shows extensive right upper lobe and perihilar air space disease consistent with pulmonary contusions, and abnormal widening of the left, and to a lesser degree the right, paraspinal lines, which is seen to better advantage on the coned-down AP view (**Fig. 99.1B**) (*arrows*). Contrast-enhanced coronal MIP CT (**Fig. 99.1C**) demonstrates a burst fracture at T11. The associated paraspinal hematoma is responsible for the widened paraspinal lines seen on radiography. The multi-focal pulmonary contusions are also seen to better advantage.

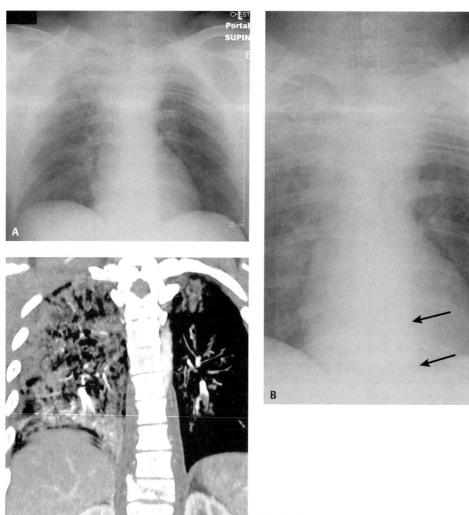

Fig. 99.1

476

■ Diagnosis

Thoracic Spine Fracture with Paraspinal Hematoma

■ Differential Diagnosis

- Other Causes of Post-Traumatic Mediastinal Hematoma (based on chest radiography)

■ Discussion

Background

Thoracic spine fractures occur in 3% of blunt chest trauma victims. Compression fractures are the *most common* injury (52%) in the thoracic spine. Fracture-dislocation injuries of the thoracic spine account for 30% of all spine injuries. These latter injuries are often clinically devastating. The most vulnerable region of the spine is the functional thoraco-lumbar spine (i.e., T9–T11). However, over 20% of patients have multi-level injuries and the injuries may be non-contiguous in up to 27% of cases, factors radiologists must keep in mind during their interpretation of trauma chest CT scans. Seventy percent of acute thoracic spine fractures may be seen on radiography. However, the conspicuity of such fractures is dependent upon many factors, including radiologic technique, patient body habitus, concomitant pulmonary contusions and hemothorax, etc. As a result, many such fractures are not appreciated.

Etiology

Most injuries result from hyperflexion and axial loading.

Clinical Findings

The prevalence of neurologic deficits in patients with thoracic spine fractures is as high as 62%, far greater than those occurring with cervical spine (32%) or lumbar spine injuries (2%). Only 12% of trauma patients with thoracic spine fracture-dislocations are neurologically intact at presentation. Chylothorax may rarely complicate thoracic spine fracture-dislocations.

Imaging Findings

Conventional Radiography

- May reveal mediastinal widening or widening of paraspinal lines (**Figs. 99.1A, 99.1B**)
- Loss of vertebral body height and/or poor definition of the pedicle(s)

MDCT

- Coronal/sagittal thoracic spine reformations demonstrate alignment and extent of fractures to better advantage; often reveal unsuspected fractures and associated complications (e.g., retropulsion) (**Figs. 99.1C, 99.2, 99.3, 99.4A, 99.4B**)
- Paraspinal hematoma, mediastinal hematoma confined to paravertebral compartment (**Figs. 99.1C, 99.4**)
- Pneumorachis (intraspinal epidural air); often associated with traumatic brain injury (especially with skull base and sinus fractures); lung injury, pneumomediastinum, pneumothorax, subcutaneous air (**Fig. 99.5**)
- 3-D volumetric images ideally display complex fractures and fracture-dislocations
- MRI indicated when neurologic deficits accompany thoracic spine fracture-dislocations

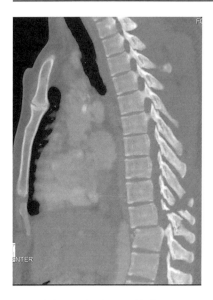

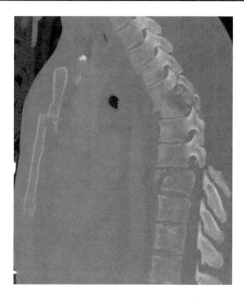

Fig. 99.2 Sagittal MIP CT (bone window) of a 45-year-old man following an 18-foot fall from a scaffold shows an acute flexion distraction injury at T10-T11 characterized by acute kyphosis with compromise of the spinal canal, an anterior corner fracture, and complete disruption of the middle and posterior columns.

Fig. 99.3 Sagittal MIP CT (bone window) of a 33-year-old man involved in a MVC with vehicular ejection shows the relationship between sternal and upper thoracic spinal injuries. All four columns of the thoracic cage are disrupted: depressed sternal fracture, flexion distraction injury at T4-T5, and disruption of the anterior, middle, and posterior columns of the thoracic spine with significant canal compromise. Note the non-contiguous concomitant injury at T8.

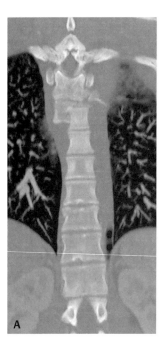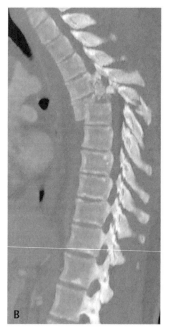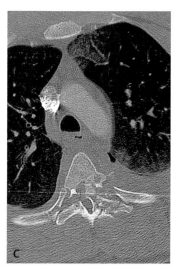

Fig. 99.4 Coronal **(A)** and sagittal **(B)** MIP with axial **(C)** CT (bone window) of a young man involved in a MVC at 75 mph with roll-over shows an acute fracture-dislocation at T3-T4 with disruption of the anterior, middle, and posterior columns and obliteration of the spinal canal. Note the extensive intracanal osseous fragments and paraspinal hematoma. The spinal cord was completely transected.

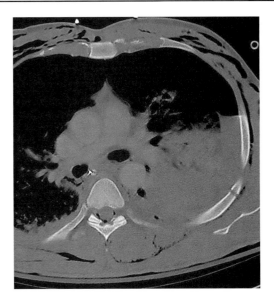

Fig. 99.5 Axial chest CT (bone window) of a 26-year-old man who fell 25 feet shows extensive subcutaneous air, foci of pneumomediastinum, left lung consolidation, left rib fractures and pneumorachis. No spine injury was detected.

Management

- Early surgical stabilization and fixation (i.e., within three days of injury) in patients with thoracic spine trauma allow earlier mobilization; reduce the incidence of atelectasis and pneumonia

Prognosis

- Prevalence of neurologic deficits with thoracic spine fractures is as high as 62%

PEARLS

- Compression fractures are the *most common* injury in the thoracic spine.
- Prevalence of neurologic deficits in patients with thoracic spine fractures is high.
- Radiologic assessment of patients with spinal trauma requires awareness of patterns of associated injuries. An important combination is that of sternal fractures and flexion distraction injuries of upper thoracic spine (T1–T6), although fractures may also occur beyond these more typical levels (**Fig. 99.3**).
- Pneumorachis is typically benign and resolves spontaneously; rarely can cause symptoms of cord compression necessitating decompressive surgery.

Suggested Reading

1. Berg EE. The sternal-rib complex. A possible fourth column in thoracic spine fractures. Spine 1993;18(13): 1916–1919
2. Chaichana KL, Pradilla G, Witham TF, Gokaslan ZL, Bydon A. The clinical significance of pneumorachis: a case report and review of the literature. J Trauma 2010;68(3):736–744
3. Gopalakrishnan KC, el Masri WS. Fractures of the sternum associated with spinal injury. J Bone Joint Surg Br 1986;68(2):178–181
4. Hills MW, Delprado AM, Deane SA. Sternal fractures: associated injuries and management. J Trauma 1993;35(1): 55–60
5. Vioreanu MH, Quinlan JF, Robertson I, O'Byrne JM. Vertebral fractures and concomitant fractures of the sternum. Int Orthop 2005;29(6):339–342

CASE 100

■ Clinical Presentation

40-year-old man involved in an all-terrain vehicle (ATV) incident with a clinical concern of possible hemo-mediastinum and acute aortic injury

■ Radiologic Findings

Contrast-enhanced axial (**Fig. 100.1A**) and sagittal oblique (**Fig. 100.1B**) chest CTA (mediastinal window) demonstrates the typical location and appearance of an acute post-traumatic aortic pseudoaneurysm. The pseudoaneurysm projects from the anteromedial aorta at the LMSB and distal to the left subclavian artery. Note the peribranch vessel and para-aortic hemomediastinum.

■ Diagnosis

Acute Post-Traumatic Aortic Injury (ATAI) with Pseudoaneurysm

■ Differential Diagnosis

None

■ Discussion

Background

ATAI from blunt trauma is a substantial cause of morbidity and mortality, occurring in approximately 0.5–2% of all non-lethal motor vehicle collisions (MVCs) and 10–20% of all high-speed deceleration fatalities. MDCT has emerged as the definitive screening modality for both diagnosis and exclusion of ATAI and great vessel in-

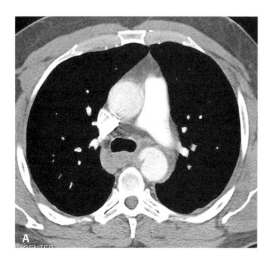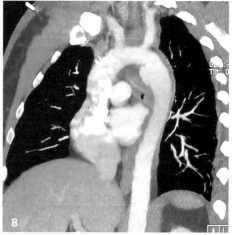

Fig. 100.1

jury without the need for conventional aortography or transesophageal echosonography. The latter are now typically only used in the infrequent setting of equivocal MDCT findings. In fact, the increased use of MDCT has led to the recognition of numerous vascular variants that may mimic acute injuries (see Case 101) as well as the diagnosis of more subtle vascular injuries, which heretofore likely went undiagnosed, often with little or no surrounding peribranch vessel or para-aortic hematoma. The increasing use of non-surgical therapies (e.g., blood pressure augmentation, endovascular stents) for both temporary and definitive management necessitates accurate localization and characterization of these otherwise lethal injuries. Thus, it is imperative that the radiologist specifically describe the:

- *Nature* of ATAI (e.g., pseudoaneurysm, intimal flap, dissection, luminal thrombosis, coarctation)
- *Diameter* of the aorta or affected branch vessel immediately proximal and distal to the injury
- *Length* of the injury along its vascular axis
- *Relationship* between the injury and the nearest arterial branch vessel
- *Congenital vascular variations* in anatomy (e.g., aberrant right subclavian artery, left vertebral artery originating off the aortic arch, right-sided aortic arch with aberrant left subclavian artery, vascular slings, etc.) and their relationship to the injury

ATAI may occur anywhere along the thoracic aorta:

- *Aortic isthmus*—within 2 cm of left subclavian artery origin: *most common* site
- *Aortic root and ascending aorta*—5–14% of autopsies with aortic injuries; rarely seen at MDCT presumably because of its lethal nature
- *Aortic arch and branch vessel*—less common. *Isolated branch vessel injuries* are more common than *aortic arch injuries* (<4% of blunt chest trauma victims), but may occur in combination with ATAI in 0–45% of patients. Brachiocephalic and common carotid arteries are the most commonly involved vessels (66–90%).
- *Mid and distal descending thoracic aorta*—1–12% of autopsies with aortic injuries. These injuries can be associated with diaphragm injury (10% cases) and adjacent thoracic spine compression fractures.
- *Minimal aortic injuries*—only affect the intima and are estimated to occur in 10% of patients with ATAI; encountered with increasing frequency. Nearly half of cases show no abnormality at conventional angiography.

Etiology

The exact mechanism of injury is not precisely known. Proposed mechanisms include shearing forces, rapid deceleration, hydrostatic forces, and the osseous pinch. Most ATAI (75–80%) results from violent deceleration, most commonly a high-speed MVC, especially head-on (50%) and lateral side-impact collisions (73%). Interestingly, various occupant restraint devices (excluding side airbags) are largely ineffective in curtailing ATAI in lateral side-impact collisions. Other potential causes include falls from height, pedestrian-automobile collisions, and crush injuries. Direct injury of the aorta may also occur due to penetration from rib and thoracic spine fractures. The nature and extent of ATAI vary widely, ranging from intimal hemorrhage to complete transection. Most injuries result from *transverse tears* and can be *segmental* (55%) or *circumferential* (45%). Tears may also be *partial* (65%) or *transmural* (35%). *Spiral* and *irregular tears* are rare. *Partial lacerations* involve the inner two walls of the aorta, resulting in a contained rupture. The adventitia may be injured in up to 40% of cases. These latter injuries are almost universally fatal because of rapid exsanguination.

Clinical Findings

Clinical signs and symptoms are nonspecific and insensitive for the diagnosis and exclusion of ATAI. Most patients have no clinical signs of aortic injury until they suddenly become hemodynamically unstable. Symptoms induced by stretching of the mediastinal connective tissues by hemomediastinum include interscapular pain, dyspnea, and hoarseness. Clinical signs of ATAI are absent in one-third of patients but when present include "pseudocoarctation syndrome" (i.e., upper extremity hypertension and lower extremity hypotension with diminished femoral pulses), external chest wall injuries, paraplegia, systolic murmur, and initial chest tube output >750 mL of blood.

There are, however, seven criteria that are useful predictors in the risk assessment of potential ATAI. The more criteria that are met, the greater the probability of ATAI (e.g., trauma patients with ≥4 criteria: 30% chance of an ATAI). These criteria include:

- Age >50 years
- Unrestrained vehicle occupant

- Systolic blood pressure <90 mm Hg
- Thoracic injury (e.g., rib fracture, pneumothorax, lung contusion, or laceration)
- Abdomino-pelvic injury requiring emergent laparotomy or with fractures of the lumbar spine and pelvis
- Long bone fractures (e.g., humerus, radius, ulna, femur, tibia, or fibula)
- Major head injury (e.g., skull fracture, intracranial hematoma, unconsciousness at time of evaluation, or intraparenchymal hemorrhage)

Imaging Findings

Chest Radiography

Primary Role

Exclusion of life-threatening injuries requiring immediate treatment (e.g., tension pneumothorax, large hemothorax, malpositioned life support devices)

Secondary Role

Indirect evidence of hemomediastinum and potential ATAI

- Abnormal aortic contour or poor definition of transverse aorta (**Fig. 100.2**)
- Superior mediastinal widening at transverse aorta level >8 cm (**Fig. 100.2**)
- Superior mediastinum ≥25% of the width of the thorax (**Fig. 100.2**)
- Opacification of aorticopulmonary window (**Fig. 100.2**)
- Rightward deviation of trachea and/or endotracheal tube (**Fig. 100.2**)
- Nasogastric tube deviation to the right of the T4 spinous process
- Thickened or poorly defined left paraspinal line
- Poor definition of descending thoracic aorta interface
- Widened right paratracheal stripe (>5 mm) (**Fig. 100.2**)
- Downward displacement of left mainstem bronchus >40° from the horizontal
- Left hemothorax and/or left apical cap
- Fractures of first and second ribs (**Fig. 100.2**)
- May be normal or deceptively underwhelming in up to 7% of proven ATAI cases
- Concomitant thoracic injuries not uncommon (e.g., pulmonary contusion, pneumothorax, hemothorax, diaphragmatic injury)

MDCT

CT imaging features of aortic and great vessel injury are categorized as *direct* or *indirect*. The *most specific direct signs* are intimal flap and luminal thrombus or debris (100%) whereas irregular aortic contour or pseudoaneurysm is the *most sensitive* (100%).

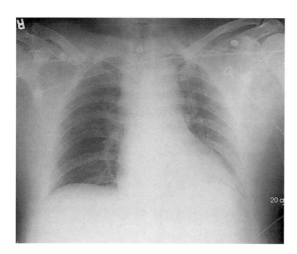

Fig. 100.2   AP trauma bay chest X-ray of a 40-year-old unrestrained driver involved in a high-speed MVC shows indirect evidence of hemomediastinum and potential ATAI, subsequently proven on MDCT. There is poor delineation of the aortic arch and opacification of the aorticopulmonary window. The superior mediastinum is widened with rightward tracheal displacement. The right paratracheal stripe is thickened. Note the displaced right clavicle fracture, fractures of bilateral first and second ribs, and additional left-sided ribs.

Direct Signs

- Pseudoaneurysm
  - Well-defined rounded bulge with irregular margins arising from anterior or anteromedial aspect of proximal descending thoracic aorta at LMSB and proximal LPA level (**Figs. 100.1A, 100.1B, 100.3, 100.4, 100.5**)
  - May involve entire circumference of aorta and may extend several centimeters in length (often better appreciated on sagittal and oblique MIP images) (**Fig. 100.3**)
  - Linear intimal flaps invariably project across the base of the traumatic pseudoaneurysm (**Figs. 100.4, 100.5**)
- Intraluminal flap
  - Torn flap of intima projecting into lumen of injured aorta (**Fig. 100.5**)
- Focal contour abnormality
  - Acute injuries can be characterized by abrupt alteration in luminal diameter or as an irregular change in shape or contour of the aorta (**Figs. 100.6, 100.7A**)
  - Contour variations more often appreciated on sagittal, coronal, and sagittal oblique MIP images
  - Aside from mild narrowing normally occurring at the isthmus, the luminal diameter of normal aorta changes very little from the LSCA take-off through the upper abdomen
- Abrupt aortic caliber change (**Figs. 100.3, 100.4, 100.5, 100.7A**)
- Coarctation
  - Aorta distal to site of injury is unusually small in caliber (**Figs. 100.7A, 100.7B**)
- Intraluminal thrombus or debris on the lacerated aortic wall
  - Thrombus may form along intimal flaps (**Fig. 100.8**), which can subsequently embolize to solid and hollow visceral organs and distal arteries of the extremities, resulting in altered perfusion and infarction
- Active contrast extravasation from injured aorta
  - Severely injured aorta, significant hemomediastinum (**Fig. 100.9**)
  - Rarely seen; affected patients rarely survive

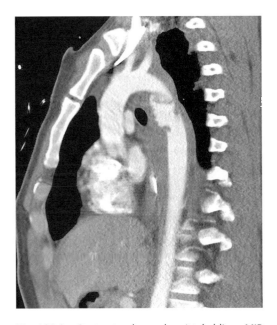

Fig. 100.3 Contrast-enhanced sagittal oblique MIP chest CT (mediastinal window) of a 30-year-old man involved in a high-speed MVC shows a severe ATAI involving the entire circumference of the aorta and extending several centimeters in length. Note the extensive mediastinal hemorrhage.

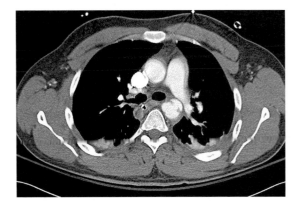

Fig. 100.4 Contrast-enhanced axial chest CT (mediastinal window) of a 28-year-old man involved in a motorcycle collision reveals a post-traumatic pseudoaneurysm of the anteromedial proximal descending thoracic aorta at the LMSB and proximal LPA level. A dominant linear intimal flap projects across the base of the traumatic pseudoaneurysm.

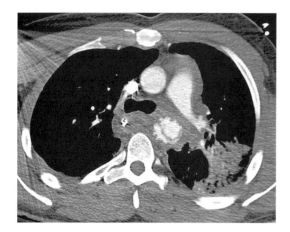

Fig. 100.5 Contrast-enhanced axial CT (mediastinal window) of a 40-year-old man involved in an ATV incident with ATAI characterized by gross irregularity in the descending aorta and an intimal flap extending from 3:00 to 11:00. Note the concomitant mediastinal hemorrhage and left upper lobe pulmonary contusion.

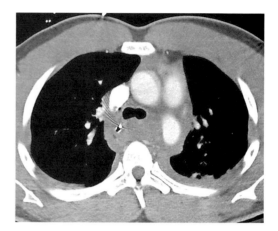

Fig. 100.6 Contrast-enhanced axial CT (mediastinal window) of a 41-year-old man involved in a MVC with ATAI manifesting as a contour abnormality in the absence of pseudoaneurysm or intimal flap. Note effacement of the medial wall of the descending aorta at the LMSB level. Also note rightward displacement of the nasogastric tube by hemomediastinum and the left hemothorax.

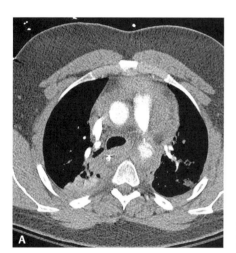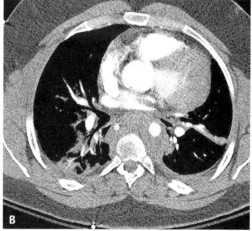

Fig. 100.7   MDCT of a 27-year-old man involved in a motorcycle collision with ATAI characterized by coarctation distal to the injury. **(A)** Contrast-enhanced axial CT (mediastinal window) shows a severe injury with an anteriorly projected pseudoaneurysm and intimal flap. The residual aortic lumen is small, compressed by the pseudoaneurysm. **(B)** Contrast-enhanced axial (mediastinal window) CT acquired several centimeters distal to the aortic injury shows a small-caliber descending aorta lumen relative to the ascending aorta at the same level. Peri-aortic hematoma is present.

Indirect Signs

- Typically accompany *direct signs* but may occur in isolation
- Subtle contour anomalies
- Hemomediastinum
- Peribranch vessel and/or peri-aortic blood (**Figs. 100.1A, 100.1B, 100.10A, 100.10B**)

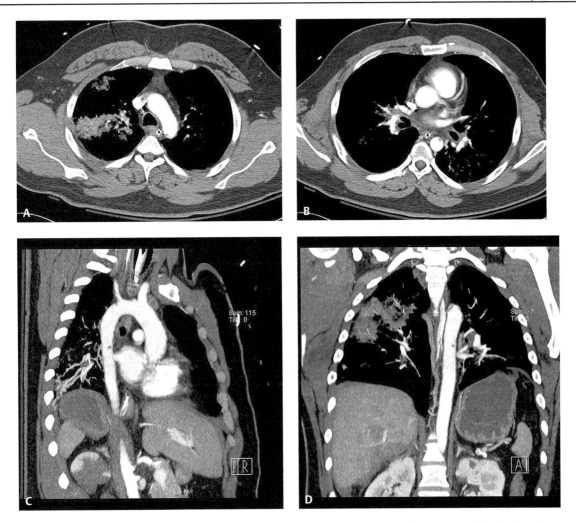

Fig. 100.8   Contrast-enhanced MDCT of a 30-year-old unrestrained man involved in a MVC with vehicular ejection and ATAI manifest by intraluminal thrombus and debris. Axial CT images at the arch **(A)** and left lower lobe bronchus **(B)** show non-contiguous foci of luminal thrombus. These foci are readily seen on the MIP sagittal oblique **(C)** and coronal **(D)** images. He was managed conservatively but experienced systemic embolization of thrombi to his kidneys and lower extremities.

MRI

- Utility in trauma patients limited
- May have a role in:
  - Further characterizing *minimal intimal injuries* or *equivocal MDCT* results
  - Follow-up studies when delayed definitive intervention is contemplated
- Evaluate for same *direct* and *indirect signs* seen on MDCT

Transcatheter Aortography

Sensitivity approaches 100%; specificity >98%; accuracy >99%

- Intimal irregularity or intraluminal filling defect
- Contrast projected outside projected aortic or branch vessel lumen (i.e., pseudoaneurysm) (**Figs. 100.11A, 100.11B**)
- Atypical or equivocal findings (1–5%)

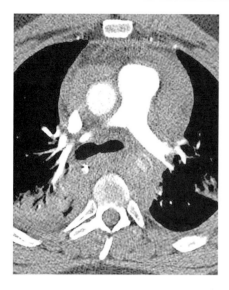

Fig. 100.9 Contrast-enhanced axial CT (mediastinal window) of a young man involved in a skydiving accident with completely transected aorta demonstrates near complete absence of opacification of the aorta at the site of injury. An amorphous blush of contrast media is seen extravasating from the transected aorta. Note the hemomediastinum. Blood is also intimately related to the ascending aorta. Bilateral pulmonary contusions are present. The patient did not survive.

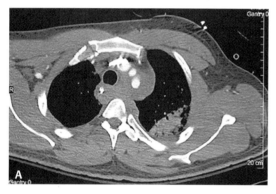
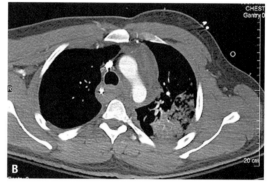

Fig. 100.10 Contrast-enhanced chest CT (mediastinal window) of a young man involved in a MVC reveals significant peribranch vessel **(A)** and para-aortic **(B)** blood and left lung contusion. Close inspection of the aorta and branch vessels in multiple planes revealed no direct signs of injury. He was managed conservatively. Follow-up MDCT (not illustrated) at two weeks and six weeks revealed gradual resorption of mediastinal blood and no evidence of vascular injury.

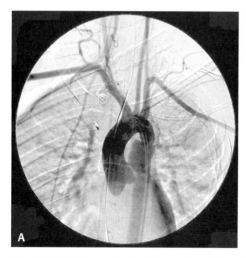
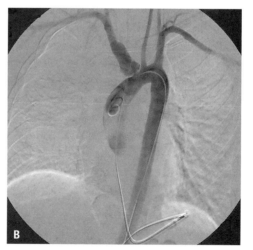

Fig. 100.11 Transcatheter left anterior oblique (LAO) **(A)** aortogram of the aortic arch of a young blunt trauma victim shows gross irregularity of the aortic lumen and a large post-traumatic pseudoaneurysm at the isthmus. Transcatheter aortogram **(B)** of a young woman involved in a MVC reveals a traumatic injury at the brachiocephalic artery origin with extension into the right subclavian artery. Note the large irregular-appearing pseudoaneurysm of the brachiocephalic artery.

- Anatomic variants (e.g., ductus diverticulum; aortic spindle; third intercostal or bronchial artery infundibulum)
- Atheromatous plaque
- Artifacts (e.g., respiratory motion; digital subtraction; mixing of contrast)

Intravascular Ultrasound (IVUS)

- Useful adjunctive modality
- High-resolution cross-sectional images of vessel wall and surrounding tissues
- Vessel wall disruption
- Intimal flap
- Focal pseudoaneurysm
- Intramural and para-aortic hematoma
- Complete transection
- Operator- and experience-dependent invasive procedure, requires arterial puncture, complete evaluation of thoracic aorta is time-consuming; incomplete visualization of brachiocephalic artery

Transesophageal Echosonography (TEE)

Sensitivity 56–99%; specificity 89–99%

- Limited role in routine screening for ATAI
- Should not be performed in lieu of evaluation for other, co-morbid injuries
- Possible adjunctive modality in equivocal MDCT cases or unstable patients
- Performed quickly at bedside or in operating room
- Aortic valve, sinotubular junction, and ascending aorta often better evaluated than with MDCT (exception: cardiac-gated studies)
- Evaluate myocardium for wall motion abnormalities; pericardial sac for fluid
- Poor visualization of distal ascending aorta and proximal arch

Management

Open Thoracotomy

- Left posterolateral thoracotomy made at the fourth or fifth intercostal space
- Appropriate location of proximal clamp placement to avoid clamping across the injury has been greatly aided by use of 2-D and 3-D reformations
- Injured segment is resected; Dacron graft placed
- Postoperative paraplegia: 10%
- Mortality rate: 15–50%
- "Clamp and sew" technique
  - Postoperative paraplegia: 16–29%
  - Hospital mortality rate: 19%
- Distal perfusion adjuncts with left heart/cardiopulmonary bypass
  - Postoperative paraplegia: 3%

Endovascular Stent-Graft Repair

- Prevents further rupture by excluding injured aorta from systemic blood pressure
- May be performed in acute setting even in patients with multisystem organ injuries
- Obviates open repair, single lung ventilation, aortic cross-clamping, cardiopulmonary bypass, systemic anticoagulation
- Procedural planning with MDCT critical for technical success (i.e., complete exclusion of vascular injury); sagittal oblique MIP or curved reformatted images are the most beneficial (**Figs. 100.12A, 100.12B**)
- Short-term complications include stroke, puncture-site bleeding, device collapse, and recurrent laryngeal nerve damage
- Morbidity: 0–20%
- Limitation: Lack of small-caliber devices for use in young patients or those with small-diameter aorta

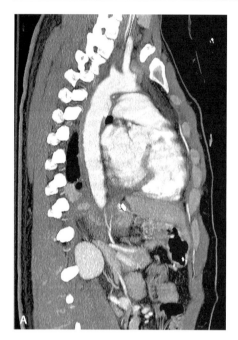 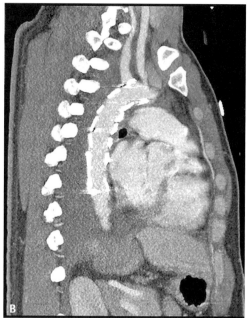

Fig. 100.12 Pre-endovascular stent-graft repair contrast-enhanced sagittal oblique MDCT (mediastinal window) **(A)** shows a typical ATAI. Post-procedural contrast-enhanced sagittal oblique MDCT (mediastinal window) **(B)** reveals a technically successful graft deployment appropriately excluding the injury from the systemic circulation and no evidence of endoleak.

Prognosis

- ATAI: high mortality rate; immediately fatal in 80–90% of cases
- Parmley et al. classic series
  - Only 20% of patients initially survived >1 hour
  - Of those survivors with undetected and untreated ATAI
    - 30% die within the first 6 hours
    - 49% die within the first 24 hours
    - 72% die by 8 days
    - 90% die by 4 months
- Williams et al. series
  - 94% mortality within 1 hour
  - 99% mortality at 24 hours if untreated
- Substantial increase in mortality following ATAI in patients with concomitant injuries of the head, chest, and abdomen
- Prompt recognition and treatment are critical for long-term survival. If detected in a timely manner, 60–80% of patients with ATAI reaching the hospital alive will survive following definitive therapy.
- Unsuspected chronic traumatic aortic pseudoaneurysm
  - Only 2% of patients with unrecognized and untreated ATAI survive long enough to form a chronic pseudoaneurysm
  - Affected patients may be asymptomatic, although 42% will develop signs or symptoms within 5 years and 85% do so within 20 years (e.g., chest pain, hoarseness, dyspnea, dysphagia, systolic murmur)
  - Chronic traumatic aortic pseudoaneurysms are at risk for rupture
  - Minimally invasive endovascular stents have recently become recognized as an effective treatment option for chronic post-traumatic pseudoaneurysms with markedly reduced morbidity and mortality
  - On imaging, a chronic post-traumatic pseudoaneurysm presents as a well-defined, often partially calcified pseudoaneurysm, located in the descending aorta at the LMSB and proximal left pulmonary artery level. Acute mediastinal hemorrhage is absent (**Fig. 100.13**).

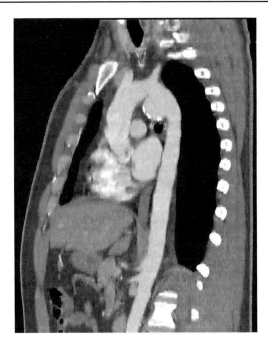

Fig. 100.13 Contrast-enhanced sagittal oblique MDCT (mediastinal window) of a 48-year-old man with complaints of non-specific chest pain reveals a chronic post-traumatic pseudoaneurysm of the thoracic aorta. Note the well-defined, partially calcified pseudoaneurysm located just distal to the left subclavian artery origin. No mediastinal hematoma is present. He had been involved in a severe boating accident with a prolonged hospitalization 20 years earlier.

PEARLS

- Lateral side-impact collisions are associated with higher mortality rates than head-on collisions, regardless of the injury severity score.
- Chest radiography may be normal or deceptively underwhelming in 7% of proven ATAI cases. In the setting of rapid deceleration force or high clinical suspicion, cross-sectional imaging is warranted regardless of radiographic findings.
- Even the "minimally" abnormal trauma bay supine chest radiograph requires further imaging. If the risk of ATAI is low based on the mechanism of injury, this can be done with an upright chest radiograph (PA view preferable). The most important radiographic observation is a well-defined aortic arch, not the absence of mediastinal widening. If the arch is not well defined, the radiograph is "abnormal" and cross-sectional imaging is indicated.
- Although most ATAIs occur at the LMSB and proximal left pulmonary artery level, radiologists should evaluate the aorta and its branch vessels in their entirety. Up to 10% of acute injuries occur elsewhere in the thoracic and proximal abdominal aorta. Additionally, non-contiguous injuries of the aorta may also occur.
- Injuries to the aortic root may occur in isolation or co-exist with injuries at the isthmus and are often associated with hemopericardium.
- Hemopericardium is an inconsistent finding in ascending aortic injuries; its absence should not be used to exclude ascending aortic injury. ECG-gated MDCT may be beneficial if the integrity of the ascending aorta is equivocal on routine MDCT.
- Little data exist on the optimal management of minimal aortic injuries; some suggest these injuries may not need intervention, and that the majority remain stable or resolve.
- Transcatheter angiography is of limited value for clarifying equivocal or *indirect* MDCT findings
- Although most ATAI are associated with mediastinal hemorrhage, subtle injuries may occur with little or no hemomediastinum. When present, hemomediastinum is most often due to bleeding from small veins and arteries, or from cervicothoracic spinal or sternal fractures and does not arise directly from injury to the aorta.
- Not infrequently, mediastinal blood dissects along the descending thoracic aorta to the diaphragm and may present as a retrocrural hematoma on abdominal CT scans. Retrocrural hematoma on trauma abdominal CT in the absence of neighboring spine trauma implies an ATAI until proven otherwise and mandates emergent imaging of the thoracic aorta to exclude such.

Suggested Reading

1. Andrassy J, Weidenhagen R, Meimarakis G, Lauterjung L, Jauch KW, Kopp R. Stent versus open surgery for acute and chronic traumatic injury of the thoracic aorta: a single-center experience. J Trauma 2006;60(4):765–771, discussion 771–772

2. Creasy JD, Chiles C, Routh WD, Dyer RB. Overview of traumatic injury of the thoracic aorta. Radiographics 1997; 17(1):27–45

3. Fishman JE, Nuñez D Jr, Kane A, Rivas LA, Jacobs WE. Direct versus indirect signs of traumatic aortic injury revealed by helical CT: performance characteristics and interobserver agreement. AJR Am J Roentgenol 1999;172(4): 1027–1031

4. Malhotra AK, Fabian TC, Croce MA, Weiman DS, Gavant ML, Pate JW. Minimal aortic injury: a lesion associated with advancing diagnostic techniques. J Trauma 2001;51(6):1042–1048

5. Parmley LF, Mattingly TW, Manion WC, Jahnke EJ Jr. Nonpenetrating traumatic injury of the aorta. Circulation 1958;17(6):1086–1101

6. Steenburg SD, Ravenel JG, Ikonomidis JS, Schönholz C, Reeves S. Acute traumatic aortic injury: imaging evaluation and management. Radiology 2008;248(3):748–762

7. Williams JS, Graff JA, Uku JM, Steinig JP. Aortic injury in vehicular trauma. Ann Thorac Surg 1994;57(3):726–730

8. Wong H, Gotway MB, Sasson AD, Jeffrey RB. Periaortic hematoma at diaphragmatic crura at helical CT: sign of blunt aortic injury in patients with mediastinal hematoma. Radiology 2004;231(1):185–189

CASE 101

■ Clinical Presentation

46-year-old man involved in a MVC with a clinical concern of hemomediastinum and potential acute traumatic aortic injury

■ Radiologic Findings

Contrast-enhanced sagittal oblique MIP CT (mediastinal window) (**Fig. 101.1**) demonstrates a focal convex bulge in the aortic isthmus consistent with a *Type III* ductus diverticulum. Note the smooth contour and obtuse margin formed with the aortic lumen and the absence of an intimal flap and hemomediastinum.

■ Diagnosis

Type III Ductus Diverticulum

■ Differential Diagnosis

None

■ Discussion

Background

The increased use of MDCT has led to the recognition of numerous vascular variants that may mimic acute aortic injuries. The most common variants include typical ductus diverticulum, atypical ductus diverticulum, aortic spindle, and branch vessel infundibula.

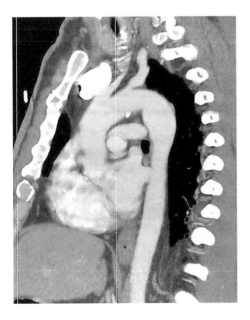

Fig. 101.1

Ductus diverticulum is a remnant of either the ductus arteriosum or the right dorsal aortic root. The most common diagnostic challenge for radiologists on trauma chest CTAs is differentiation of a post-traumatic aortic isthmus pseudoaneurysm from a normal *Type III* ductus diverticulum. Both aortic entities occur in roughly the same anatomic location, often leading to diagnostic confusion. There are four distinct variations in the contour of the aortic isthmus as follows:

Type I—concave contour

Type II—mild straightening or convexity without a discrete bulge

Type III—discrete focal bulge referred to as the ductus diverticulum (**Fig. 101.1**)

Atypical ductus diverticulum—often causes even more diagnostic confusion; characterized superiorly by a shorter, steeper slope and inferiorly by a more typical, gentler slope (**Fig. 101.2**)

Aortic spindle manifests as fusiform dilatation of the aorta immediately distal to the isthmus (i.e., region between the left subclavian artery origin and point of attachment of the ligamentum arteriosum) (**Fig. 101.3**).

Infundibula of the aortic *branch vessels*, including the brachiocephalic artery, bronchial artery, intercostal arteries (i.e., most commonly the right third), left common carotid, and left subclavian arteries, may simulate acute traumatic injuries or pseudoaneurysms. Infundibula are recognized by their triangular anatomic morphology, smooth margins, and the presence of a vessel emanating from their apex (**Fig. 101.4**).

Imaging Features

MDCT/MRI

Type III Ductus Diverticulum

- Best appreciated on sagittal and sagittal oblique MIP CT images (**Fig. 101.1**)

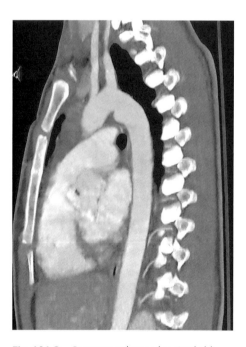

Fig. 101.2 Contrast-enhanced sagittal oblique MIP CT (mediastinal window) of 27-year-old man involved in a MVC shows an *atypical ductus diverticulum*. This focal convex bulge in the aortic isthmus shows a shorter, steeper slope superiorly and a gentler-appearing slope inferiorly. Margins appear smooth and uninterrupted. No mediastinal hemorrhage is present.

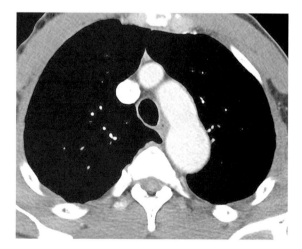

Fig. 101.3 Contrast-enhanced axial CT (mediastinal window) of a 26-year-old man involved in a MVC demonstrates an aortic spindle. Note the characteristic mild, fusiform enlargement of the distal aortic arch and the absence of hemomediastinum.

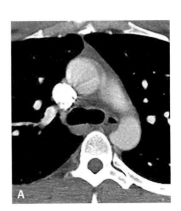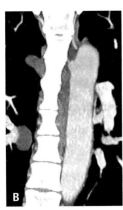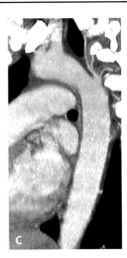

Fig. 101.4 Contrast-enhanced axial **(A)**, coronal MIP **(B)**, and sagittal oblique **(C)** (mediastinal window) CT of a young man involved in a MVC reveals the typical appearance of a prominent right third intercostal-bronchial artery infundibulum. The triangular morphology and smooth anatomic margins and the presence of a vessel emanating from its apex differentiate this normal anatomic structure from an acute injury.

- Focal convex bulge; smooth contour; obtuse angle with aortic lumen (**Fig. 101.1**).
- Intimal flaps and hemomediastinum not present (**Fig. 101.1**)
- In contrast, post-traumatic pseudoaneurysm manifests as an irregular out-pouching from aortic lumen, displaying more acute margins. Intimal flaps and mediastinal hemorrhage are usually present (**Figs. 100.1, 100.3, 100.4, 100.5, 100.7**).
  - On axial CT images, *ductus diverticulum* demonstrates a smooth transition between contiguous slices, whereas *post-traumatic pseudoaneurysm* is variable in shape with sharp and more irregular margins

Atypical Ductus Diverticulum

- Shorter, steeper slope superiorly, and more typical, gentler slope inferiorly
- Smooth uninterrupted margins aid in differentiation from true post-traumatic aortic pseudoaneurysm (**Fig. 101.2**)

Aortic Spindle

- Fusiform dilatation of aorta immediately distal to isthmus (**Fig. 101.3**)
- Mild, fusiform enlargement of distal aortic arch (**Fig. 101.3**)
- MPR/MIP images acquired along the vascular axis are helpful supplements; reveal normal caliber aortic arch and proximal descending thoracic aorta

Branch Vessel Infundibula

- Recognized by triangular or conical anatomic morphology (**Fig. 101.4A**)
- Smooth margins (**Fig. 101.4A**)
- Presence of a vessel emanating from their apex (**Fig. 101.4C**)
- MIP/3-D reformations-useful confirmatory images; delineate origin and course of the vessel related to the infundibulum (**Fig. 101.4B, 101.4C**)

Management

- Represent anatomic variations in normal anatomy, no management indicated

Prognosis

- Not applicable

PEARLS

- Radiologists must be mindful of normal anatomic variants that may simulate acute aortic injury.

Suggested Reading

1. Goodman PC, Jeffrey RB, Minagi H, Federle MP, Thomas AN. Angiographic evaluation of the ductus diverticulum. Cardiovasc Intervent Radiol 1982;5(1):1–4
2. Grollman JH. The aortic diverticulum: a remnant of the partially involuted dorsal aortic root. Cardiovasc Intervent Radiol 1989;12(1):14–17
3. Macura KJ, Corl FM, Fishman EK, Bluemke DA. Pathogenesis in acute aortic syndromes: aortic aneurysm leak and rupture and traumatic aortic transection. AJR Am J Roentgenol 2003;181(2):303–307

CASE 102

■ Clinical Presentation

84-year-old woman trapped in a house fire two and a half weeks earlier with burns over 30% of total body surface area, ongoing hypoxia, and inability to be weaned from ventilator support

■ Radiologic Findings

AP chest exam (**Fig. 102.1A**) shows heterogeneous, multi-focal, primarily peripheral, patchy air space opacities and consolidations throughout both lungs. A mid-line tracheostomy and left upper extremity PICC are seen. Sequential unenhanced CT images through the upper, mid, and lower lung zones (lung window) (**Figs. 102.1B, 102.1C, 102.1D, 102.1E, 102.1F**) demonstrate patchy, multi-focal ground glass opacities and areas of crazy paving in non-dependent lung, areas of more frank consolidation in dependent lung, and intervening areas of normal lung. Bronchial and bronchiolar dilatation is seen in some foci of affected lung. Note the dependent layering bilateral pleural effusions.

■ Diagnosis

Diffuse Alveolar Damage (DAD) with Acute Respiratory Distress Syndrome (ARDS)

■ Differential Diagnosis

- Aspiration Pneumonia
- Various Heath Care–Related or Ventilator-Acquired Pneumonias
- Other Causes of Non-Cardiogenic Pulmonary Edema
- Diffuse Alveolar Hemorrhage

■ Discussion

Background

Diffuse alveolar damage (DAD) is a form of acute lung injury that progresses through two and sometimes three phases. The *exudative (acute) phase* occurs during the first week after the onset of lung injury and is characterized by damage to type 1 pneumocytes and endothelial cells with exudation of plasma proteins into the alveolar interstitium and spaces. The *proliferative (organizing) phase* begins at the end of the first week after lung injury, during which time the inflammatory exudate organizes and there is extensive proliferation of type 2 pneumocytes and fibroblasts. The *fibrotic (chronic) phase* develops in patients who survive three to four weeks on a ventilator and is characterized by extensive lung remodeling by dense fibrous tissue. The clinical syndrome associated with DAD histology is the *acute respiratory distress syndrome (ARDS)*.

Etiology

ARDS is associated with a wide array of precipitating clinical events (**Table 102.1**). More than 60 possible causes of ARDS have been identified and the list continues to grow. The *most common risk factor* for ARDS is sepsis. The *most common* direct lung injury associated with ARDS is aspiration of gastric contents. Several

495

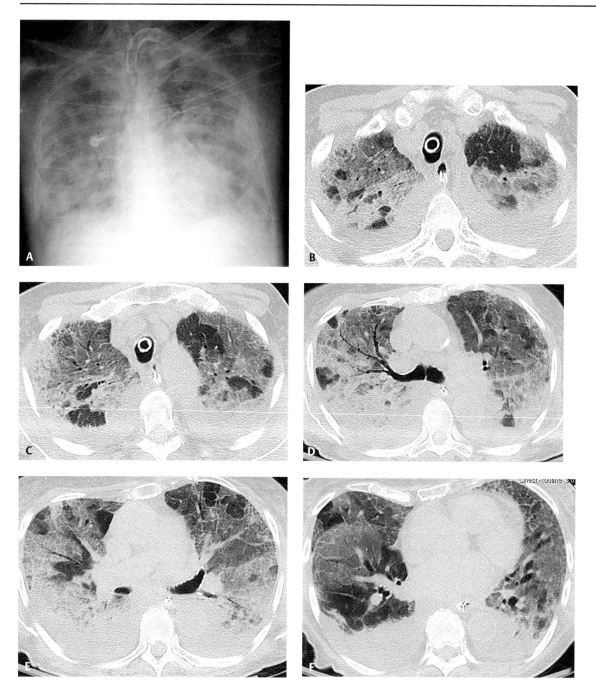

Fig. 102.1

factors increase the risk of ARDS after an inciting event: advanced age, female sex (only in trauma patients), cigarette smoking, and alcohol use. For any underlying precipitant, increasingly severe illness as predicted by a severity scoring system (e.g., Acute Physiology and Chronic Health Evaluation [(APACHE)] increases the risk of ARDS.

Clinical Findings

A prospective study performed in King County, Washington, from April 1999 through July 2000 found the age-adjusted incidence of ARDS was 86.2 per 100,000 person-years. The same study found the incidence increased with age, reaching 306 per 100,000 person-years for patients aged 75–84 years. Based on these sta-

Table 102.1 Potential Clinical Precipitants of ARDS

Infection	Trauma	Drugs	Metabolic Disturbances	Other
Severe bacterial pneumonia	Lung contusion	Amiodarone	Pancreatitis	Aspiration gastric contents
Bacteremia	Head trauma	Azathioprine	Uremia	Burns
PCP	Non-thoracic trauma	Bleomycin		Idiopathic (AIP)
Viral pneumonia	Fat emboli syndrome	Busulfan		Inhalation injury
Fungal pneumonia		Cocaine		Massive transfusion
		Cyclophosphamide		Near drowning
		Methotrexate		Shock
		Nitrofurantoin		Toxic shock syndrome
		Pencillamine		
		Vinblastine		

tistics, it is estimated that 190,600 cases occur in the United States annually, associated with 74,500 deaths. The onset of ARDS is rapid, usually occurring within 24–48 hours of the precipitating event. The first clinical symptoms are tachypnea and dyspnea, which coincide with hypoxemia (refractory to supplemental oxygen) and decreased PaO_2. Respiratory failure and non-cardiogenic pulmonary edema ensue. The North American–European Consensus Conference definition of ARDS includes acute onset of illness, bilateral air space opacities on chest radiography, PaO_2/FIO_2 (fraction of inspired oxygen) ratio <200, PACW*p* <18 mm Hg, and no clinical evidence of left heart failure.

Imaging Findings

Chest Radiography

First 12–24 Hours from Clinical Onset of Respiratory Failure

- Decreased lung volume
- Otherwise normal unless concomitant aspiration or pneumonia

After 12–24 Hours from Clinical Onset of Respiratory Failure

- Patchy air space consolidation; rapidly becomes confluent and diffuse (**Fig. 102.1A**)
- Consolidation more severe in peripheral lung (**Fig. 102.1A**)
- Small intervening regions of normal lung (**Fig. 102.1A**)
- Air bronchograms; frequent (**Fig. 102.1A**)
- Septal lines and pleural effusions; uncommon

5–7 days on Mechanical Ventilation

- Gradual replacement of consolidated lung by less dense, ground glass disease
- Small rounded areas of lucency or thin-walled cystic air spaces (barotrauma)

2–3 weeks on Mechanical Ventilation

- Reticular opacities from fibrosis become apparent

MDCT

- Patchy areas of ground glass opacity, crazy paving; and frank consolidation (**Figs. 102.1B, 102.1C, 102.1D, 102.1E, 102.1F**)

- Usually most marked in dependent lung zones (**Fig. 102.1B, 102.1C, 102.1D, 102.1E, 102.1F**)
- Foci of bronchial and bronchiolar dilation or bronchiectasis in affected lung (**Fig. 102.1B, 102.1C, 102.1D, 102.1E, 102.1F**)
- Intervening areas of uninvolved lung (**Fig. 102.1B, 102.1C, 102.1D, 102.1E, 102.1F**)
- Small unilateral or bilateral pleural effusions (<50%) (**Fig. 102.1B, 102.1C, 102.1D, 102.1E, 102.1F**)

Management

- Supportive therapy directed at maintaining adequate tissue oxygenation and perfusion; treating hemodynamic instability; minimizing risk of ventilator-associated lung injury; avoiding infectious complications
- Non-invasive ventilation
  - Full face mask attached to ventilator delivering continuous positive airway pressure (CPAP) with or without ventilator breaths or inspiratory pressure support (i.e., noninvasive positive-pressure ventilation [NIPPV]) in patients with less severe ARDS may be beneficial
- Mechanical ventilation
  - Maintain oxygen saturations (85–90%) while avoiding oxygen toxicity and complications of mechanical ventilation
  - May promote development of acute lung injury
- Prone positioning
  - 60–75% patients—significantly improved oxygenation when placed prone (e.g., recruitment-dependent lung zones, increased functional residual capacity, improved diaphragmatic excursion, improved ventilation-perfusion matching, increased cardiac output)
  - Improvement in oxygenation is rapid
  - May allow reductions in FIO_2 or level of CPAP
  - No survival benefit exists

Prognosis

- Mortality rate 50%; most deaths due to sepsis or multisystem organ failure
- Radiographic abnormalities generally begin to improve over 10–14 days in those patients who survive; more protracted course not uncommon
- Patient survivors; radiographic abnormalities may completely resolve and normal lung function recovered; alternatively may develop pulmonary fibrosis

PEARLS

- Correlation between radiographic findings and severity of hypoxemia is highly variable.

Suggested Reading

1. Bernard GR, Artigas A, Brigham KL, et al. The American-European Consensus Conference on ARDS. Definitions, mechanisms, relevant outcomes, and clinical trial coordination. Am J Respir Crit Care Med 1994;149(3 Pt 1):818–824

2. Gattinoni L, Pelosi P, Suter PM, Pedoto A, Vercesi P, Lissoni A. Acute respiratory distress syndrome caused by pulmonary and extrapulmonary disease. Different syndromes? Am J Respir Crit Care Med 1998;158(1):3–11

3. Rubenfeld GD, Caldwell E, Peabody E, et al. Incidence and outcomes of acute lung injury. N Engl J Med 2005;353(16): 1685–1693

4. Travis WD, Colby TV, Koss MN, Rosado-de-Christenson ML, Müller NL, King TE. Diffuse parenchymal lung diseases. In: Atlas of Nontumor Pathology: Non-Neoplastic Disorders of the Lower Respiratory Tract. Washington, DC: Armed Forces Institute of Pathology; 2001;89–101

CASE 103

■ Clinical Presentation

86-year-old man with new onset of dyspnea and non-productive cough developing five days following vertebroplasty of a symptomatic L1-L2 compression fracture. Respiratory failure developed over the following several days.

■ Radiologic Findings

PA (**Fig. 103.1A**) and lateral (**Fig. 103.1B**) chest radiographs demonstrate diffuse ground glass and reticular opacities throughout the right lung with associated volume loss. Unenhanced chest CT through the upper (**Figs. 103.1C, 103.1D**), mid (**Fig. 103.1E**), and lower (**Fig. 103.1F**) lung zones (lung window) reveal a diffuse "crazy-paving" pattern throughout the right lung with some foci of intervening normal lung. Mild bronchial and bronchiolar dilatation is seen in the affected lung. Subtle foci of ground glass and reticular opacities are present in the peripheral left lung. Unenhanced CT (mediastinal window) through the mid-thorax (**Fig. 103.1G**) and upper abdomen (**Fig. 103.1H, 103.1I**) shows high-attenuation polymethylmethacrylate in the anteromedial basal and lateral basal arterial divisions of the left lower lobe (**Fig. 103.1F**) and also emanating out from the L1 vertebroplasty site, with linear tracts extending into the paravertebral and extradural venous plexus into the right renal vein (**Figs. 103.1H, 103.1I**).

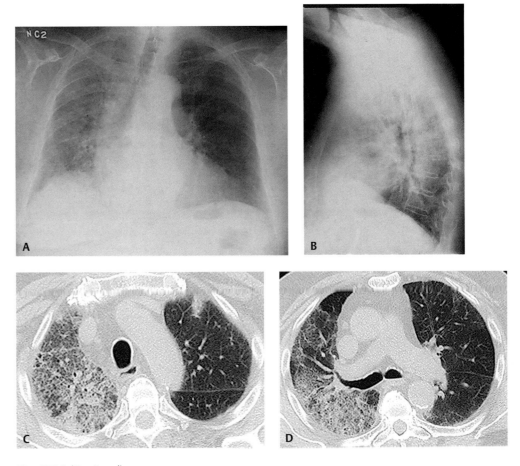

Fig. 103.1 (Continued)

499

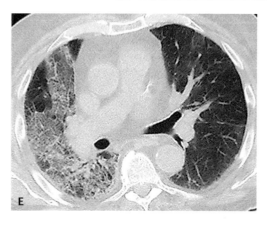
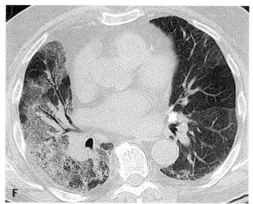
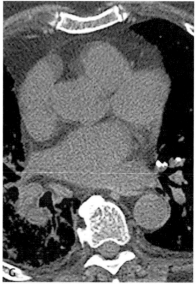
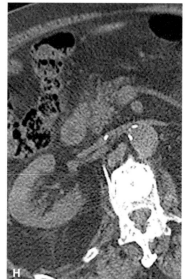
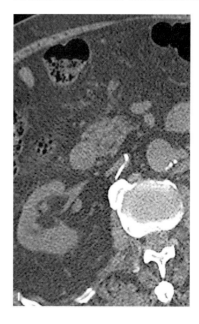

Fig. 103.1 *(Continued)*

■ Diagnosis

Fat Emboli Syndrome Complicated by ARDS Following Vertebroplasty

■ Differential Diagnosis

- Acute Interstitial Pneumonia (AIP)/Acute Respiratory Distress Syndrome (ARDS)
- Infection
  - ∘ Various bacteria
  - ∘ *Mycoplasma*
  - ∘ PCP/CMV
- Non-Cardiogenic Pulmonary Edema
- Diffuse Alveolar Hemorrhage
- Eosinophilic Pneumonia
- Alveolar Proteinosis
- Adenocarcinoma in-situ (formerly known as Bronchioloalveolar Cell Carcinoma [BAC])

■ Discussion

Background

Vertebroplasty is a percutaneous image-guided procedure in which polymethylmethacrylate (PMMA) bone cement is injected into a compression fracture sequela of osteoporosis or neoplastic disease. The procedure successfully strengthens and stabilizes the affected vertebral body, alleviates pain, and prevents further collapse. However, the vertebral body is highly vascularized, and because the intraosseous vertebral veins freely communicate via a valveless paravertebral and extradural venous plexus, leakage of cement into the circulation frequently occurs. This same phenomenon explains the presence of "paradoxical" metastasis (e.g., breast and prostate cancer) with no direct line of spread. Adverse consequences of vertebroplasty may include (1) release of chemical microemboli that activate the inflammatory cascade, increasing vascular permeability and ARDS (**Figs. 103.1C, 103.1D, 103.1E, 103.1F**); (2) chemical macroemboli with cement thromboemboli (**Figs. 103.1G, 103.1H, 103.1I, 103.2A, 103.2B, 103.2C**); and (3) fat emboli syndrome—vertebral body fat mobilized and embolized to the pulmonary circulation during injection of the bone cement, causing a chemical pneumonitis (**Figs. 103.1A, 103.1B, 103.1C, 103.1D, 103.1E, 103.1F, 103.1G, 103.1H, 103.1I**).

   Fat emboli occur when fat enters the circulation following trauma (e.g., long bone or pelvic trauma), surgery (e.g., intramedullary nailing of long bone fractures; liposuction) or childbirth. Most affected patients have mild or no symptoms and the chest X-ray is often normal. *Fat emboli syndrome* (FES) is distinct from the presence of fat emboli and is characterized by various clinical signs and symptoms and may be complicated by respiratory distress, respiratory failure, ARDS, and death.

Etiology

In addition to the clinical scenarios outlined above, FES has been described following total joint arthroplasty, external cardiac massage, spontaneous vertebral body compression fractures, and bone biopsy, and with acute sickle cell crisis.

Clinical Findings

Symptoms usually occur one to three days after the injury and may include hypoxia (96%); mental status changes (59%); petechial skin rash (33%); fever with temperature higher than 39°C (70%); tachycardia (heart rate >120 beats per minute) (93%); thrombocytopenia (platelet count <150 × 10⁹/L) (37%); and unexplained anemia (67%). Only the petechial skin rash was absent in this particular patient. However, both the BAL fluid and urine analysis were markedly positive for lipid-laden macrophages. A contrast-enhanced CT for pulmonary embolism performed two days later revealed extensive pulmonary emboli throughout the left lung. It was postulated the pulmonary emboli may have "protected" the left lung from sequelae of the fat and MMPA cement emboli and resultant ARDS.

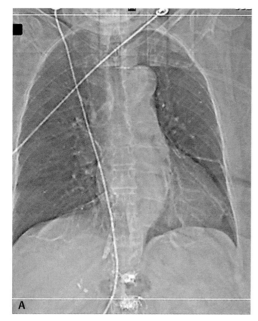

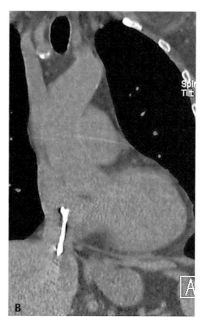

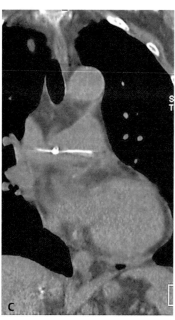

Fig. 103.2 Digital CT scout **(A)** demonstrates high-density bone cement at the vertebroplasty sites in the proximal lumbar spine and a vertically oriented linear focus of similar density overlying the expected location of the inferior vena cava. Unenhanced coronal MIP CT (mediastinal window) confirms embolized bone cement in the inferior vena cava **(B)** and in the main pulmonary artery **(C)**

Imaging Findings

Chest Radiography

- Resembles ARDS of any cause (**Figs. 103.1A, 103.1B**) (also see Case 102)
- Absence of cardiac enlargement and signs of pulmonary venous hypertension (**Figs. 103.1A, 103.1B**) (also see Case 102)
- Pleural effusions typically absent (**Figs. 103.1A, 103.1B**)
- Survivors: resolution usually takes 7–10 days; occasionally up to four weeks

MDCT

- Resembles ARDS of any cause (**Fig. 103.1C, 103.1D, 103.1E, 103.1F**) (also see Case 102)
- Nodular calcifications may evolve in branches of pulmonary arteries over time

Management

- Most effective prophylactic measure: reduce long bone fractures soon after injury
- Maintenance of intravascular volume: shock exacerbates lung injury caused by FES
- Albumin and balanced electrolyte solution recommended for volume resuscitation: restore blood volume and bind fatty acids; may decrease extent of lung injury
- Steroid prophylaxis for high-risk patients: may reduce the incidence

Prognosis

- Mortality rate of FES is approximately 5–15%

PEARLS

- FES is a diagnosis of exclusion and is based on clinical criteria.
- Clinically apparent FES is unusual, often masked by associated injuries in more severely injured patients.

Suggested Reading

1. Bulger EM, Smith DG, Maier RV, Jurkovich GJ. Fat embolism syndrome. A 10-year review. Arch Surg 1997;132(4): 435–439

2. Padovani B, Kasriel O, Brunner P, Peretti-Viton P. Pulmonary embolism caused by acrylic cement: a rare complication of percutaneous vertebroplasty. AJNR Am J Neuroradiol 1999;20(3):375–377

3. Vasconcelos C, Gailloud P, Martin JB, Murphy KJ. Transient arterial hypotension induced by polymethylmethacrylate injection during percutaneous vertebroplasty. J Vasc Interv Radiol 2001;12(8):1001–1002

4. Yoo KY, Jeong SW, Yoon W, Lee J. Acute respiratory distress syndrome associated with pulmonary cement embolism following percutaneous vertebroplasty with polymethylmethacrylate. Spine 2004;29(14):E294–E297

Section VIII

Diffuse Lung Disease

OVERVIEW OF DIFFUSE LUNG DISEASE

■ Introduction

Diffuse lung disease (DLD), also referred to as diffuse parenchymal lung disease (DPLD) or interstitial lung disease (ILD), collectively encompasses more than 200 diseases which affect the lung by a combination of interstitial inflammation, granulomatous inflammation, and/or fibrosis. The incidence of DLD is approximately 50 per 100,000, or 1 in 2,000 persons. This heterogeneous group of diseases is classified under one heading because of similar clinical, radiologic, and pathophysiologic features. DLD may manifest in an acute, subacute, or chronic manner. Although DLD cases may be sequelae of various occupational and environmental exposures, drug reactions, granulomatous disorders, and mixed connective tissue disorders, the vast majority are idiopathic. Most patients with DLD present in one of three manners: (1) progressive dyspnea or dyspnea on exertion, often with a nonproductive cough; (2) respiratory symptoms in the setting of a known concomitant disease (e.g., rheumatoid arthritis); and (3) abnormal chest radiography acquired for unrelated reasons. The physical examination is frequently abnormal but nonspecific. DLD is often characterized by basilar crackles or "Velcro rales." Most cases of DLD demonstrate a restrictive pattern with reductions in total lung capacity (TLC), functional residual capacity (FRC), and residual volume (RV) on pulmonary function studies. A pattern of airflow obstruction is more often seen with sarcoidosis, lymphangioleiomyomatosis, hypersensitivity pneumonitis, or chronic obstructive lung disease with superimposed ILD. Severe reductions in diffusing capacity for carbon monoxide (DLCO) suggest DLD combined with emphysema, Langerhans' cell histiocytosis, lymphangioleiomyomatosis, or advanced idiopathic pulmonary fibrosis.

The diagnosis of DLD is often first suggested based on an abnormal chest radiograph. However, chest radiography may be normal in 10% of patients. The most common radiographic abnormality is a nonspecific reticular pattern. HRCT is acquired to further characterize the nature and extent of disease, assess response to therapy, and guide potential lung biopsy in problematic cases.

Approach to HRCT Interpretation

HRCT interpretation requires (1) understanding the *secondary pulmonary lobule (SPL)* anatomy, (2) recognizing how the SPL is affected by disease, (3) identifying the dominant pattern of disease affecting the SPL, (4) characterizing the distribution of disease, and (5) identifying concomitant findings.

Secondary Pulmonary Lobule Anatomy

The *secondary pulmonary lobule (SPL)* represents the smallest discrete portion of lung surrounded by connective tissue. It is polyhedral, averages 1.0–2.5 cm in size, is supplied by 3–5 terminal bronchioles, and contains 5–15 pulmonary acini (**Fig. VIII.1**). *Central core structures* include the centrilobular bronchus and its accompanying pulmonary artery and lymphatics that course along the bronchovascular bundle toward the center of the SPL. Diseases affecting the airways involve this portion of the SPL (i.e., aspiration, centrilobular emphysema, hypersensitivity pneumonitis, infection, inhalational diseases, and respiratory bronchiolitis). *Peripheral structures* include the interlobular septa, which are continuous with the pleural surface, pulmonary veins, and lymphatics (**Fig. VIII.1**). Diseases affecting the pulmonary veins or lymphatics involve this portion of the SPL (i.e., pulmonary edema, sarcoidosis, and lymphangitic carcinomatosis).

Disease Patterns

The *specific pattern of disease* involving the SPL is useful in narrowing the differential diagnosis. Although several patterns of disease may coexist, invariably one of four dominant patterns is observed: (1) *lines* or *reticular opacities* (i.e., interlobular, intralobular, smooth, or nodular); (2) *nodules* (e.g., centrilobular, perilymphatic, or random) (**Fig. VIII.2**); (3) areas of *increased attenuation* (i.e., ground glass and consolidation) (**Fig. VIII.3**); and (4) areas of *decreased attenuation* (e.g., emphysema, cystic lung disease, bronchiectasis, and honeycombing) (**Fig. VIII.4**).

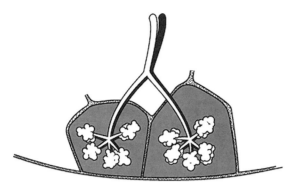

Fig. VIII.1 Secondary pulmonary lobule (*artist's illustration*). Two individual lobules abut the visceral pleura surface. Each is fed by a terminal bronchiole that divides into respiratory bronchioles and then into alveolar ducts to supply the acini. Central core and peripheral structures are illustrated.

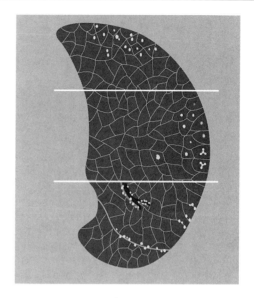

Fig. VIII.2 Artist's illustration showing three dominant nodular patterns of disease that may affect the SPL: random (upper one-third), centrilobular/tree-in-bud (middle one-third), and perilymphatic (lower one-third). See text for further description.

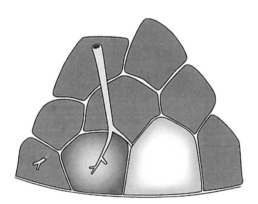

Fig. VIII.3 Artist's illustration contrasting a normal SPL (far left) with those affected by varying degrees of increased attenuation. Whereas visualization of the central core structures is preserved with ground glass (center SPL), these structures are no longer conspicuous with consolidation (far right SPL).

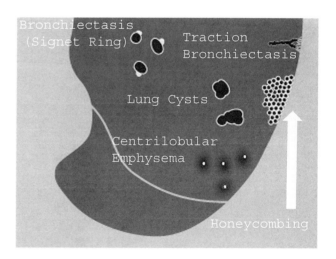

Fig. VIII.4 Artist's illustration demonstrating various patterns of decreased attenuation on HRCT. See text for description.

Reticular Patterns

Well-defined polygons or secondary pulmonary lobules are seen with *interlobular septal thickening* (**Table VIII.1**). A network of disorganized lines within individual SPLs reflects *intralobular septal thickening* and is the hallmark of fibrosis (**Table VIII.1**). *Reticular opacities* may also appear *smooth* or *nodular* (**Table VIII.2**).

Table VIII.1 HRCT Patterns of Disease: Lines or Reticular Opacities, Differential Diagnostic Considerations

Interlobular Septal Lines	Intralobular Septal Lines§
Pulmonary edema	Idiopathic pulmonary fibrosis
Viral infections	Pulmonary edema*
Lymphangitic carcinomatosis	Atypical infections*
Acute eosinophilic pneumonia	
Sarcoidosis*	
Amyloidosis*	
Kaposi sarcoma*	

* Less frequently observed pattern
§ Hallmark of fibrosis

Table VIII.2 HRCT Patterns of Disease: Lines or Reticular Opacities, Differential Diagnostic Considerations

Smooth	Nodular
Pulmonary edema	Sarcoidosis
Lymphangitic carcinomatosis	Lymphangitic carcinomatosis
Lymphoma	Lymphoma
Pulmonary alveolar proteinosis	Silicosis

Nodular Patterns

Centrilobular nodules are evenly spaced and spare the outer 3–5 mm of lung along the costal pleura (**Fig. VIII.2**). This pattern suggests airway dissemination of disease, as with endobronchial spread of tuberculosis or nontuberculous mycobacteria, and bacterial bronchopneumonia but may also occur with respiratory bronchiolitis in heavy smokers and with hypersensitivity pneumonitis. *Perilymphatic nodules* are located along the costal pleura, fissural surfaces, and bronchovascular bundles (**Fig. VIII.2**). Such nodules do not spare the outer 5 mm of lung. *Random nodules* occur everywhere and may occur in association with centrilobular and perilymphatic nodules (**Fig. VIII.2**). This pattern more often occurs with miliary (*Mycobacterium tuberculosis*, nontuberculous mycobacteria, fungal) infections or hematogenous spread of disease (metastases). These nodules tend to be more uniform in size when infection is the underlying cause and more variable in size with neoplastic disease (**Table VIII.3**). *Tree-in-bud* represents a specific *centrilobular nodular pattern* characterized by a combination of nodules and branching structures resembling a tree budding in the springtime. This appearance is created by dilated and mucus- or pus-filled impacted centrilobular bronchioles and occurs most commonly with endobronchial spread of various infections (**Fig. VIII.5**, **Table VIII.4**).

Table VIII.3 HRCT Patterns of Disease: Nodules, Differential Diagnostic Considerations

Centrilobular	Perilymphatic	Random
Infection	Sarcoidosis	Miliary infections
Aspiration	Lymphoproliferative disorders	Hematogenous metastases
Inhalation lung disease	Lymphangitic carcinomatosis	Sarcoidosis*
Hypersensitivity pneumonitis	Silicosis	Pulmonary Langerhans' cell histiocytosis
Respiratory bronchiolitis	Coal worker's pneumoconiosis	
Adenocarcinoma in-situ*		
Early pulmonary Langerhans' cell histiocytosis*		
Pulmonary edema*		

* Less frequently observed pattern

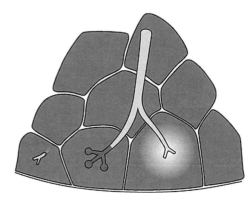

Fig. VIII.5   Artist's illustration contrasting a normal SPL (far left) with those demonstrating centrilobular ground glass opacity (far right SPL) and the combination of centrilobular nodules (buds) and impacted bronchioles (tree) forming so-called tree-in-bud opacities (middle SPL).

Table VIII.4   HRCT Patterns of Disease: Tree-in-Bud Opacities, Differential Diagnostic Considerations

Infection	Non-infection
M. tuberculosis	Asthma
Nontuberculous mycobacteria	Cystic fibrosis
Bacterial bronchopneumonia	Allergic bronchopulmonary aspergillosis
Aspiration	Bronchiectasis

Patterns of Increased Attenuation

Ground glass (**Fig. VIII.3**) creates areas of increased attenuation with preservation of underlying broncho-vascular bundles and can be differentiated from *mosaic perfusion* by comparing relative vessel diameters in affected and unaffected regions (**Table VIII.5**). The pulmonary vessels are similar in size with the former but discrepant with the latter. *Mosaic perfusion* results from differential blood flow and may occur with vascular obstruction (e.g., chronic pulmonary thromboembolic disease) and small airways disease. Air trapping on expiratory images differentiates the latter category from the former (**Table VIII.6**). The presence or absence of edema or pleural fluid can further stratify the *ground glass* differential into "wet" and "dry" categories (**Table VIII.7**). *Consolidation* (**Fig. VIII.3**) causes increased attenuation that obscures visualization of underlying bronchovascular bundles and in many cases is a further progression of diseases that cause ground glass (**Table VIII.5**), that is, replacement of intra-alveolar air by pus, fluid, blood, tumor, or fibrosis.

Crazy paving is a specific pattern of increased attenuation created by a combination of ground glass with superimposed interlobular septal thickening. Numerous diseases may manifest with this pattern (**Table VIII.8**). *Ground glass nodules* represent poorly defined, fuzzy, or smudgy centrilobular or air space nodules. This pattern has a limited differential (**Table VIII.9**).

Table VIII.5   HRCT Patterns of Disease: Areas of Increased Attenuation, Differential Diagnostic Considerations

Acute Ground Glass	Chronic Ground Glass	Acute Consolidation	Chronic Consolidation
Edema	COP/BOOP	Edema	COP/BOOP
ARDS	Chronic eosinophilic pneumonia	ARDS	Chronic eosinophilic pneumonia
Hemorrhage	Adenocarcinoma in-situ	Hemorrhage	Adenocarcinoma in-situ
Pneumonia*	Hypersensitivity pneumonitis	Pneumonia§	Lipoid pneumonia
Acute eosinophilic pneumonia	Pulmonary alveolar proteinosis	Acute eosinophilic pneumonia	Pulmonary alveolar proteinosis
Early XRT	UIP/NSIP (fibrosis)	AIP	UIP/NSIP (fibrosis)
			Lymphoma
			Alveolar sarcoidosis

*Pneumonias include bacterial, *Mycoplasma*, various viral infections, and *Pneumocystis Jiroveci*.
§ Pneumonias include bacterial, *Mycoplasma*, and *Pneumocystis jiroveci*.

Table VIII.6   HRCT Patterns of Disease: Mosaic Perfusion, Differential Diagnostic Considerations

Vascular Obstruction (No Air Trapping)	Small Airways Disease (Air Trapping)
Chronic pulmonary thromboemboli	Reactive airways disease
	Constrictive bronchiolitis
	Hypersensitivity pneumonitis

Table VIII.7   HRCT Patterns of Disease: Ground Glass Opacities, Differential Diagnostic Considerations

Wet Disease	Dry Disease
Pulmonary edema	*Pneumocystis jiroveci*
Acute lung injury	Cytomegalovirus
	Acute hypersensitivity pneumonia
	Pulmonary hemorrhage syndrome
	Respiratory bronchiolitis–interstitial lung disease (RB-ILD)
	Desquamative interstitial pneumonia
	Nonspecific interstitial pneumonia

Table VIII.8   HRCT Patterns of Disease: Crazy Paving, Differential Diagnostic Considerations

Edema	Infection	Organizing Pneumonia	Neoplasm	Other
Cardiogenic	*Pneumocystis jiroveci*	COP/BOOP	AIS	Hemorrhage
ARDS	*Mycoplasma*			Pulmonary alveolar proteinosis
AIP	Bacterial			Sarcoidosis
	Viral			NSIP
				Subacute XRT
				Lipoid pneumonia

Table VIII.9   HRCT Patterns of Disease: Smudgy Centrilobular Nodules, Differential Diagnostic Considerations

Respiratory bronchiolitis (RB)*
Respiratory bronchiolitis–interstitial lung disease (RB-ILD)*
Hypersensitivity pneumonitis (subacute)§
Inhalation lung disease

* Usually seen only in smokers
§ Uncommon in smokers

Patterns of Decreased Attenuation

Four major causes of decreased attenuation on HRCT are:

(1) *Emphysema. Centrilobular emphysema* involves preservation of the centrilobular artery and absence of a perceptible wall. This pattern is more often seen in the upper lobes and superior segments of the lower lobes and is associated with tobacco abuse. This is easily differentiated from *paraseptal emphysema*, which occurs adjacent to the pleura and interlobar fissures and may be associated with bullae formation, and *panlobular emphysema*, which involves the entire SPL and has a predilection for the lower lobes.

(2) *Lung cysts*, which vary in size and shape, and demonstrate a thin perceptible wall (≤4 mm) but no centrilobular artery. *Cavities*, alternatively, have more irregular-appearing walls >4 mm in thickness.

(3) *Honeycombing*, which represents replacement of normal lung by 0.3–1.0 cm juxtapleural cystic spaces in several contiguous layers whose walls are composed of varying amounts of fibrous tissue. Honeycombing is associated with varying degrees of architectural distortion.

(4) *Bronchiectatic airways*, which vary in size and shape, have definable walls, and parallel an accompanying artery (**Fig. VIII.4**, **Table VIII.10**).

Table VIII.10   HRCT Patterns of Disease: Areas of Decreased Attenuation, Differential Diagnostic Considerations

Emphysema	Cystic Disease	Honeycomb	Bronchiectasis
Centrilobular (tobacco abuse/exposure)	Pneumatoceles (*Pneumocystis jiroveci*)	UIP MCTD* Asbestosis Drug reaction Chronic HP§ Idiopathic	Infection
Paraseptal (isolated or associated with centrilobular)	Langerhans' cell histiocytosis		Immune deficiency syndromes IgG, IgE, IgA, HIV
Panlobular (α-1-antiprotease deficiency and smokers with advanced emphysema)	Lymphangioleiomyomatosis		Cystic fibrosis
	Lymphocytic interstitial pneumonia		MCTD*
			Chronic bronchitis and COPD
			Asthma (ABPA)
			XRT

* MCTD (mixed connective tissue disorders) more commonly including scleroderma and rheumatoid arthritis.
§ Chronic HP (chronic or end-stage hypersensitivity pneumonitis)

Zonal Distribution

Various DLDs have a predilection for affecting either the *upper* or *lower lung zone* (**Table VIII.11**). Likewise, there may be preferential involvement of either the *central* or *axial compartment* of the lung (i.e., bronchovascular bundles) or the *peripheral compartment* (outer 1.0 cm of the lung) (**Table VIII.12**). The particular *zone* or *compartment* involved may be useful in narrowing the differential diagnosis (**Tables VIII.11, VIII.12**).

Table VIII.11   HRCT Patterns of Disease: Zonal Distribution, Differential Diagnostic Considerations

Upper Lung Zone	Lower Lung Zone
Centrilobular emphysema	Pulmonary edema
Respiratory bronchiolitis (RB) Respiratory bronchiolitis-ILD	Aspiration
Sarcoidosis	UIP Mixed connective tissue disorders* Asbestosis Drug reaction Chronic hypersensitivity pneumonitis Idiopathic
Silicosis	
Coal worker's pneumoconiosis	
Langerhans' cell histiocytosis	
Chronic hypersensitivity pneumonitis	

* Mixed connective tissue disorders more commonly include scleroderma and rheumatoid arthritis.

Table VIII.12 HRCT Patterns of Disease: Compartmental Distribution, Differential Diagnostic Considerations

Central Compartment	Peripheral Compartment
Sarcoidosis	COP/BOOP
Bronchitis	Chronic eosinophilic pneumonia
	Hematogenous metastases
	UIP Mixed connective tissue disorders* Asbestosis Drug reaction Chronic hypersensitivity pneumonitis Idiopathic

Concomitant Findings

The presence of various concomitant imaging findings (e.g., lymphadenopathy, pleural effusion, pneumothorax, pleural plaques, and osseous lesions) is often helpful and can be used to narrow the differential diagnosis. Examples are provided in **Table VIII.13**.

The application of these five principles to the diagnostic interpretation of HRCT scans is illustrated in the cases that follow in this section.

Table VIII.13 HRCT Patterns of Disease: Concomitant Findings, Differential Diagnostic Considerations

Lymphadenopathy	Effusion	Pneumothorax	Plaques	Osseous Lesions
M. tuberculosis	M. tuberculosis	PLCH•	Asbestos exposure	Metastatic disease
Nontuberculous mycobacteria	Pulmonary edema	LAM§		PLCH•
Sarcoidosis				
Lung carcinoma				
Lymphangitic carcinomatosis	Lymphangitic carcinomatosis			
Progressive systemic sclerosis	LAM§			
Silicosis*	Asbestosis			
Coal worker's pneumoconiosis*				

* Rarely observed.
§ LAM: lymphangioleiomyomatosis.
• PLCH: pulmonary Langerhans' cell histiocytosis.

Suggested Readings

1. Lynch DA, Brown KK, Lee JS, et al. Imaging of diffuse infiltrative lung disease. In: Lynch DA, Newell JD Jr, Lee JS eds. Imaging of Diffuse Lung Disease. Hamilton, Ontario: Decker; 2000

2. Smithuis R, van Delden O, Schaefer-Prokop C. HRCT Part I; Basic Interpretation. Radiology Department of the Rijnland Hospital, Leiderdorp and the Academical Medical Centre, the Netherlands. Publication date: 24-12-2006. http://www.radiologyassistant.nl/en/42d94cdOc326b; accessed 28 July 2009

3. Webb WR. High Resolution Lung CT. Interactive Radiology Series CD-ROM. UCSF Radiology Postgraduate Education. Lippincott Williams and Wilkins; 2000

4. Webb WR, Müller NL, Naidich DP. In: High-Resolution CT of the Lung, 3rd ed. Philadelphia: Lippincott Williams and Wilkins; 2001

CASE 104

■ Clinical Presentation

50-year-old woman with persistent fever, progressive dyspnea, and non-productive cough for several weeks despite antibiotics for presumed community-acquired pneumonia

■ Radiologic Findings

Baseline frontal chest X-ray (**Fig. 104.1A**) reveals mild hypoaeration but is otherwise unremarkable. Follow-up chest X-ray eight days later (**Fig. 104.1B**) shows bilateral, patchy ground glass and subtle reticular opacities. The heart is not enlarged. Lung volumes remain mildly diminished. Chest CT (lung window) through the upper (**Fig. 104.1C**), mid (**Figs. 104.1D, 104.1E**), and lower (**Figs. 104.1E, 104.1F**) lung zones performed two days later demonstrates bilateral ground glass opacities with sparing of some secondary pulmonary lobules, resulting in a geographic appearance to the lungs. Smooth septal thickening, intralobular lines, and ground glass result in a "crazy paving" pattern. Mild bronchial dilatation is present. Patient required mechanical ventilator support two days later. Subsequent open lung biopsy confirmed the diagnosis.

■ Diagnosis

Acute Interstitial Pneumonia (AIP)

■ Differential Diagnosis

- Permeability Edema
- Diffuse Pneumonia
- Diffuse Alveolar Hemorrhage
- Acute Hypersensitivity Pneumonitis

■ Discussion

Background

The idiopathic interstitial pneumonias (IIP) are the most common group of diffuse parenchymal lung diseases. They were recently reclassified by a multidisciplinary panel of experts in a collaborative effort by the American Thoracic Society (ATS), the European Respiratory Society (ERS), and the American College of Chest Physicians (ACCP). The new classification includes seven distinct clinico-pathologic entities: (1) idiopathic pulmonary fibrosis (IPF) or cryptogenic fibrosing alveolitis (CFA); (2) non-specific interstitial pneumonia (NSIP); (3) cryptogenic organizing pneumonia (COP); (4) acute interstitial pneumonia (AIP); (5) lymphocytic interstitial pneumonia (LIP); (6) respiratory bronchiolitis–interstitial lung disease (RB-ILD); and (7) desquamative interstitial pneumonitis (DIP).

Acute interstitial pneumonia (*AIP*) is an uncommon and fulminant form of lung injury of unknown etiology that usually occurs in previously healthy persons and produces histologic findings of diffuse alveolar damage (DAD). Previously called Hamman-Rich syndrome, it was originally thought to be rapidly progressive UIP but is now recognized as a distinct clinico-pathologic entity and is much less common than UIP. Because the clinical presentation is acute and the histologic features are identical to those of ARDS, AIP is also often referred to as idiopathic ARDS.

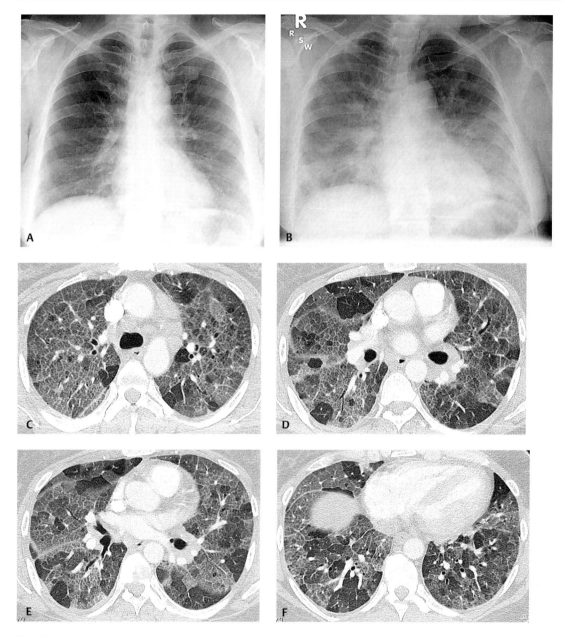

Fig. 104.1

Etiology

The etiology of AIP is unknown.

Clinical Findings

Patients are typically younger than those with UIP, with an average age at presentation of 50–60 years (range 7–83 years), and the clinical course is more acute. Affected patients often have a prodromal illness associated with symptoms of a viral upper respiratory tract infection (URI). Clinical symptoms include dry cough, fever, and dyspnea, which rapidly progresses in severity, followed by hypoxemia and respiratory failure necessitating mechanical ventilation.

Imaging Findings

Chest Radiography

- Progressive diffuse bilateral air space consolidations with air bronchograms (similar to ARDS) (**Figs. 104.1A, 104.1B**)
- Consolidation often initially patchy; rapidly becomes confluent and diffuse (**Figs. 104.1A, 104.1B**)
- May have either upper or lower lobe predominance (**Figs. 104.1A, 104.1B**)
- Lung volumes usually decreased (**Figs. 104.1A, 104.1B**)

MDCT/HRCT

Early Stages

- Geographic pattern of diseased and normal lung (**Figs. 104.1C, 104.1D, 104.1E, 104.1F**)
- Bilateral ground glass opacities; patchy or diffuse or occasionally peripheral (**Figs. 104.1C, 104.1D, 104.1E, 104.1F**)
- Areas of consolidation; patchy or confluent; involve mainly dependent lung
- Focal sparing of lung lobules (**Figs. 104.1C, 104.1D, 104.1E, 104.1F**)
- Smooth septal thickening and intralobular lines superimposed on ground glass opacities ("crazy paving" pattern) (**Figs. 104.1C, 104.1D, 104.1E, 104.1F**)
- Lymphadenopathy and pleural effusion; uncommon

Later Stages (>7 days after onset)

- Architectural distortion
- Traction bronchiectasis
- Juxtapleural honeycombing; involves <10% of lung parenchyma
- Thickening of bronchovascular bundles and interlobular septa

Management

- Supportive
- Corticosteroids may benefit some patients

Prognosis

- Mortality rate: 60–90%
- May develop severe parenchymal fibrosis, without progression in post-recovery period (unlike UIP)
- Survivors may have significant functional abnormalities
- Extent of ground glass opacity or consolidation without traction bronchiolectasis or bronchiectasis is greater in survivors than in non-survivors
- Extent of either ground glass opacity or consolidation combined with traction bronchiolectasis or bronchiectasis is greater in non-survivors

PEARLS

- Patients with AIP are often initially misdiagnosed with severe community-acquired pneumonia but fail to respond to broad-spectrum antibiotic therapy.
- Diagnosis requires negative bacterial, viral, and fungal cultures, and exclusion of other causes of ARDS.
- Integrating biopsy results with clinical, laboratory, and microbiologic findings is necessary to establish the final diagnosis.

Suggested Reading

1. American Thoracic Society; European Respiratory Society. American Thoracic Society/European Respiratory Society International Multidisciplinary Consensus Classification of the Idiopathic Interstitial Pneumonias. This joint statement of the American Thoracic Society (ATS), and the European Respiratory Society (ERS) was adopted by the ATS board of directors, June 2001, and by the ERS Executive Committee, June 2001. Am J Respir Crit Care Med 2002;165(2): 277–304

2. Ichikado K, Suga M, Müller NL, et al. Acute interstitial pneumonia: comparison of high-resolution computed tomography findings between survivors and nonsurvivors. Am J Respir Crit Care Med 2002;165(11):1551–1556

3. Travis WD, Colby TV, Koss MN, Rosado-de-Christenson ML, Müller NL, King TE Jr. Diffuse parenchymal lung diseases. In: King DW, ed. Atlas of Nontumor Pathology: Non-Neoplastic Disorders of the Lower Respiratory Tract. First Series. Fascicle 2. Washington, DC: The American Registry of Pathology; 2001:103–106

4. Vourlekis JS, Brown KK, Cool CD, et al. Acute interstitial pneumonitis. Case series and review of the literature. Medicine (Baltimore) 2000;79(6):369–378

5. Webb WR, Muller NL, Naidich DP. The idiopathic interstitial pneumonia. In: High-Resolution CT of the Lung, 4th ed. Philadelphia: Lippincott, Williams & Wilkins; 2009:206–209

CASE 105

■ Clinical Presentation

46-year-old woman, non-smoker, complaining of dyspnea and cough over the past six to eight months

■ Radiologic Findings

PA (**Fig. 105.1A**) chest radiograph demonstrates subtle bilateral ground glass and reticular opacities most pronounced in the mid- and lower lung zones. Coronal (**Fig. 105.1B**) and axial (**Figs. 105.1C, 105.1D, 105.1E, 105.1F**) CT (lung window) confirms the presence of primarily lower lobe patchy ground glass opacities and mild reticulation without significant fibrosis. Note the relative juxtapleural sparing by ground glass in the dorsal regions of the lower lobes. Open lung biopsy confirmed the diagnosis.

■ Diagnosis

Non-Specific Interstitial Pneumonia (NSIP); Cellular Pattern

■ Differential Diagnosis

- Acute Interstitial Pneumonia (AIP)
- Cryptogenic Organizing Pneumonia (COP)
- Desquamative Interstitial Pneumonia (DIP)
- Hypersensitivity Pneumonitis (HP)
- Respiratory Bronchiolitis–Interstitial Lung Disease (RB-ILD)
- Usual Interstitial Pneumonia (UIP)

■ Discussion

Background

Non-specific interstitial pneumonia (NSIP) is one of the chronic idiopathic interstitial pneumonias (IIPs). Katzenstein first described NSIP in 1994. The term is used for cases of interstitial pneumonia in which diagnostic features of UIP, DIP, AIP, or COP are not present. NSIP accounts for 14–35% of biopsies performed for chronic interstitial pneumonia. Pathologically and radiologically, NSIP is characterized by two patterns of lung involvement. The *cellular pattern of NSIP* is predominantly an inflammatory process of plasma cells and lymphocytes and is characterized by more of a ground glass pattern on CT/HRCT, The *fibrotic pattern of NSIP* is characterized by collagen accumulation and fibrosis of the alveolar septa, interlobular septa, peribronchiolar tissues, and visceral pleura and manifests with greater reticulation, traction bronchiectasis and bronchiolectasis, interlobular septal thickening, and irregular interfaces on CT/HRCT.

Etiology

NSIP may be idiopathic, but more commonly occurs as a pulmonary manifestation of mixed connective tissue or collagen vascular disease, drug-induced lung disease, hypersensitivity pneumonia, or chronic interstitial lung disease complicating diffuse alveolar damage.

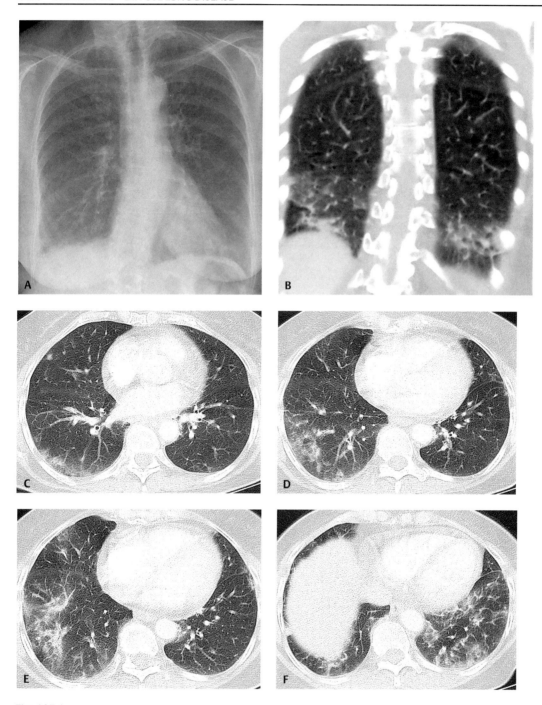

Fig. 105.1

Clinical Findings

Affected patients often present with symptoms similar to IPF. The most common symptom is exertional dyspnea. Patients may also have cough and fever. The duration of symptoms ranges from six months up to three years. Crackles are frequently heard on auscultation. PFTs often reveal a restrictive defect with reduced DLCO. The median age at presentation is 40–50 years, approximately 10 years younger than patients with IPF.

Imaging Findings

Chest Radiography

- Normal: 10–15%
- Ground glass opacities or consolidation; predominantly involving lower lung zones (most common) (**Fig. 105.1A**)
- Predominant reticular pattern in other cases
- Combination of interstitial and air space disease (**Fig. 105.1A**)

MDCT/HRCT

- Ground glass opacities often with basal and peripheral predominance (approximately 100%) (**Figs. 105.1B, 105.1C, 105.1D, 105.1E, 105.1F**)
- ± associated irregular linear or reticular opacities (50–100%) (**Figs. 105.2A, 105.2B**)
- Reticular opacities often associated with other findings of mild fibrosis; traction bronchiectasis, traction bronchiolectasis, interlobular septal thickening, intralobular septal thickening, irregular interfaces (**Figs. 105.3A, 105.3B**)
- Honeycombing; mild involving <10% of parenchyma (10–30%)
- Centrilobular nodules; uncommon
- Abnormalities may be diffuse; lower lung zone predominant (60–90%); peripheral lung (50–70%); relative sparing of immediate juxtapleural dorsal lung in lower lobes (64%)
- Mediastinal lymph node enlargement (80%)
  - 10–15 mm short axis diameter
  - Usually involves one or two nodal stations, most commonly lower right paratracheal (4R) and subcarinal (7)

Management

- NSIP is a common reaction pattern to various medications; associated with mixed connective tissue and collagen vascular disorders (e.g., scleroderma) and hypersensitivity pneumonia. Before a diagnosis of idiopathic NSIP can be made, these other conditions must be excluded.
- Definitive diagnosis of NSIP requires open lung biopsy
- Corticosteroids

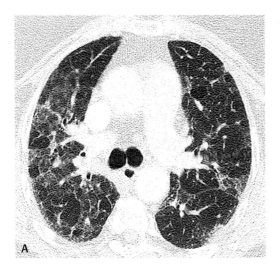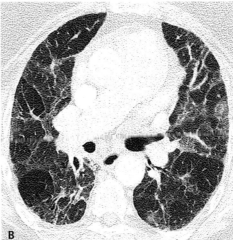

Fig. 105.2   HRCT of a 47-year-old woman with dermatomyositis and exertional dyspnea with biopsy-proven mixed cellular and fibrotic NSIP shows a combination of peripheral ground glass and abnormal reticular opacities with mild fibrosis and architectural distortion.

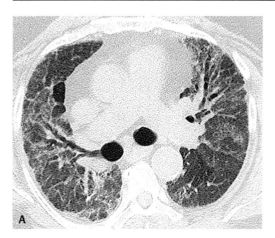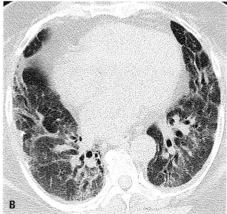

Fig. 105.3 Fibrotic NSIP in a 71-year-old woman. CT (lung window) shows extensive interlobular and intralobular interstitial thickening and traction bronchiectasis. Mild ground glass is present but primarily in the regions of reticulation. Note the relative juxtapleural sparing of the dorsal region of the left lower lobe **(B)**.

Prognosis

- *Cellular NSIP*—better prognosis and more steroid responsive than *fibrotic NSIP*
  - ○ *Cellular NSIP*—excellent prognosis
  - ○ *Fibrotic NSIP*—median survival ranges from 6 to 14 years
- NSIP prognosis much better than that for IPF (median survival 2.5–3.5 years)
- Patients may develop an abrupt worsening or deterioration of symptoms due to infection, acute PTE, heart failure, or idiopathic acute exacerbation or accelerated disease similar to that seen with UIP-IPF. Characteristic imaging findings include extensive ground glass or consolidation on the background of reticulation.

PEARLS

- Patients with only ground glass opacities typically have *cellular NSIP* and are more likely to improve with steroids and have a better long-term prognosis.
- Patients with ground glass opacities, reticulation, and traction bronchiectasis may have *cellular* or *fibrotic NSIP*; the greater the fibrosis, the poorer the response to steroids and the worse the long-term prognosis.
- Diagnosis often requires open lung biopsy, but even histologic evidence of NSIP does not establish a definitive diagnosis; such findings may occur with mixed connective tissue disorders, drug-induced lung disease and hypersensitivity pneumonitis.

Suggested Reading

1. American Thoracic Society; European Respiratory Society. American Thoracic Society/European Respiratory Society International Multidisciplinary Consensus Classification of the Idiopathic Interstitial Pneumonias. This joint statement of the American Thoracic Society (ATS) and the European Respiratory Society (ERS) was adopted by the ATS board of directors, June 2001, and by the ERS Executive Committee, June 2001. Am J Respir Crit Care Med 2002;165(2): 277–304

2. Kim DS, Collard HR, King TE Jr. Classification and natural history of the idiopathic interstitial pneumonias. Proc Am Thorac Soc 2006;3(4):285–292

3. Silva CIS, Müller NL, Hansell DM, Lee KS, Nicholson AG, Wells AU. Nonspecific interstitial pneumonia and idiopathic pulmonary fibrosis: changes in pattern and distribution of disease over time. Radiology 2008;247(1):251–259

4. Travis WD, Colby TV, Koss MN, Rosado-de-Christenson ML, Müller NL, King TE Jr. Idiopathic interstitial pneumonia and other diffuse parenchymal lung diseases. In: King DW, ed. Atlas of Nontumor Pathology: Non-Neoplastic Disorders of the Lower Respiratory Tract, fascicle 2, series 1. Washington, DC: American Registry of Pathology and Armed Forces Institute of Pathology; 2001:49–231

5. Webb WR, Müller NL, Naidich DP. The idiopathic interstitial pneumonias. In: High-Resolution CT of the Lung, 4th ed. Philadelphia: Lippincott, Williams & Wilkins; 2009:189–196

CASE 106

■ Clinical Presentation

58-year-old woman complaining of progressive shortness of breath

■ Radiologic Findings

Unenhanced chest CT axial (**Figs. 106.1A, 106.1B, 106.1C, 106.1D**; lung window) and coronal (**Figs. 106.1E**; lung window) images demonstrate bilateral symmetric ground glass and smooth reticular opacities diffusely throughout the lungs without a zonal predilection. The involved regions of lung parenchyma are sharply demarcated from adjacent normal lung. This combination of ground glass with reticular opacities creates a pattern of disease called "crazy paving." Note the preservation of lung volume and the absence of lymphadenopathy and pleural effusion.

■ Diagnosis

Pulmonary Alveolar Proteinosis

■ Differential Diagnosis

- Edema
  - Cardiogenic
  - ARDS
  - Acute Interstitial Pneumonia (AIP)
- Infection
  - *Pneumocystis jiroveci* Pneumonia
  - Viral Pneumonia
  - *Mycoplasma* Pneumonia
  - Bacterial Pneumonia
- Organizing Pneumonia
  - Bronchiolitis Obliterans Organizing Pneumonia (BOOP)/Cryptogenic Organizing Pneumonia (COP)
- Neoplasia
  - Adenocarcinoma in-situ
- Other
  - Hemorrhage
  - Pulmonary Alveolar Proteinosis
  - Sarcoidosis
  - Non-Specific Interstitial Pneumonia (NSIP)
  - Lipoid Pneumonia
  - Subacute Radiation Therapy–Related Pneumonitis (XRT)

■ Discussion

Background

Pulmonary alveolar proteinosis (PAP) is a rare lung disorder (estimated prevalence of 1 case per 100,000 population) characterized by the abnormal accumulation of lipid-rich granular eosinophilic material within the alveoli.

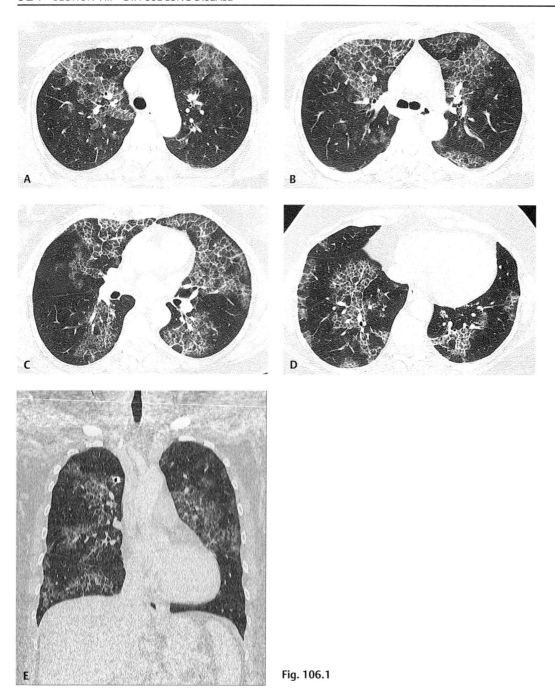

Fig. 106.1

Etiology

The etiology is unknown. However, three forms are recognized. These include primary (idiopathic), secondary, and congenital varieties. *Primary PAP* is the most common form, accounting for 90% of cases, and occurs in isolation. *Secondary PAP* (5–10%) occurs with the industrial inhalation of mineral dusts (e.g., silica, titanium oxide, aluminum) and insecticides, various hematologic malignancies, and immunodeficiency syndromes, including AIDS. An association with cigarette smoking has also been suggested. *Congenital PAP* is rare (2%). Affected neonates are deficient in surfactant-associated protein B (SP-B).

Clinical Findings

Most patients presenting with PAP are 20–50 years old and have a gradual onset of symptoms, including persistent dry cough, progressive dyspnea, fatigue, malaise, weight loss, low-grade fever, and/or night sweats. Expectoration of gelatinous material has been reported. However, up to 30% of affected patients are asymptomatic, even in the setting of profoundly abnormal chest radiography. Physical exam findings may include fine end-inspiratory crackles. PFTs often reveal impaired diffusion and mild to moderate restrictive physiology. PAP is four times more common in males than females.

Imaging Findings

Chest Radiography

- Bilateral, symmetric, patchy, and diffuse ground glass opacities and consolidations
- Nodular or reticular opacities
- Lower lobe predilection
- Relative sparing of costophrenic angles and apices
- Preserved lung volumes
- Lymphadenopathy and pleural effusion; rare

MDCT/HRCT

- Diffuse, patchy, bilateral ground glass with superimposed smooth reticular opacities or septal thickening ("crazy paving" pattern) (**Figs. 106.1A, 106.1B, 106.1C, 106.1D, 106.1E**)
- Areas of affected lung sharply demarcated from adjacent uninvolved or normal lung (**Figs. 106.1A, 106.1B, 106.1C, 106.1D, 106.1E**)
- Multifocal nodules or confluent areas of consolidation may occur with concomitant superimposed infection

Management

- Depends on degree of physiological impairment, underlying concomitant diseases or associated factors and presence of coexisting infection(s)
- Indications for mechanical removal of the lipoproteinaceous-rich material from the alveoli by bilateral, sequential whole lung lavage with isotonic NaCl solution, and/or repeated lobar lavage via bronchoscopy include:
  - Alveolar-arterial oxygen gradient ≥40 mm Hg
  - PaO_2 <65 mm Hg
  - Dyspnea and hypoxemia at rest or with exercise
- Lung transplantation reserved for:
  - Adult patients with end-stage interstitial fibrosis and complicating cor pulmonale
  - Congenital PAP

Prognosis

- Overall prognosis for *primary PAP* is very good
- Often dramatic clinical improvement and remission with one-time whole-lung lavage
- Relapses may necessitate repeat lavage(s); often have poorer outcome, complicated by
  - Interstitial fibrosis
  - Respiratory failure
  - Cor pulmonale
- Complicating lung infections include:
  - *N. asteroides*
  - *M. tuberculosis*
  - *Mycobacterium avium-intracellulare*
  - *Aspergillus* sp.
  - *Pneumocystis jiroveci*
  - *Candida*

○ *C. neoformans*
○ *H. capsulatum*
○ Cytomegalovirus

PEARLS

- *Primary PAP* may occur in isolation.
- Thirty percent of patients are asymptomatic, even with profoundly abnormal chest radiography.
- Whole lung lavage is the treatment of choice in *primary PAP*.
- "Crazy paving" pattern is not pathognomonic of PAP but has a broad differential diagnosis that requires clinical and laboratory correlation to appropriately narrow the alternatives.

Suggested Reading

1. Frazier AA, Franks TJ, Cooke EO, Mohammed TL, Pugatch RD, Galvin JR. From the archives of the AFIP: pulmonary alveolar proteinosis. Radiographics 2008;28(3):883–899, quiz 915

2. Holbert JM, Costello P, Li W, Hoffman RM, Rogers RM. CT features of pulmonary alveolar proteinosis. AJR Am J Roentgenol 2001;176(5):1287–1294

3. Rossi SE, Erasmus JJ, Volpacchio M, Franquet T, Castiglioni T, McAdams HP. "Crazy-paving" pattern at thin-section CT of the lungs: radiologic-pathologic overview. Radiographics 2003;23(6):1509–1519

4. Parker MS, Rosado-de-Christenson ML, Abbott GF. Diffuse lung disease. In: Teaching Atlas of Chest Imaging. New York: Thieme Medical Publishers, Inc.; 2006:455–458

5. Travis WD, Colby TV, Koss MN, Rosado-de-Christenson ML, Müller NL, King TE Jr. Idiopathic interstitial pneumonia and other diffuse parenchymal lung diseases. In: King DW, ed. Atlas of Nontumor Pathology: Non-Neoplastic Disorders of the Lower Respiratory Tract, fascicle 2, series 1. Washington, DC: American Registry of Pathology and Armed Forces Institute of Pathology; 2001:49–231

CASE 107

■ Clinical Presentation

43-year-old woman undergoing treatment for rheumatoid arthritis presents with dry cough and pleuritic chest pain

■ Radiologic Findings

PA chest radiograph (**Fig. 107.1**) demonstrates bilateral asymmetric peripheral upper lobe predominant consolidations, more pronounced in the right upper lobe. Contrast-enhanced chest CT (lung window) (**Figs. 107.2, 107.3**) shows bilateral peripheral nodular non-segmental consolidations with intrinsic air bronchograms affecting predominantly the upper lobes. The symptoms and radiographic abnormalities resolved after a change in drug therapy was instituted.

■ Diagnosis

Eosinophilic Pneumonia

■ Differential Diagnosis

- Infection (tuberculosis, other bacteria)
- Cryptogenic Organizing Pneumonia (COP)
- Multicentric Adenocarcinoma
- Pulmonary Lymphoma

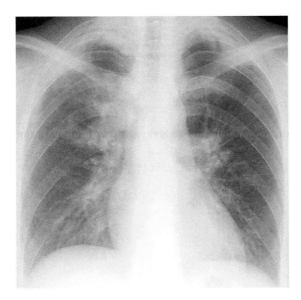

Fig. 107.1

527

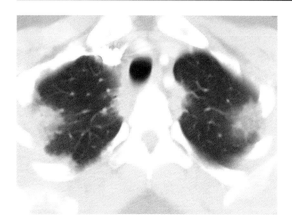

Fig. 107.2

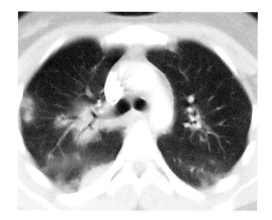

Fig. 107.3

■ Discussion

Background

Eosinophilic lung diseases are a diverse group of disorders characterized by pulmonary abnormalities associated with peripheral blood eosinophilia, tissue eosinophilia, and/or increased eosinophils in bronchoalveolar lavage (BAL) fluid.

Etiology

Eosinophilic pneumonias can be divided into diseases of unknown etiology and those of known causes. The former include simple (Loeffler syndrome), acute, and chronic eosinophilic pneumonias and idiopathic hypereosinophilic syndrome. Eosinophilic lung diseases of known cause include allergic bronchopulmonary fungal disease (typically aspergillosis), bronchocentric granulomatosis, parasitic infections, and eosinophilic lung disease secondary to drug reaction. Eosinophilic vasculitides include Churg-Strauss syndrome and allergic angiitis. In addition, several other diseases are associated with eosinophilia, including asthma, various infections, neoplasms, and collagen vascular disorders. Specific diseases that may produce minor eosinophilia include rheumatoid arthritis, Wegener granulomatosis, idiopathic pulmonary fibrosis, and pulmonary Langerhans' cell histiocytosis.

Clinical Findings

Patients with *simple eosinophilic pneumonia* (SEP) or *Loeffler syndrome* (LS) have minimal or absent pulmonary symptoms, and their pulmonary disease resolves spontaneously within one month. *Acute eosinophilic pneumonia* (AEP) is characterized by a rapid onset of fever, myalgias, pleuritic pain, and hypoxemia, often progressing to respiratory failure and requiring mechanical ventilation. *Chronic eosinophilic pneumonia* (CEP) has an insidious onset, with cough, fever, dyspnea, weight loss, and asthma. It affects middle-aged adults and women more commonly than men. *Idiopathic hypereosinophilic syndrome* is a systemic disorder with preferential involvement of the heart and central nervous system that affects patients in the third and fourth decades of life, with a reported male-to-female ratio of 7:1. Lung involvement is seen in 40% of affected patients and pleural effusions occur in 50%.

Eosinophilic lung disease may manifest as an allergic reaction to fungal antigens (usually *Aspergillus* sp.) in patients with asthma, peripheral eosinophilia, and central bronchiectasis. It may also manifest with constitutional symptoms, fever, and respiratory complaints in patients with parasitic infestations. Mild to fulminant respiratory symptoms associated with eosinophilic pneumonia may develop in patients undergoing drug therapy with drugs like methotrexate, nitrofurantoin, salicylates, sulfonamides, and many others. Patients with eosinophilic pneumonia respond promptly to corticosteroid therapy, a factor that helps confirm the diagnosis.

Imaging Findings

Chest Radiography

Simple Eosinophilic Pneumonia (SEP)

- Non-segmental, multi-focal migratory parenchymal consolidations; may exhibit a peripheral distribution; rarely single or multiple pulmonary nodules; resolution within one month

Acute Eosinophilic Pneumonia (AEP)

- Bilateral reticular and alveolar opacities, pleural effusions, patchy ground glass opacities, may undergo rapid progression to diffuse air space disease

Chronic Eosinophilic Pneumonia (CEP)

- Bilateral non-segmental air space consolidations with a subpleural distribution in up to 60% of cases
- Predilection for the upper and middle lung zones; rarely nodules and pleural effusions

Eosinophilic Pneumonia Secondary to Drug Reaction

- Peripheral consolidations (**Fig. 107.1**), reticular and nodular opacities, lymphadenopathy and pleural effusion

Eosinophilic Pneumonia Secondary to Parasitic Infestation

- Fine diffuse reticular and nodular opacities with a lower lung zone predilection

MDCT/HRCT

- Peripheral distribution of air space disease (**Figs. 107.2, 107.3, 107.4**) (may not be evident on radiography)
- Patchy peripheral ground glass opacities and consolidations with a middle and upper lung zone predilection in SEP and CEP (**Figs. 107.4, 107.5**)
- Non-segmental air space disease (**Fig. 107.5**)
- Band-like peripheral linear opacities in CEP, particularly with chronic or treated disease (**Fig. 107.5**)
- Ground glass opacity (may be diffuse) with superimposed smooth interlobular septal thickening in AEP
- Single or multiple nodular opacities; may exhibit surrounding ground glass
- Reticular opacities; mixed alveolar and reticular opacities
- Pleural effusion
- Lymphadenopathy in drug-induced eosinophilic pneumonia and rarely in CEP

Management

- Corticosteroids: prompt symptom relief and resolution of radiologic abnormalities
- Treatment of underlying conditions in cases of secondary eosinophilic pneumonia
  - Antibiotics in parasitic disease
  - Steroids
  - Drug withdrawal in drug-induced disease

Prognosis

- Generally favorable
- Spontaneous disease resolution or cure following first course of steroids in patients with SEP and AEP and in many patients with CEP
- Common recurrences in CEP; may result in steroid dependence

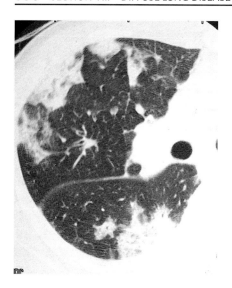

Fig. 107.4 Unenhanced HRCT (lung window) targeted at the right lung of a patient with chronic eosinophilic pneumonia demonstrates the peripheral distribution of multifocal non-segmental right lung consolidations.

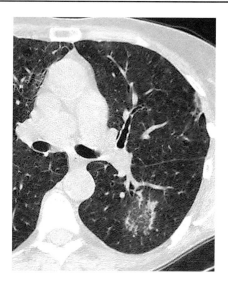

Fig. 107.5 Coned-down HRCT (lung window) of a patient with recurrence of chronic eosinophilic pneumonia demonstrates multifocal patchy air space disease affecting predominantly the left lower lobe. Note subpleural band-like opacities in the peripheral portions of the left and right upper lobes.

Suggested Reading

1. Jeong YJ, Kim K-I, Seo IJ, et al. Eosinophilic lung diseases: a clinical, radiologic, and pathologic overview. Radiographics 2007;27(3):617–637, discussion 637–639

2. Johkoh T, Müller NL, Akira M, et al. Eosinophilic lung diseases: diagnostic accuracy of thin-section CT in 111 patients. Radiology 2000;216(3):773–780

3. Travis WD, Colby TV, Koss MN, Rosado-de-Christenson ML, Müller NL, King TE Jr. Idiopathic interstitial pneumonia and other diffuse parenchymal lung diseases. In: King DW, ed. Atlas of Nontumor Pathology: Non-Neoplastic Disorders of the Lower Respiratory Tract, fasc 2, ser 1. Washington, DC: American Registry of Pathology and Armed Forces Institute of Pathology; 2001:49–231

CASE 108

■ Clinical Presentation

42-year-old man, cigarette smoker, with increasing dyspnea for several months

■ Radiologic Findings

HRCT (lung window) (**Figs. 108.1A, 108.1B**) demonstrates extensive bilateral areas of ground glass attenuation, irregular juxtapleural linear opacities consistent with mild fibrosis, and traction bronchiectasis.

■ Diagnosis

Desquamative Interstitial Pneumonia (DIP)

■ Differential Diagnosis

- Chronic Hypersensitivity Pneumonitis
- Pulmonary Drug Toxicity
- Pulmonary Hemorrhage
- Eosinophilic Pneumonia

■ Discussion

Background

Desquamative interstitial pneumonia (DIP) is a rare idiopathic interstitial pneumonia that occurs almost exclusively in current or former smokers and is characterized histologically by diffuse, marked intra-alveolar accumulation of macrophages and minimal interstitial fibrosis. It is considered part of a histopathologic spectrum of smoking-related interstitial lung diseases that includes pulmonary Langerhans' cell histiocytosis and respiratory bronchiolitis–associated interstitial lung disease (RB-ILD). The term *desquamative* is a misno-

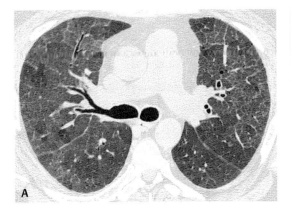
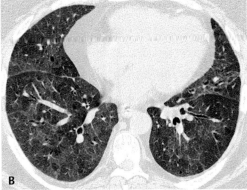

Fig. 108.1

mer based on the previous but erroneous concept that the intra-alveolar cells represent desquamated pneumocytes. Some authors have suggested that a more technically correct terminology for DIP would be alveolar macrophage pneumonia. The incidence of DIP is much lower than that of usual interstitial pneumonia (UIP). The diagnosis of DIP requires open or thoracoscopic lung biopsy.

Etiology

The etiology of DIP is unknown, but the majority of affected patients are current or former cigarette smokers. A similar histopathologic pattern has been described in metabolic diseases, drug reactions, connective tissue disorders, and cases of dust inhalation.

Clinical Findings

Patients are typically younger, present with more acute pulmonary symptoms, and have more mild pulmonary function abnormalities than those with UIP. Patients with DIP typically present with cough and dyspnea. Pulmonary function tests typically reveal a restrictive pattern and hypoxemia.

Imaging Findings

Chest Radiography

- Normal (3–22% of patients)
- Bilateral, symmetric ground glass opacification
- Bibasilar, irregular linear opacities
- Lower lung zone predominance
- Preserved lung volumes
- Nodules and honeycombing (10%)

MDCT/HRCT

- Diffuse ground glass opacity (100%) (**Figs. 108.1A, 108.1B, 108.2**)
- Subpleural and lower lobe predominance (**Figs. 108.1A, 108.1B, 108.2**)
- May have mild peripheral reticulation and architectural distortion (50%) (**Fig. 108.2**)
- Traction bronchiectasis, honeycombing uncommon
- Small cysts (microcysts) (32–75%) (**Fig. 108.2**)

Management

- Cessation of smoking
- Corticosteroids

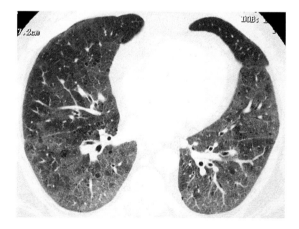

Fig. 108.2 Unenhanced HRCT (lung window) of a 34-year-old man with an 18-year history of cigarette smoking and increasing dyspnea for 1 year shows extensive bilateral ground glass opacities and irregular juxtapleural linear opacities consistent with mild fibrosis. Small cystic areas (microcysts) are seen bilaterally, an uncommon but recognized feature of DIP. The combination of ground glass opacity and small cysts is suggestive of DIP.

Prognosis

- 5- and 10-year survival of 95.2% and 69.6%, respectively (better than other ILDs)
- Progression to end-stage fibrosis in some patients

PEARLS

- DIP is part of the spectrum of smoking-related interstitial lung disease.
- Characteristic HRCT findings: bilateral ground glass opacity with lower lobe predominance, with or without associated mild reticulation.
- Findings of proximal acinar (centrilobular) emphysema may also be present, as most patients with DIP are current or former cigarette smokers.

Suggested Reading

1. Desai SR, Ryan SM, Colby TV. Smoking-related interstitial lung diseases: histopathological and imaging perspectives. Clin Radiol 2003;58(4):259–268

2. Hansell DM, Nicholson AG. Smoking-related diffuse parenchymal lung disease: HRCT-pathologic correlation. Semin Respir Crit Care Med 2003;24(4):377–392

3. Ryu JH, Colby TV, Hartman TE, Vassallo R. Smoking-related interstitial lung diseases: a concise review. Eur Respir J 2001;17(1):122–132

4. Hansell DM, Lynch DA, McAdams HP, Bankier AA. Inhalational lung disease. In: Hansell DM, Lynch DA, McAdams HP, Bankier AA, ed. Imaging of Diseases of the Chest, 5th ed. Philadelphia: Mosby Elsevier; 2010:451–504

5. McAdams HP, Rosado-de-Christenson ML, Wehunt WD, Fishback NF. The alphabet soup revisited: the chronic interstitial pneumonias in the 1990s. Radiographics 1996;16(5):1009–1033, discussion 1033–1034

CASE 109

■ Clinical Presentation

31-year-old woman with cough, dyspnea, and weight loss

■ Radiologic Findings

Unenhanced chest CT (lung window) (**Figs. 109.1A, 109.1B**) reveals bilateral, patchy ground glass opacities and thin-walled cysts that are more extensive in the lower lobes. There is mild interlobular septal thickening (**Fig. 109.1B**). A 1.0 cm nodule is also seen in the left lower lobe (**Fig. 109.1A**).

■ Diagnosis

Lymphocytic Interstitial Pneumonia (LIP)
(Biopsy of left lower lobe nodule revealed amyloid deposition)

■ Differential Diagnosis

Immunocompetent Patients

* Nonspecific Interstitial Pneumonia (NSIP)
* Hypersensitivity Pneumonitis (HP)
* Various Drug Reactions
* Sarcoidosis
* Low-grade B-Cell Lymphoma; Mucosal-Associated Lymphoid Tissue (MALT)
* Lymphangitic Carcinomatosis

Patients with HIV-AIDS

* *Pneumocystis jiroveci* Pneumonia
* *Mycobacterium avium-intracellulare* Complex Infection
* Fungal Pneumonia

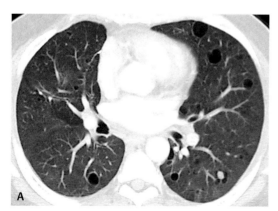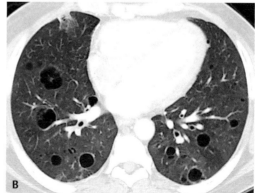

Fig. 109.1

■ Discussion

Background

Lymphoid interstitial pneumonia (LIP) is a rare form of interstitial pneumonia characterized by diffuse infiltration of the alveolar septa by dense lymphocytic infiltration. It has been regarded as part of the spectrum of pulmonary lymphoproliferative disorders, ranging in severity from such benign entities as follicular bronchiolitis to low-grade lymphoma. LIP is a non-neoplastic entity that may be distinguished from lymphoma by immunologic stains. Most patients with LIP have underlying autoimmune disease or immunodeficiency (e.g., Sjögren syndrome, AIDS). Conditions associated with LIP include collagen vascular and autoimmune diseases, systemic immunodeficiency states, drug-induced injury, and infection (other than HIV). LIP may also occur as a complication of bone marrow transplantation. Idiopathic LIP is extremely rare.

Etiology

The etiology and pathogenesis are varied. An immunologic basis for LIP is postulated because of the association of LIP with other immunologic disorders (e.g., AIDS and Sjögren syndrome). Some cases likely represent a form of hypersensitivity pneumonitis, whereas other cases may be caused by viral infection (e.g., HIV, Epstein-Barr).

Clinical Findings

LIP is most often seen in HIV(+) children and is considered an AIDS-defining diagnosis in children less than 13 years of age. Less than 1% of HIV-infected adults develop LIP. Adults who are not infected with HIV and develop LIP often have underlying autoimmune disease, most commonly Sjögren syndrome. Approximately 1% of adults with Sjögren syndrome have LIP, whereas up to 25% of adults with LIP have Sjögren syndrome. Whether LIP is idiopathic or related to an underlying systemic disease, most adults with LIP are women in the fourth to seventh decades of life who present with cough and/or dyspnea (50–80%), and 60% of patients have dysproteinemia and hypergammaglobulinemia. B-cell lymphoma may develop in patients with LIP, especially those with Sjögren syndrome; 5% of patients with LIP develop disseminated malignant lymphoma. Recent reports have described the concurrence of LIP, Sjögren syndrome, and nodular amyloid deposition.

Imaging Findings

Chest Radiography

- Preserved lung volume
- Non-specific bilateral reticular-nodular and ground glass opacities with or without consolidation
- Lower lung zone predilection
- Nodular pattern and lymphadenopathy more common in AIDS patients
- Rare pleural effusions

MDCT/HRCT

- Diffuse, bilateral, patchy areas of ground glass opacity (**Fig. 109.1B**) and/or poorly defined centrilobular nodules (100%) (**Figs. 109.1A, 109.1B**)
- Small juxtapleural nodules (86%) (**Fig. 109.2**)
- Peribronchovascular bundle thickening (86%)
- Mild interlobular septal thickening (82%) (**Fig. 109.1B**)
- Thin-walled cystic airspaces (68%) (**Figs. 109.1A, 109.1B, 109.2**)
- Less common: larger nodules, 1–3 cm diameter

Management

- Immunocompetent patients: corticosteroids with variable response
- Immunocompromised patients with AIDS and progressive symptoms: highly active antiretroviral therapy (HAART)

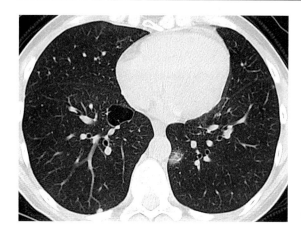

Fig. 109.2 Unenhanced chest CT demonstrates a patchy area of ground glass opacity in the left lower lobe and a thin-walled cyst and subpleural nodule in the right lower lobe.

Prognosis

- Variable clinical course; spontaneous remissions reported
- Death within five years in one-third to one-half of affected immunocompetent adult patients from infectious complications secondary to immunosuppressive drug therapy, respiratory insufficiency, or malignant lymphoma
- Most immunocompromised patients with AIDS and LIP have mild disease that may spontaneously resolve
- Rarely, LIP may evolve into lymphoma

PEARLS

- Cystic air spaces are seen more commonly in LIP (82%) than in lymphoma (2%).
- Air space consolidation is seen more commonly in lymphoma (66%) than in LIP (18%).
- Nodules measuring 10–30 mm are seen more commonly in lymphoma (41%) than in LIP (6%).
- Pleural effusions are seen more commonly in lymphoma.
- Nodules detected on HRCT in patients with LIP may represent amyloid deposits.

Suggested Reading

1. Do KH, Lee JS, Seo JB, et al. Pulmonary parenchymal involvement of low-grade lymphoproliferative disorders. J Comput Assist Tomogr 2005;29(6):825–830

2. Mueller-Mang C, Grosse C, Schmid K, Stiebellehner L, Bankier AA. What every radiologist should know about idiopathic interstitial pneumonias. Radiographics 2007;27(3):595–615

3. Lynch DA, Travis WD, Müller NL, et al. Idiopathic interstitial pneumonias: CT features. Radiology 2005;236(1): 10–21

4. Travis WD, Galvin JR. Non-neoplastic pulmonary lymphoid lesions. Thorax 2001;56(12):964–971

5. Honda O, Johkoh T, Ichikado K, et al. Differential diagnosis of lymphocytic interstitial pneumonia and malignant lymphoma on high-resolution CT. AJR Am J Roentgenol 1999;173(1):71–74

CASE 110

■ Clinical Presentation

56-year-old woman treated for presumed community-acquired pneumonia for the last two months without improvement complains of dyspnea, persistent non-productive cough, and recent 8 pound weight loss.

■ Radiologic Findings

PA (**Fig. 110.1A**) and lateral (**Fig. 110.1B**) chest radiographs demonstrate bilateral perihilar and upper lobe non-segmental consolidations. HRCT (**Figs. 110.1C, 110.1D, 110.1E, 110.1F**) reveals patchy bilateral consolidations and ground glass opacities with a peribronchial distribution. Pleural tails extend out from the opacities to the chest wall. Bronchial wall thickening and dilatation can be seen.

■ Diagnosis

Cryptogenic Organizing Pneumonia (COP)

■ Differential Diagnosis

- Acute Interstitial Pneumonia (AIP)
- Non-Specific Interstitial Pneumonia (NSIP)
- Chronic Eosinophilic Pneumonia
- Sarcoidosis
- Chronic Aspiration
- Diffuse Alveolar Damage (DAD)
- Desquamative Interstitial Pneumonia (DIP)

■ Discussion

Background

Organizing pneumonia (*OP*) is histologically characterized by intraluminal plugs of granulation tissue within alveolar ducts and surrounding alveoli, with associated chronic inflammation in the surrounding lung. Because granulation tissue polyps are also present in the respiratory bronchioles, OP is also called *bronchiolitis obliterans with organizing pneumonia* (*BOOP*). Because the clinical, functional, radiologic, and HRCT features of this interstitial lung disease are primarily the result of an organizing pneumonia, the American Thoracic Society/European Respiratory Multidisciplinary Consensus Classification Committee has proposed *cryptogenic organizing pneumonia* (*COP*) as an alternative designation in idiopathic cases. The exact incidence and prevalence are unknown. The diagnosis is usually made on open lung biopsy.

Etiology

Most cases of OP are idiopathic (COP). Numerous conditions may be associated with an OP- or BOOP-like reaction, including but not limited to collagen vascular diseases, pulmonary infection (e.g., HIV, *Pneumocystis* pneumonia, *Mycoplasma* pneumonia), inflammatory bowel disease, hypersensitivity pneumonitis, drug toxicity, vasculitides (e.g., Wegener granulomatosis), intravenous drug abuse (e.g., cocaine), drug reactions, toxic fume inhalation, and lung and chest wall irradiation.

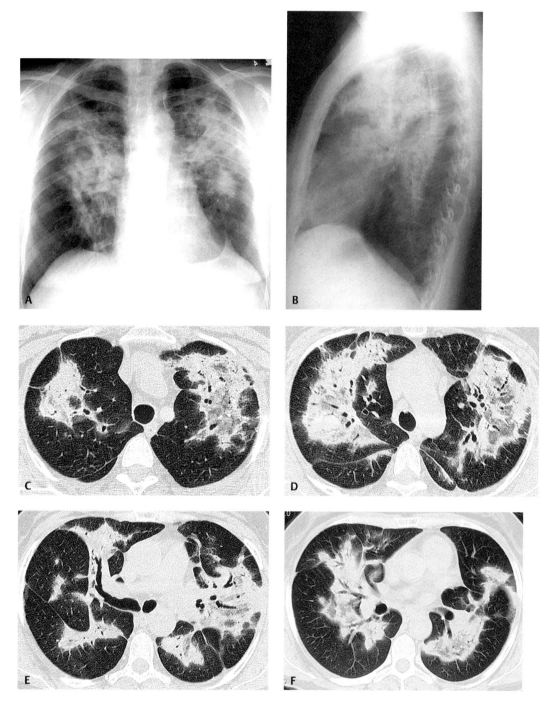

Fig. 110.1

Clinical Findings

Patients affected with COP typically present in the fifth or sixth decade of life with symptoms of non-resolving community-acquired pneumonia. Most patients have had symptoms for two or three months and complain of persistent non-productive cough. Dyspnea, malaise, and low-grade fever are not uncommon. Flu-like illness may herald the onset of COP. Weight loss of less than 10 pounds is common. Inspiratory crackles may be heard, but wheezing is rare. PFTs often show a restrictive pattern and DLCO is reduced. Hypoxemia is usually present. Fifty percent of patients with COP have leukocytosis.

Imaging Findings

Chest Radiography

- Non-specific
- Patchy, non-segmental, unilateral or bilateral consolidations (**Figs. 110.1A, 110.1B**)
- Irregular reticular opacities less common
- Small nodular opacities with or without air space consolidations

MDCT/HRCT

Multiple Patterns

Alveolar Opacities

- Patchy consolidation, varying from a few centimeters to the entire lobe; often admixed with ground glass opacities (80–90%) (**Figs. 110.1C, 110.1D, 110.1E, 110.1F**)
- Air bronchograms common; bronchial wall thickening or dilatation in affected lung (**Figs. 110.1C, 110.1D, 110.1E, 110.1F**)
- Bilateral; often symmetric; juxtapleural and or peribronchial in distribution (60–80%); lower lung zone predilection (**Figs. 110.1C, 110.1D, 110.1E, 110.1F**)
- Ground glass/consolidation peripheral edge of radiation therapy port in those select patients
- Ground glass/consolidation may be migratory and wax and wane over weeks to months (similar to eosinophilic pneumonia)
- *Reverse halo* or *atoll sign*—central ground glass opacity surrounded by denser consolidation at least 2 mm thick (20%)
- Parenchymal bands (25%)
- Lung volumes preserved

Nodules

- Centrilobular nodules 1–10 mm diameter (30–50%)
- No zonal predilection

Mass

- Larger nodules or masses; two to eight per patient
  - 8 mm to 5 cm diameter
  - Irregular (88%) or spiculated (35%) margins
  - Air bronchograms (45%)
  - Pleural tails (50%)
  - Vessels converge on lesion edge (80%)
- Upper lung zone predilection (60%)
- Juxtapleural (40%); peripheral bronchovascular (33%); peripheral (30%)
- Satellite nodules (55%)

Perilobular Pattern

- Poorly defined linear opacities located in periphery of SPL (60%)
- Greater in thickness than linear opacities seen with thickened interlobular septa
- Polygonal or arcade appearance
- Predilection for mid and lower lung zones

Reticular Interstitial Pattern (10%)

- Mimics IPF/NSIP
- Irregular linear opacities; honeycombing uncommon

Mediastinal Lymphadenopathy (20–40%)

- Right paratracheal
- Subcarinal

Pleural

- Small pleural effusion(s) (10–30%) or pleural thickening (33%)

Management

- Complete recovery and radiographic normalization in two-thirds of patients treated with corticosteroids
- Persistent disease: one-third of patients despite corticosteroid therapy
- Cytotoxic drugs (e.g., cyclophosphamide, azathioprine) for corticosteroid failures; limited success

Prognosis

- Dramatic clinical response with improvement in days or weeks
- Relapses common two or three months after steroid withdrawal
- Worse prognosis in patients with primarily interstitial opacities

PEARLS

- Presence of consolidation is associated with greater likelihood of corticosteroid response.
- Consolidation is a more common pattern seen in immunocompetent patients (91%), whereas nodules are more commonly seen in immunocompromised patients (55%).
- IPF and COP/BOOP can appear clinically and functionally similar. Duration of symptoms and response to steroids in patients with COP aid in differentiation.
- Consolidation and a paucity of reticular opacities differentiate COP from UIP on imaging.

Suggested Reading

1. American Thoracic Society; European Respiratory Society. American Thoracic Society/European Respiratory Society International Multidisciplinary Consensus Classification of the Idiopathic Interstitial Pneumonias. This joint statement of the American Thoracic Society (ATS) and the European Respiratory Society (ERS) was adopted by the ATS board of directors, June 2001, and by the ERS Executive Committee, June 2001. Am J Respir Crit Care Med 2002;165(2): 277–304

2. Gurney JW, Winer-Muram HT, Rosado-de-Christenson ML, et al. Cryptogenic organizing pneumonia. In: Specialty Imaging-HRCT of the Lung: Anatomic Basis, Imaging Features, Differential Diagnosis. Salt Lake City: Amirsys, Inc.; 2009: 96–101

3. Kim SJ, Lee KS, Ryu YH, et al. Reversed halo sign on high-resolution CT of cryptogenic organizing pneumonia: diagnostic implications. AJR Am J Roentgenol 2003;180(5):1251–1254

4. Webb WR, Müller NL, Naidich DP. The idiopathic interstitial pneumonias. In: High-Resolution CT of the Lung, 4th ed. Philadelphia: Lippincott, Williams & Wilkins; 2009:200–206

5. Zompatori M, Poletti V, Battista G, Diegoli M. Bronchiolitis obliterans with organizing pneumonia (BOOP), presenting as a ring-shaped opacity at HRCT (the atoll sign). A case report. Radiol Med (Torino) 1999;97(4):308–310

CASE 111

■ Clinical Presentation

34-year-old man with recent sore throat, chills, and fever, subsequently developed hematuria, dysuria, cough, dyspnea, hemoptysis, and respiratory failure

■ Radiologic Findings

AP chest radiograph (**Fig. 111.1A**) reveals diffuse bilateral air space opacities. Chest CT (lung window), coronal reformatted image (**Fig. 111.1B**), and axial images (**Figs. 111.1C, 111.1D**) reveal diffuse bilateral ground glass opacity and patchy areas of consolidation.

■ Diagnosis

Diffuse Alveolar Hemorrhage; Goodpasture Syndrome

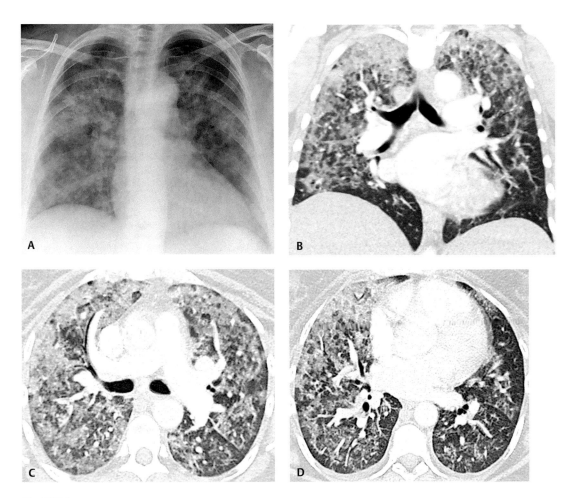

Fig. 111.1

541

■ Differential Diagnosis

- Idiopathic Pulmonary Hemorrhage
- Other Diffuse Pulmonary Hemorrhage Syndromes
  ○ Wegener Granulomatosis
  ○ Henoch-Schonlein Purpura
  ○ Microscopic Polyangiitis Pauci–Immune Glomerulonephritis
  ○ Systemic Lupus Erythematosus
- Sequela of Drug Therapy
  ○ Drug-Induced Coagulopathy
  ○ Penicillamine; Nitrofurantoin; Amiodarone
- Crack Cocaine Abuse
- Environmental Exposures
  ○ Paraquat (Zeneca Ag Products, Wilmington, DE)
  ○ Pesticides
  ○ Leather Conditioners
  ○ Isocyanates
- Bone Marrow and Heart-Lung Transplantation
- Dieulafoy Disease (e.g., endobronchial vascular malformation)

■ Discussion

Background

Diffuse alveolar hemorrhage (DAH) is characterized by extensive intra-alveolar hemorrhage. DAH may be acute, chronic, recurrent, idiopathic, or associated with a variety of systemic disorders.

Etiology

Goodpasture syndrome is an anti–basement membrane antibody disease (ABMABD) that affects the lung alone in 10% of patients (e.g., DAH), the kidneys alone in 20–40% of patients (e.g., glomerulonephritis), and both organ systems in 60–80% of patients.

Clinical Findings

Most patients with DAH experience acute dyspnea, which may progress to respiratory failure, and hemoptysis. However, hemoptysis may be absent even with severe intra-alveolar hemorrhage. Uveitis, fever, arthralgias, arthritis, and dermatologic leukocytoclastic vasculitis may be clues to the diagnosis. Elevated erythrocyte sedimentation rate (ESR), elevated white blood count, falling hematocrit levels, and impaired renal function may be seen. Elevated serum antineutrophil cytoplasmic antibody (ANCA) to myeloperoxidase may be seen, depending on the underlying systemic disease. Hypoxemia is invariably present and often severe, and affected patients may require ventilatory support. Most patients with Goodpasture syndrome are young Caucasian men presenting with recent viral illness, cough, fever, respiratory alkalosis, hemoptysis (80–90%), and renal disease (e.g., azotemia, hematuria, proteinuria, granular casts). Alternatively, Goodpasture syndrome may occur in elderly women with kidney disease. The mean age at presentation is 35 years, and men are affected two to nine times as often as women. Over 90% of patients have antiglomerular basement membrane antibodies. Recurrent episodes of pulmonary hemorrhage may be associated with the development of interstitial fibrosis and eventual respiratory failure.

Imaging Findings

Chest Radiography

- Patchy or diffuse bilateral ground glass opacities or frank consolidation (**Fig. 111.1A**)
- Widespread or perihilar/basilar opacities gradually resolve over two to three weeks after cessation of hemorrhage
- Following acute hemorrhage, replacement of air space opacities by interstitial opacities or septal thickening

MDCT/HRCT

- Patchy or diffuse ground glass opacity or consolidation (**Figs. 111.1B, 111.1C, 111.1D, 111.2, 111.3**)
- Sparing of subpleural lung may occur (**Fig. 111.3**)
- Ill-defined centrilobular nodules (**Fig. 111.3**)
- Interlobular septal thickening may develop over several days (**Figs. 111.2, 111.3**)
- Crazy paving pattern (**Figs. 111.2, 111.3**)

Management

- Directed toward underlying systemic disease
- Intravenous corticosteroids: acute fulminant disease
- Immunosuppressive therapy (e.g., cyclophosphamide, azathioprine)
- ABMABD: Plasmapheresis to remove circulating antibodies and immunosuppressive agents
- Renal transplantation for patients who develop end-stage renal disease

Prognosis

- Fulminant clinical course
- Pulmonary fibrosis resulting from repeated hemorrhage
- Long-term survival in over 50% of patients with Goodpasture syndrome; dialysis dependence common
- Mean survival of three to five years in patients with idiopathic pulmonary hemorrhage
- Death from massive pulmonary hemorrhage (25%)
- Persistent active disease with repeated hemoptysis, complicating pulmonary fibrosis, and cor pulmonale (25%)
- Persistent anemia and dyspnea (25%)
- Recovery without recurrence (25%)

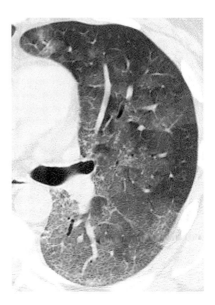

Fig. 111.2 Chest CT demonstrates patchy ground glass opacity and areas of mild interlobular septal thickening ("crazy paving" pattern).

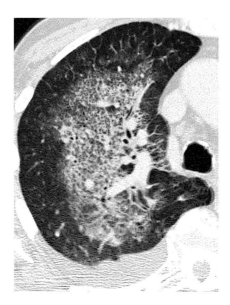

Fig. 111.3 Chest CT demonstrates patchy ground glass opacity and mild interlobular septal thickening that is seen as an isolated finding in the medial aspect of the right upper lobe, and elsewhere in combination with the ground glass opacity (i.e., "crazy paving" pattern). There is relative sparing of the peripheral lung.

- Diffuse pulmonary hemorrhage should be suspected when imaging studies reveal the acute onset of bilateral, diffuse, or predominantly basilar consolidation in an anemic patient.
- Within 48 hours of the onset of diffuse alveolar hemorrhage, intralobular and smooth interlobular septal thickening may develop within areas of ground glass ("crazy paving" pattern).
- Repeated episodes of pulmonary hemorrhage may lead to fibrosis.

Suggested Reading

1. Travis WD. Pathology of pulmonary vasculitis. Semin Respir Crit Care Med 2004;25(5):475–482

2. Jara LJ, Vera-Lastra O, Calleja MC. Pulmonary-renal vasculitic disorders: differential diagnosis and management. Curr Rheumatol Rep 2003;5(2):107–115

3. Travis WD, Colby TV, Koss MN, et al. Reactive lymphoid lesions. In: King DW, ed. Atlas of Nontumor Pathology: Non-Neoplastic Disorders of the Lower Respiratory Tract, first series, fascicle 2. Washington, DC: American Registry of Pathology; 2002:176–186

4. Primack SL, Miller RR, Müller NL. Diffuse pulmonary hemorrhage: clinical, pathologic, and imaging features. AJR Am J Roentgenol 1995;164(2):295–300

5. Ball JA, Young KR Jr. Pulmonary manifestations of Goodpasture's syndrome. Antiglomerular basement membrane disease and related disorders. Clin Chest Med 1998;19(4):777–791, ix

CASE 112

■ Clinical Presentation

55-year-old man with progressive dyspnea on exertion

■ Radiologic Findings

Contrast-enhanced chest CT (lung window, **Figs. 112.1A, 112.1C, 112.1E**; mediastinal window, **Figs. 112.1B, 112.1D, 112.1F**) demonstrates interlobular septal and fissural thickening and calcification, juxtapleural and pleural calcification, and profuse micronodular calcifications throughout both lungs. Note the preferential involvement of the peripheral secondary pulmonary lobule, producing sharply defined polygonal calcific opacities.

■ Diagnosis

Pulmonary Alveolar Microlithiasis (PAM)

■ Differential Diagnosis

- Amyloidosis (diffuse septal form)
- Granulomatous Infection
  - Miliary Tuberculosis
  - Disseminated Fungal Disease
- Sarcoidosis (micronodules more profuse in upper lobes; rarely calcify)
- Silicosis (micronodules more profuse in upper lobes)
- Talcosis (upper lobe nodules; aggregate into perihilar masses)
- Metastatic Ossification Chronic Renal Failure (calcifications larger; less well defined)
- Idiopathic Ossification (elderly men; calcifications not as pronounced)

■ Discussion

Background

Pulmonary alveolar microlithiasis (PAM) is a rare disorder characterized by accumulation of calcium phosphate calcospherites within the alveolar spaces.

Etiology

The etiology is unknown. A familial occurrence (autosomal recessive) has been noted in approximately 50% of reported cases.

Clinical Findings

Most patients (70%) are asymptomatic despite grossly abnormal chest radiography acquired for unrelated reasons. The most common symptom is dyspnea on exertion. Patients may develop a non-productive cough and on occasion may expectorate microliths. As the disease progresses, respiratory insufficiency may develop. The average age at presentation is 35 years (range 20–50 years). Sporadic cases are more common in men, whereas familial cases are more common in women. Serum calcium and phosphorus levels are usually normal.

545

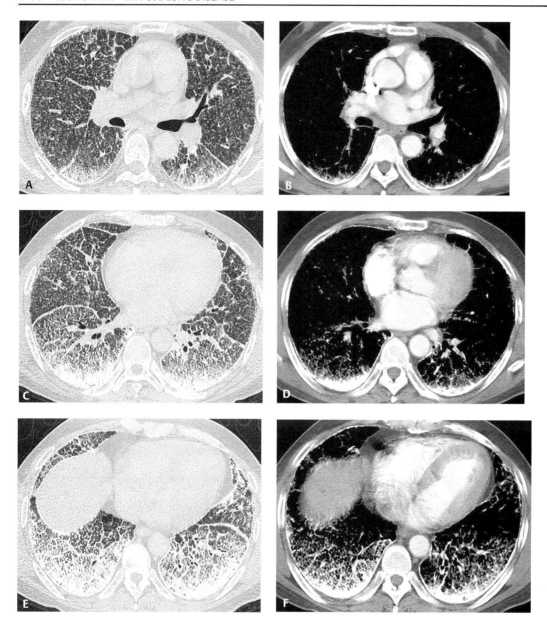

Fig. 112.1

Imaging Findings

Chest Radiography

- Dense lungs (out of proportion to clinical symptoms) (**Figs. 112.2A, 112.2B**)
  - May silhouette heart border and diaphragm (**Figs. 112.2A, 112.2B**)
- Calcifications often more dense medially than laterally
- *Sandstorm sign*—diffuse miliary calcifications distributed through lungs (**Figs. 112.2A, 112.2B**)
- *Black pleural line* (**Fig. 112.2B**)
- ± Apical bulla

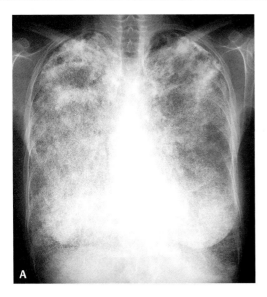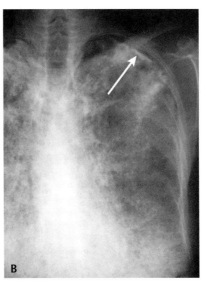

Fig. 112.2   PA chest radiograph **(A)** and coned-down view of the left lung **(B)** demonstrate dense diffuse bilateral micronodular parenchymal opacities with confluence and calcification in the lung apices. Note the *black pleural line* (*arrow*) adjacent to the apical calcification.

MDCT/HRCT

- Early disease: ground glass/reticulation predominant finding; precedes calcification
- Discrete micronodular calcifications (0.2–3 mm) (**Figs. 112.1A, 112.1C, 112.1E**) superimposed on ground glass may create a "crazy paving" pattern
- Micronodular calcifications may become confluent, forming areas of consolidation
- Two patterns of calcospherite distribution
  - Diffuse, but gradient of calcospherite deposition greatest in lung bases and dorsal juxtapleural aspect of lung; symmetric (**Figs. 112.1A, 112.1C, 112.1E**)
  - Anterolateral aspect of middle lobe, lingula, and anterior upper lobes
- Perilobular (**Figs. 112.1A, 112.1C, 112.1E**) and centrilobular distribution of calcifications
- Calcifications may be associated with interlobular septa and bronchovascular bundles (50%) (**Figs. 112.1A, 112.1C, 112.1E**)
- Intraparenchymal cysts; paraseptal and centrilobular emphysema; juxtapleural cysts (latter etiology of *black pleural line*)
- Reticular opacities; interstitial; thickening (50%)
- Pleural calcifications (20%); fissural calcification (90%) (**Figs. 112.1A, 112.1C, 112.1E**)

Scintigraphy

- Intense pulmonary uptake of Tc-99m-MDP

Management

- No known treatment
- Bronchoalveolar lavage ineffective
- Steroids and chelating agents ineffective
- Disodium etidronate; inhibits microcrystal hydroxyapatite, reversing micolithiasis in some patients
- Lung transplant; end-stage lung disease

Prognosis

- Slow progression over time
- Respiratory failure; pulmonary artery hypertension; cardiac failure may develop

PEARLS

- No other pulmonary disease has a radiologic pattern as characteristic and diagnostic.
- Lack of association between radiologic and clinical findings is more pronounced in PAM than in any other condition.

Suggested Reading

1. Gurney JW, Winer-Muram HT, Rosado-de-Christenson ML, et al. Alveolar microlithiasis In: Specialty Imaging-HRCT of the Lung: Anatomic Basis, Imaging Features, Differential Diagnosis. Salt Lake City: Amirsys, Inc.; 2009:296–299

2. Deniz O, Ors F, Tozkoparan E, et al. High resolution computed tomographic features of pulmonary alveolar microlithiasis. Eur J Radiol 2005;55(3):452–460

3. Marchiori E, Gonçalves CM, Escuissato DL, et al. Pulmonary alveolar microlithiasis: high-resolution computed tomography findings in 10 patients. J Bras Pneumol 2007;33(5):552–557

4. Webb WR, Müller NL, Naidich DP. High-resolution computed tomography findings of lung disease. In: High-Resolution CT of the Lung, 4th ed. Philadelphia: Lippincott, Williams & Wilkins; 2009:133

CASE 113

■ Clinical Presentation

41-year-old man with mental retardation. CT scan was acquired to evaluate a suspected lung mass identified on outside chest radiography (not available).

■ Radiologic Findings

Contrast-enhanced chest CT (**Fig. 113.1A**, mediastinal window; **Fig. 113.1B**, lung window) through the right middle lobe demonstrates a focal mass-like region of consolidation with a mild degree of surrounding ground glass. Note the low-attenuation regions in the consolidation. Contrast-enhanced chest CT (**Fig. 113.1C**, mediastinal window; **Fig. 113.1D**, lung window) through the lower lobes demonstrates mass-like regions of basilar consolidation containing low-attenuation areas and surrounding ground glass. Mild interlobular septal thickening is seen in the right base. A calcified nodule is present in the right lung base. Corresponding chest CT images with deposited regions of interest reveal attenuation coefficients ranging between –80 HU in the left lower lobe (**Fig. 113.1E**) and –44 HU in the right lower lobe (**Fig. 113.1F**). The attenuation coefficients in the right middle lobe consolidation were estimated at –68 HU (not illustrated).

■ Diagnosis

Exogenous Lipoid Pneumonia

■ Differential Diagnosis

- Endogenous Lipoid Pneumonia—in the setting of proximal or distal airway obstruction
- Pseudolipoid Pneumonia—an air bubble artifact associated with collapse of air spaces
- Infection
- Primary Lung Cancer
- Pulmonary Lymphoma
- Other Fat-Containing Lesions

Differential Diagnosis: Other Intrathoracic Fat-Containing Lesions

- Hamartoma
- Lipoma
- Liposarcoma
- Germ Cell Tumors
- Mediastinal Lipomatosis
- Thymolipoma
- Diaphragmatic Hernias, Fat Herniation

■ Discussion

Background

Exogenous lipid pneumonia (ELP) is an uncommon cause of parenchymal consolidation secondary to chronic aspiration or inhalation of animal, vegetable, or petroleum-based oils or fats.

549

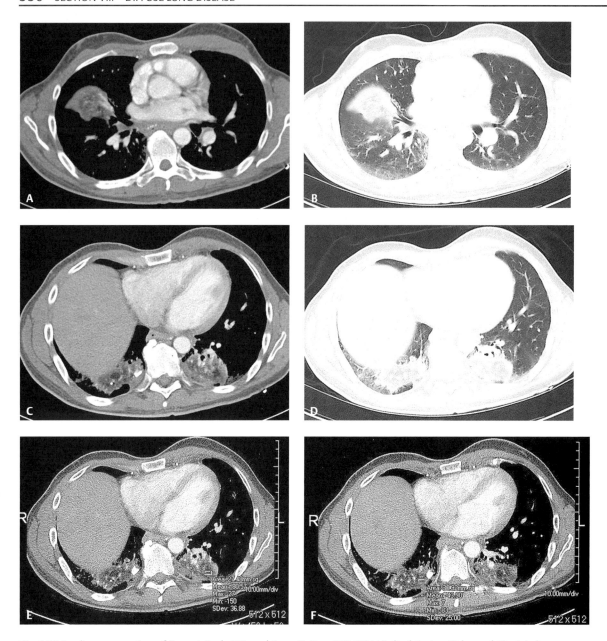

Fig. 113.1   *(Images courtesy of Susan J. Back, MD, and Roger Tutton, MD, VCU Medical Center; Richmond, Virginia.)*

Etiology

Mineral oil is the most common irritant and has the ability to inhibit the cough reflex and ciliary motility, resulting in a "silent" inhalation. ELP is more common in the elderly, young children, and debilitated patients. Two-thirds of patients have a predisposition to aspiration from swallowing dysfunction, structural esophageal abnormalities, or altered consciousness. Infants with feeding difficulties may aspirate oil used as a lubricant. Elderly patients with constipation may aspirate oil ingested as a laxative. Other potential sources include oil-based nose drops, camphor and eucalyptus oil-based cough suppressants and nasal decongestants, lip gloss, and petroleum jelly applied to the face and nose for various reasons. Aspiration of animal oils may be associated with ingestion of milk or milk products, and cod liver and shark liver oil. Most vegetable oil aspirations occur during eating or with regurgitation of gastric contents. Pure vegetable oil aspiration is uncommon. An unusual form of ELP is seen in "fire eaters" who use liquid paraffin to help generate the fire. The pathogenesis of mineral and vegetable oil–related fibrosis is unknown, but the release of lysosomal enzymes by lipid-laden macrophages may be responsible. Animal fats hydrolyzed by lung lipases into fatty acids may cause acute hemorrhagic pneumonitis.

Clinical Findings

Most patients with mineral oil–related ELP are asymptomatic and present as an incidental radiologic finding. The most frequent signs and symptoms associated with animal and vegetable oil–related ELP mirror those of acute bronchopneumonia and include fever (39%), weight loss (34%), cough (64%), dyspnea (50%), and crepitations (45%). Lung function is usually normal or shows a restrictive pattern. DLCO is frequently diminished. BAL fluid often shows non-specific increases in lymphocytes, eosinophils, multi-nucleated giant cells containing lipid droplets, and large numbers of lipid-laden macrophages. This latter finding is highly suggestive of chronic aspiration or lipoid pneumonia.

Imaging Findings

Radiography

- Variable patterns depending on the volume and nature of aspirate
- Preferential involvement of dependent lung zones
- Cavitation in cases of secondary anaerobic infection
- Acute aspiration of large amounts of animal oil:
  - Extensive ground glass opacities and/or
  - Frank regions of consolidation
- Aspiration of mineral oil:
  - Ground glass opacities
  - Septal lines
  - Lung mass resembling primary lung cancer
- Aspiration of vegetable oil:
  - Inconspicuous
  - Atelectasis
  - Variable-size, poorly defined nodular opacities

MDCT/HRCT

- Preferential involvement of dependent lung zones
- Ground glass opacities
  - Initial pattern (50%) with centrilobular or panlobular distribution due to aspiration
- Ground glass and interstitial opacities forming "crazy paving pattern" (33%)
  - Develops over two to four weeks
- Patchy unilateral or bilateral air space consolidation(s) (90%) (**Figs. 113.1, 113.2**)
- Consolidation with internal low or fat attenuation (–10 to –150 HU) (i.e., attenuation less than chest wall musculature but greater than subcutaneous fat) (80%) (**Figs. 113.1A, 113.1C, 113.1E, 113.1F, 113.2B**)
- Centrilobular nodules
- Foci of calcification; rare (**Figs. 113.1C, 113.1E, 113.1F**)
- Chronic cases: juxtapleural pulmonary fibrosis; architectural distortion, honeycombing; volume loss

MRI

- High signal intensity on both T1- and T2-weighted images (i.e., lipid content)
- Chemical shift/in-phase/out-of-phase imaging useful to make a specific diagnosis

PET

- FDG-PET scans reveal standard uptake values (SUV) suggestive of malignancy (**Figs. 113.2C, 113.2D**)

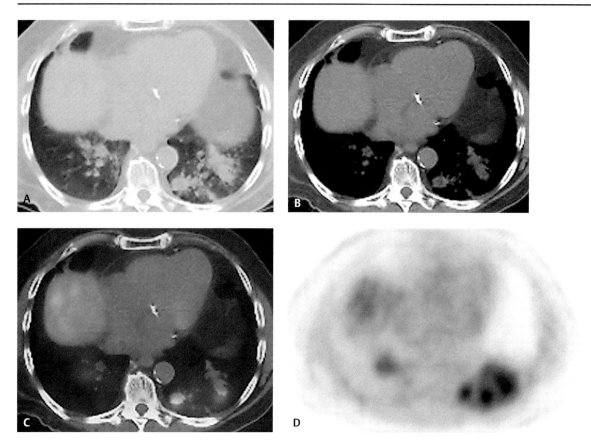

Fig. 113.2   Unenhanced chest CT (lung window, **A**; mediastinal window, **B**) of a 50-year-old man with colon cancer and suspected pulmonary metastases demonstrates ill-defined, spiculated nodular areas of mass-like consolidation and centrilobular nodules in the posterobasal segments of both lower lobes. Regions of low or fat attenuation can be seen in the areas of consolidation **(B)**. Fused transverse PET/CT images **(C,D)** show focal increased uptake of ¹⁸F-FDG in the areas of basilar disease, suggesting neoplasia. (*See color insert following page 108.*) Diagnosis: false-positive FDG-PET from biopsy-proven lipoid pneumonia.

Management

- Mainstay: removal of offending agent
- Correction of underlying defects or abnormalities predisposing to aspiration
- Oral steroids; helpful in select cases
- Prednisone and whole lung lavage; may be successful in cases of diffuse ELP

Prognosis

- May be complicated by superimposed infection; should be suspected when cavitary nodules are present
- Increased risk of infection with nontuberculous mycobacteria (e.g., *Mycobacterium fortuitum*, *Mycobacterium chelonae*) and of developing primary lung cancer
- Clinical course and outcome of animal and vegetable oil aspiration: similar to that of aspiration of gastric contents

PEARLS

- ELP predominantly affects the lower lobes; posterior segments of upper lobes, superior segments of lower lobes, and middle lobes are affected less often.

- ELP may mimic primary and secondary lung neoplasia; appropriate diagnosis is dependent upon recognition of fat or low-attenuation areas in the consolidation.
- Increased risk of infection with *Mycobacterium fortuitum* and *Mycobacterium chelonae* and of developing primary lung cancer.
- ELP-avid F-18-fluorodeoxyglucose (FDG) uptake on positron emission tomography (PET) imaging; mimics neoplasia (false positive).

Suggested Reading

1. Fox BD, Shechtman I, Shitrit D, Bendayan D, Kramer MR. A "fat chance" it's malignant: lipoid pneumonia simulating lung cancer on PET scan. Thorax 2007;62(5):464

2. Gaerte SC, Meyer CA, Winer-Muram HT, et al. Fat containing lesions of the chest. Radiographics 2002;22:S61–S78

3. Kitchen JM, O'Brien DE, McLaughlin AM. Perils of fire eating. An acute form of lipoid pneumonia or fire eater's lung. Thorax 2008;63(5):401–439

4. Mokhlesi B, Angulo-Zereceda D, Yaghmai V. False-positive FDG-PET scan secondary to lipoid pneumonia mimicking a solid pulmonary nodule. Ann Nucl Med 2007;21(7):411–414

5. Travis WD, Colby TV, Koss MN, Rosado-de-Christenson ML, Müller NL, King TE Jr. Diffuse parenchymal lung diseases. In: King DW, ed. Atlas of Nontumor Pathology: Non-Neoplastic Disorders of the Lower Respiratory Tract, fascicle 2, series 1. Washington, DC: American Registry of Pathology and Armed Forces of Pathology; 2001:187–196

6. Zanetti G, Marchiori E, Gasparetto TD, Escuissato DL, Soares Souza A Jr. Lipoid pneumonia in children following aspiration of mineral oil used in the treatment of constipation: high-resolution CT findings in 17 patients. Pediatr Radiol 2007;37(11):1135–1139

CASE 114

■ Clinical Presentation

52-year-old woman with dyspnea and uveitis

■ Radiologic Findings

PA (**Fig. 114.1**) and lateral (**Fig. 114.2**) chest radiographs demonstrate profuse bilateral small pulmonary nodules most numerous in the upper and middle lung zones in association with symmetrical bilateral hilar lymphadenopathy. HRCT (**Figs. 114.3, 114.4**) reveals diffuse bilateral multi-focal micronodules distributed along perilymphatic areas, subpleural regions, interlobular septa, and bronchovascular bundles

■ Diagnosis

Sarcoidosis

■ Differential Diagnosis

- Pulmonary Infection
- Silicosis
- Lymphoproliferative Disorder
- Pulmonary Metastases

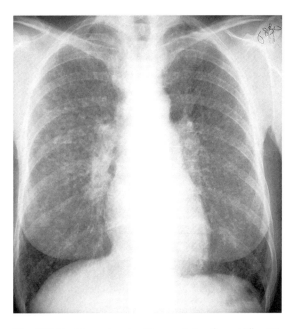

Fig. 114.1 *(Reproduced with permission from Miller BH, Rosado de Christenson ML, McAdams HP, Fishback NF. Thoracic Sarcoidosis: Radiologic-Pathologic Correlation. RadioGraphics 1995;15:421–437.)*

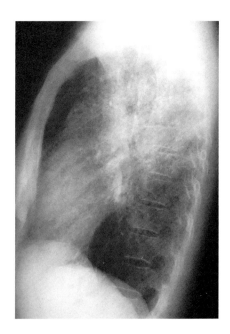

Fig. 114.2

554

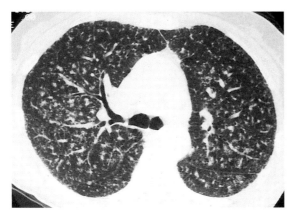

Fig. 114.3

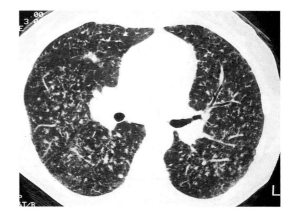

Fig. 114.4

■ Discussion

Background

Sarcoidosis is a systemic granulomatous disease that frequently affects the lung and the lymphatic system. The diagnosis is established based on typical clinical and radiologic findings supported by histologic evidence of non-caseating epithelioid granulomas in more than one organ.

Etiology

The etiology of sarcoidosis remains unknown. An abnormal immune-mediated response to a yet unidentified antigen has been postulated.

Clinical Findings

Most affected patients are under the age of 40 years, with a peak incidence between 20 and 29 years. Annual incidence in the United States is 35.5 per 100,000 persons for African Americans and 10.9 per 100,000 for Caucasians. High disease prevalences are also reported in Swedes and Danes. *Löfgren syndrome* is an acute form of sarcoidosis characterized by fever, polyarthralgias, erythema nodosum and bilateral hilar lymphadenopathy. *Heerfordt syndrome* is the association of fever, parotid enlargement, facial palsy, and anterior uveitis. Lupus pernio is a chronic form of sarcoidosis typified by indurated plaques and raised discoloration of the central face and ears.

Approximately 50% of patients with sarcoidosis are asymptomatic. Symptomatic patients may present with dry cough, dyspnea, chest pain, and hemoptysis. Non-specific symptoms are also reported, including constitutional symptoms, fatigue, weight loss, malaise, and fever. Pulmonary function studies may reveal restrictive abnormalities and decreased DLCO, but obstructive abnormalities can be seen with endobronchial sarcoidosis. Laboratory abnormalities include elevation of serum angiotensin converting enzyme (ACE), decreased blood serum CD4 to CD8 ratios, and hypercalcemia due to increased intestinal calcium absorption and activation of vitamin D by the sarcoid granulomas. Approximately 20% of patients develop pulmonary fibrosis, which may lead to pulmonary insufficiency and pulmonary hypertension.

Imaging Findings

Chest Radiography

Radiographic Staging System

- ∘ Stage 0: normal chest radiographs
- ∘ Stage 1: hilar and/or mediastinal lymphadenopathy
- ∘ Stage 2: lymphadenopathy and parenchymal abnormalities (**Figs. 114.1, 114.2, 114.5A**)

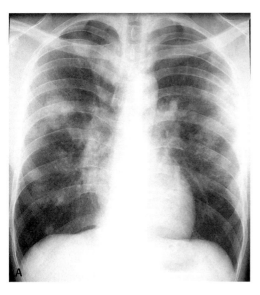
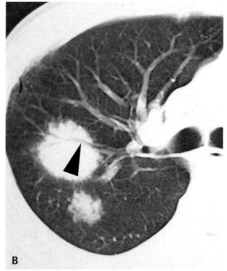

Fig. 114.5 PA chest radiograph **(A)** of a young woman with cough demonstrates bilateral ill-defined nodular opacities and bilateral hilar and subcarinal lymphadenopathy. Coned-down chest CT (lung window) **(B)** shows multifocal bilateral nodules and masses with a central distribution and intrinsic air bronchograms (*arrow*).

- ◦ Stage 3: parenchymal abnormalities, no visible lymphadenopathy
- ◦ Stage 4: upper lobe fibrosis, volume loss, hilar retraction, cystic change (**Figs. 114.6A, 114.7**)
- Intrathoracic lymphadenopathy
  - ◦ 80% of patients at presentation, typically bilateral and symmetric
  - ◦ Classic triad of right paratracheal and bilateral hilar lymphadenopathy, so-called 1-2-3 sign or *Garland triangle*
  - ◦ Bilateral hilar lymphadenopathy with or without mediastinal lymphadenopathy (95%) (**Figs. 114.1, 114.5A**)
  - ◦ Aortopulmonary window lymphadenopathy (76%)
  - ◦ Common involvement of 4R, 5, 7, 10R, 11R, 11L ATS lymph node stations; more conspicuous on CT
  - ◦ Calcified lymph nodes with chronicity of disease; 20% after 10 years (**Fig. 114.7**); may demonstrate *eggshell* pattern of calcification
- Pulmonary involvement
  - ◦ Bilateral, symmetric small nodular and reticular opacities with a predilection for the upper and middle lung zones (**Figs. 114.1, 114.2**)
  - ◦ Nodular (so-called alveolar or nummular) sarcoidosis: multi-focal nodules and/or masses with or without air bronchograms (**Fig. 114.5A**)
  - ◦ Rarely focal opacity, pleural effusion, pneumothorax, atelectasis, cavitation
  - ◦ Central upper lobe–predominant fibrosis with volume loss, hilar retraction, and cystic change; may be complicated by mycetoma (**Figs. 114.6A, 114.7**)

MDCT/HRCT

- Bilateral small discrete or irregular nodules with perilymphatic distribution (**Figs. 114.3, 114.4**): along subpleural regions, interlobular septa, bronchi, and vessels
- Miliary nodules
- Ground glass opacities, large nodules, and masses with perilymphatic distribution; may exhibit air bronchograms (**Fig. 114.5B**)
- *Sarcoid galaxy sign*—large nodular opacities with satellite micronodules
- Perihilar opacities radiating from the hilum with irregular edges, with or without air bronchograms
- Mosaic attenuation and air trapping on expiratory images
- Lymphadenopathy: bilateral, symmetric; may exhibit amorphous, punctate, and *eggshell* pattern of calcification

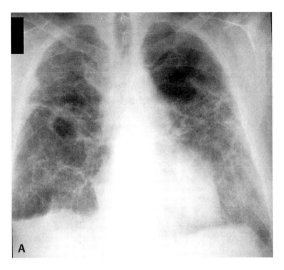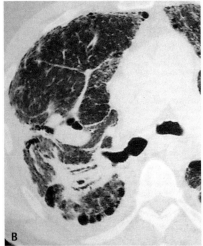

Fig. 114.6   PA chest radiograph **(A)** of a 49-year-old man with end-stage sarcoidosis demonstrates bilateral diffuse coarse central linear opacities, architectural distortion, and volume loss. Coned-down HRCT (lung window) **(B)** shows central architectural distortion, a right perihilar conglomerate mass, and posterior hilar retraction, traction bronchiectasis, and peripheral honeycomb lung. Note subtle perilymphatic micronodules in the subpleural and septal regions of the right lung.

- Pulmonary fibrosis: central and upper lobe distribution, architectural distortion, traction bronchiectasis, large cystic spaces, honeycomb lung (**Fig. 114.6B**)
    - Conglomerate central masses with superior/posterior hilar displacement
    - Peripheral honeycomb lung, bullae, and cystic spaces; may be complicated by saprophytic mycetoma

Scintigraphy

- Gallium-67 imaging; high sensitivity for active disease, low specificity
- Gallium-67 uptake patterns suggestive of sarcoidosis:
    - "Lambda" distribution: homogeneous uptake in hilar, infrahilar, and paratracheal lymph nodes
    - "Panda" distribution: bilateral symmetrical lacrimal gland and parotid gland uptake

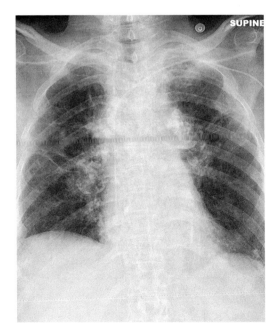

Fig. 114.7   Frontal chest radiograph of a 52-year-old man with end-stage sarcoidosis shows low lung volumes, central architectural distortion, and bilateral hilar and mediastinal lymphadenopathy. The enlarged lymph nodes exhibit "eggshell" calcifications.

Management

- Treatment of cardiac, ocular, central nervous system, and splenic involvement
- Corticosteroids; symptom relief, resolution of radiologic abnormalities, improved function
- Cytotoxic agents, chlorambucil, cyclophosphamides, and antimalarials
- Response to therapy does not prevent recurrence

Prognosis

- Favorable prognosis:
  - Acute presentation
  - Löfgren syndrome
  - Erythema nodosum
- Poor prognosis:
  - Insidious onset
  - Lupus pernio
  - Extrathoracic organ involvement
  - Pulmonary fibrosis
  - Non-Caucasian patient
- Two-thirds of patients have remission or stable disease
- 20% of patients develop chronic disease with pulmonary fibrosis
- Mortality approximately 5%
  - Pulmonary fibrosis
  - Cor pulmonale
  - Cardiac/central nervous system involvement, renal failure, pulmonary hemorrhage from mycetoma

Suggested Reading

1. Criado E, Sánchez M, Ramírez J, et al. Pulmonary sarcoidosis: typical and atypical manifestations at high-resolution CT with pathologic correlation. Radiographics 2010;30(6):1567–1586

2. Koyama T, Ueda H, Togashi K, Umeoka S, Kataoka M, Nagai S. Radiologic manifestations of sarcoidosis in various organs. Radiographics 2004;24(1):87–104

3. Statement on sarcoidosis. Joint Statement of the American Thoracic Society (ATS), the European Respiratory Society (ERS) and the World Association of Sarcoidosis and Other Granulomatous Disorders (WASOG) adopted by the ATS Board of Directors and by the ERS Executive Committee, February 1999. Am J Respir Crit Care Med 1999;160(2): 736–755

4. Travis WD, Colby TV, Koss MN, Rosado-de-Christenson ML, Müller NL, King TE Jr. Idiopathic interstitial pneumonia and other diffuse parenchymal lung diseases. In: King DW, ed. Atlas of Nontumor Pathology: Non-Neoplastic Disorders of the Lower Respiratory Tract, fasc 2, ser 1. Washington, DC: American Registry of Pathology and Armed Forces Institute of Pathology; 2001:49–231

CASE 115

■ Clinical Presentation

51-year-old female non-smoker with progressive dyspnea over the last several months

■ Radiologic Findings

PA (**Fig. 115.1A**) and lateral (**Fig. 115.1B**) chest radiographs reveal bilateral perihilar ground glass opacities and ill-defined subcentimeter nodular opacities. Note the preservation of lung volume and the absence of pulmonary edema, pleural effusions, and lymphadenopathy. Chest CT (**Figs. 115.1C, 115.1D, 115.1E, 115.1F, 115.1G, 115.1H**) (lung window) demonstrates mosaic perfusion and diffuse, patchy, ground glass opacities with innumerable ill-defined, "fuzzy" centrilobular nodules. Note the lobular areas of hypoattenuated lung parenchyma (**Figs. 115.1D, 115.1E, 115.1H**)

■ Diagnosis

Subacute Hypersensitivity Pneumonitis (Bird Fancier's Lung)

■ Differential Diagnosis

- Respiratory Bronchiolitis (RB) (cigarette smokers)
- Respiratory Bronchiolitis–Interstitial Lung Disease (RB-ILD) (cigarette smokers)
- Desquamative Interstitial Pneumonia (DIP) (cigarette smokers)
- *Pneumocystis jiroveci* Pneumonia (immunocompromised patients)

■ Discussion

Background

Hypersensitivity pneumonitis (HP), also known as extrinsic allergic alveolitis (EAA), is an immunologic reaction to inhaled organic antigens (e.g., animal proteins, bacteria, fungi, and various chemicals) that produces a diffuse interstitial granulomatous lung disease that varies in its intensity, clinical presentation, and natural history.

Etiology

There are a variety of known antigens as indicated above. Most exposures are occupational or recreational in nature. Farmer's lung and bird fancier's lung are the most common forms of HP. *Farmer's lung* results from exposure to a bacterium in moldy hay and most often demonstrates upper lung zone predominance. *Bird fancier's lung* results from chronic exposure to proteins from bird feathers, serum, or excrement, and most often demonstrates mid–lung zone predominance. This particular patient had six exotic birds at home that were imported from overseas. Her symptoms gradually developed over the first two months after having brought the birds into her home.

Clinical Findings

HP has been classified into acute, subacute, and chronic forms although patients tend to present clinically with subacute or chronic disease. Patients with *acute HP* present with a sudden onset of flu-like symptoms (e.g., fevers, chills, malaise, cough, and shortness of breath) within a few hours of heavy exposure to the

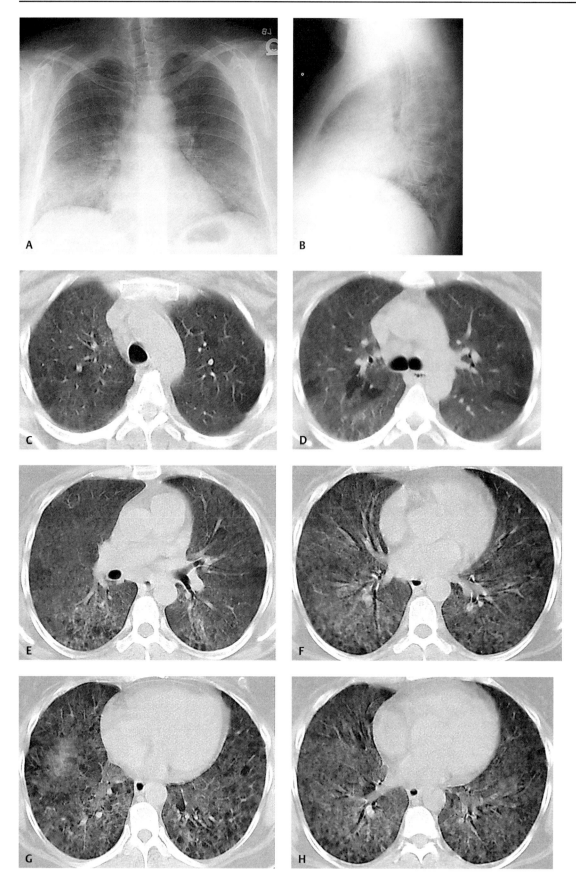

Fig. 115.1 *(Images courtesy of Nicole M. Kelleher-Linkonis, MD, VCU Medical Center, Richmond, Virginia.)*

antigen. *Subacute HP* is somewhat more insidious. Affected patients become symptomatic with cough and dyspnea over a period of days or weeks following intermittent and continuous exposure to low-dose antigens. *Chronic HP* presents following very-low-level antigenic exposures for a prolonged period of time with progressive dyspnea.

Imaging

Chest Radiography

Acute

- Abnormal in only 10% of patients
- Non-specific fine nodular or reticulonodular pattern
- Mid- to lower lobe predominance
- Consolidation rare

Subacute

- Most often abnormal (90%) (**Figs. 115.1A, 115.1B**)
- Small, poorly defined subcentimeter or miliary nodules (**Figs. 115.1A, 115.1B**)
- Diffuse ground glass opacities (**Figs. 115.1A, 115.1B**)
- Diffuse or middle and lower lobe predominance (**Figs. 115.1A, 115.1B**)
- Preservation of lung volume (**Figs. 115.1A, 115.1B**)

Chronic

- Fibrotic changes (reduced lung volumes)
- Coarse, irregular, linear opacities
- Variable distribution: upper, mid, or lower lung
- Honeycombing with advanced cases (mimicking IPF)
- Usually no lymphadenopathy or pleural disease

MDCT/HRCT

Acute and Subacute

- Patchy or diffuse bilateral ground glass opacities (100%) with associated poorly defined subcentimeter nodules and mosaic perfusion (80%) (**Figs. 115.1C, 115.1D, 115.1E, 115.1F, 115.1G, 115.1H**)
- Fuzzy or ill-defined centrilobular nodules (70%) (**Figs. 115.1C, 115.1D, 115.1E, 115.1F, 115.1G, 115.1H**)
- Most prominent mid- to lower lungs; costophrenic angles commonly spared (or less severely involved) (**Figs. 115.1C, 115.1D, 115.1E, 115.1F, 115.1G, 115.1H**)
- Air trapping on expiratory imaging (95%)
- Lobular areas of hypoattenuated lung parenchyma (**Figs. 115.1D, 115.1E, 115.1H**)
- *Head cheese sign:* geographic ground glass attenuation + normal lung + mosaic perfusion + air trapping
- Thin-walled lung cysts (10%); nearly always seen in conjunction with diffuse ground glass opacities
- Mediastinal lymphadenopathy (50%); nodes <20 mm short axis diameter
- Pleural effusion rare

Chronic

- Background of subacute findings
  - Centrilobular nodules (60%); usually ground glass attenuation
  - Mosaic perfusion (60%) (**Figs. 115.2A, 115.2B**)
- Lung cysts (30%); nearly always seen in association with ground glass opacities
- Fibrosis
  - Irregular linear opacities (40%) (**Figs. 115.2A, 115.2B**)
  - Traction bronchiectasis (20%) (**Figs. 115.2A, 115.2B**)
  - Honeycombing (50%)

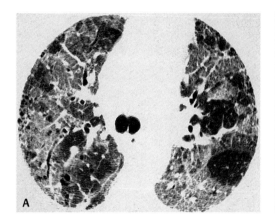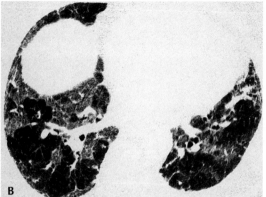

Fig. 115.2 HRCT (lung window) of a patient with chronic HP demonstrates a background mosaic perfusion pattern with patchy ground glass opacities, reticular opacities, and traction bronchiectasis most pronounced in the mid to upper lung zones. Note the relative paucity of fibrosis in the extreme lower lobes.

- Architectural distortion and volume loss
- Emphysema (20%); patients with HP tend to be non-smokers

Management

- Cessation of exposure to and/or removal from the responsible antigen
- Steroids

Prognosis

- Following cessation of antigen exposure: symptoms and imaging abnormalities should resolve (acute and subacute cases)
- Continued antigen exposure: progression to fibrosis and irreversible lung damage

PEARLS

- The two most common forms of HP are *farmer's lung* and *bird fancier's lung.*
- HP may also result from exposure to organisms growing in stagnant water (e.g., swimming pools, hot tubs [i.e., "hot tub" lung];, central heating systems).
- High index of suspicion and inquisition about potential environmental, occupation, and recreational exposures is critical in making the diagnosis.
- Normal chest radiography with a marked, diffusely abnormal CT is commonly seen.

Suggested Reading

1. Gurney JW, Winer-Muram HT, Rosado-de-Christenson ML, et al. Hypersensitivity pneumonitis. In: Specialty Imaging: HRCT of the Lung-Anatomic Basis, Imaging Features, Differential Diagnosis. Salt Lake City: Amirys, Inc.; 2009:148–159

2. Silva CI, Churg A, Müller NL. Hypersensitivity pneumonitis: spectrum of high-resolution CT and pathologic findings. AJR Am J Roentgenol 2007;188(2):334–344

3. Silva CI, Müller NL, Lynch DA, et al. Chronic hypersensitivity pneumonitis: differentiation from idiopathic pulmonary fibrosis and nonspecific interstitial pneumonia by using thin-section CT. Radiology 2008;246(1):288–297

4. Webb WR, Müller NL, Naidich DP. Hypersensitivity pneumonitis and eosinophilic lung diseases. In: High-Resolution CT of the Lung, 4th ed. Philadelphia: Lippincott, Williams & Wilkins; 2009:335–347; 357–358

CASE 116

■ Clinical Presentation

70-year-old man, non-smoker, with non-productive cough, increasing dyspnea, and fatigue

■ Radiologic Findings

Chest CT coronal anterior (**Fig. 116.1A**) and posterior (**Fig. 116.1B**) with accompanying right (**Fig. 116.1C**) and left (**Fig. 116.1D**) parasagittal MIP images demonstrate mild reduction in lung volume and a diffuse, chronic, interstitial fibrotic process that more extensively involves the posterior lung and lower lobes. HRCT axial CT images through the upper (**Fig. 116.1E**), mid (**Figs. 116.1F, 116.1G**), and lower lobes (**Figs. 116.1G, 116.1H**) reveal irregular septal and non-septal reticular opacities, architectural distortion characterized by traction bronchiectasis and bronchiolectasis, and honeycombing. Although all lobes are involved to some degree, the findings predominantly affect the paraseptal and juxtapleural regions of the lower lobes.

■ Diagnosis

Usual Interstitial Pneumonia (UIP); (Idiopathic Pulmonary Fibrosis) (IPF)
aka Cryptogenic Fibrosing Alveolitis

■ Differential Diagnosis

- Mixed Connective Tissue and Collagen Vascular Disorders with IPF
- Recurrent Bouts of Aspiration
- Chronic Pulmonary Drug Toxicity
- Asbestosis
- Chronic Hypersensitivity Pneumonitis
- Fibrosing NSIP

■ Discussion

Background

Usual interstitial pneumonia (UIP) is the most common of the idiopathic interstitial pneumonias (IIPs). It is a histologic pattern of chronic fibrosing interstitial pneumonia that may be idiopathic (idiopathic interstitial pneumonia, IPF) or may be a manifestation of various connective tissue disorders (e.g., rheumatoid arthritis, scleroderma), cytotoxic (e.g., bleomycin, busulfan, cyclophosphamide, methotrexate) and non-cytotoxic (e.g., amiodarone, gold salts, nitrofurantoin, oxygen) pulmonary drugs, or asbestosis. HRCT is accurate in the diagnosis of UIP. In one study, 47% of observers rendered a high-confidence diagnosis of UIP based on clinical findings alone, 79% with the addition of radiographic data, and 88% with the addition of HRCT. While HRCT is more sensitive than chest radiography, a normal HRCT does not exclude UIP, although this occurs in less than 10% of cases. Transbronchial biopsy cannot be used to establish the diagnosis but is useful in excluding alternative diagnoses (e.g., infection, malignancy, COP, eosinophilic pneumonia, sarcoidosis).

Etiology

The cause of UIP-IPF remains unknown. A role for genetic factors is supported by the findings of familial cases (e.g., Hermansky-Pudlak syndrome). Cigarette smoking results in a 1.6–2.3-fold increased risk of developing pulmonary fibrosis. Long-term exposure to metal or wood dusts is also an independent risk factor.

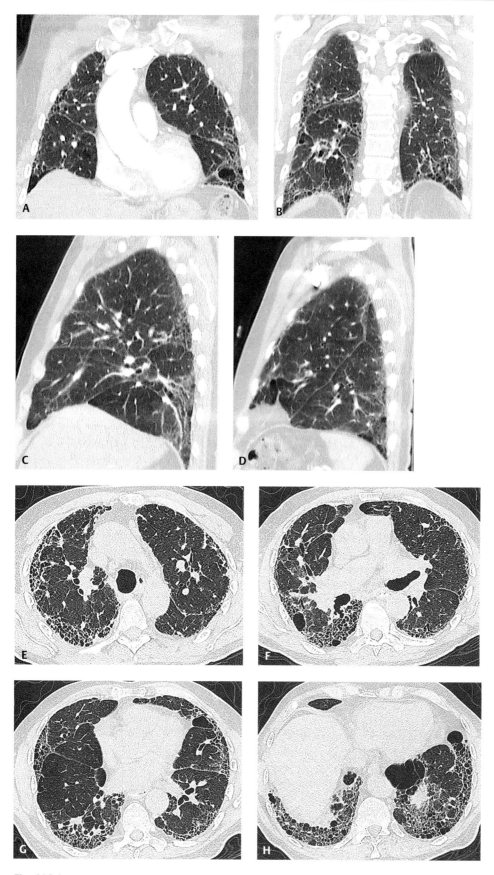

Fig. 116.1

Clinical Findings

The prevalence of IPF is 20.2 cases per 100,000 persons per year for males and 13.2 cases per 100,000 persons per year for females. The incidence is estimated as 10.7 cases per 100,000 persons per year for males and 7.4 cases per 100,000 persons per year for females, and increases with increasing age. Patients often present between 50 and 70 years of age, and two-thirds of patients are over 60 years old at presentation. The typical patient complains of an insidious onset of exertional dyspnea and non-productive cough. Weight loss, fever, fatigue, and myalgias are occasional concomitant concerns. Symptoms have usually been present for 12–18 months before patients seek medical attention. Physical signs may include tachypnea, increased work of breathing, "Velcro" rales (i.e., bibasilar, late, inspiratory, fine crackles). Digital clubbing is a late manifestation in 45–70% of patients. Pulmonary hypertension may develop as the disease progresses. PFTs show reduced TLC, FRC, RV, and DLCO. Resting blood gases reveal hypoxemia and respiratory alkalosis.

Imaging Findings

Radiography

- Normal (<10% of cases)
- Bilateral, symmetric, irregular linear opacities; reticular pattern (**Figs. 116.2A, 116.2B**)
- ± concomitant ground glass opacities, reduced lung volumes, and honeycombing
- Abnormalities may be diffuse; most commonly affect lower lobes (80% of cases) (**Figs. 116.2A, 116.2B**)

MDCT/HRCT

Early Findings

- Fine, irregular lines within SPL (intralobular linear opacities)
- Irregular interlobular septal thickening
- Irregular pleural thickening
- Irregular interfaces between lung parenchyma and bronchovascular bundles

Typical Findings

- Fibrosis and progressive lung parenchyma architectural distortion (**Figs. 116.1A, 116.1B, 116.1C, 116.1D, 116.1E, 116.1F, 116.1G, 116.1H**)
- Traction bronchiectasis and bronchiolectasis (**Figs. 116.1A, 116.1B, 116.1C, 116.1D, 116.1E, 116.1F, 116.1G, 116.1H**)

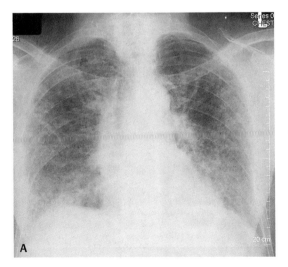
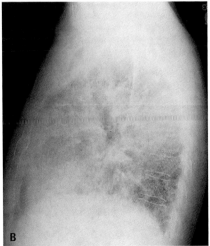

Fig. 116.2 PA **(A)** and lateral **(B)** chest radiographs of a 56-year-old man with UIP and exertional dyspnea show a reduction in lung volume and bilateral, symmetric, irregular linear opacities creating a background coarse reticular pattern. Note the areas of traction bronchiectasis and architectural distortion.

- Honeycombing (**Figs. 116.1A, 116.1B, 116.1C, 116.1D, 116.1E, 116.1F, 116.1G, 116.1H**)
- Predominance of paraseptal, peribronchiolar, basal, and juxtapleural abnormalities (**Figs. 116.1A, 116.1B, 116.1C, 116.1D, 116.1E, 116.1F, 116.1G, 116.1H**)
- Reduction in lung volume
- Common mild mediastinal lymph node enlargement
  - Lower right paratracheal (4R) and subcarinal (7) node stations, most commonly
  - Short axis diameters range between 10 and 21 mm
  - More prevalent with severe lung disease; associated with progression of fibrosis
- Foci of ground glass correlate with active alveolitis (70% of cases) or fibrosis beyond the resolution of the CT scan
- Rarely, punctate calcified nodules (pulmonary ossification) within the areas of fibrosis.

Management

- Conventional management: suppression of inflammation to prevent progression of ground glass opacities to fibrosis with corticosteroids
- Aggressive immunosuppressive and cytotoxic treatment regimens have largely failed to reduce morbidity and mortality
- Lung transplantation in select patients
- Future therapies aimed at preventing or inhibiting the fibroproliferative response and promoting alveolar reepithelialization

Prognosis

Typical Patient

- Slowly progressive course over years
- Mortality rate: 3.3 (men) and 2.5 (women) per 100,000 population
- Mean length of survival from time of diagnosis: 3.2–5.0 years
- Respiratory failure most common cause of death (40%)
- Other causes of death include heart failure, lung cancer, pulmonary infection, cor pulmonale, ischemic heart disease, and pulmonary emboli

Accelerated UIP-IPF (**Figs. 116.3A, 116.3B, 116.3C, 116.3D, 116.3E, 116.3F**)

- Small percentage of affected patients
- Accelerated decline or acute exacerbation of underlying disease
- Rapid downhill course; acute increase in dyspnea; fulminant respiratory failure
- Usually refractory to therapy; very poor prognosis; death often within 1 week
- New juxtapleural or patchy ground glass/air space opacities (**Figs. 116.3A, 116.3B, 116.3C, 116.3D, 116.3E, 116.3F**)

PEARLS

- Irregular linear opacities, honeycombing, and traction bronchiectasis indicate fibrosis and predict a poor response to therapy.
- Combined with clinical and radiographic findings, HRCT can render a high-confidence diagnosis of UIP, obviating open lung biopsy in many cases.
- Fibrosing NSIP can be difficult to differentiate from UIP. UIP tends to be primarily paraseptal, juxtapleural, or peribronchiolar in distribution. This pattern is less often seen with fibrosing NSIP (see Case 105). Accurate differentiation is based primarily on histology (i.e., fibrosing NSIP lacks temporal heterogeneity).
- Acute exacerbation or acceleration of the underlying disease process most often results in fulminant respiratory failure and death.

Suggested Reading

1. Attili AK, Kazerooni EA, Gross BH, Flaherty KR, Martinez FJ. Thoracic lymph node enlargement in usual interstitial pneumonitis and nonspecific-interstitial pneumonitis: prevalence, correlation with disease activity and temporal evolution. J Thorac Imaging 2006;21(4):288–292

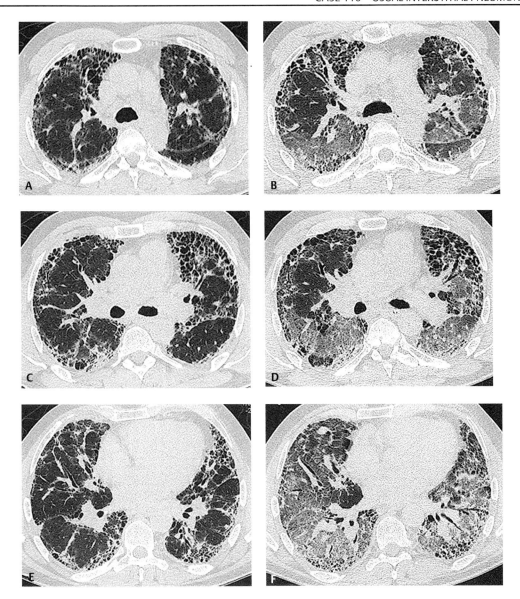

Fig. 116.3   Baseline HRCT images through the upper **(A)**, mid **(C)**, and lower **(E)** lung zones of a 53-year-old man with known advanced UIP show reduced lung volumes, extensive fibrosis, architectural distortion with traction bronchiectasis and bronchiolectasis, and juxtapleural honeycombing. Follow-up HRCT at roughly the same anatomic regions **(B–F)** performed 17 months later when he presented with acutely worsening breathlessness reveals not only progressive fibrosis, traction bronchiectasis, and honeycombing but widespread patchy ground glass opacities consistent with an acute exacerbation and acceleration of the underlying disease. Fulminant respiratory failure and death ensued over the next five days. Autopsy confirmed the above findings and excluded concomitant infection and alveolar hemorrhage

2. Bnà C, Zompatori M, Poletti V, et al. Differential diagnosis between usual interstitial pneumonia (UIP) and nonspecific interstitial pneumonia (NSIP) assessed by high-resolution computed tomography (HRCT). Radiol Med (Torino) 2005;109(5-6):472–487

3. Elliot TL, Lynch DA, Newell JD Jr, et al. High-resolution computed tomography features of nonspecific interstitial pneumonia and usual interstitial pneumonia. J Comput Assist Tomogr 2005;29(3):339–345

4. Travis WD, Colby TV, Koss MN, Rosado de Christenson ML, Müller NL, King TE Jr. Diffuse parenchymal lung diseases. In: King DW, ed. Atlas of Nontumor Pathology: Non-Neoplastic Disorders of the Lower Respiratory Tract, first series, fascicle 2. Washington, DC: American Registry of Pathology; 2002:59–73

5. Souza CA, Müller NL, Flint J, Wright JL, Churg A. Idiopathic pulmonary fibrosis: spectrum of high-resolution CT findings. American Journal of Roentgenology 2005;185(6):1531–1539

CASE 117

■ Clinical Presentation

41-year-old man with long-standing history of tobacco abuse since age 11, complaining of worsening cough and progressive dyspnea over the past 18 months

■ Radiologic Findings

HRCT (**Figs. 117.1A, 117.1B, 117.1C, 117.1D**) demonstrates profuse poorly defined subtle centrilobular nodules primarily in the upper lung zones (**Figs. 117.1A, 117.1B**) and a background of diffuse, patchy ground glass throughout both lungs with a mid and upper lung zone predominance (**Figs. 117.1A, 117.1B, 117.1C, 117.1D**). Mild bronchial wall thickening is present. Expiratory images (not provided) demonstrated multifocal lobular areas of air trapping. Subsequent open lung biopsy confirmed the diagnosis.

■ Diagnosis

Respiratory Bronchiolitis–Interstitial Lung Disease (RB-ILD)

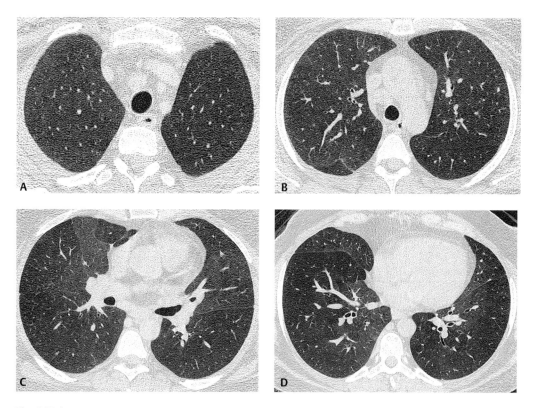

Fig. 117.1

568

■ Differential Diagnosis

- Desquamative Interstitial Pneumonitis (DIP)
- Acute-Subacute Hypersensitivity Pneumonitis (HP)
- Pulmonary Langerhans' Cell Histiocytosis (PLCH)

■ Discussion

Background

Respiratory bronchiolitis (RB) (*smoker's bronchiolitis*) is a common but incidental histologic finding in asymptomatic cigarette smokers. Symptomatic smokers presenting with symptoms mimicking interstitial lung disease are diagnosed with *respiratory bronchiolitis–interstitial lung disease (RB-ILD)*. RB, RB-ILD, and desquamative interstitial pneumonia (DIP) (see Case 108) are part of the spectrum of smoking-related interstitial lung diseases. Any given patient with a significant history of tobacco abuse may exhibit overlapping clinical and histopathologic features of all three diseases as well as centrilobular emphysema (see Case 28). The incidence and prevalence of RB and RB-ILD are unknown, and there is no sexual predilection.

Etiology

The cause and pathogenesis are unknown, but RB and RB-ILD are strongly related to tobacco abuse.

Clinical Findings

Patients with RB-ILD are usually young. The mean age at presentation is 36 years. Signs and symptoms include: chronic cough and progressive dyspnea over 1–2 years and bibasilar, end-inspiratory crackles. Rales are coarser than those heard in other interstitial lung diseases and may be heard throughout inspiration and sometimes into early expiration. Most patients are current heavy smokers, with more than 30 pack-years of abuse. On occasion, RB-ILD is diagnosed in former smokers and in persons exposed to secondhand smoke or fumes. PFTs may be normal. Alternatively, these studies may reveal an increased residual volume or mixed obstructive-restrictive pattern. Mild hypoxemia and mild to moderate reduction in DLCO have also been reported.

Imaging Findings

Chest Radiography

- Normal in 20–30% of patients
- Bronchial wall thickening
- Diffuse ground glass opacities or poorly defined fine reticular or reticulonodular opacities; diffuse or exhibits lower lung zone predominance

MDCT/HRCT

Respiratory Bronchiolitis (RB)

- Normal, most often
- Poorly defined centrilobular nodules (3–5 mm) (75%) and multifocal ground glass opacities (38%) (**Figs. 117.1A, 117.1B, 117.1C, 117.1D**)
  - Diffuse or patchy (**Figs. 117.1A, 117.1B, 117.1C, 117.1D**)
  - Predilection to involve mid and upper lung zones (**Figs. 117.1A, 117.1B, 117.1C, 117.1D**)
- Centrilobular emphysema (56%)

Respiratory Bronchiolitis–Interstitial Lung Disease (RB-ILD)

- May be normal
- Poorly defined centrilobular nodules (71%) and groundglass opacities (67%)
  - Diffuse (**Figs. 117.1A, 117.1B, 117.1C, 117.1D**)

- ◦ More profuse in upper lung zones (53%) (**Figs. 117.1A, 117.1B, 117.1C, 117.1D**)
- ◦ Middle or lower lung zones (20%) (**Figs. 117.1A, 117.1B, 117.1C, 117.1D**)
- ◦ Even distribution (27%)
- ◦ Tree-in-bud
- Bronchial wall thickening (90%) (**Figs. 117.1B, 117.1D**)
- Upper lobe centrilobular emphysema; usually mild (57%)
- Intralobular linear opacities and honeycombing due to fibrosis (<25%)
  - ◦ Mild
  - ◦ Lower lung zones
- Patchy areas of hypoattenuation (38%) with lower lobe predominance
- Air trapping on expiratory images

Management

- Cessation of smoking; improves symptoms and PFTs; decrease in ground glass opacities and centrilobular nodules on follow-up HRCT
- Non-compliant patients who continue to smoke and remain symptomatic may benefit from corticosteroid therapy

Prognosis

- Favorable clinical course and excellent prognosis in most compliant patients
  - ◦ Progression to pulmonary fibrosis, respiratory failure, or death; not been reported
- Precursor to chronic airway disease or centrilobular emphysema in some patients

PEARLS

- Diagnosis requires history of tobacco abuse, appropriate clinical signs and symptoms, and lung biopsy that reveals RB-ILD and excludes other diffuse parenchymal lung diseases.

Suggested Reading

1. Heyneman LE, Ward S, Lynch DA, Remy-Jardin M, Johkoh T, Müller NL. Respiratory bronchiolitis, respiratory bronchiolitis-associated interstitial lung disease, and desquamative interstitial pneumonia: different entities or part of the spectrum of the same disease process? AJR Am J Roentgenol 1999;173(6):1617–1622

2. Park JS, Brown KK, Tuder RM, Hale VA, King TE Jr, Lynch DA. Respiratory bronchiolitis-associated interstitial lung disease: radiologic features with clinical and pathologic correlation. J Comput Assist Tomogr 2002;26(1):13–20

3. Travis WD, Colby TV, Koss MN, Rosado-de-Christenson ML, Müller NL, King TE Jr. Reactive lymphoid lesions. In: King DW, ed. Atlas of Nontumor Pathology: Non-Neoplastic Disorders of the Lower Respiratory Tract. First Series. Fascicle 2. Washington, DC: The American Registry of Pathology; 2002:106–109

4. Webb WR, Müller NL, Naidich DP. The idiopathic interstitial pneumonias. In: High-Resolution CT of the Lung, 4th ed. Philadelphia: Lippincott, Williams & Wilkins; 2009:209–212

CASE 118

■ Clinical Presentation

32-year-old man with AIDS, cough, and dyspnea

■ Radiologic Findings

Coned-down PA chest radiograph (**Fig. 118.1A**) demonstrates bilateral, symmetric, poorly defined nodular opacities measuring up to 3.0 cm in diameter with a predominantly perihilar distribution. The bronchovascular bundles appear thickened. Chest CT (lung window) (**Figs. 118.1B, 118.1C**) from another patient with a similar history reveals ill-defined and irregular or "flame-shaped" nodular opacities in a predominantly perihilar and peribronchovascular bundle distribution.

■ Diagnosis

Kaposi sarcoma

■ Differential Diagnosis

- Lymphoma
- Metastatic Disease

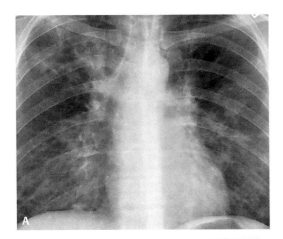

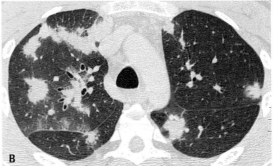

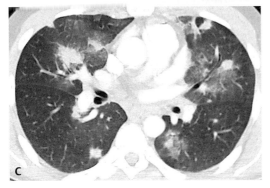

Fig. 118.1

571

- *Pneumocystis jiroveci* Pneumonia
- *Mycobacterium tuberculosis* Infection; Nontuberculous Mycobacterial Infection
- Other Bacterial and Fungal Pulmonary Infections

■ Discussion

Background

Kaposi sarcoma (KS) is a multicentric malignant neoplasm that originates from vascular and lymphatic endothelial cells. It occurs in 15–20% of HIV-infected male homosexuals, and in 1–3% of other HIV-infected individuals. The incidence of KS as an AIDS-defining illness has been decreasing over the last decade and is distinctly reduced in HIV-infected patients receiving antiretroviral therapy (ART). Cutaneous or visceral KS usually precedes lung involvement.

Etiology

There seems to be an association between infection with human herpesvirus 8 DNA and the development of KS. The HIV regulatory protein (transactivator target, TAT), important for viral replication, is also likely responsible for the proliferation of KS cells.

Clinical Findings

Most patients with pulmonary KS are symptomatic and typically complain of dyspnea and cough. Blood-streaked sputum in a patient with cutaneous KS suggests endobronchial involvement. Endobronchial lesions may also be associated with focal wheezing on auscultation. Concomitant opportunistic infections (e.g., *Pneumocystis jiroveci* pneumonia) are not uncommon. KS lesions have a unique appearance on bronchoscopy. The lesions appear as irregularly shaped, flat, or slightly raised violaceous or bright-red plaques, located at the bifurcations of segmental and large subsegmental bronchi.

Imaging Findings

Chest Radiography

- Bilateral, symmetric, poorly defined nodular or linear opacities in a predominantly perihilar distribution (**Fig. 118.1A**)
- Nodules ranging between 0.5 and 3.0 cm in diameter; tendency to coalesce (**Fig. 118.1A**)
- Bronchovascular bundle thickening (**Fig. 118.1A**); may progress to perihilar consolidation
- Interlobular septal thickening (e.g., Kerley B-lines)
- Pleural effusions (30–70%); exudative and serous or serosanguineous
- Hilar and/or mediastinal lymphadenopathy (5–15%)

MDCT/HRCT

- Ill-defined, irregular, "flame-shaped" or spiculated nodules in a predominantly perihilar and peribronchovascular distribution (85%) (**Figs. 118.1B, 118.1C**)
- Larger nodules may contain air bronchograms and/or surrounding rim of ground glass opacity (*halo sign*) (**Figs. 118.1B, 118.1C**)
- Thickening of bronchovascular bundles (81%) (**Figs. 118.1B, 118.1C**)
- Interlobular septal thickening (38%) (**Fig. 118.1C**)
- Areas of ground glass attenuation (23%) or parenchymal consolidation (35%) (**Figs. 118.1B, 118.1C**)
- Pleural effusions (35%)
- Hilar and/or mediastinal lymphadenopathy (15–50%)

MRI

- Parenchymal lesions: high signal on T1WI; low signal on T2WI
- Marked increased signal on T1WI after Gadolinium administration

Management

- Regression after highly active antiretroviral therapy (HAART)
- Combination chemotherapy; paclitaxel

Prognosis

- Poor: Median survival 2–10 months
- Poor prognostic indicators:
  - Pleural effusion
  - Severe breathlessness
  - CD4 counts <100 × 10^6 cells /L
  - Absence of cutaneous lesions
  - Previous opportunistic infection
  - Low white blood count or hemoglobin

PEARLS

- Irregular nodules greater than 1.0 cm in diameter in a peribronchovascular distribution strongly suggest this diagnosis in HIV-infected patients.
- Focal and/or multifocal ground glass opacities or consolidations are often secondary to concomitant infection with *Pneumocystis jiroveci* pneumonia.

Suggested Reading

1. Hansell DM, Lynch DA, McAdams HP, Bankier AA. The immunocompromised patient. In: Hansell DM, Lynch DA, McAdams HP, Bankier AA, ed. Imaging of Diseases of the Chest, 5th ed. Philadelphia: Mosby Elsevier; 2010:295–384

2. Cheung MC, Pantanowitz L, Dezube BJ. AIDS-related malignancies: emerging challenges in the era of highly active antiretroviral therapy. Oncologist 2005;10(6):412–426

3. Boiselle PM, Aviram G, Fishman JE. Update on lung disease in AIDS. Semin Roentgenol 2002;37(1):54–71

4. Cannon MJ, Dollard SC, Black JB, et al. Risk factors for Kaposi's sarcoma in men seropositive for both human herpesvirus 8 and human immunodeficiency virus. AIDS 2003;17(2):215–222

5. Kobayashi M, Takaori-Kondo A, Shindo K, Mizutani C, Ishikawa T, Uchiyama T. Successful treatment with paclitaxel of advanced AIDS-associated Kaposi's sarcoma. Intern Med 2002;41(12):1209–1212

CASE 119

■ Clinical Presentation

58-year-old woman with untreated adenocarcinoma of the left lung diagnosed three months earlier and who refused treatment returns with complaints of increasing dyspnea.

■ Radiologic Findings

PA (**Fig. 119.1A**) and lateral (**Fig. 119.1B**) chest X-rays reveal abnormal irregularly thickened septal linear opacities throughout both lungs. Although the cardiomediastinal silhouette is enlarged, there is no evidence of heart failure. The vascular pedicle is not widened and vascular clarity is maintained. Note the left upper lobe mass and the right hilar lymphadenopathy. HRCT images through the upper, mid, and lower lung zones (**Figs. 119.1C, 119.1D, 119.1E, 119.1F**) acquired three weeks later following the onset of respiratory failure demonstrate profuse smooth and nodular thickening of the interlobular septa of multiple SPLs in both lungs. Asymmetric thickening of the bronchovascular bundles are seen in the right lung (**Figs. 119.1E, 119.1F**). The right pleural effusion proved to be malignant. Note the left upper lobe mass (**Fig. 119.1D**).

■ Diagnosis

Lymphangitic Carcinomatosis; Primary Lung Adenocarcinoma

■ Differential Diagnosis

- Pulmonary Edema
- Sarcoidosis
- Coal Worker's Pneumoconiosis (CWP)
- Lymphocytic Interstitial Pneumonia (LIP)
- Idiopathic Pulmonary Fibrosis (IPF)
- Pulmonary Lymphoma

■ Discussion

Background

Pulmonary lymphangitic carcinomatosis (PLC) refers to the proliferation and spread of tumor in the pulmonary lymphatics. Virtually any metastatic neoplasm can demonstrate lymphangitic spread. The *most common* primary neoplasms associated with PLC are adenocarcinomas that originate in the lung, breast, stomach, pancreas, and prostate. PLC also occurs in patients with carcinomas of the thyroid and cervix, and with metastatic adenocarcinoma from an unknown primary site.

Etiology

PLC typically results from hematogenous spread of neoplasm to the lung with subsequent interstitial and lymphatic invasion. Direct lymphatic spread of tumor from mediastinal and hilar nodes may also occur.

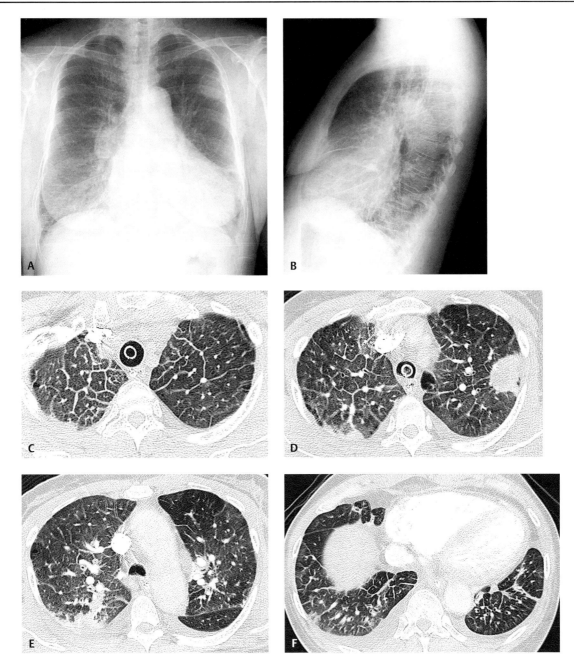

Fig. 119.1

Clinical Findings

The most common clinical manifestation is dyspnea. Although initially insidious, it progresses rapidly and may result in severe respiratory distress in a few weeks time. Some affected patients may also complain of cough.

Imaging Findings

Chest Radiography

- Normal; 30–50% of patients with pathologically proven PLC
- Coarse bronchovascular markings with predominant perihilar and basal distribution (**Figs. 119.2A, 119.2B**)

- Bilateral, unilateral, single lobe involvement (**Figs. 119.1A, 119.1B, 119.2A, 119.2B**)
- Septal lines (i.e., Kerley B-lines) usually present (i.e., simulates pulmonary edema) (**Figs. 119.1A, 119.1B**)
- Coarse reticulonodular pattern (**Fig. 119.2B**)
- Hilar and mediastinal lymphadenopathy (20–40%) (**Figs. 119.1A, 119.1B, 119.2A, 119.2B**)
- Pleural effusion (30–50%) (**Figs. 119.2A, 119.2B**)

MDCT/HRCT

- Smooth or nodular peribronchovascular interstitial thickening (**Figs. 119.1C, 119.1D, 119.1E, 119.1F, 119.2C, 119.2D, 119.2E**)
- Smooth or nodular interlobular septal and/or visceral pleural thickening (**Figs. 119.1C, 119.1D, 119.1E, 119.1F, 119.2C, 119.2D, 119.2E**)

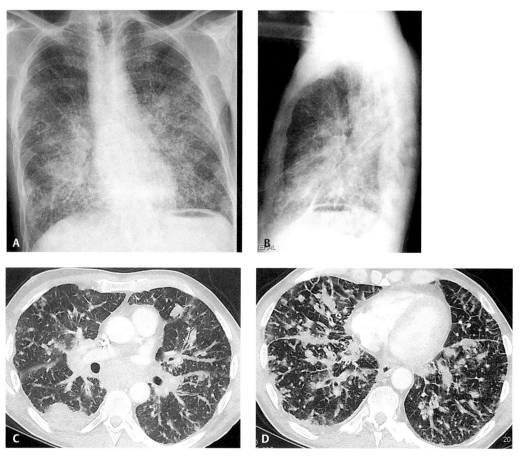

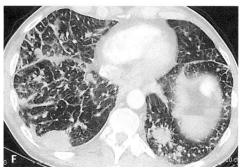

Fig. 119.2 PA **(A)** and lateral **(B)** chest X-rays of a 55-year-old man with metastatic renal cell cancer and PLC show profuse reticulo-nodular opacities throughout both lungs, coarse bronchovascular bundle thickening, and a loculated posterolateral pleural effusion. Note the right paratracheal, hilar, and subcarinal lymphadenopathy. Chest CT through the mid and lower lung zones **(C–E)** (lung window) demonstrates profuse but asymmetric smooth and nodular interlobular septal thickening of multiple SPLs in both lungs, right more so than left. Marked bronchovascular bundle thickening and prominent subpleural interstitium and centrilobular structures can be seen. A dominant spiculated metastatic nodule is present in the left lower lobe. Note the loculated right effusion and extensive sub-carinal and right hilar lymphadenopathy.

- Prominence of centrilobular structures (**Figs. 119.2C, 119.2D, 119.2E**)
- Characteristic septal thickening outlining distinct secondary pulmonary lobules (i.e., polygonal arcades) (**Figs. 119.1C, 119.1D, 119.1E, 119.1F, 119.2C, 119.2D, 119.2E**)
- Asymmetric diffuse, patchy, or unilateral parenchymal involvement (50%) (**Figs. 119.1C, 119.1D, 119.1E, 119.1F, 119.2C, 119.2D, 119.2E**)
- Preservation of normal lung architecture (i.e., no architectural distortion or fibrosis) (**Figs. 119.1C, 119.1D, 119.1E, 119.1F, 119.2C, 119.2D**)
- Hilar and mediastinal lymphadenopathy (40%) (**Figs. 119.2C, 119.2D, 119.2E**)
- Pleural effusion (30%) (**Figs. 119.1E, 119.1F, 119.2C, 119.2E**)

Management

- Supportive and directed toward the underlying malignancy

Prognosis

- Usually poor
- Up to 50% of affected patients die within 3 months
- Only 15% of affected patients survive more than 6 months

PEARLS

- Preservation of lung architecture is an important CT finding used to differentiate PLC from other causes of diffuse parenchymal lung disease.
- If architectural distortion or fibrosis is present, another diagnosis should be considered.

Suggested Reading

1. Honda O, Johkoh T, Ichikado K, et al. Comparison of high resolution CT findings of sarcoidosis, lymphoma, and lymphangitic carcinoma: is there any difference of involved interstitium? J Comput Assist Tomogr 1999;23(3): 374–379

2. Webb WR, Müller NL, Naidich DP. Diffuse pulmonary neoplasms and pulmonary lymphoproliferative diseases. In: High-Resolution CT of the Lung. 4th ed. Philadelphia: Lippincott Williams and Wilkins; 2009:241–247

CASE 120

■ Clinical Presentation

38-year-old woman smoker with cough and dyspnea

■ Radiologic Findings

PA chest radiograph (**Fig. 120.1**) demonstrates normal lung volume without visible pulmonary abnormalities. HRCT (**Figs. 120.2, 120.3**) shows subtle bilateral upper lobe–predominant small pulmonary cysts with nodular irregular cyst walls and scattered small nodules with ill-defined borders (**Fig. 120.2**). Note the relative sparing of the lung bases (**Fig. 120.3**).

■ Diagnosis

Pulmonary Langerhans' Cell Histiocytosis

■ Differential Diagnosis

* Infection
* Emphysema
* Bronchiectasis
* Lymphangioleiomyomatosis

■ Discussion

Background

Pulmonary Langerhans' cell histiocytosis (PLCH) is a chronic, progressive interstitial lung disease that results from abnormal non-malignant proliferation of monoclonal Langerhans' cells. Multiple organs may be affected, including bone, pituitary gland, mucous membranes, skin, lymph nodes, and liver.

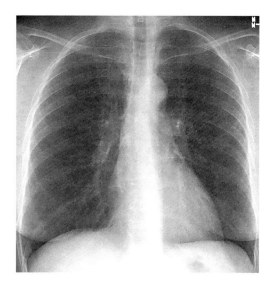

Fig. 120.1

578

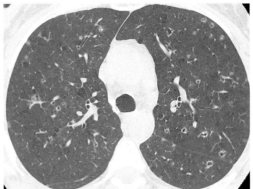

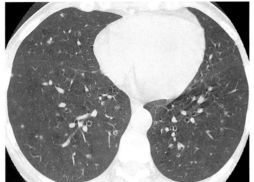

Fig. 120.2

Fig. 120.3

Etiology

The exact etiology of PLCH has not been established. An immune response to an exogenous antigen has been postulated as an etiologic factor, as the disease is strongly associated with cigarette smoking. PLCH has been described in association with malignant neoplasia, specifically lung cancer and Hodgkin lymphoma.

Clinical Findings

Affected patients are typically adult smokers in the third and fourth decades of life. There may be a slight female predominance. Symptomatic patients may present with dyspnea, cough, and fatigue. Patients with spontaneous pneumothorax secondary to PLCH may present with acute chest pain. Constitutional symptoms, weight loss and fever have also been described. Pulmonary function studies may show obstructive, restrictive, or mixed abnormalities. Most patients have a decreased DLCO. A small percentage of patients are entirely asymptomatic and diagnosed incidentally because of an abnormal chest radiograph. Bone lesions occur in 4–13% of patients with PLCH; 20% involve the ribs and may be seen on chest radiography.

Imaging Findings

Chest Radiography

- Upper and mid lung predominance of pulmonary abnormalities; sparing of lung bases
- Normal or increased lung volumes (**Fig. 120.1**)
- Diffuse bilateral symmetrical small nodules with irregular contours; measuring up to 10 mm in size
- Bilateral reticular and nodular opacities; pulmonary cysts measuring up to 2–3 cm
- Normal chest radiography (**Fig. 120.1**)
- Spontaneous secondary pneumothorax
- Rarely lymphadenopathy, consolidation, focal lung disease

MDCT/HRCT

- Upper lobe–predominant abnormalities with sparing of lung bases (**Figs. 120.2, 120.3**)
- Characteristic combination of nodules and cysts with normal intervening lung parenchyma (**Figs. 120.2, 120.3**)
- Centrilobular small nodules with irregular borders (**Figs. 120.2, 120.3, 120.4, 120.5**)
- Solid nodules or nodules with central low attenuation (intrinsic cavitation)
- Cysts of variable size, often with bizarre shapes; thin, thick, or irregular/nodular cyst walls (**Figs. 120.2, 120.5, 120.6**)
- Visualization of spontaneous secondary pneumothorax

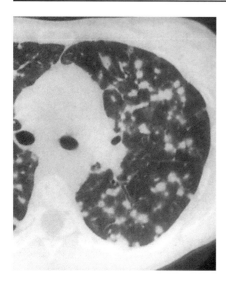

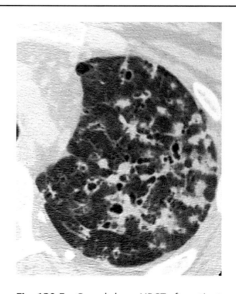

Fig. 120.4 Coned-down unenhanced chest CT (lung window) of a patient with PLCH demonstrates profuse pulmonary nodules with irregular borders measuring up to 10 mm predominantly affecting the upper and mid-lung zones.

Fig. 120.5 Coned-down HRCT of a patient with PLCH demonstrates a combination of pulmonary cysts and coalescent lung nodules. Note the nodular thickening of the cyst walls and the irregular contours of the lung nodules.

Management

- Cessation of smoking
- Corticosteroids, chemotherapeutic agents
- Lung transplantation in selected cases

Prognosis

- Spontaneous remission in approximately 25% of cases
- Clinical and radiologic stability in 50% of cases
- Progression to end-stage lung disease (particularly with continued cigarette smoking); may develop pulmonary hypertension and respiratory failure

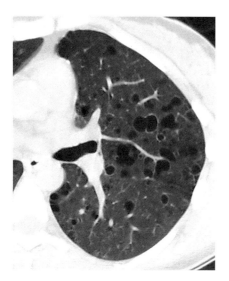

Fig. 120.6 Coned-down unenhanced chest CT (lung window) of a patient with PLCH shows upper lung–predominant thin-walled small cysts with irregular shapes. There were no pulmonary nodules and there was relative sparing of the lung bases.

PEARLS

- Cysts may be the only HRCT imaging finding of PLCH, but in most cases small nodules are also present.

Suggested Reading

1. Abbott GF, Rosado-de-Christenson ML, Franks TJ, Frazier AA, Galvin JR. From the archives of the AFIP: pulmonary Langerhans cell histiocytosis. Radiographics 2004;24(3):821–841

2. Leatherwood DL, Heitkamp DE, Emerson RE. Best cases from the AFIP: Pulmonary Langerhans cell histiocytosis. Radiographics 2007;27(1):265–268

CASE 121

■ Clinical Presentation

34-year-old woman with dyspnea

■ Radiologic Findings

PA chest radiograph (**Fig. 121.1**) demonstrates increased lung volumes without other radiographic abnormality or evidence of interstitial lung disease. HRCT (**Figs. 121.2, 121.3**) reveals profuse, uniform, bilateral, small thin-walled cysts affecting both lungs.

■ Diagnosis

Lymphangioleiomyomatosis

■ Differential Diagnosis

- Pulmonary Langerhans' Cell Histiocytosis (PLCH)
- *Pneumocystis jiroveci* Pneumonia
- Emphysema

■ Discussion

Background

Lymphangioleiomyomatosis (LAM) is a rare idiopathic disease that affects women of childbearing age and is characterized by abnormal proliferation of smooth muscle cells (LAM cells) along lymphatics in the chest and abdomen but also along vessels and bronchi in the lung. Lymphatic involvement can lead to chylous pleural effusions and/or ascites.

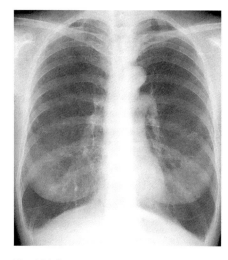

Fig. 121.1

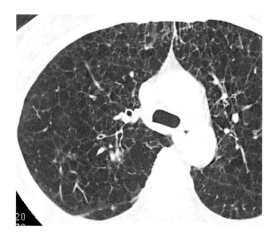

Fig. 121.2

582

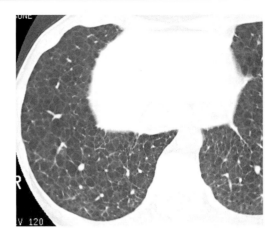

Fig. 121.3

Etiology

Unknown

Clinical Findings

LAM occurs almost exclusively in women of childbearing age who are between 20 and 40 years of age at the onset of symptoms or at the time of diagnosis. Most patients complain of dyspnea, but also cough and chest pain. Hemoptysis and wheezing are less common. Pulmonary function tests reveal obstructive or mixed abnormalities. Pneumothorax, hemoptysis, and chylothorax are associated complications. Approximately 1% of patients with tuberous sclerosis have pulmonary involvement with identical clinical, radiologic, and pathologic findings. Renal angiomyolipomas develop in 60% of patients, characteristically those with tuberous sclerosis.

Imaging Findings

Chest Radiography

- Diffuse bilateral reticular opacities, may represent visualization of pulmonary cysts; interlobular septal thickening
- Cystic air spaces, hyperinflation, pneumothorax
- Pleural effusion may be chylous
- Normal chest radiograph in 20% of patients (**Fig. 121.1**)
- Normal to large lung volumes (**Fig. 121.1**)

MDCT/HRCT

- Thin-walled cysts (0.2–2.0 cm) with intervening normal lung parenchyma; typically rounded shapes but other shapes observed with extensive lung involvement (**Figs. 121.2, 121.3, 121.4, 121.5A**)
- Diffuse bilateral distribution of cysts throughout both lungs (upper and lower lungs equally affected) (**Figs. 121.2, 121.3, 121.5A**)
- Pleural effusion; typically chylous, may exhibit low attenuation (**Figs. 121.4, 121.5A**)
- Pneumothorax (**Fig. 121.5A**)
- Lymphadenopathy
- Rarely, patchy ground glass opacity and small nodules
- Incidental visualization of abdominal abnormalities; including abdominal ascites, lymphadenopathy, abdominal lymphangiomyomas, and renal angiomyolipomas (**Fig. 121.5B**)

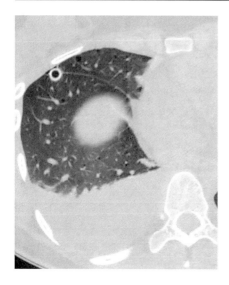

Fig. 121.4 Coned-down unenhanced chest CT (lung window) of a woman with LAM who presented with a right hydropneumothorax demonstrates a moderate right pleural effusion (which proved to be chylous) and a few scattered small thin-walled lung cysts most numerous in the middle lobe. Note the right anterior intrafissural pleural drain.

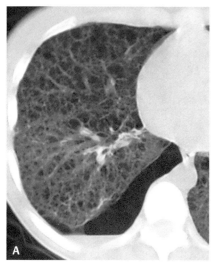
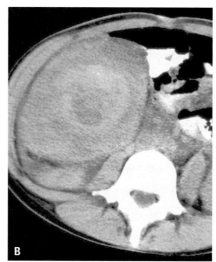

Fig. 121.5 Coned-down unenhanced chest CT (lung window) **(A)** of a woman with tuberous sclerosis and lymphangioleiomyomatosis demonstrates profuse right-sided uniform thin-walled pulmonary cysts. Note associated right-sided hydropneumothorax. Coned-down unenhanced abdomen CT (soft-tissue window) **(B)** shows a large heterogeneous mass in the right renal fossa representing severe spontaneous hemorrhage within a right renal angiomyolipoma.

Management

- Hormonal manipulation may improve or stabilize disease; oophorectomy, luteinizing hormone releasing hormone analogue, and most typically progesterone
- Lung transplantation

Prognosis

- Variable; frequent disease progression; influenced by extent of pulmonary involvement
- Median survival from time of diagnosis: 8–10 years
- Recurrence reported in transplanted lungs

PEARLS

- Cysts of *LAM* are usually more regular in size and shape than cysts of *PLCH*.
- *LAM* typically involves both lungs diffusely; *PLCH* characteristically spares the lung bases.
- Nodules are not a typical features of *LAM* but are common in *PLCH*.
- Pleural effusions are common in *LAM* but are uncommon in *PLCH*.
- *Emphysema* can be distinguished from *LAM* by the polygonal shape of the affected pulmonary lobule in emphysema and the presence of a central dot representing the core lobular artery in the emphysematous lobule.
- The so-called cysts of centrilobular emphysema have no perceptible walls. *LAM* cysts have thin, perceptible walls.

Suggested Reading

1. Abbott GF, Rosado-de-Christenson ML, Frazier AA, Franks TJ, Pugatch RD, Galvin JR. From the archives of the AFIP: lymphangioleiomyomatosis: radiologic-pathologic correlation. Radiographics 2005;25(3):803–828

2. Attili AK, Kazerooni EA. Case 116: lymphangioleiomyomatosis. Radiology 2007;244(1):303–308

CASE 122

■ Clinical Presentation

57-year-old man with long-standing cardiac dysrhythmias on anti-arrhythmic pharmacotherapy who now complains of dyspnea on exertion, dry cough, and weakness

■ Radiologic Findings

Unenhanced chest CT (lung window) (**Figs. 122.1A, 122.1C, 122.1E**) demonstrates patchy ground glass opacities in both lungs and focal mass-like regions of consolidation in the lingula, left lower lobe, and lateral segment right middle lobe. Corresponding mediastinal windows (**Figs. 122.1B, 122.1D**) reveal the focal areas of consolidation are higher in attenuation (89 HU and 87 HU, respectively) than the soft tissues (38 HU). Unenhanced CT through the liver (**Figs. 122.1F**) shows it is also higher in attenuation than normal.

■ Diagnosis

Amiodarone Pulmonary Toxicity ("Amiodarone Lung")

■ Differential Diagnosis

- Cryptogenic Organizing Pneumonia (COP)
- Pulmonary Fungal Disease
- Primary and Secondary Lung Neoplasia

■ Discussion

Background

Amiodarone is a tri-iodinated benzofuran derivative used to treat refractory tachyarrhythmias. Amiodarone contains 37% iodine by weight, has a long half-life (58 days), accumulates in the lung, and may cause a form of drug-induced lung injury that develops acutely, within a few days of initial use, or more than 10 years later, while the patient is on chronic therapy. The precise incidence of pulmonary toxicity is unknown but it is estimated to occur in 5–7% of patients, 5–10% of whom die as a result. Risk factors for pulmonary toxicity include high cumulative dose (more than 400 mg/day), duration of use over two months, increased age, and preexisting pulmonary disease. Amiodarone also accumulates in the liver, spleen, muscles, adipose tissue, and skin.

Clinical Findings

Two distinct clinical presentations of pulmonary toxicity have been described. The *most common* is characterized by the insidious onset of dyspnea on exertion, dry cough, weight loss, weakness, and sometimes fever. These patients most often exhibit an interstitial pattern of disease radiographically. One-third of patients have a more acute presentation that may mimic infection, pulmonary edema, or thromboembolism clinically and radiographically. The most specific test of amiodarone pulmonary toxicity is a dramatically decreased diffusing capacity (DLCO) on PFTs. Manifestations of extrapulmonary toxicity include blue-gray skin discoloration, vortex corneal keratopathy (90%), hypothyroidism (<26%), hyperthyroidism (5%), hepatic dysfunction, muscle weakness, and peripheral neuropathy.

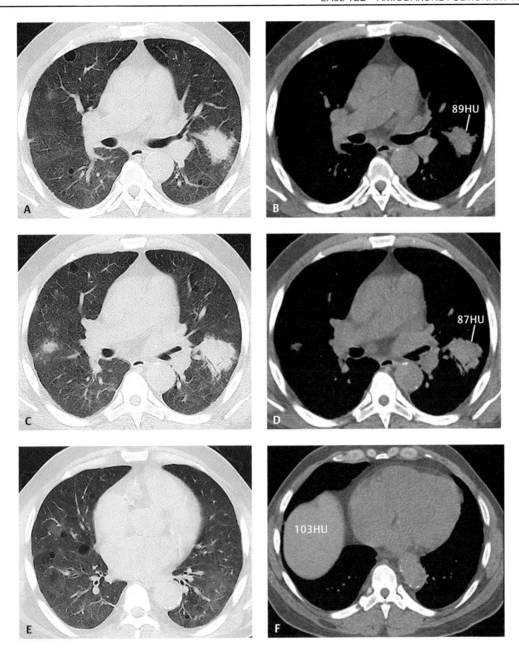

Fig. 122.1

Imaging Findings

Chest Radiography

- Diffuse bilateral reticular opacities
- Bilateral areas of consolidation; peripheral and predominantly upper lobes (resembles chronic eosinophilic pneumonia)
- Focal consolidations and nodules; less common
- ± pleural thickening
- Pleural effusion; uncommon (exudative)

MDCT/HRCT

- Ground glass opacities (**Figs. 122.1A, 122.1C, 122.1E**)
- Focal or diffuse areas of consolidation
- Reticular opacities
- Conglomerate mass(es); less common (**Figs. 122.1A, 122.1B, 122.1C, 122.1D**)
- Consolidations/masses contain foci of attenuation greater than soft tissue (82–175 HU) (73%) (**Figs. 122.1A, 122.1B, 122.1C, 122.1D**)
- Increased attenuation of liver or spleen (91%) and myocardium (18%) (**Fig. 122.1F**)
- ± Increased attenuation of mediastinal lymph nodes

Management

- Cessation of amiodarone therapy
- Corticosteroids
- Three months after cessation of amiodarone treatment, follow-up CT in this particular patient (not illustrated) showed near-complete resolution of disease

Prognosis

- Usually good response to drug cessation and corticosteroids
- Irreversible pulmonary fibrosis may develop in some cases
- 5–10% of patients who develop pulmonary toxicity die as a sequela

PEARLS

- Increased liver attenuation on CT is also present in patients treated with amiodarone without pulmonary toxicity.

Suggested Reading

1. Camus P, Martin WJ II, Rosenow EC III. Amiodarone pulmonary toxicity. Clin Chest Med 2004;25(1):65–75 Review
2. Fabiani I, Tacconi D, Grotti S, et al. Amiodarone-induced pulmonary toxicity mimicking acute pulmonary edema. J Cardiovasc Med (Hagerstown) 2011;12(5):361–365
3. Papiris SA, Triantafillidou C, Kolilekas L, Markoulaki D, Manali ED. Amiodarone: review of pulmonary effects and toxicity. Drug Saf 2010;33(7):539–558
4. Poll LW, May P, Koch JA, Hetzel G, Heering P, Mödder U. HRCT findings of amiodarone pulmonary toxicity: clinical and radiologic regression. J Cardiovasc Pharmacol Ther 2001;6(3):307–311

CASE 123

■ Clinical Presentation

63-year-old man with Sjögren syndrome and abnormal chest radiography (not illustrated)

■ Radiologic Findings

Unenhanced chest CT (**Figs. 123.1A, 123.1B, 123.1C, 123.1D, 123.1E, 123.1F**) demonstrates a combination of variable-size thin-walled cysts, bulla, and nodules throughout both lungs. Some nodules are well defined whereas others are irregular. Several nodules contain eccentric calcifications (*arrows*) and others abut the cystic lesions (*arrowhead*).

■ Diagnosis

Nodular Parenchymal Amyloidosis with Lymphoid Interstitial Pneumonia (LIP)

■ Differential Diagnosis

*   Granulomatous Disease
*   Metastatic Lung Cancer
*   Rheumatoid Nodules

■ Discussion

Background

Amyloidosis is a generic term that describes a group of disorders characterized by extracellular deposition of abnormal insoluble protein and protein derivatives that show apple green birefringence when stained with Congo red and viewed with polarized light.

Etiology

There are two distinct classes based on the type of amyloid deposited. *Primary amyloid light (AL) chain disease* is characterized by extracellular deposition of immunoglobulin light chains produced by plasma cells (i.e., plasma cell dyscrasia) and is responsible for most clinically significant cases with respiratory disease. *Secondary amyloid A (AA) chain disease* is most commonly seen in association with rheumatoid arthritis, but is also associated with other chronic inflammatory disorders (e.g., inflammatory bowel disease, chronic systemic inflammatory disorders, and chronic pulmonary infections) as well as Sjögren syndrome and lymphoid interstitial pneumonia (LIP) (see Case 109).

Clinical Findings

Amyloidosis may be defined by anatomical extent as either *localized* (20%) or *systemic* (80%). *Localized amyloidosis* results from focal deposition of AL proteins and usually causes symptoms. *Systemic amyloidosis* results from deposition of AL proteins in multiple organ systems, including the lungs. In these latter cases, amyloid deposition is an incidental finding that only rarely causes symptoms. Respiratory system involvement occurs only with *primary* and not *secondary amyloidosis*. Thoracic amyloidosis most often manifests with cardiac involvement (restrictive cardiomyopathy). Involvement in order of frequency then includes the *airways* (i.e.,

589

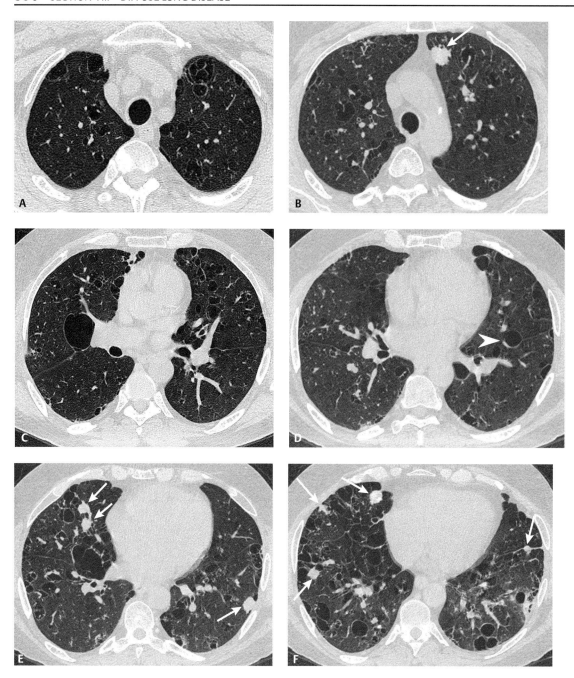

Fig. 123.1

tracheobronchial tree) (see Case 22), the *lung parenchyma* (solitary or multiple nodules), the *interstitium* (diffuse alveolar septal thickening), and the *mediastinal* and *hilar lymph nodes* (i.e., lymphadenopathy). Approximately one to five cases are diagnosed per 100,000 population. The median latency between clinical presentation of chronic inflammatory disorders and clinically significant amyloidosis is 20 years.

Imaging Findings

Chest Radiography

- Most cases; normal

Localized Amyloidosis

- Tracheobronchial disease: stenosis; atelectasis; consolidation (see Case 22)
- Nodular parenchymal amyloidosis: solitary or multiple nodules/masses

Primary Systemic Amyloidosis

- Reticular or reticulonodular pattern
- Nodules and interlobular septal thickening (mimicking sarcoidosis or miliary tuberculosis)
- Abnormal areas may calcify or rarely ossify

MDCT/HRCT

Nodules (localized disease)

- Solitary (60%)
- Multiple; usually <10 in number (**Figs. 123.1B, 123.1E, 123.1F**)
- Peripheral or juxtapleural (**Figs. 123.1B, 123.1E, 123.1F**)
- May follow bronchovascular bundles
- Vary from well defined to irregular in nature (**Figs. 123.1B, 123.1E, 123.1F**)
- 0.5–15 cm diameter (**Figs. 123.1B, 123.1E, 123.1F**)
- Calcification (20–50%); often eccentric (**Figs. 123.1B, 123.1E, 123.1F**)
- Cavitation; rare
- No architectural distortion

Diffuse Septal Form

- Least common form of lung involvement (systemic disease)
- Interlobular smooth septal thickening (**Fig. 123.2**)
- Bronchovascular bundle thickening (**Fig. 123.2**)
- Associated centrilobular, random, perilymphatic nodules
- Nodules may aggregate into larger masses
- Non-specific ground glass opacities (**Fig. 123.2**)
- Traction bronchiectasis
- Hilar and or mediastinal lymphadenopathy; eccentric calcifications
- Diffuse thin-walled cysts/bullae; usually part of Sjögren syndrome and LIP (**Figs. 123.1A, 123.1B, 123.1C, 123.1D, 123.1E, 123.1F**)

Lymphadenopathy

- Common in primary type with systemic disease; most commonly lymphoplasmacytic lymphoma or Waldenstrom macroglobulinemia
- Usually mediastinal and hilar; often multiple nodal groups
- Stippled; diffuse; "eggshell" pattern of calcification
- 50% of patients have concomitant parenchymal disease

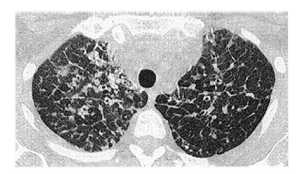

Fig. 123.2 HRCT demonstrates the diffuse septal form of primary amyloidosis from underlying systemic disease characterized by smooth as well as nodular septal thickening and thickening of bronchovascular bundles. Conglomerate lobular ground glass nodules are forming in the right upper lobe. *(Images courtesy of Daniel A. Henry, MD, VCU Medical Center, Richmond, Virginia.)*

Pleura

- Thickening; focal pleural calcification; effusion (latter usually sequela of cardiac involvement)

Differential Diagnosis of Small Calcified Interstitial Nodules on HRCT

- Infectious granulomatous disease
- Sarcoidosis
- Coal worker's pneumoconiosis
- Talcosis
- Fat embolism syndrome
- Alveolar microlithiasis
- UIP-IPF
- Amyloidosis

Management

- Directed at underlying cause in systemic disease

Prognosis

Primary Amyloidosis

- One-third of patients eventually diagnosed with multiple myeloma or B-cell lymphoma
- 10–15% of patients with multiple myeloma or B-cell lymphoma develop primary amyloidosis
- Median survival: 1.5 years

Secondary Amyloidosis

- Median survival: 4.5 years

PEARLS

- One-third of patients with *primary amyloidosis* develop multiple myeloma or B-cell lymphoma
- Ten to 15% of patients with multiple myeloma or B-cell lymphoma develop *primary amyloidosis.*
- *Secondary amyloidosis* does not cause pulmonary disease; usually it is an incidental finding.
- Diffuse septal form of the disease is the *least common* form of lung involvement.
- Lymphadenopathy should prompt investigation for lymphoplasmacytic lymphoma or Waldenstrom macroglobulinemia.
- Nodules abutting cysts suggests an association of nodular amyloidosis in patients with known LIP (**Figs. 123.1A, 123.1B, 123.1C, 123.1D, 123.1E, 123.1F**).

Suggested Readings

1. Aylwin AC, Gishen P, Copley SJ. Imaging appearance of thoracic amyloidosis. J Thorac Imaging 2005;20(1): 41–46

2. Calatayud J, Candelas G, Gómez A, Morado C, Trancho FH. Nodular pulmonary amyloidosis in a patient with rheumatoid arthritis. Clin Rheumatol 2007;26(10):1797–1798

3. Gurney JW, Winer-Muram HT, Rosado-de-Christenson ML, et al. Amyloidosis, lung. In: Specialty Imaging-HRCT of the Lung: Anatomic Basis, Imaging Features, Differential Diagnosis. Salt Lake City: Amirsys, Inc.; 2009:270–275

4. Webb WR, Müller NL, Naidich DP. Miscellaneous infiltrative lung disease. In: High-Resolution CT of the Lung, 4th ed. Philadelphia: Lippincott, Williams & Wilkins; 2009:485–489

Section IX

Occupational Lung Disease

OVERVIEW OF OCCUPATIONAL LUNG DISEASE

The tracheobronchial tree and lung parenchyma may be injured by a variety of inhaled agents, most commonly cigarette smoke, with its potential to cause tracheitis, bronchitis, and bronchiolitis of the airways, and to incite inflammatory and destructive changes in the lung parenchyma.

Several occupations have the potential to expose individuals to other forms of inhalational lung disease. Prior to our current knowledge regarding the dangers of occupational exposure, workers moved freely and without environmental protection through work sites where silica and asbestos, for example, were widespread and freely disseminated. Today, the danger of such exposures is well recognized and federal regulations have brought about a steep decline in the incidence of high exposure to those agents. But today's patient population often includes older individuals who were part of the former work force, and present-day radiologists can expect to encounter additional cases of occupational lung disease throughout their years of professional practice.

In addition to silica and asbestos, there are other workplace exposures that may affect the airways and lungs. Farmers, for example, may develop a striking hypersensitivity reaction to hay; and metal workers working with hard metal grinding tools may develop an unusual interstitial lung disease with debilitating effects.

The Occupational Safety and Health Administration (OSHA) under the United States Department of Labor establishes and monitors safety standards for the workplace that have had a beneficial effect upon the incidence and severity of occupational lung disease. Some of the more commonly encountered cases of occupational lung disease are discussed in this section.

CASE 124

■ Clinical Presentation

80-year-old man with increasing dyspnea

■ Radiologic Findings

Coned-down PA chest radiograph (**Fig. 124.1A**) demonstrates small bilateral well-defined nodules (1–6 mm) and coalescent nodular opacities (>1 cm) that predominantly involve the upper and mid lung zones. There is bilateral upper lobe parenchymal distortion. Chest CT (lung window) (**Figs. 124.1B, 124.1C**) shows bilateral upper lobe spiculated masses, small well-defined nodules, and larger irregular opacities in the dorsal aspect of both upper lobes.

■ Diagnosis

Silicosis; complicated

■ Differential Diagnosis

- Coal Worker's Pneumoconiosis
- Sarcoidosis
- Tuberculosis

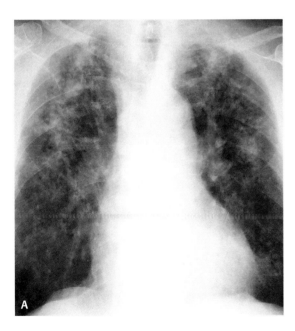
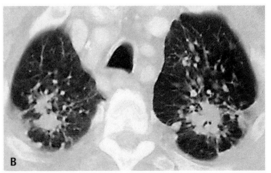
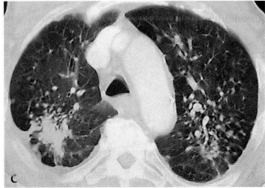

Fig. 124.1

■ Discussion

Background

The term *pneumoconiosis* refers to the accumulation of dust in the lungs and the tissue reaction to its presence. The most frequently encountered inorganic dusts are silica, asbestos, coal, iron, and beryllium, and accumulation occurs most commonly through inhalation during occupational exposure. Silicosis is a chronic occupational lung disease characterized by pulmonary nodules that may coalesce to form lung masses and may progress to pulmonary fibrosis in patients with a history of inhalation of crystalline free silica. Criteria for the diagnosis of silicosis are (1) appropriate exposure history, (2) radiologic findings consistent with silicosis, and (3) absence of other diseases to explain the radiologic findings. *Simple silicosis* refers to cases in which small silicotic nodules (<10 mm) are present and larger, conglomerate opacities are not demonstrated. It occurs in 10–20% of exposed workers. *Complicated silicosis* refers to progression of disease with larger nodules which coalesce to form conglomerate masses (>1 cm) in a process called progressive massive fibrosis (PMF). Complicated silicosis occurs in 1–2% of exposed workers.

Etiology

The most important factors in the development of silicosis are the intensity and duration of exposure to silica. The most abundant source of crystalline silica is quartz, and exposure is most common in rock mining, quarrying, stone cutting, sandblasting, and ceramics. Pathogenetic factors include the size, shape, and concentration of dust particles, duration of exposure, and individual patient susceptibility. Relatively low levels of exposure result in classic chronic silicosis. Silica particles are ingested by alveolar macrophages; when the macrophages eventually break down, enzymes and other products are released and the silica particles become available for re-ingestion by other macrophages. This repeating cycle explains the progression of silicosis, despite cessation of exposure to silica dust. A rare, generalized form of *alveolar proteinosis* (silicoproteinosis; syn. acute silicosis) may occur in individuals who experience a massive exposure to silica dust in enclosed spaces (e.g., sandblasters). In those individuals, the normal clearing mechanisms are overwhelmed, and silica particles are taken up by type II pneumocytes. *Silicoproteinosis* is a rapidly progressive condition that may result in death from respiratory failure within 1–2 years.

Clinical Findings

Patients with *simple silicosis* are typically asymptomatic. In cases of *complicated silicosis*, dyspnea usually occurs and typically develops following a latency period of 10–20 years. Individuals with *silicoproteinosis* (acute silicosis) may develop symptoms within a few weeks or months of exposure. Patients with silicosis have an increased susceptibility to infection with *Mycobacterium tuberculosis*, atypical mycobacteria, and fungi. The development of fever or weight loss in a patient with silicosis is suggestive of concomitant infection, especially by *M. tuberculosis*.

Imaging Features

Chest Radiography

- Small, well-circumscribed nodules, typically 2–5 mm (**Figs. 124.1A, 124.2A, 124.6**)
- Large opacities (>1 cm) typically in middle portion or peripheral upper lobes; eventual hilar migration with resultant emphysematous lung between mass and pleura (**Figs. 124.1A, 124.3, 124.4, 124.6**)
- Predominant upper and posterior lung zone involvement (**Figs. 124.1A, 124.3, 124.4, 124.6**)
- Frequent hilar and mediastinal lymphadenopathy; often calcified (peripheral "eggshell" pattern of calcification in 5%) (**Figs. 124.5A, 124.6**)
- Cavitation of PMF, apical pleural thickening, or rapid changes in the radiographic abnormalities (**Fig. 124.6**)

MDCT/HRCT

- Small (2–5 mm) ill-defined or well-defined (centrilobular and subpleural) nodules (**Figs. 124.1B, 124.1C**)
- Reticular opacities (**Figs. 124.1B, 124.1C**)
- Diffuse distribution with upper lobe and posterior predominance (**Figs. 124.1B, 124.1C, 124.2B**)
- Conglomerate irregular masses; may show central areas of cavitation (**Figs. 124.1B, 124.1C**)
- Focal centrilobular emphysema

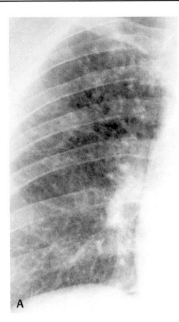

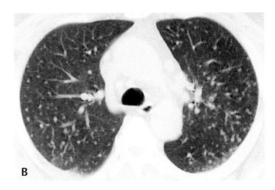

Fig. 124.2 Coned down PA chest radiograph **(A)** of a 72-year-old man with simple silicosis demonstrates diffuse small pulmonary nodules that involve both lungs with a predominant upper lung zone distribution. Chest CT **(B)** demonstrates small (2–5 mm) well-defined (centrilobular and subpleural) nodules.

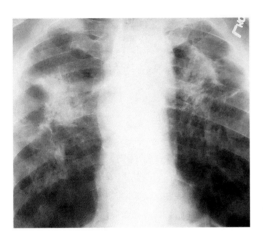

Fig. 124.3 Coned-down PA chest radiograph of a 67-year-old man with complicated coal worker's pneumoconiosis demonstrates irregular spiculated conglomerate masses in the upper lung zones with peripheral emphysema and subtle nodularity.

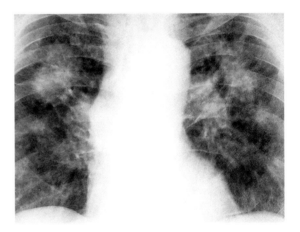

Fig. 124.4 Coned-down PA chest radiograph of a 62-year-old man with complicated silicosis demonstrates bilateral conglomerate masses predominantly involving the upper lung zones.

- Irregular or cicatricial emphysema
- Lymph node enlargement or calcification; may exhibit peripheral pattern of calcification (i.e., "eggshell") (**Fig. 124.5B**)

Management

- Cessation of exposure

Prognosis

- Simple silicosis: good
- Advanced complicated silicosis: significantly increased mortality rates
- Recent decrease in mortality rates (from 1.5 deaths per million population in 1990 to 1.17 in 1999) reported by the Centers for Disease Control and Prevention

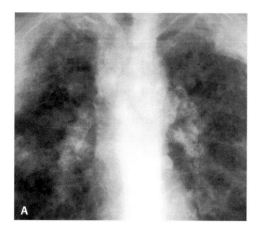
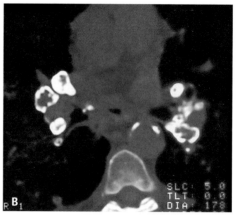

Fig. 124.5 PA chest radiograph **(A)** of a 58-year-old man with complicated silicosis demonstrates multiple bilateral pulmonary nodules, conglomerate masses, and bilateral hilar lymphadenopathy with peripheral ("eggshell") calcification. Unenhanced chest CT (mediastinal window) **(B)** shows dense peripheral ("eggshell") calcification in bilateral hilar lymph nodes.

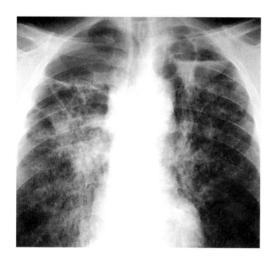

Fig. 124.6 Coned-down PA chest radiograph of a 64-year-old man with complicated silicosis and active tuberculosis (silicotuberculosis) demonstrates multiple small nodules predominantly involving the upper and middle lung zones with conglomerate opacities and biapical bullae. Note bilateral hilar and mediastinal lymphadenopathy with peripheral calcification ("eggshell") in aortico-pulmonary lymph nodes. An air-fluid level developed in the left apical bulla and prompted further evaluation, which resulted in the diagnosis of silicotuberculosis.

PEARLS

- 1980 International Labor Office (ILO) International Classification of Radiographs of the Pneumoconioses is a system used worldwide to record radiographic findings related to the inhalation of dusts. A set of 22 standard radiographs that demonstrate increasing profusion of round and irregular opacities are compared with the radiograph being evaluated, and a standardized scoring system is used. A CT scoring system similar to the ILO system is now being employed by several European countries.
- Tuberculosis is a serious complication of silicosis and should be suspected when nodular opacities increase in size rapidly or cavitate, if apical pleural thickening develops, or when there is a relatively rapid change in other radiographic abnormalities (**Fig. 124.6**).
- Silicoproteinosis (acute silicosis) manifests as bilateral diffuse or perihilar air space consolidation or ground glass opacities.
- Radiographic and CT features of coal worker's pneumoconiosis (CWP) are nearly identical. The prevalence of CWP has decreased since 1970, when federal mandates were established to reduce coal dust levels.

Suggested Reading

1. Hansell DM, Lynch DA, McAdams HP, et al. Inhalational lung disease. In: Hansell DM, Lynch DA, McAdams HP, Bankier AA, ed. Imaging of Diseases of the Chest. 5th ed. Philadelphia: Mosby Elsevier; 2010:451–504

2. Kim JS, Lynch DA. Imaging of nonmalignant occupational lung disease. J Thorac Imaging 2002;17(4):238–260

3. Laga AC, Allen T, Cagle PT. Silicosis. In: Cagle PT, ed. Color Atlas and Text of Pulmonary Pathology. Philadelphia: Lippincott Williams & Willkins; 2005:397–399

4. National Institute for Occupational Safety and Health (NIOSH). Silicosis and related exposures. In: The Work-Related Lung Disease Surveillance Report, 2002. Washington, DC: U.S. Department of Health and Human Services (Centers for Disease Control and Prevention); 2003

5. Rosenman KD, Reilly MJ, Kalinowski DJ, Watt FC. Silicosis in the 1990s. Chest 1997;111(3):779–786

CASE 125

■ Clinical Presentation

68-year-old man with cough and dyspnea recently retired after a 35-year career in the insulation manufacturing industry

■ Radiologic Findings

HRCT (modified lung window) (**Figs. 125.1A, 125.1B**) demonstrates peripheral lower lobe architectural distortion with subpleural dot-like opacities (**Fig. 125.1A**), subpleural lines (**Figs. 125.1A, 125.1B**), and parenchymal bands (**Fig. 125.1A**) and additional findings of fibrosis with irregular interlobular septal thickening, intralobular interstitial thickening, irregular interfaces, and traction bronchiectasis or bronchiolectasis (**Figs. 125.1A, 125.1B**).

■ Diagnosis

Asbestosis

■ Differential Diagnosis

- Idiopathic Pulmonary Fibrosis
- Connective Tissue Lung Disease (scleroderma, rheumatoid arthritis)
- Drug Toxicity
- Post-Irradiation Pneumonitis

■ Discussion

Background

Inhalation of asbestos fibers is associated with a variety of pleural and parenchymal lung diseases, including pleural effusion, pleural plaques, rounded atelectasis, mesothelioma, asbestosis, and an increased inci-

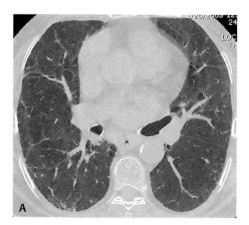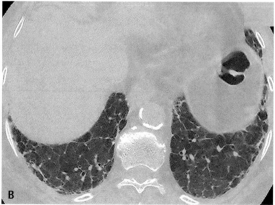

Fig. 125.1

dence of lung cancer (**Table 125.1**). Asbestos fibers are naturally occurring fibrous silicates that have been widely used in industry because of their heat-resistant properties. They are usually categorized as chrysotile (serpentine) or amphibole (needle-like) fibers. Chrysotile fibers are more easily cleared from the lung and less strongly associated with carcinogenesis than the amphibole fibers. Asbestos fibers may be found within alveoli and have been isolated from the pleura, omentum, and mesentery. Pulmonary parenchymal fibrosis initially occurs in and around the respiratory bronchioles, preferentially occurring in the lower lobes and adjacent to visceral pleura, where asbestos fibers are known to accumulate.

Etiology

Most urban-dwelling individuals have been exposed to asbestos as a frequent component of ambient air. High levels of exposure are associated with some occupations: asbestos mining and processing, working with asbestos cement, shipbuilding, construction, manufacture of insulation, handling brake lining and friction products, and production of floor tiles. Asbestosis occurs almost exclusively in individuals exposed to high concentrations of asbestos mineral fibers, often occurring over the course of many years. Federal regulations established in the late 1970s led to a sharp decline in high exposures to asbestos.

Clinical Findings

Affected patients complain of cough and dyspnea. Pulmonary function tests demonstrate restrictive lung disease, and patients become hypoxic with exercise. Auscultation reveals basal crackles or rales. Asbestos bodies may be found in bronchoalveolar lavage specimens, indicating asbestos exposure, but are not diagnostic of asbestosis. Lung cancer occurs in a significantly larger number of asbestos-exposed individuals than in the general population. The risk of lung cancer increases with the severity of exposure to asbestos and with the presence of asbestosis. It occurs 50–100 times more frequently in asbestos-exposed individuals who smoke than in the non-smoking, non-exposed population. Asbestos-related lung cancers occur most frequently in the lower lobes, corresponding to the distribution of asbestosis.

Imaging Findings

Chest Radiography

- Fine to medium reticular opacities predominantly involving the peripheral aspects of the lower lobes (**Fig. 125.2**)
- Pleural plaques (**Fig. 125.2**)
- Coarse reticulation and honeycomb lung (advanced cases)
- Normal chest radiograph in 26% of proven cases

MDCT/HRCT

- Subpleural dot-like opacities (**Figs. 125.1A, 125.4**)
- Subpleural lines (**Figs. 125.1A, 125.1B, 125.3, 125.4**)
- Parenchymal bands (**Fig. 125.1A**)
- Findings of fibrosis; irregular interlobular septal thickening, intralobular interstitial thickening, irregular interfaces, traction bronchiectasis or bronchiolectasis (**Figs. 125.1A, 125.1B, 125.3, 125.4**)
- Predominance of findings in dorsal aspects of lower lobes (**Figs. 125.1A, 125.1B, 125.4**)

Table 125.1 Thoracic Manifestations of Asbestos Fiber Exposure

Pulmonary Manifestations	Pleural Manifestations
Primary lung cancer	Pleural effusion
Rounded atelectasis	Non-calcified plaques
Asbestosis	Calcified plaques
	Diffuse pleural thickening
	Diffuse malignant mesothelioma

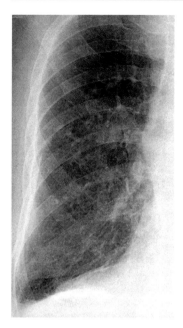

Fig. 125.2 Coned-down PA chest radiograph demonstrates reticular opacities that predominantly involve the peripheral lower lung zones. Calcified pleural plaques are seen on the mid pleural surfaces and along the diaphragm.

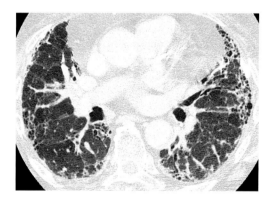

Fig. 125.3 HRCT (lung window) of a 72-year-old man with asbestosis shows advanced findings of fibrosis with irregular interlobular septal thickening, intralobular reticulation, subpleural lines, honeycombing, and a calcified pleural plaque along the left costal pleura.

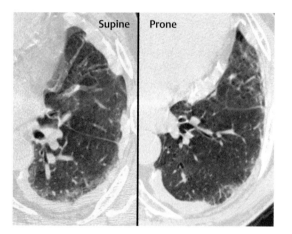

Fig. 125.4 Composite HRCT (lung window) of a 69-year-old man with asbestosis obtained in the supine position (*left*) demonstrates subpleural ground glass opacity that partly obscures the underlying lung parenchyma. Prone HRCT image at the same level (*right*) reveals findings of fibrosis characteristic of asbestosis (irregular interlobular septal thickening, intralobular interstitial thickening, and subpleural lines) with extensive partially calcified pleural plaques.

- Honeycomb lung (advanced disease) (**Fig. 125.3**)
- Parietal pleural thickening or plaques (**Figs. 125.3, 125.4**)
- Earliest abnormalities posterior and basal (may require prone HRCT imaging) (**Fig. 125.4**)

Management

- None

Prognosis

- Slow progression; may occur in the absence of further exposure
- Increasing dyspnea with advancing imaging abnormalities
- Increase in asbestosis-related deaths in recent decades (annual age-adjusted death rate of 0.54 per million population in 1968 to 6.88 per million in 2000) reported by Centers for Disease Control and Prevention

PEARLS

- Pathologic diagnosis of asbestosis requires demonstration of asbestos bodies in association with interstitial fibrosis with or without visceral pleural fibrosis.
- Imaging features of asbestosis may be indistinguishable from idiopathic pulmonary fibrosis (IPF) and other diseases manifesting with a usual interstitial pneumonia (UIP) pattern on HRCT.
- Presence of parietal pleural thickening in association with interstitial fibrosis that is peripheral and predominant in the lower lung zones is highly suggestive of asbestosis.
- Prone HRCT is most sensitive for detecting early findings of asbestosis and distinguishes it from dependent atelectasis in the dorsal lung (**Fig. 125.4**).

Suggested Reading

1. Hansell DM, Lynch DA, McAdams HP, et al. Inhalational lung disease. In: Hansell DM, Lynch DA, McAdams HP, Bankier AA, ed. Imaging of Diseases of the Chest, 5th ed. Philadelphia: Mosby Elsevier; 2010:451–504

2. Webb WR, Müller NL, Naidich DP. Diseases characterized primarily by linear and reticular opacities. In: Webb WR, Müller NL, Naidich DP, eds. High-Resolution CT of the Lung, 3rd ed. Philadelphia: Lippincott Williams and Wilkins; 2001:236–244

3. Akira M, Yamamoto S, Yokoyama K, et al. Asbestosis: high-resolution CT-pathologic correlation. Radiology 1990; 176(2):389–394

4. Kim JS, Lynch DA. Imaging of nonmalignant occupational lung disease. J Thorac Imaging 2002;17(4):238–260

CASE 126

■ Clinical Presentation

37-year-old man with acute dyspnea

■ Radiologic Findings

HRCT (lung window) (**Figs. 126.1A, 126.1B**) demonstrates patchy bilateral diffuse ground glass opacity

■ Diagnosis

Farmer's Lung; Hypersensitivity Pneumonitis

■ Differential Diagnosis

- *Pneumocystis jiroveci* Pneumonia
- Desquamative Interstitial Pneumonia (DIP)
- Pulmonary Drug Toxicity
- Alveolar Proteinosis

■ Discussion

Background

Farmer's lung is an occupational lung disease caused by exposure to moldy hay and inhalation of the associated antigen. Farmer's lung was one of first recognized forms of hypersensitivity pneumonitis, a group of diseases characterized by an abnormal immunologic reaction to specific antigens in a variety of organic dusts. A long list of other forms of hypersensitivity pneumonitis now exists, including bird fancier's lung, mushroom worker's lung, and detergent worker's lung. A striking similarity in the clinical, pathologic, and imaging features of these entities suggests a common pathogenesis (see Case 115). Hypersensitivity pneumonitis may develop acutely or may occur as a subacute or chronic disease, depending on the duration of exposure and individual patient susceptibilities.

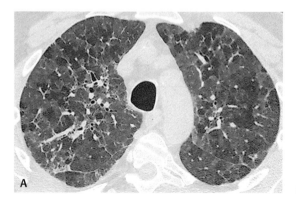 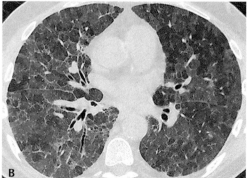

Fig. 126.1 *(Images courtesy of Jud W. Gurney MD, University of Nebraska Hospital, Omaha, Nebraska.)*

Etiology

Farmer's lung is caused by hypersensitivity to inhaled microorganisms (thermophilic actinomycetes) that grow in moldy hay. Affected patients are typically farmers who are exposed during the seasonal use of hay for feeding cattle.

Clinical Findings

Patients with farmer's lung are typically 40–50-year-old men who present with acute dyspnea after working with stored hay used for cattle feeding. Most cases occur during the winter or early spring (January–March). Affected patients typically present with fever, chills, cough, and dyspnea. Criteria for establishing the diagnosis of farmer's lung and other forms of hypersensitivity pneumonitis are summarized in **Table 126.1**.

Imaging Features

Chest Radiography

- Ground glass opacities or ill-defined consolidation
- Interstitial linear/nodular opacities

MDCT/HRCT

Subacute

- Patchy or diffuse ground glass opacity (**Figs. 126.1A, 126.1B**)
- Small centrilobular nodular opacities
- Mosaic perfusion (lobular areas of decreased attenuation) (**Figs. 126.1A, 126.1B**)
- Air trapping on expiratory scans

Chronic

- Fibrosis without zonal predominance
- Ground glass opacity or centrilobular nodules
- Patchy distribution

Management

- Cessation of exposure

Table 126.1 Criteria for Diagnosis of Farmer's Lung and Other Forms of Hypersensitivity Pneumonitis

Exposure to organic dust of sufficiently fine particle size to allow deep penetration into lung
Dyspnea; often associated with cough, fever, and malaise occurring within hours after exposure to offending antigen
Auscultatory crackles over both lung bases
Diffuse ground glass opacities or ill-defined small nodules on imaging studies
Reduced vital capacity on pulmonary function tests (PFTs)
Serum precipitins against suspected antigen
Increased T-lymphocytes and increased levels of immunoglobulins on bronchoalveolar lavage
Bronchiolitis and interstitial pneumonitis on lung biopsy; occasional granuloma formation
Resolution of symptoms after cessation of exposure to relevant antigen

Prognosis

- Good with prompt cessation of exposure; resolution of radiographic abnormalities within 10 days to three months
- Poor with repeated or continued exposure; progression to interstitial fibrosis

PEARLS

- Extent of ground glass opacities seen in patients with hypersensitivity pneumonitis does *not* correlate with the results of PFTs, which may show restriction or obstruction.

Suggested Reading

1. Adler BD, Padley SPG, Müller NL, Remy-Jardin M, Remy J. Chronic hypersensitivity pneumonitis: high-resolution CT and radiographic features in 16 patients. Radiology 1992;185(1):91–95

2. Cormier Y, Brown M, Worthy S, Racine G, Müller NL. High-resolution computed tomographic characteristics in acute farmer's lung and in its follow-up. Eur Respir J 2000;16(1):56–60

3. Glazer CS, Rose CS, Lynch DA. Clinical and radiologic manifestations of hypersensitivity pneumonitis. J Thorac Imaging 2002;17(4):261–272

4. Hansell DM, Lynch DA, McAdams HP, et al. Inhalational lung disease. In: Hansell DM, Lynch DA, McAdams HP, Bankier AA, ed. Imaging of Diseases of the Chest, 5th ed. Philadelphia: Mosby Elsevier; 2010:451–504

5. Hansell DM, Wells AU, Padley SPG, Müller NL. Hypersensitivity pneumonitis: correlation of individual CT patterns with functional abnormalities. Radiology 1996;199(1):123–128

CASE 127

▪ Clinical Presentation

43-year-old man with cough and dyspnea

▪ Radiologic Findings

HRCT (lung window) (**Figs. 127.1A, 127.1B**) demonstrates peripheral areas of ground glass opacity involving the upper, middle, and lower lung zones with fine, peripheral, and subpleural reticulation. An area of traction bronchiectasis is demonstrated in the left mid lung (**Fig. 127.1A**).

▪ Diagnosis

Hard Metal Pneumoconiosis (Cobalt-Related)

▪ Differential Diagnosis

- Desquamative Interstitial Pneumonia (DIP)
- Interstitial Lung Disease of Other Etiologies
- Immunoglobulin (IgE)-Mediated Asthma
- Hypersensitivity Pneumonitis (HP)

▪ Discussion

Background

In the 1960s, Liebow originally classified giant cell interstitial pneumonia (GIP) as one of the idiopathic interstitial pneumonias. Today, it is recognized as an uncommon interstitial lung disease caused by exposure to hard metal. Hard metal pneumoconiosis is related to exposure to metals used primarily to grind, drill, cut, and polish other metals. Occupational exposure may occur during those activities or during the hard metal manufacture. Occupations associated with exposure to hard metal include diamond polishing, saw and drill grinding, oil well drilling, and armor plating.

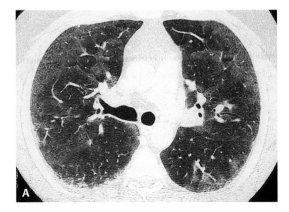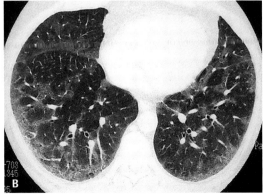

Fig. 127.1

609

Etiology

Hard metal pneumoconiosis (syn. giant cell interstitial pneumonia) is caused by exposure to hard metal, an alloy that consists primarily of tungsten, carbon, and cobalt. Animal studies suggest that cobalt is the constituent of hard metal that causes pulmonary disease. Diamond polishers are exposed to high levels of cobalt alone and develop interstitial lung disease identical to that which occurs in hard metal workers.

Clinical Findings

Affected patients present with cough, dyspnea, wheezing, and allergic-type asthma and have a suggestive occupational exposure. Pulmonary function tests reveal both restrictive and obstructive lung disease, often with decreased diffusing capacity. The diagnosis is usually confirmed by work history and analysis of lung tissue for metals by energy-dispersive X-ray analysis or other techniques.

Imaging Features

Chest Radiography

- Diffuse reticular and nodular opacities
- Lymphadenopathy
- Upper and middle zone–predominant distribution; may resemble sarcoidosis
- Small cystic spaces representing honeycombing in advanced cases
- Normal chest radiograph in some cases

MDCT/HRCT

- Bilateral ground glass opacities (**Figs. 127.1A, 127.1B**)
- Variable appearance; may resemble NSIP, UIP, or sarcoidosis
- Findings of fibrosis or UIP (**Figs. 127.1A, 127.1B**)
- Traction bronchiectasis (**Fig. 127.1A**)
- Peripheral cystic spaces
- Spontaneous pneumothorax

Management

- Removal from offending workplace exposure
- Corticosteroids

Prognosis

- Progressive symptoms leading to respiratory failure, which may be fatal

Suggested Reading

1. Enriquez LS, Mohammed TL, Johnson GL, Lefor MJ, Beasley MB. Hard metal pneumoconiosis: a case of giant-cell interstitial pneumonitis in a machinist. Respir Care 2007;52(2):196–199

2. Gotway MB, Golden JA, Warnock M, et al. Hard metal interstitial lung disease: high-resolution computed tomography appearance. J Thorac Imaging 2002;17(4):314–318

3. Kim KI, Kim CW, Lee MK, et al. Imaging of occupational lung disease. Radiographics 2001;21(6):1371–1391

Section X

Adult Cardiovascular Disease

CASE 128

■ Clinical Presentation

44-year-old man presenting to the emergency department following an 18-hour transcontinental air flight with chest pain and shortness of breath

■ Radiologic Findings

Chest CTPA (mediastinal window) (**Figs. 128.1A, 128.1B, 128.1C, 128.1D, 128.1E, 128.1F**) demonstrates extensive filling defects involving virtually every branch of the pulmonary arterial circuit. The right heart, and right ventricle in particular, is enlarged and there is inward bowing of the interventricular septum consistent with right heart strain.

■ Diagnosis

Acute Pulmonary Thromboembolic Disease

■ Differential Diagnosis

None

■ Discussion

Background

Acute pulmonary thromboembolism (PTE) is responsible for 2–7% of acute care hospital deaths, and the *third most common* cause of cardiovascular death, after myocardial ischemia and stroke. However, PTE is not a disease in and of itself but a complication of underlying venous thrombosis (VTE). The average annual incidence of VTE is 1 per 1,000 (United States), with approximately 250,000 incident cases occurring annually. Autopsy studies show an equal number of patients with PTE-VTE unsuspected or not diagnosed antemortem. Thus, an estimated 650,000 to 900,000 cases of fatal and nonfatal PTE-VTE occur annually in the United States alone.

Etiology

Normally in the venous system there is a dynamic balance between the formation and subsequent lysis of microthrombi that allows for local hemostasis in response to injury but prevents uncontrolled propagation of thrombus. Certain pathologic conditions allow microthrombi to escape the fibrinolytic system, propagate, and potentially embolize into the pulmonary arterial circuit as pulmonary emboli. Ninety percent of such pulmonary emboli originate from lower extremity deep veins. Predisposing VTE is induced by inflammation of the vessel wall, venous stasis, and hypercoagulable states (i.e., Virchow triad). Clinical risk factors for PTE-VTE are directly related to one or more of these components and are summarized in **Table 128.1**.

Clinical Findings

Diagnosis of PTE poses a challenge for both clinicians and radiologists because the signs and symptoms are nonspecific. The *classic triad* of pleuritic chest pain, dyspnea, and hemoptysis is neither sensitive nor specific and occurs in less than 20% of patients. Additionally, many patients are relatively asymptomatic. Physical

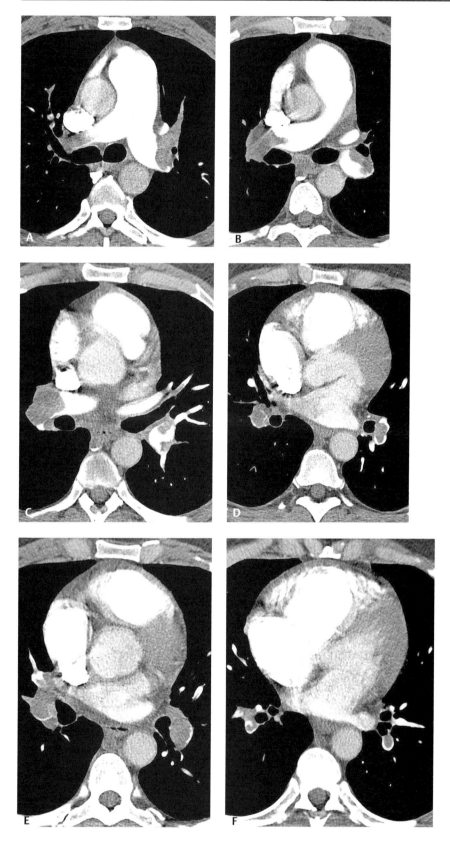

Fig. 128.1

Table 128.1   Clinical Risk Factors for Developing PTE-VTE

| Hereditary | Acquired | | | | |
	Prolonged Immobilization	Acute Illness	Neoplasia	Pregnancy	Other
Protein C deficiency	Trauma	ICU	Chemotherapy	Peri-partum	OCP*
Protein S deficiency	Recent surgery	Heart failure		Post-partum	Long-term catheters
Anti-thrombin III deficiency	Burns	AIDS (lupus anticoagulant)			Pacemakers
Factor V leiden	Fractures	Acute MI			Advanced age
Plasminogen or plasminogen activator abnormalities	Obesity	New-onset atrial fibrillation			Previous PTE-VTE
Fibrinogen abnormalities	Spinal cord injuries	Polycythemia			High-dose estrogen therapy
	Travel	SLE			Varicose veins

Abbreviation: OCP,* oral contraceptives

signs may include tachypnea; rales, pleural rub, or new wheezing; tachycardia; S_3 or S_4 gallop; new murmur; accentuated second heart sound; fever; diaphoresis; lower extremity edema; and cyanosis. Massive pulmonary embolism may be associated with hypotension due to acute cor pulmonale. Patients with PTE may have an abnormally high A-a gradient, and right ventricular strain on ECG. D-dimer levels may be elevated with PTE-VTE. D-dimer is a degradation product of plasmin-mediated proteolysis of cross-linked fibrin and is considered *positive* when >500 ng/mL. However, levels may be falsely elevated in numerous clinical settings (e.g., severe trauma, recent surgery, infection, neoplasia, rheumatoid factor, and advanced age).

Imaging Findings

Chest Radiography

- Primary role: exclude other causes of a particular patient's signs and symptoms; guide V/Q scan interpretation
- 10–15% of symptomatic patients with angiographically proven PTE—normal chest X-ray
- Over 24–72 hours, initially normal chest radiograph may begin to demonstrate atelectasis, small pleural effusion, and ipsilateral diaphragmatic elevation
- After 24–72 hours, one-third of patients with proven PTE develop focal air space opacities indistinguishable from pneumonia

Chest Radiography: Thromboembolism without Infarction

- Peripheral oligemia (i.e., *Westermark* sign) (**Fig. 128.2A**)
- Enlargement of a major pulmonary artery (i.e., *Fleischner* sign) (**Fig. 128.2A**)
- Abrupt tapering of the occluded vessel (i.e., *knuckle* sign)
- Volume loss and ipsilateral diaphragmatic elevation
- Cardiac enlargement

Chest Radiography: Thromboembolism with Hemorrhage or Infarction

- 15% of acute PTE—complicated by pulmonary infarction
- Any of the above signs and peripheral parenchymal consolidation (i.e., *Hampton hump*) (**Figs. 128.3A, 128.3B**)
- Early infarcts

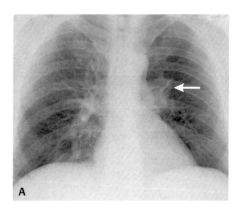
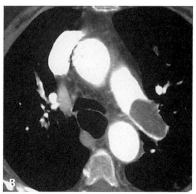

Fig. 128.2 PA chest radiograph **(A)** of a 46-year-old man complaining of chest pain shows preserved lung volumes, a hyperlucent left hemithorax, a disproportionately enlarged left pulmonary artery (*Fleischner* sign), and diffuse oligemia of the ipsilateral thorax (*Westermark* sign). Contrast-enhanced chest CT (mediastinal window) **(B)** reveals a large soft-tissue attenuation acute PTE occluding and expanding the left pulmonary artery. *(Images courtesy of Laura E. Heyneman, MD, University of North Carolina, Wilmington, North Carolina.)*

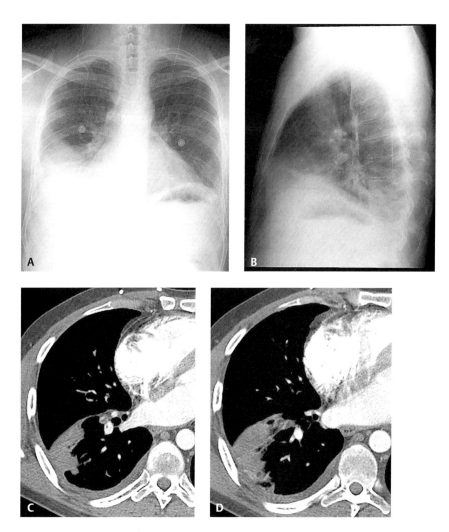

Fig. 128.3 PA **(A)** and lateral **(B)** chest radiographs of a 33-year-old man three days following abdominal and pelvic surgery for testicular cancer and now complaining of right-sided pleuritic chest pain shows a focal peripheral region of consolidation in the right lower lobe and a small pleural effusion. Contrast-enhanced chest CT (mediastinal window) **(C,D)** reveals segmental arterial filling defects in the right lower lobe and a peripheral infarct in that vascular territory as well as the small effusion. Diagnosis: acute PTE with infarct.

- Often appears as ill-defined parenchymal opacities or as a homogeneous peripheral wedge-shaped opacity (**Figs. 128.3A, 128.3B**)
- Base contiguous with visceral pleura; apex points toward hilum (**Figs. 128.3A, 128.3B**)
- Most infarcts located in the costophrenic sulcus of right lower lobe and involve one or two segments (**Figs. 128.3A, 128.3B**)
- Opacities range from 3 to 5 cm in diameter; may develop in as little as 10 hours following the vascular occlusion (**Figs. 128.3A, 128.3B**)
- Air bronchograms and cavitation rare (**Figs. 128.3A, 128.3B**)
- Small ipsilateral pleural effusion (30–50%) (**Figs. 128.3A, 128.3B**)

Ventilation-Perfusion Scintigraphy

Normal V/Q Scan

- No perfusion defects seen
- 2% of patients with PTE have this pattern; 4% of patients with this pattern have PTE

Low-Probability V/Q Scan

- Small perfusion defects, regardless of number, ventilation findings, or chest X-ray findings
- Perfusion defects substantially smaller than chest X-ray abnormality in same area
- Matching perfusion and ventilation defects <75% of one lung zone or <50% of one lung; normal or nearly normal chest X-ray
- Single segmental perfusion defect and normal chest X-ray, regardless of ventilation match or mismatch
- Nonsegmental perfusion defects
- 16% of patients with PTE have this pattern; 14% of patients with this pattern have PTE

Intermediate Probability V/Q Scan

- Any V/Q abnormality not otherwise classified
- 40% of patients with PTE have this pattern; 30% of patients with this pattern have PTE

High-Probability V/Q Scan (**Fig. 128.4**)

- ≥2 segmental or larger perfusion defects; normal chest X-ray; normal ventilation
- ≥2 segmental or larger perfusion defects; chest X-ray abnormalities and ventilation defects substantially smaller than perfusion defects
- ≥2 subsegmental + 1 large segmental perfusion defect; normal chest X-ray; normal ventilation
- ≥4 subsegmental perfusion defects; normal chest X-ray; normal ventilation
- 41% of patients with PTE have this pattern; 87% of patients with this pattern have PTE

Duplex Ultrasonography

- Clinical suspicion can be supported by demonstrating deep venous thrombosis (DVT)
- Normal, patent veins easily and completely compressible with transducer pressure; alternatively, adjacent muscular arteries resistant to compression
- Thrombosed veins (DVT) are not compressible and do not completely collapse with transducer pressure
- Negative duplex scan does not exclude potential DVT; the site of DVT may be inaccessible or not visualized in up to two-thirds of patients with PTE

Catheter Pulmonary Angiography

Direct signs

- Intraluminal filling defects or abrupt vascular cut-offs (**Fig. 128.5**)

Indirect (Non-Specific) signs

- Diminished capillary staining or delayed opacification

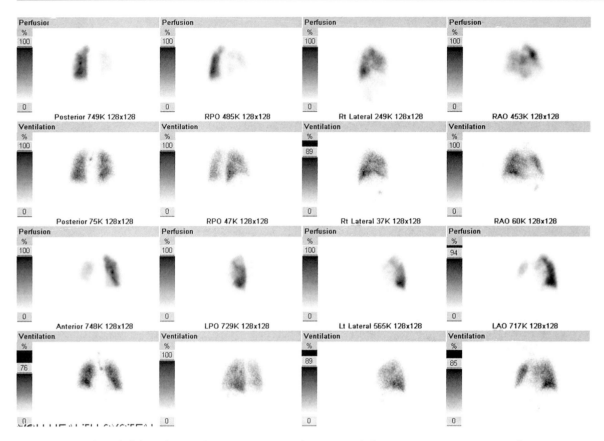

Fig. 128.4   High-probability V/Q scan (Tc99m DTPA aerosol; 1.2 mCi inhalation; Tc99m MAA 3.5 mCi IV) on a 62-year-old man with dyspnea and pleuritic chest pain. Globally diminished tracer uptake in the right lung compared with the left. Partially mismatched perfusion defect in the apicoposterior segment LUL and a mismatched perfusion defect in the posterobasal segment and possibly anterobasal segment LLL. Mismatched tracer activity is seen in the anterior segment LUL and lingula.

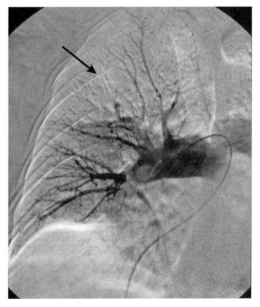

Fig. 128.5   Digital subtraction angiogram demonstrates right upper lobe oligemia, a large clot in the proximal upper lobe pulmonary artery, and scattered smaller emboli in the right middle and lower lobe arteries. Note the peripheral wedge-shaped area of non perfusion or oligemia (*arrow*) (i.e., *Westermark* sign).

MDCT Pulmonary Angiography (CTPA)

- New gold standard for ruling in or ruling out diagnosis of PTE

Diagnostic Criteria (Direct Signs)

- Complete arterial occlusion with failure to opacify entire lumen; artery may be enlarged in comparison with pulmonary arteries of the same order of branching (**Figs. 128.1A, 128.1B, 128.1C, 128.1D, 128.1E, 128.1F, 128.6A, 128.6B**)
- Central arterial filling defect surrounded by contrast media (**Figs. 128.1A, 128.1B, 128.1C, 128.1D, 128.1E, 128.1F**)
- Peripheral intraluminal filling defect; acute angle with arterial wall (**Figs. 128.1D, 128.1E, 128.1F**)

Indirect Signs

- Atelectasis; often subsegmental
- Small pleural effusion
- Oligemia of affected segment
- Pulmonary hemorrhage or infarct (**Figs. 128.3C, 128.3D, 128.7**)
- Right heart strain (**Fig. 128.6B**)
  - Right ventricular dilatation (right ventricular cavity wider than left ventricular cavity in short axis); ± reflux of contrast media into hepatic veins
  - Deviation of interventricular septum toward left ventricle

Potential CT Pitfalls

- Confusing hilar and infrahilar lymph nodes with vascular filling defects
- Poor vessel opacification and motion artifact mimicking or obscuring filling defects
- Increased noise (i.e., quantum mottle) in obese patients
- Obscuration of vessels by adjacent regions of parenchymal consolidation
- Segmental or subsegmental bronchial mucus plugs

Indirect CT Venography (ICTV)

- Performed in conjunction with CTPA once contrast media has passed through deep venous system of pelvis and lower extremities
- Complete or partial filling defect with enlargement of the vein (**Figs. 128.8A, 128.8B**)
- Dense rim enhancement due to contrast staining of the vasa vasorum, and perivenous soft-tissue edema (**Figs. 128.8A, 128.8B**)
- Isolated pelvic DVT is uncommon

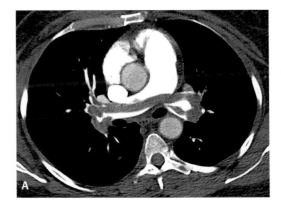 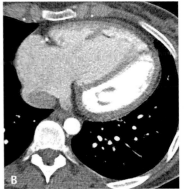

Fig. 128.6 CTPA (mediastinal window) reveals a "saddle" embolus involving the main lobar divisions of each lung with extension into the proximal segmental branches **(A)**. More inferiorly, the right ventricle is enlarged with inward displacement of the interventricular septum, indicating right heart strain **(B)**.

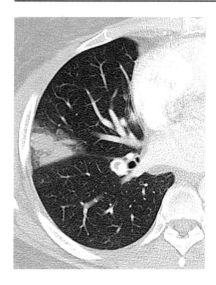

Fig. 128.7 CTPA (lung window) of a 36-year-old man with protein C deficiency shows indirect evidence of acute PTE manifest by a wedge-shaped infarct in the lateral segment RML.

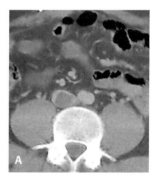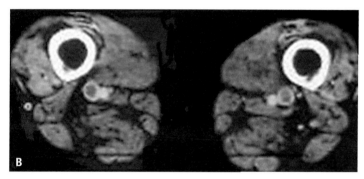

Fig. 128.8 Select ICTV images through the lower abdomen and lower extremities of a 33-year-old man with testicular cancer and suspected PTE reveals thrombus in the iliac system **(A)** and both popliteal veins **(B)**.

Advantages of ICTV

- Determination of overall clot burden
- Road map for therapy (e.g., IVC filter placement)
- Determination of contributing factors (e.g., pelvic mass)

Disadvantage of ICTV

- Increased radiation dose to gonads

Management

- Anticoagulation
- Thrombolysis and/or thrombectomy in select patients (i.e., extensive PTE; concomitant moderate to severe right ventricular dysfunction despite preserved systemic arterial pressure)
- IVC filter deployment; contraindications to anticoagulation therapy

Prognosis

- One-third of patients with PTE will have recurrent emboli
- Mortality massive PTE (i.e., systolic arterial pressure <90 mm Hg; 4% patients): between 30% and 60%; majority of deaths occur in the first one or two hours

- Mortality for patients with non-massive PTE (i.e., systolic arterial pressure ≥90 mm Hg; 96% of patients): <5% in the first three to six months of anticoagulation therapy
- Shock Index (Heart Rate ÷ Systolic Blood Pressure) >1 used as a predictor of in-hospital deterioration of patients diagnosed with acute PTE
- Troponin levels commonly elevated in acute PTE, especially in patients with significant clot burden and right heart dysfunction (**Fig. 128.6B**); associated with worse short-term and long-term prognosis and up to fivefold increase in mortality

PEARLS

- Most important clinically identifiable risk factor for PTE-VTE is prior history of such.
- Considerable advantage of CTPA over both V/Q scan and catheter pulmonary angiography: ability to depict other conditions that clinically mimic PTE (e.g., aortic dissection, pneumothorax, pleural or pericardial disease, pneumonia, lung abscess, pneumomediastinum, esophageal rupture, mediastinitis, pulmonary fibrosis, and neoplastic disease). Such alternative diagnoses have been reported in 11–70% of CTPA examinations performed for clinically suspected acute PTE.
- Paradoxical systemic arterial embolism (PSAE) is a rare complication of PTE (2%). PSAE requires passage of venous thrombus into the arterial circulatory system through a right-to-left shunt, most commonly a patent foramen ovale (PFO). Complications include stroke, myocardial infarction, and showering of thrombi to kidneys, superior mesenteric artery, and lower extremities. PFO may be confirmed by an echosonographic bubble study.

Suggested Reading

1. Grifoni S, Olivotto I, Cecchini P, et al. Short-term clinical outcome of patients with acute pulmonary embolism, normal blood pressure, and echocardiographic right ventricular dysfunction. Circulation 2000;101(24):2817–2822
2. Nazaroğlu H, Ozmen CA, Akay HO, Kilinç I, Bilici A. 64-MDCT pulmonary angiography and CT venography in the diagnosis of thromboembolic disease. AJR Am J Roentgenol 2009;192(3):654–661
3. Sandler DA, Martin JF. Autopsy proven pulmonary embolism in hospital patients: are we detecting enough deep vein thrombosis? J R Soc Med 1989;82(4):203–205
4. Silverstein MD, Heit JA, Mohr DN, Petterson TM, O'Fallon WM, Melton LJ III. Trends in the incidence of deep vein thrombosis and pulmonary embolism: a 25-year population-based study. Arch Intern Med 1998;158(6):585–593
5. Patel S, Kazerooni EA. Helical CT for the evaluation of acute pulmonary embolism. AJR Am J Roentgenol 2005;185(1):135–149
6. Tapson VF. Acute pulmonary embolism. N Engl J Med 2008;358(10):1037–1052

CASE 129

■ Clinical Presentation

72-year-old man with past history of PTE and DVT presents with progressive dyspnea on exertion and fatigue

■ Radiologic Findings

Chest CTPA (mediastinal window) (**Figs. 129.1A, 129.1B, 129.1C, 129.1D, 129.1E**) demonstrates a peripheral, crescent-shaped intraluminal defect with obtuse angles along the left main lobar pulmonary artery's posterior wall (**Fig. 129.1A**) and the lateral wall of the proximal descending left pulmonary artery (**Fig. 129.1B**). The obtuse margins of the intraluminal filling defect relative to the left pulmonary artery are readily appreciated on the MIP sagittal (**Fig. 129.1C**) (*black arrowhead*), coronal (**Fig. 129.1D**) (*white arrow*), and sagittal oblique (**Fig. 129.1E**) (*white arrow*) images. Compare the relative size of the main pulmonary artery (MPA) and ascending aorta. The MPA is not enlarged.

■ Diagnosis

Chronic Pulmonary Thromboembolic Disease

■ Differential Diagnosis

Pulmonary Angiosarcoma

■ Discussion

Background

PTE may be *acute* (≤2 weeks from initial event) or *chronic* (more long-standing, occurring weeks, months, or years after the acute event). Most acute emboli undergo fibrinolysis within 10–21 days and resolve spontaneously or under the course of medical therapy. Complete resolution may take several months in some patients. In a small percentage of patients, pulmonary emboli fail to resolve and become organized into fibrous tissue, resulting in chronic pulmonary thromboembolic disease (CPTE).

Clinical Findings

CPTE obstructs blood flow through the lungs, increasing pulmonary artery pressures (PAP). In some cases, the PAP may approach or exceed systemic arterial pressures. Affected patients may complain of dyspnea on exertion or fatigue. Later on, patients may experience syncope and angina, and develop pulmonary artery hypertension (PAH), right heart enlargement, and eventual right heart failure (i.e., cor pulmonale).

Pulmonary artery sarcoma (PAS) is a rare tumor frequently misdiagnosed as CPTE and is almost uniformly fatal, with reported survival times of a few months to a few years. Surgical resection is the single most effective modality for short-term palliation. The reported age at presentation ranges from 13 to 86 years, although most cases occur in middle age. PASs most often arise from the posterior wall of the MPA trunk. However, tumors may also arise from the right pulmonary artery (RPA), left pulmonary artery (LPA), pulmonary valve (PV), and right ventricular outflow tract (RVOT). Symptoms and signs such as weight loss, fever, anemia, and digital clubbing may suggest the correct diagnosis. Additional clinical findings include absence of risk factors for DVT, high

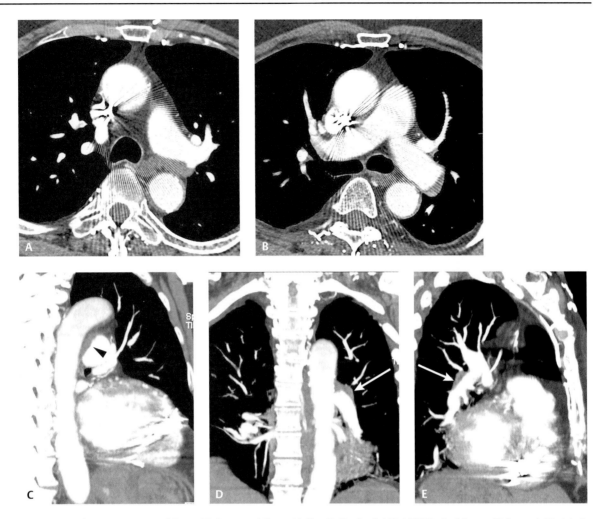

Fig. 129.1   *(Images courtesy of Susan W. Bennett, MD, and Jeffery D. Settles II, MD, VCU Medical Center, Richmond, Virginia.)*

sedimentation rate, nodular parenchymal opacities on CT (i.e., metastases), and failure to respond to anticoagulation. Unfortunately, none of these clinical features definitively excludes the possibility of CPTE.

Imaging Findings

Chest Radiography

- Normal
- Features of pulmonary artery hypertension (see Case 130)

CTPA

Direct Signs of CPTE

- Complete occlusion of a vessel that is smaller than adjacent patent vessels
  - Vessel cut-off from *CTPE* has a *convex* margin with respect to contrast column (i.e., "pouch" defect) (**Fig. 129.2**)
  - Vessel cut-off from *acute PTE* is *concave* with respect to contrast column due to the trailing edge of thrombus
  - Decrease in vessel diameter distal to the complete obstruction from thrombus contraction

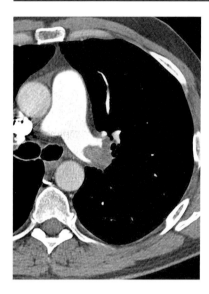

Fig. 129.2 Chest CTPA of a 45-year-old man with progressive dyspnea and CPTE. Large eccentric thrombus completely occludes the distal left pulmonary artery and demonstrates a *convex* margin with respect to contrast column (i.e., "pouch" defect).

- Nonobstructive Filling Defects
  - Organized thrombus may cause intimal irregularities, bands and webs, abrupt vessel narrowing, and subsequent pulmonary artery stenosis (**Fig. 129.3**)
- Intimal Irregularities
  - Broad-based, smoothly marginated opacities; create obtuse angles with vessel wall (**Fig. 129.3**)
  - Unilateral or bilateral
- Bands and Webs (**Fig. 129.4**)
  - *Bands*
    - Delicate ribbon-like structures anchored to vessel wall at two ends with a free unattached midportion
    - Range from 0.3 to 2 cm in length and from less than 0.1 to 0.3cm in width
    - Often oriented along long axis of vessel
  - *Webs*
    - Descriptive term for bands that have branches and form networks of varying complexity (**Fig. 129.4**)
  - *Bands* and *webs* appear as thin lines surrounded by contrast media on CTPA or catheter pulmonary angiography (**Fig. 129.4**)

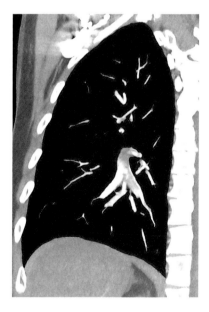

Fig. 129.3 Chest CTPA of a 47-year-old man with persistent dyspnea following acute PTE four months earlier reveals non-obstructing eccentric thrombus with irregularity and narrowing of the vessel lumen in the right lower lobe, consistent with CPTE.

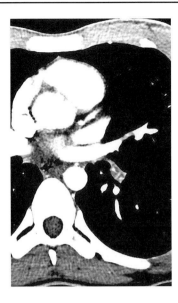

Fig. 129.4 Chest CTPA of a 20-year-old man with protein S deficiency and CTPE. Note the partially thrombosed left lower lobe segmental artery and enhancing "dot-like" areas of vascular recanalization and the obliquely oriented linear band or web.

- Abrupt Vessel Narrowing
  - Often the result of recanalization (**Fig. 129.5**)
  - Abrupt convergence of contrast media that leads to a thin column of intravascular contrast media more distally (**Fig. 129.5**)

Indirect Signs of CPTE

- Post-Stenotic Dilatation or Aneurysm
  - Nonspecific; commonly occurs
- Tortuous Pulmonary Vessels
  - Also seen with PAH
- Enlargement of Main Pulmonary Artery (MPA)
  - Diameter ≥33 mm: precapillary, capillary, and post-capillary PAH; commonly identified in PAH secondary to CPTE
- Enlargement of Bronchial Arteries (BA) (**Fig. 129.6**)

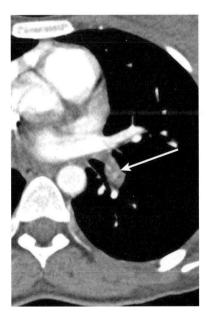

Fig. 129.5 CPTE in the same patient as in **Fig. 129.4**. Chest CTPA further down the left lower lobe pulmonary artery shows a small recanalized pulmonary artery with contrast media in the central lumen (*arrow*).

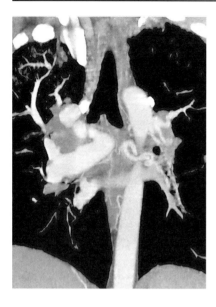

Fig. 129.6 Coronal CPTE in a 29-year-old man with sickle cell disease and progressive dyspnea reveals eccentric thrombus in the pulmonary arterial circuit and serpiginous collateral bronchial artery dilatation in the pericarinal region and along the left lower lobe bronchus.

- Mosaic Perfusion Pattern (**Figs. 129.7A, 129.7B**)
  - Affected arteries small relative to accompanying bronchi (**Figs. 129.7A, 129.7B**)
  - Unaffected arteries often larger than accompanying bronchi
- Airway Abnormalities (**Figs. 129.7A, 129.7B**)
  - Cylindrical bronchiectasis (64%) (**Figs. 129.7A, 129.7B**)
  - Bronchial wall thickening (12%) (**Figs. 129.7A, 129.7B**)

V/Q Lung Scintigraphy in Chronic Thromboembolic Pulmonary Hypertension (CTEPH)

- Characteristically read as high probability (unlike those of PPH)
- Asymmetric segmental or larger mismatched perfusion defects; often leads to underestimation of extent of central thromboembolism
- CPTE may also manifest with predominantly unilateral hypoperfusion or occlusion on radionuclide scans

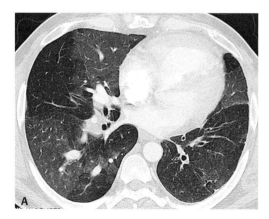
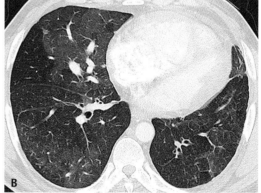

Fig. 129.7 CPTE in a 40-year-old man with dyspnea and pulmonary artery pressures calculated at 90 mm Hg. CTPA (lung window) shows a mosaic perfusion pattern. Blood vessels in hypoattenuated regions of lung are smaller in caliber than those in adjacent regions of hyperattenuated lung. Mild cylindrical bronchiectasis and bronchial wall thickening are seen. Note the right ventricular enlargement, right ventricular hypertrophy, and displacement of the interventricular septum toward the left ventricle from elevated right heart pressures.

Primary Pulmonary Artery Sarcoma (Angiosarcoma)

CTPA/MRA (Figs. 129.8A, 129.8B, 129.8C)

- Mimics CPTE and vice versa (**Figs. 129.8A, 129.B, 129.8C**)
- Most often arises from dorsal surface of MPA; may involve LPA, RPA, PV, RVOT
- Gd-DTPA-MRI: Enhancement of intraluminal filling defect may differentiate tumor from non-enhancing CPTE
- ^{18}F-FDG-PET: PAS usually FDG-avid; organized thrombus is not.

Management

- Some patients with proximal chronic thromboembolic pulmonary hypertension (CTEPH) may benefit from pulmonary endarterectomy; surgical mortality rate 8.7%
- Other patients may require lung or combined heart-lung transplantation
- Most patients are not suitable candidates for definitive surgical therapy (e.g., coexistence of distal pulmonary embolism; decompensated cor pulmonale; COPD; underlying neoplasia) and can only be treated medically; (i.e., indefinite anticoagulation)

Prognosis

- Variable; primary prognostic factors are mPAP (mean pulmonary artery pressure); coexistence of COPD and exercise intolerance; 32% mortality rate over 19 months
- Clinically relevant CTEPH occurs in 0.01% of CPTE patients
- Pulmonary artery pressure—most important risk factor in CPTE
  - Positive correlation between mortality and mPAP ≥30 mm Hg
  - mPAP <30 mm Hg; relatively good prognosis
  - 20% survival rate over a period of two years with mPAP >50 mm Hg

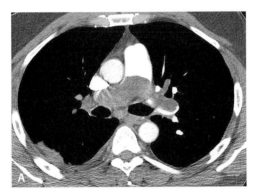
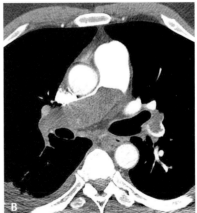
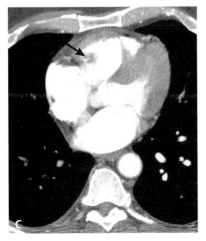

Fig. 129.8   CTPA of a 56-year-old man diagnosed with presumed CPTE demonstrates extensive filling defects in the MPA, LPA, RPA, and extension into segmental divisions. Subsequent endovascular biopsy confirmed the diagnosis of extensive primary pulmonary artery sarcoma. Note the metastasis in the right ventricle **(C)** (*arrow*).

- Diagnosis of CPTE should be considered in all dyspneic patients with no other clinical explanation for their symptoms.
- Non-invasive diagnosis of CPTE can be obtained with CTPA.
- HRCT findings of CTEPH include combination of mosaic lung attenuation and marked regional variation in segmental vessels; this helps distinguish CTEPH from the more diffuse pattern of findings in PPH and other causes of PAH. Cylindrical bronchiectasis adjacent to stenotic or obstructed pulmonary arterial segments occurs in two-thirds of patients with CTEPH.
- After pulmonary thromboendarterectomy, a form of noncardiogenic pulmonary edema described as "reperfusion edema" may manifest as patchy, bilateral perihilar alveolar opacities.
- Other causes of BA enlargement besides CTEPH include congenital vascular anomalies, bronchiectasis, acute or chronic lung abscesses, and mycobacterial and fungal infections.
- PAS—rare tumor frequently misdiagnosed as CPTE. Gd-DTPA-MRI and or PET may be useful in differentiating this tumor from thrombus. Patients often present without symptom resolution despite therapeutic anticoagulation.

Suggested Reading

1. Lewczuk J, Piszko P, Jagas J, et al. Prognostic factors in medically treated patients with chronic pulmonary embolism. Chest 2001;119(3):818–823

2. Lozada JCLP, Torstenson G. Chronic pulmonary embolism mimicking pulmonary angiosarcoma. Radiology Case Reports. [Online] 2008:148

3. Mattoo A, Fedullo PF, Kapelanski D, Ilowite JS. Pulmonary artery sarcoma: a case report of surgical cure and 5-year follow-up. Chest 2002;122(2):745–747

4. Remy-Jardin M, Remy J, Louvegny S, Artaud D, Deschildre F, Duhamel A. Airway changes in chronic pulmonary embolism: CT findings in 33 patients. Radiology 1997;203(2):355–360

5. Wittram C, Kalra MK, Maher MM, Greenfield A, McLoud TC, Shepard JA. Acute and chronic pulmonary emboli: angiography-CT correlation. AJR Am J Roentgenol 2006;186(6, Suppl 2):S421–S429

CASE 130

■ Clinical Presentation

72-year-old man with progressive dyspnea, repeated syncopal episodes, and medically refractory chronic pulmonary thromboembolic disease

■ Radiologic Findings

PA (**Fig. 130.1A**) and lateral (**Fig. 130.1B**) chest radiographs demonstrate marked enlargement of the central pulmonary and interlobar arteries with sharply tapered or pruned peripheral vessels. The cardiac silhouette is enlarged. The enlarged right heart encroaches upon the retrosternal clear space on the lateral exam (**Fig. 130.1B**). Subsequent catheter pulmonary angiography (not illustrated) confirmed CPTE.

■ Diagnosis

Chronic Thromboembolic Disease Pulmonary Hypertension (CTEPH)

■ Differential Diagnosis

- Idiopathic Pulmonary Artery Dilatation
  - Young women
  - Unilateral enlargement of main and left pulmonary artery
  - No pressure gradient
- Pulmonary Valve Stenosis
  - Unilateral enlargement of main and left pulmonary artery
  - Left upper lobe vessels larger than counterpart right upper lobe vessels
- Pulmonary Artery Sarcoma (see Case 129)

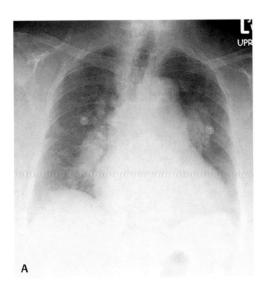 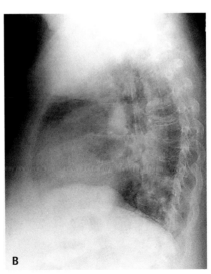

Fig. 130.1

629

■ Discussion

Background

Pulmonary artery hypertension (PAH) is defined by an elevated mPAP >25 mm Hg at rest (>30 mm Hg during exercise) and is classified by vascular changes affecting either the *precapillary* (arterial) or *postcapillary* (venous) pulmonary circulation. The latter occurs between the capillary bed and the left atrium.

Etiology

The vascular changes may be *idiopathic*, as in *primary pulmonary hypertension* (PPH) (i.e., *precapillary* level in the absence of an identifiable cause), but more commonly represent a *secondary* response to alterations in pulmonary blood flow. The *postcapillary* counterpart to PPH is pulmonary venoocclusive disease (PVOD), a rare idiopathic condition that diffusely affects the postcapillary pulmonary circulation but is characterized by normal pulmonary capillary wedge pressures (PCWP). Both *precapillary* and *postcapillary* pulmonary hypertension are regarded as *secondary* (SPH) when a cause can be established (**Table 130.1**).

Clinical Findings

Pulmonary Artery Hypertension

Precapillary hypertension creates a hemodynamic pattern of elevated right atrial pressure, increased mPAP, increased pulmonary vascular resistance, normal PCWP, and decreased cardiac output. *Postcapillary hypertension* is characterized by elevated right atrial pressure, increased resistance, and normal or elevated PCWP. Patients present with progressive dyspnea (60%), fatigue, angina, syncope, cor pulmonale, and Raynaud phenomenon. Women are affected three times as often as men. Onset of symptoms is typically in youth or middle age. Patients with portal hypertension (with or without liver disease), collagen vascular disease, HIV-AIDS, or a history of aminorex fumarate (an appetite suppressant) ingestion have an increased risk. Additionally, pregnant or postpartum patients and those using oral contraceptives may also be at increased risk.

Pulmonary Venoocclusive Disease (PVOD)

In addition to the hemodynamic derangements of PAH discussed above, PVOD is associated with normal or variably elevated PCWP. Normal left atrial and left ventricular pressures are characteristic and help exclude

Table 130.1 Potential Causes of Pulmonary Artery Hypertension

Primary (Precapillary or Arterial) Pulmonary Hypertension	Primary (Postcapillary or Venous) Pulmonary Hypertension
Idiopathic	Pulmonary venoocclusive disease (PVOD)
Secondary (precapillary or arterial) pulmonary hypertension	Secondary (postcapillary or venous) pulmonary hypertension
Congenital left-to-right cardiac shunt (e.g., ASD, Eisenmenger physiology)	Pulmonary capillary hemangiomatosis
CPTE	Focal venous constriction (e.g., congenital venous stenosis, fibrosing mediastinitis)
Tumor embolism (e.g., breast cancer, gastric cancer, renal cell, right atrial sarcoma, hepatoma)	Obstructive left atrial mass (e.g., left atrial neoplasia, myxoma, mitral stenosis, left ventricular failure)
Infection (e.g., HIV-AIDS, schistosomiasis)	Compromised pulmonary venous drainage (e.g., anomalous pulmonary venous connections)
IVDA (e.g., talc and other foreign body embolization)	
Chronic interstitial lung disease (end-stage) or chronic emphysema	
Portal hypertension	
Chronic alveolar hypoxia	

cardiac disease as the cause of venous hypertension. Patients present with progressive dyspnea, hemoptysis, and antecedent flulike symptoms. One-third of cases occur in children. There is a slight male predominance in adult patients. PVOD may be associated with pregnancy, bone marrow transplantation, or drug toxicity (e.g., carmustine, bleomycin, mitomycin). The clinical presentation and radiographic findings are suggestive of interstitial lung disease often leading to a delay in diagnosis.

Imaging Findings

Precapillary Pulmonary Hypertension

Chest Radiography

- Insidious clinical onset; minimal early radiographic findings

Advanced PPH or SPH

Chest Radiography

- Central arterial enlargement (i.e., enlarged MPA and hilar vessels) (**Figs. 130.1A, 130.1B**)
- Sharply tapered or pruned peripheral vessels (**Figs. 130.1A, 130.1B**)
- Right-sided heart hypertrophy and chamber dilatation (**Figs. 130.1A, 130.1B**)
- Dilatation right interlobar pulmonary artery (**Figs. 130.1A, 130.1B**)
  - >16 mm men
  - >14 mm women

Advanced PPH or SPH

MDCT/HRCT

Pulmonary Vasculature

- MPA diameter: measured in scan plane of bifurcation, at a right angle to its long axis and lateral to ascending aorta (**Fig. 130.2**)
  - MPA diameter ≥29 mm (87% sensitivity; 89% specificity for predicting PAH)
  - Specificity approximately 100%: MPA diameter ≥29 mm accompanied by a segmental artery to bronchus ratio greater than 1:1 in three of four pulmonary lobes
  - Ratio of MPA diameter to ascending aorta diameter greater than one (rPA >1); strong correlation with elevated mPAP, particularly in patients <50 years of age

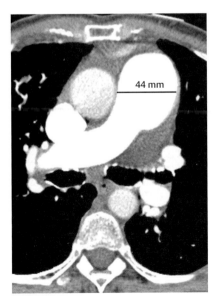

Fig. 130.2 Axial CTPA on a 55-year-old man with precapillary PAH demonstrates marked enlargement of the MPA, estimated at 44 mm in diameter. The MPA is much larger in diameter than the adjacent ascending aorta.

44 mm

- Abrupt tapering of peripheral vessels
- Intimal calcification of pulmonary arteries with severe long-standing disease
- In situ intraluminal thrombus (**Figs. 130.3A, 130.3B**)
- ± bronchial collaterals (**Figs. 130.3A, 130.3B**)

Cardiac

- Right ventricular dilatation, wall thickening, and or hypertrophy (**Fig. 130.4**)
- Reversal of septal curvature (**Fig. 130.4**)
- Right atrium dilatation (**Fig. 130.4**)
- Reflux of contrast media into dilated suprahepatic IVC and proximal hepatic veins
- Pericardial thickening and or effusion (>50%) (**Fig. 130.4**)

Lung Parenchyma

- Mosaic pattern of lung attenuation (**Figs. 130.5A, 130.5B, 130.5C**)
  - Suggesting regional variations in parenchymal perfusion (**Figs. 130.5A, 130.5B, 130.5C**)
  - High-attenuation areas (normal lung): larger-caliber vessels; low-attenuation areas (abnormal lung): smaller-caliber vessels (**Figs. 130.5A, 130.5B, 130.5C**)
- Centrilobular nodules; usually ground glass in attenuation

Postcapillary Pulmonary Hypertension

MDCT/HRCT

Additional findings beyond those of precapillary hypertension:

- Septal thickening
- Centrilobular nodules
- Pleural effusions
- Mediastinal lymphadenopathy

Pulmonary Venoocclusive Disease (PVOD)

Chest Radiography (Non-Specific)

- Features of PAH; enlarged pulmonary arteries (100%) (**Figs. 130.6A, 130.6B**)
- Non-specific basilar interstitial opacities (**Figs. 130.6A, 130.6B**)
- Cardiomegaly (90%); normal-size left atrium

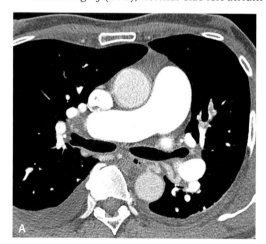
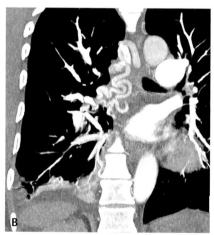

Fig. 130.3   Axial **(A)** and coronal MPR **(B)** CTPA of a 45-year-old man with CTEPH. Note the disproportionate enlargement of the MPA relative to the ascending aorta and recruitment of large pericarinal bronchial collaterals. Chronic thrombus is seen in the left upper lobe segmental artery. Pleural effusions are present. *(Images courtesy of Daniel A. Henry, MD, VCU Medical Center, Richmond, Virginia.)*

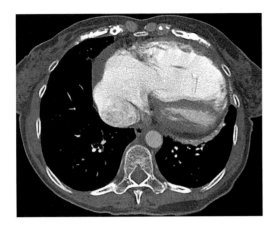

Fig. 130.4   Axial CTPA of a 45-year-old woman with progressive dyspnea and precapillary PAH shows marked enlargement of both the right atrium and right ventricle, right ventricular wall thickening, gross deviation of the interventricular septum with compression of the left ventricle, and a small pericardial effusion.

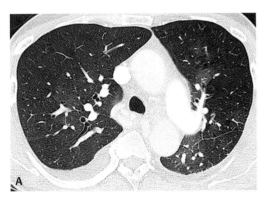

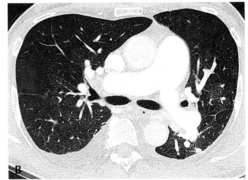

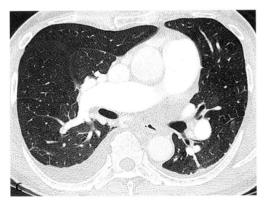

Fig. 130.5   Axial chest CT images (lung window) of the same patient shown in **Fig. 130.3** reveal the lung parenchymal changes seen with precapillary PAH—namely, mosaic perfusion reflecting regional variations in lung perfusion. Note the small-caliber vessels in the hypoattenuated lung relative to the normal hyperattenuated lung.

Pulmonary Venoocclusive Disease

MDCT/HRCT

Pulmonary Vasculature

- Enlarged main and central pulmonary arteries (**Fig. 130.6C**)
- Normal-caliber pulmonary veins

Cardiac

- Dilated right atrium and right ventricle
- Thickened right ventricular wall
- Normal-size left atrium and left ventricle
- Small pericardial effusion (nearly 100%)

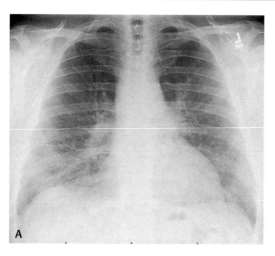

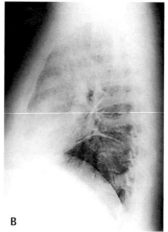

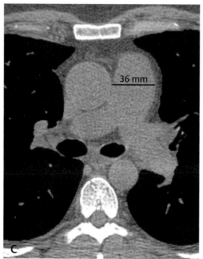

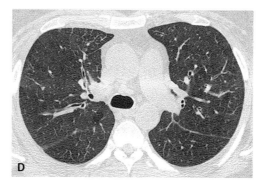

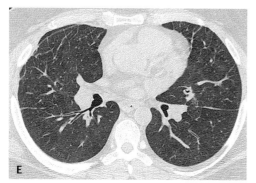

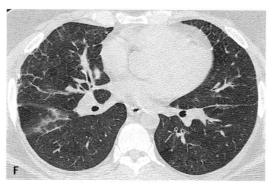

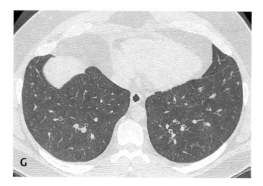

Fig. 130.6 50-year-old man with progressive dyspnea and biopsy-proven PVOD. PA **(A)** and lateral **(B)** radiographs show bibasilar interstitial opacities and an upper limit normal-size cardiomediastinal silhouette. Lung volumes are preserved. Unenhanced CT **(C)** (mediastinal window) reveals a dilated MPA estimated at 36 mm. Accompanying lung windows **(D–G)** demonstrate patchy ground glass opacities, interlobular septal thickening, and peribronchovascular thickening with normal size pulmonary veins. The lack of centrilobular nodules and right heart enlargement is somewhat atypical. *(Images courtesy of Alpha A. Fowler, III, MD, and Janet Pinson, NP, VCU Medical Center, Richmond, Virginia.)*

Mediastinum

- Mild lymphadenopathy (50%); 15 ± 5 mm

Lung Parenchyma

- Ground glass opacities (nearly 100%) (**Figs. 130.6D, 130.6E, 130.6F, 130.6G**)
  ○ Centrilobular (65%); most specific pattern
  ○ Other patterns include geographic, diffuse, mosaic, patchy, and perihilar
- Smooth, interlobular septal thickening (80%) (**Figs. 130.6D, 130.6E, 130.6F, 130.6G**)
- Peribronchovascular thickening (**Figs. 130.6D, 130.6E, 130.6F, 130.6G**)

Complications of sustained precapillary PAH include

- Central arterial thrombosis
- Premature atherosclerosis of central elastic and muscular pulmonary arteries
- Aneurysmal dissection of pulmonary arteries
- Hypertrophy and dilatation of the right heart chambers

Prognosis

PAH

- No cure; most patients succumb two to five years following diagnosis

PVOD

- Potentially fatal pulmonary edema may be induced by administration of vasodilator therapy for presumed PAH
- Disease usually fatal within three years of diagnosis

Management

PAH

- Oxygen of little benefit
- Therapeutic agents include vasodilators, calcium channel blockers, anticoagulants, and diuretics to counteract the unfavorable hemodynamics
- Lung or combined heart-lung transplantation may be performed according to organ availability and the patient's clinical status

PVOD

- Treatment with anticoagulants; limited success
- Single or double lung transplantation may prolong life expectancy

PEARLS

- One to 5% of patients with acute PTE develop CTEPH, which may mimic PPH clinically.
- Two to 26% of patients with neoplasia develop microscopic tumor emboli to the pulmonary circulation; diagnosis is frequently missed antemortem. Cor pulmonale in such patients is an ominous sign; death often ensues within 4–12 weeks of onset. Gastric cancer is the *most common* clinically occult neoplasm to embolize and produce PAH.
- Cardiopulmonary schistosomiasis is the *most common* cause of *secondary* PAH worldwide (e.g., *Schistosoma mansoni* infection). Infestation is endemic in the Middle East, Africa, South America, and the Caribbean. Disease may be seen in travelers and immigrants entering the United States from endemic areas.
- Bronchial artery dilatation and tortuosity may be seen in up to 77% of MDCTs in patients with CTEPH; statistically significant predictor of patient survival immediately following thromboendarterectomy.

- PVOD is suggested radiographically when features of PAH are accompanied by diffuse pulmonary interstitial edema and a normal-size left atrium. Presence of centrilobular ground glass nodular opacities or smooth septal thickening in patients with PAH predicts life-threatening pulmonary edema if treated with vasodilators.

Suggested Reading

1. Alunni JP, Degano B, Arnaud C, et al. Cardiac MRI in pulmonary artery hypertension: correlations between morphological and functional parameters and invasive measurements. Eur Radiol 2010;20(5):1149–1159

2. Cummings KW, Bhalla S. Multidetector computed tomographic pulmonary angiography: beyond acute pulmonary embolism. Radiol Clin North Am 2010;48(1):51–65

3. Devaraj A, Wells AU, Meister MG, Corte TJ, Wort SJ, Hansell DM. Detection of pulmonary hypertension with multidetector CT and echocardiography alone and in combination. Radiology 2010;254(2):609–616

4. Frazier AA, Franks TJ, Mohammed TL, Ozbudak IH, Galvin JR. From the Archives of the AFIP: pulmonary veno-occlusive disease and pulmonary capillary hemangiomatosis. Radiographics 2007;27(3):867–882

5. Froelich JJ, Koenig H, Knaak L, Krass S, Klose KJ. Relationship between pulmonary artery volumes at computed tomography and pulmonary artery pressures in patients with and without pulmonary hypertension. Eur J Radiol 2008;67(3):466–471

CASE 131

■ Clinical Presentation

53-year-old man presenting to the Emergency Department with an acute onset of chest pain, hypoxia and shortness of breath

■ Radiologic Findings

AP (**Fig. 131.1A**) and lateral (**Fig. 131.1B**) chest radiograph demonstrates an enlarged cardiomediastinal silhouette; widened vascular pedicle; peripheral vascular engorgement; bilateral parahilar ground glass opacities, right greater than left; and bilateral pleural effusions, again right greater than left. Abnormal thickening of the posterior wall of the bronchus intermedius is seen on the lateral exam (**Fig. 131.1B**). Baseline PA (**Fig. 131.1C**) chest radiograph from five months earlier for comparison is grossly normal.

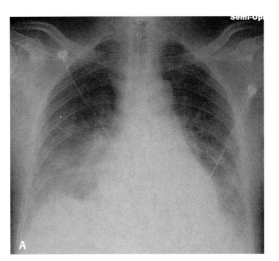
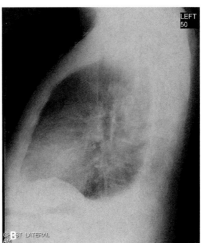
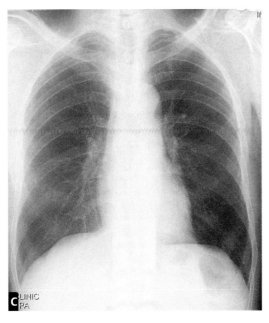

Fig. 131.1

637

■ Diagnosis

Increased Hydrostatic Pressure Pulmonary Edema; Acute Myocardial Infarction

■ Differential Diagnosis

- Increased Hydrostatic Pressure Pulmonary Edema of Other Etiologies
- Mixed Edema: Simultaneous Increased Hydrostatic Pressure and Permeability Changes

■ Discussion

Background

Pulmonary edema results from the abnormal accumulation of fluid in the extravascular compartments of the lung. The relative amounts of intravascular and extravascular fluid are determined by the permeability of capillary membranes and the oncotic pressure. Pathophysiologic alterations in either will result in accumulation of fluid in the lung and edema. Pulmonary edema is divided into four main categories: (1) increased hydrostatic pressure edema, (2) permeability edema with diffuse alveolar damage (DAD), (3) permeability edema without DAD, and (4) mixed edema from simultaneous increased hydrostatic pressure and permeability changes (e.g., neurogenic pulmonary edema, reperfusion pulmonary edema, pulmonary edema following lung transplantation, re-expansion pulmonary edema, post-pneumonectomy edema, post–lung volume reduction edema). The variable clinical manifestations and radiologic patterns of pulmonary edema are summarized in **Table 131.1**.

Etiology

There are two pathophysiologic and radiologic phases of *increased pressure hydrostatic pulmonary edema*. These are *interstitial edema* and *alveolar flooding*. These phases are similar for left-sided heart failure and volume overload, the *most common* causes of increased pressure hydrostatic edema in both ICU and emergency department patients. The intensity and duration of these phases is related to the degree of increased pressure, which is determined by the ratio of hydrostatic to oncotic pressures. *Interstitial edema* occurs with an increase of 15–25 mm Hg in mean transmural arterial pressure. *Alveolar flooding* occurs with increases in transmural pressures >25 mm Hg.

Clinical Findings

Pulmonary artery catheters are often used to assess and monitor hydrostatic pressure in critically ill patients. Pulmonary capillary wedge pressure (PCWP) reflects left atrial pressure and correlates well with the radiologic manifestations of heart failure and pulmonary venous hypertension. The PCWP can often be predicted on the basis of the radiologic findings by the application of the "rule of 6's" as depicted in **Table 131.2**. However, in acute heart failure, a "lag time" is often seen between increased PCWP and radiologic manifestations of edema. Similarly, radiographic features of edema may lag behind clinically resolving pulmonary edema and reductions in PCWP. In approximately 10% of cases, the radiograph will demonstrate a central pattern of edema. This *bat wing pattern* generally occurs with the rapid onset of severe heart failure (e.g., acute mitral insufficiency associated with papillary muscle rupture, massive infarction, septic endocarditis with valve leaflet destruction) or renal failure (**Fig. 131.2A, 131.2B**).

Imaging Findings

Radiography

- Increased cardiothoracic ratio (**Fig. 131.1A**)
- Increased vascular pedicle width (**Fig. 131.1A**)
  - >70 mm supine chest radiography
  - Measuring vascular pedicle: Draw vertical line paralleling left subclavian artery origin off transverse aorta; draw horizontal line extending from this line to lateral border of superior vena cava as it crosses right main bronchus

Table 131.1   Radiologic Patterns of Pulmonary Edema Based on Clinical Scenario

Clinical Scenario	Typical Radiologic Pattern
Negative pressure (post-obstruction)	Septal lines Peribronchial cuffing Central alveolar edema (severe cases) Normal cardiac size
Chronic pulmonary thromboemboli	Sharply demarcated areas of increased ground glass attenuation associated with dilated pulmonary arteries
Pulmonary venoocclusive disease	Large pulmonary arteries Diffuse interstitial edema Numerous Kerley lines Peribronchial cuffing Dilated right ventricle
Stage I near drowning	Kerley lines Peribronchial cuffing Patchy perihilar air space consolidations
Following cytokine administration	Bilateral, symmetric interstitial edema Thickened septal lines Peribronchial cuffing Absence of alveolar opacities Small pleural effusions
High altitude	Central interstitial edema Peribronchial cuffing Ill-defined vessels Patchy asymmetric air space opacities (spare apex and lung cortex)
Neurogenic	Bilateral, homogeneous central air space consolidations (predominant in apices) Normal heart size No pleural effusion No Kerley lines
Reperfusion	Heterogeneous air space consolidations (predominant in areas distal to recanalized vessels)
Re-expansion	Mild air space consolidation (involving the entire ipsilateral lung; less commonly ipsilateral lobe or segment)
Post–lung transplant	Diffuse, confluent alveolar opacities Normal heart size Normal vascular axes

Table 131.2   "Rule of 6's" Correlation between Radiologic Findings of Increased Hydrostatic Pressure Edema and Pulmonary Capillary Wedge Pressure (PCWP)

PCWP (mm Hg)	CXR Findings
6–12	Normal
12–18	Cephalization of pulmonary blood flow
18–24	Early loss of definition of segmental and subsegmental vessel clarity Mild enlargement of peribronchovascular spaces Kerley lines Subpleural effusions Central migration of edema Progressive blurring of lobar and hilar vessels Peribronchial cuffing
24–30	Alveolar flooding Air space or acinar nodular opacities Frank air space consolidations

- Cephalization of blood flow (**Fig. 131.3**)
- Discrepant arterial to bronchial ratios (**Figs. 131.4A, 131.4B**)
- Kerley B-lines (septal reticular opacities) (**Figs. 131.5A, 13.5B, 131.5C**)
- Central migration of edema; progressive blurring lobar/hilar vessels (**Figs. 131.6A, 131.6B**)
- Alveolar flooding/frank air space consolidation (**Figs. 131.2A, 131.2B**)
- Pleural effusion (**Figs. 131.3, 131.7A, 131.7B**)
- Asymmetric distribution of increased hydrostatic pressure pulmonary edema (**Figs. 131.8A, 131.8B**)
  - Morphologic changes in lung parenchyma (emphysema, fibrosis)
  - Hemodynamic factors (mitral regurgitation)
  - Gravitational (preferential patient positioning)

MDCT

- Ground glass opacity; diffuse; patchy; geographic; often shows gravitational predominance (**Fig. 131.9**)
- Occasional mild centrilobular ground glass opacities (**Figs. 131.10A, 131.10B**)
- Interlobular septal thickening; linear or reticular opacities 1–5 mm thick; smooth and uniform (**Figs. 131.10A, 131.10B**)
- Peribronchovascular interstitial thickening resulting in apparent bronchial wall thickening (**Figs. 131.9, 131.10A, 131.10B**)
- Increased vascular diameter; dilatation of pulmonary arteries and veins (**Figs. 131.9, 131.10A, 131.10B**)
- Thickening of interlobar fissures; unilateral right or bilateral pleural effusions (**Fig. 131.11**)

Management

- Directed toward underlying cause
- High pulmonary pressures: diuretics/fluid restriction
- Supplemental oxygen
  - Non-rebreather often adequate in early stages; ineffective once pulmonary edema develops
  - CPAP; endotracheal intubation, and ventilation with positive end-expiratory pressure (PEEP): once pulmonary edema develops
- Pharmacotherapy
  - Workload reduction
  - Correction of dysrhythmias
  - Positive inotropic agents
  - Mobilization of fluid

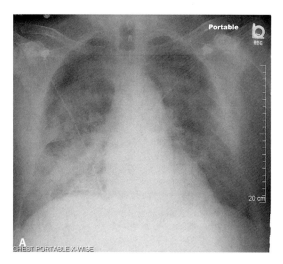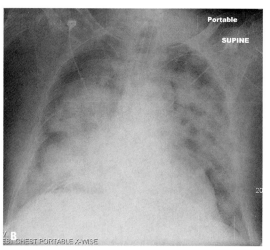

Fig. 131.2 AP **(A)** chest radiograph of a 61-year-old man with severe heart failure from acute mitral insufficiency and papillary muscle rupture shows a *bat wing pattern* of central, nongravitational pulmonary edema. As is often seen with acute mitral regurgitation, the edema asymmetrically involves the right lung. AP **(B)** chest radiograph six hours later shows rapid but asymmetric progression of edema. He experienced progressive respiratory failure requiring intubation. Emergent mitral valve replacement was subsequently performed.

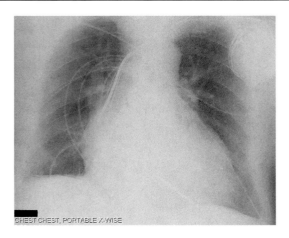

Fig. 131.3   AP chest radiograph of a 56-year-old man with increased hydrostatic pressure pulmonary edema from early heart failure shows cephalization of blood flow. Note the upper lobe vessels are larger in diameter than the lower lobe vessels. A right subpulmonic pleural effusion is also present.

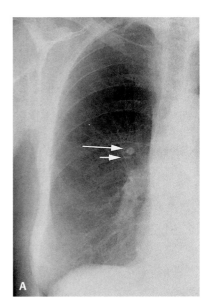
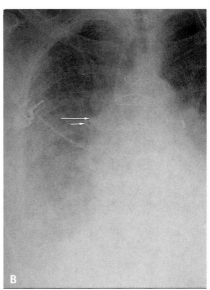

Fig. 131.4   Coned-down AP chest radiograph **(A)** showing the normal relationship of the right upper lobe anterior segmental artery (*long white arrow*) and its accompanying bronchus (*short white arrow*) (1:1). Coned-down AP chest radiograph **(B)** of a 79-year-old woman with cardiogenic shock and increased hydrostatic pressure pulmonary edema with discrepant arterial to bronchial ratios. Note the relative size of the right upper lobe anterior segmental artery (*long white arrow*) and its accompanying bronchus (*short white arrow*) (>1:1). Peribronchial cuffing is also seen.

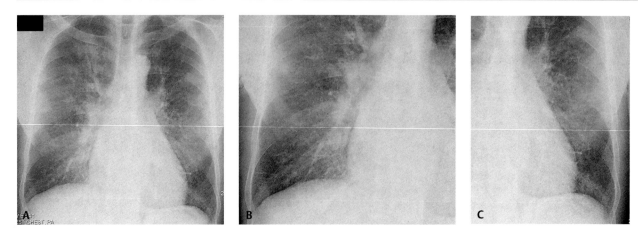

Fig. 131.5   AP chest radiograph **(A)** of a 54-year-old woman with increased hydrostatic pressure pulmonary edema from an acute myocardial infarction. Bilateral septal reticular opacities at the costophrenic angles seen to better advantage on the accompanying coned-down right **(B)** and left **(C)** radiographs.

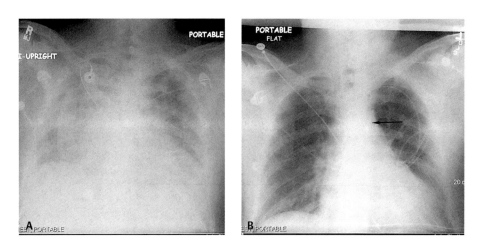

Fig. 131.6   AP chest radiograph **(A)** of a 60-year-old man with antecedent coronary artery disease and abrupt onset of florid heart failure following severe myocardial infarction shows bilateral perihilar ground glass opacities with partial silhouetting and blurring of the central vasculature. Note the marked improvement following deployment of the intra-aortic balloon pump (*arrow*) **(B)**.

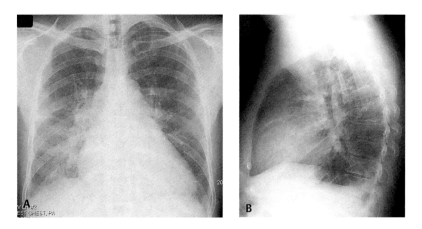

Fig. 131.7   PA **(A)** and lateral **(B)** chest radiographs of a 53-year-old man with COPD, coronary artery disease, and acute parvovirus-related myocarditis demonstrates radiographic features of increased hydrostatic pressure pulmonary edema—specifically, enlargement of the cardiomediastinal silhouette, diminished vascular clarity, perihilar ground glass and septal reticular opacities, and bilateral pleural effusion.

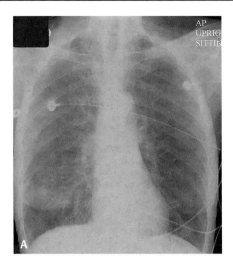
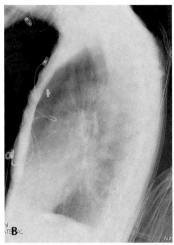

Fig. 131.8   PA **(A)** and lateral **(B)** chest radiographs of a 74-year-old man with advanced emphysema and acute myocardial infarction shows an asymmetric pattern of increased hydrostatic pressure pulmonary edema. The decreased vascular clarity and abnormal septal reticular opacities preferentially involve the right hemithorax as a result of the underlying emphysema.

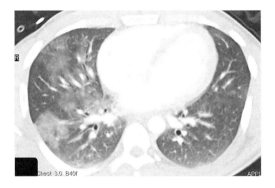

Fig. 131.9   Chest CT (lung window) shows diffuse, patchy ground glass opacities asymmetrically distributed in the right hemithorax. Note thickened peribronchovascular bundles in the right lower lobe and prominent septal veins in the left lower lobe.

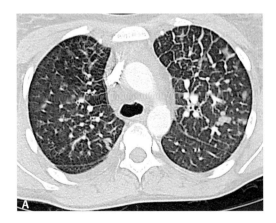
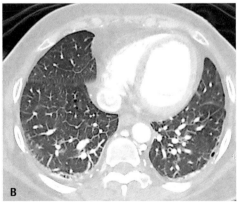

Fig. 131.10   Chest CT (lung window) shows centrilobular ground glass opacities in the left upper lobe **(A)**. Peribronchovascular interstitial thickening, septal linear opacities, prominent septal veins, and dilated pulmonary arteries and veins are also seen **(A,B)**.

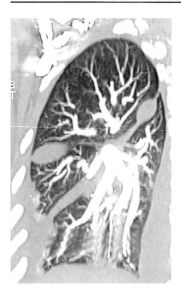

Fig. 131.11 Sagittal MIP chest CT (lung windows) reveals thickening of the right horizontal and oblique interlobar fissures and accompanying localized pleural fluid collections (i.e., pseudotumors or vanishing tumors) in the same.

Prognosis

- Dependent on underlying cause

PEARLS

- Vascular pedicle width is not affected by phase of respiration. However, patient rotation will affect vascular pedicle width. It is reduced with right anterior oblique (RAO) rotation and accentuated with left anterior oblique rotation (LAO).
- Increased hydrostatic pressure pulmonary edema results from abnormal increase in extravascular water secondary to elevated pressure in the pulmonary circulation (e.g., heart failure) or intravascular volume (e.g., volume overload).
- Most frequent cause of asymmetric increased hydrostatic pressure edema is COPD. Asymmetric patterns of edema may also occur in end-stage tuberculosis, sarcoidosis, asbestosis, and pulmonary fibrosis of other causes.
- Edema associated with mitral regurgitation preferentially affects the right upper lobe because of impaired flow directed into the right upper lobe pulmonary vein.

Suggested Reading

1. Gluecker T, Capasso P, Schnyder P, et al. Clinical and radiologic features of pulmonary edema. Radiographics 1999;19(6):1507–1531, discussion 1532–1533

2. Ketai LH, Godwin JD. A new view of pulmonary edema and acute respiratory distress syndrome. J Thorac Imaging 1998;13(3):147–171

3. Storto ML, Kee ST, Golden JA, Webb WR. Hydrostatic pulmonary edema: high-resolution CT findings. AJR Am J Roentgenol 1995;165(4):817–820

CASE 132

■ Clinical Presentation

21-year-old woman who developed severe laryngospasm following extubation, necessitating reintubation

■ Radiologic Findings

AP chest radiograph (**Fig. 132.1A**) acquired six hours before extubation shows an appropriately positioned endotracheal tube, slight decrease in vascular clarity, and mild basilar hypoaeration. AP chest radiograph (**Fig. 132.1B**) acquired roughly 20 minutes following the onset of post-extubation laryngospasm reveals slightly diminished but largely unchanged vascular clarity and basilar hypoaeration. AP chest exam (**Fig. 132.1C**) obtained 30 minutes following reintubatation and subsequent relief of the laryngospasm demonstrates significant decrease in vascular clarity and central, perihilar ground glass opacities, right greater than left, consistent with pulmonary edema.

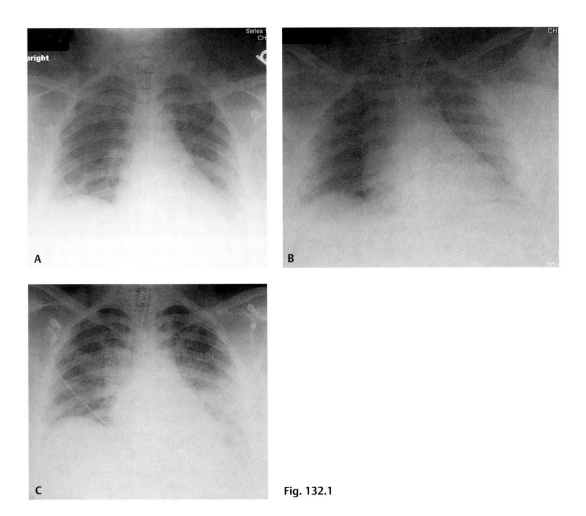

Fig. 132.1

■ Diagnosis

Post-Obstructive (Negative Pressure) Pulmonary Edema

■ Differential Diagnosis

- Increased Hydrostatic Pressure Pulmonary Edema of Other Etiologies
- Aspiration

■ Discussion

Background

Post-obstructive negative pressure pulmonary edema (NPPE) is a mixed form of edema (see discussion in Case 131) produced by forceful inspiration against an obstructed upper airway (Müller maneuver). The struggle to inhale against an obstruction causes high "negative" intrathoracic pressure, increasing venous return, which pulls fluid from the pulmonary capillary bed into the alveoli. An obstruction that prevents both inspiration and expiration may create high "positive" intrathoracic pressure, impairing the development of edema initially. Edema then develops following relief of the obstruction as the intrathoracic pressure suddenly drops. The exact incidence of NPPE is unknown. However, it has been estimated that pulmonary edema develops in 11% of patients requiring emergent intervention for acute upper airway obstruction.

Etiology

Risk factors for NPPE include obesity with obstructive sleep apnea, anatomically difficult intubations, ET tube manipulations, biting of the ET tube, presence of airway lesions, patients undergoing oral maxillofacial surgical procedures, suffocation and/or choking from an impacted foreign body, strangulation, epiglottitis, laryngospasm, and angioedema. Young athletes may be at increased risk because of their ability to generate significant negative intrathoracic pressures. Likewise, pediatric patients are at increased risk because of their extremely compliant chest walls and ability to generate large negative intrathoracic pressures.

Clinical Findings

NPPE usually manifests acutely but can develop several hours later. Signs and symptoms of respiratory distress are often present. Frothy, pink sputum is the hallmark. Tachycardia, hypertension, and diaphoresis may be present. Rales and wheezing from fluid-compressed airways may be heard on auscultation.

Imaging Findings

Chest Radiography

Similar to that of increased hydrostatic pressure pulmonary edema

- Septal lines
- Peribronchial cuffing
- Central or diffuse alveolar opacities in severe cases (**Fig. 132.1C**)
- Cardiothoracic ratio is usually normal; differentiates from overhydration edema
- Resolution over two to three days

Management

- Reverse hypoxia
  - Maintain airway
  - Supplemental oxygen

- ○ Failure of oxygenation to improve in non-intubated patients: immediate intubation; positive-pressure ventilation and positive end-expiratory pressure
  - ○ Failure of oxygenation to improve in intubated patients: positive end-expiratory pressure should be administered
- Decrease fluid volume in the lungs; use of diuretics is controversial

Prognosis

- Prompt diagnosis and treatment markedly improve patient prognosis and significantly decrease morbidity and mortality

PEARLS

- Most common causes of post-obstructive NPPE are an impacted foreign body, laryngospasm, epiglottitis, and strangulation.
- NPPE usually manifests acutely but can develop several hours later.
- Frothy, pink sputum is the hallmark of NPPE.

Suggested Reading

1. Cascade PN, Alexander GD, Mackie DS. Negative-pressure pulmonary edema after endotracheal intubation. Radiology 1993;186(3):671–675

2. Davidson S, Guinn C, Gacharna D. Diagnosis and treatment of negative pressure pulmonary edema in a pediatric patient: a case report. AANA J 2004;72(5):337–338

3. Gluecker T, Capasso P, Schnyder P, et al. Clinical and radiologic features of pulmonary edema. Radiographics 1999;19(6):1507–1531, discussion 1532–1533

CASE 133

■ Clinical Presentation

53-year-old man with tension pneumothorax following a new central line placement

■ Radiologic Findings

AP chest radiograph (**Fig. 133.1A**) reveals a right-sided tension pneumothorax, marked leftward mediastinal shift, and left lower lobe volume loss. AP chest radiograph 24 hours later (**Fig. 133.1B**) immediately following chest tube placement shows relief of the pneumothorax. However, right perihilar, upper lobe, and lower lobe air space consolidations are now present. AP chest radiograph 10 hours following the chest tube placement (**Fig. 133.1C**) shows progressive right perihilar air space consolidation, air bronchograms, ipsilateral lower lobe volume loss, and a right pleural effusion.

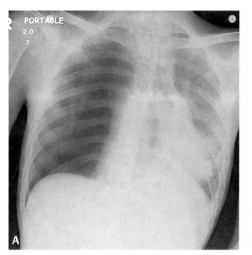
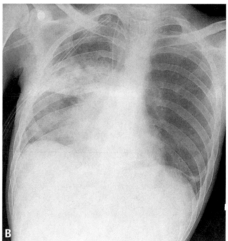
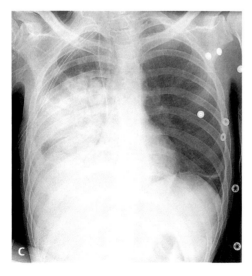

Fig. 133.1

648

■ Diagnosis

Re-Expansion Pulmonary Edema

■ Differential Diagnosis

- Cardiogenic Pulmonary Edema
- Aspiration
- Alveolar Hemorrhage
- Pulmonary Infection

■ Discussion

Background

Re-expansion pulmonary edema (RxPE) is a mixed form of edema (see discussion in Case 131) resulting from a simultaneous increase in hydrostatic pressure and some degree of diffuse alveolar damage with permeability changes. This rare form of acute lung injury usually follows rapid reinflation of collapsed lung parenchyma, with an incidence of up to 1% following evacuation of pleural air or fluid. In most cases, the affected lung has been collapsed for three or more days. RxPE may also be related to the volume of the intrathoracic space occupied by fluid, air, or mass; the presence of bronchial obstruction; the application of excessive suction to the tracheobronchial tree during bronchoscopy and suctioning with a tracheal catheter; alterations of pulmonary artery pressure; and the removal of large extrathoracic lesions (i.e., abdominal masses) that may have compressed the thoracic cavity.

Etiology

The pathophysiology is complex and not completely understood. However, it has been postulated that rapid lung expansion following prolonged parenchymal collapse (three to seven days) causes a rapid increase in blood flow to the affected lung and concurrent alveolar distension. This is associated with increases in pulmonary capillary pressure, hydrostatic pressure, pressure-induced alveolar-capillary membrane disruption, increased capillary permeability, and resultant leakage of fluid and protein into the lung, causing pulmonary edema, hypoxia, and hypoxia-induced heart failure.

Clinical Findings

The rapid removal of an extrapulmonary thoracic space-occupying lesion (e.g., pleural air, fluid, or mass) that has been associated with a period of prolonged lung collapse is the *most common* clinical scenario in which RxPE occurs. Affected patients may be asymptomatic, experience minimal symptoms, or develop life-threatening hypoxia, hemodynamic instability, and death. When present, symptoms usually appear within 1–2 hours following rapid pulmonary re-expansion but may not occur until 24–48 hours later. Signs and symptoms vary but may include dyspnea, chest pain, cough with or without pink frothy sputum, cyanosis, rales, fever, nausea, vomiting, tachycardia, hypotension, and respiratory failure.

Imaging Findings

Chest Radiography

- Pulmonary edema
  - Unilateral (93%)
  - Bilateral (7%)
  - Contralateral (1%)
- Reticular or interstitial opacities (**Fig. 133.2**)
- Kerley B-lines (**Fig. 133.2**)
- Ground glass opacities and/or consolidations (**Figs. 133.1B, 133.1C**)
- Air bronchograms (**Fig. 133.1C**)

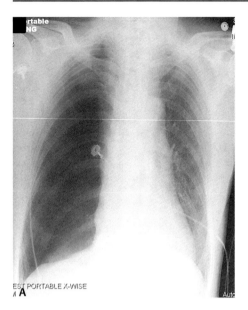
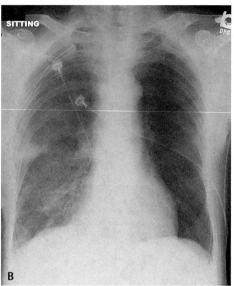

Fig. 133.2 AP chest radiograph **(A)** of a 63-year-old man who presented to the Emergency Department after several days of non-resolving pleuritic chest pain shows a spontaneous right-sided tension pneumothorax. Decompression of the pneumothorax relieved the chest pain. However, four hours later he began experiencing significant dyspnea. AP chest exam at that time **(B)** demonstrates an asymmetric pulmonary edema pattern involving the right hemithorax. Note the ipsilateral perihilar ground glass and reticular opacities consistent with RxPE.

Management

- Supplemental oxygen
- Ventilatory support
  - Non-invasive
  - Invasive
- Hemodynamic monitoring
- ± Vasopressor and or inotropic agents
- Guarded diuresis
- Lateral decubitus positioning: affected side up may reduce intrapulmonary shunting and improve oxygenation
- Reduce negative pressure applied to the affected pleural space, if doing so will not create intrathoracic tension physiology

Prognosis

- Usually persists clinically for as long as one or two days; may take up to five to seven days to resolve
- Unpredictable path from spontaneous resolution to fatal respiratory failure may occur
- Mortality as high as 21%

PEARLS

- The most effective clinical approach is prevention. It is critical that the interventional radiologist or treating clinician be aware of the chronicity and estimated volume of the space-occupying extrathoracic pulmonary process. Each drainage procedure should not evacuate >1,000–1,500 mL at a time if the process has been present for ≥3 days. If pleural pressures are carefully monitored during the procedure and do not exceed –20 cm H$_2$O, it is possible to evacuate larger quantities of pleural fluid or air.
- More than 80% of cases of RxPE occur in patients with prolonged duration of lung collapse (≥3days). However, RxPE has been reported after the evacuation of pneumothoraces present for only a few hours.

Suggested Reading

1. Gluecker T, Capasso P, Schnyder P, et al. Clinical and radiologic features of pulmonary edema. Radiographics 1999;19(6):1507–1531, discussion 1532–1533

2. Heller BJ, Grathwohl MK. Contralateral reexpansion pulmonary edema. South Med J 2000;93(8):828–831

3. Stawicki SP, Sarani B, Braslow BM. Reexpansion pulmonary edema. OPUS 12 Scientist 2008;2(2):29–31

4. Tariq SM, Sadaf T. Images in clinical medicine. Reexpansion pulmonary edema after treatment of pneumothorax. N Engl J Med 2006;354(19):2046

CASE 134

■ Clinical Presentation

40-year-old woman found down and unresponsive following a heroin drug overdose

■ Radiologic Findings

AP chest radiograph (**Fig. 134.1**) demonstrates an upper limit normal heart size for the depth of inspiration, bilateral perihilar ground glass opacities, and diminished vascular clarity with poorly defined pulmonary vessels, and dependent layering left pleural effusion.

■ Diagnosis

Heroin-Induced Pulmonary Edema

■ Differential Diagnosis

- Increased Hydrostatic Pressure Pulmonary Edema of Other Etiologies
- Permeability Edema with Diffuse Alveolar Damage (DAD)
- Permeability Edema without Diffuse Alveolar Damage (DAD)
- Aspiration

■ Discussion

Background

Pulmonary edema directly associated with an overdose of opiates occurs almost exclusively with heroin but may also occur with the use of cocaine and "crack" (**Fig. 134.2**). Heroin-induced pulmonary edema complicates 15% of heroin overdose cases. Both cardiogenic and non-cardiogenic pulmonary edema have been

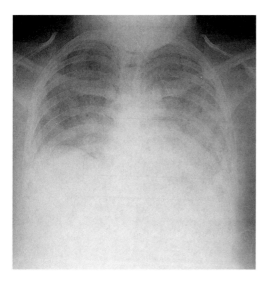

Fig. 134.1

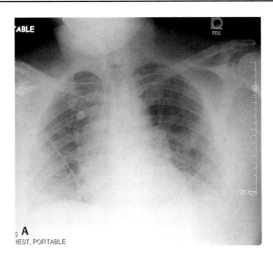
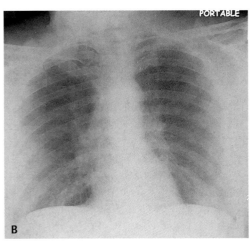

Fig. 134.2   AP chest radiograph **(A)** of a 42-year-old man with crack cocaine–induced pulmonary edema shows diminished vascular clarity and bilateral perihilar ground glass opacities with a normal-size heart. The perihilar opacities quickly resolve and the vascular clarity returns to normal over the ensuing two days **(B)**.

reported with intravenous cocaine abuse and crack cocaine smoking. Pulmonary edema is seen in 77–85% of cocaine-related deaths at autopsy.

Etiology

Unlike cocaine, heroin has no adverse effects on cardiac function. *Heroin* directly depresses the medullary respiratory center of the brain, causing hypoxia and acidosis, resulting in permeability edema without DAD. The pathogenesis of *cocaine-induced pulmonary edema* is more complex. Cocaine does have deleterious effects on the heart and may cause myocardial ischemia and infarction, dysrhythmias, and dilated cardiomyopathy, resulting in cardiogenic pulmonary edema. However, cocaine also damages the pulmonary capillary endothelium, resulting in increased permeability edema.

Clinical Findings

Heroin overdose victims often lie motionless for hours or even days before receiving medical attention. As a result, the pulmonary edema often demonstrates a gravity-dependent distribution. Victims may also suffer crush injuries with associated muscle damage and rhabdomyolysis with resultant kidney damage. Pulmonary complications resulting from *cocaine* abuse depend on the method of administration (i.e., oral, nasal, intravenous), dose size, frequency of use, and the presence of associated contaminants and particles. Respiratory symptoms are common after crack cocaine use and include cough with production of carbonaceous sputum, chest pain, dyspnea, hemoptysis, wheezing, and asthma exacerbation. Cocaine-induced ischemic organ injury affects the liver, kidneys, bowel, myocardium, central nervous system, and placenta.

Imaging Findings

Chest Radiography

Heroin-Induced Pulmonary Edema

- Often indistinguishable from other forms of pulmonary edema without DAD
- Peribronchial cuffing
- Marked asymmetric distribution of edema associated with gravity dependency
- Diminished vascular clarity with ill-defined pulmonary vessels (**Fig. 134.1**)
- Widespread, patchy, bilateral air space consolidations (**Fig. 134.1**)
- May be complicated by edema due to volume overload associated with renal failure
- Rapid resolution within one or two days if not complicated by renal failure or aspiration

Cocaine-Induced Pulmonary Edema

- Normal-size heart and cardiothoracic ratio (**Figs. 134.2A, 134.2B**)
- Bilateral perihilar / fairly symmetric interstitial or alveolar opacities (**Figs. 134.2A, 134.2B**)
- Resolves within 24–72 hours in the absence of cardiopulmonary complications (**Figs. 134.2A, 134.2B**)

Prognosis

- Heroin-induced pulmonary edema: overall mortality rate of 10%
- Crack-cocaine pulmonary edema usually resolves within 24–72 hours in the absence of cardiac damage
- Additional cardiopulmonary complications of cocaine and crack-cocaine abuse include eosinophilic lung disease; pulmonary fibrosis; pulmonary hypertension; alveolar hemorrhage; asthma exacerbation; barotrauma; thermal airway injury; hilar lymphadenopathy; emphysema; pulmonary infarction; bronchiolitis obliterans; cocaine-induced Churg-Strauss vasculitis; silicosis

Suggested Reading

1. Gluecker T, Capasso P, Schnyder P, et al. Clinical and radiologic features of pulmonary edema. Radiographics 1999;19(6):1507–1531, discussion 1532–1533

2. Laposata EA. Cocaine-induced heart disease: mechanisms and pathology. J Thorac Imaging 1991;6(1):68–75

3. Restrepo CS, Carrillo JA, Martínez S, Ojeda P, Rivera AL, Hatta A. Pulmonary complications from cocaine and cocaine-based substances: imaging manifestations. Radiographics 2007;27(4):941–956

CASE 135

■ Clinical Presentation

67-year-old man with a history of remote CABG presents with increasing substernal and chest pain

■ Radiologic Findings

AP chest radiograph (**Fig. 135.1A**) shows an 8.0 cm left-sided focal convex mediastinal mass overlying the aortic pulmonary window contiguous with and in close proximity to the thoracic aorta. Remote CABG surgical changes are evident. Patchy air space disease is seen in the right upper lobe. MDCTA axial (**Fig. 135.1B**), coronal (**Fig. 135.1C**), sagittal (**Fig. 135.1D**), and 3-D color volume-rendered (**Fig. 135.1E**) images confirm the mediastinal mass is a large saccular aneurysm off the transverse aorta. Note the abundant mural thrombus, displaced intimal calcifications, and extensive atheromatous plaque in the aorta. Right upper lobe air space disease is also seen.

■ Diagnosis

Thoracic Aorta Aneurysm

■ Differential Diagnosis

- Saccular Aneurysm Sequelae of Ruptured Penetrating Ulcer or Plaque
- Saccular Aneurysm Sequelae of Remote Blunt Trauma/Missed ATAI (**Fig. 100.13**)
- Coronary Artery Bypass Graft Aneurysm
- Other Non-Vascular Mediastinal Masses (based on chest radiography alone)

■ Discussion

Background

Dimensions of the normal thoracic aorta at various anatomic regions are summarized in **Table 135.1**. An *aneurysm* is a focal, abnormal, irreversible dilatation of a vessel greater than 50% of that of the adjacent normal vessel lumen. Thoracic aortic aneurysms (TAAs) may be classified as either *true aneurysms* (contain all three layers of aortic wall) or *false aneurysms* (pseudoaneurysms) (contained only by adventitial or periadventitial tissues). *True aneurysms* are usually associated with *fusiform* dilatation of the aorta (80%) and are most commonly due to atherosclerosis. *False aneurysms* are typically saccular and are most commonly due to trauma, penetrating atherosclerotic ulcers, or infection (**Figs. 135.1A, 135.1B, 135.1C, 135.1D, 135.1E**).

Etiology

Seventy percent of TAAs result from atherosclerosis and most involve the descending aorta. Other possible causes of TAAs are listed in **Table 135.2**. Non-syphilitic infection of the arterial wall with subsequent aneurysm formation is called a *mycotic aneurysm*. Mycotic aneurysms are usually saccular, contain eccentric thrombus, and have a propensity to involve the ascending aorta.

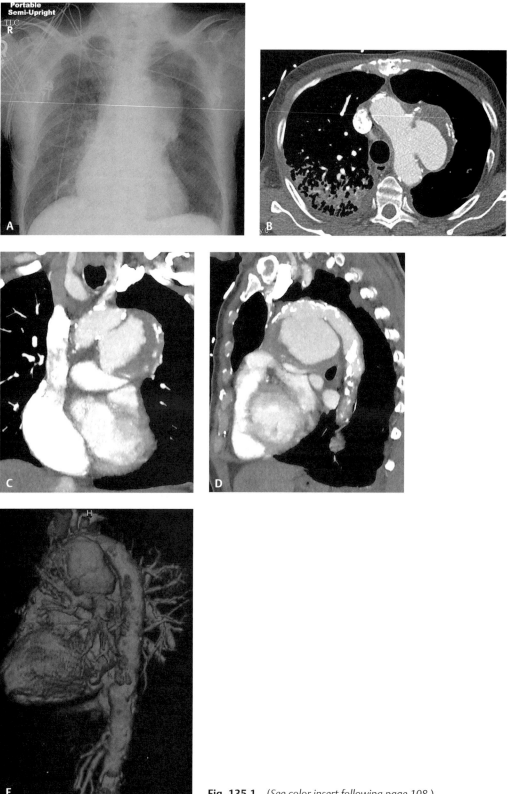

Fig. 135.1 (*See color insert following page 108.*)

Table 135.1   Normal Thoracic Aorta Dimensions

Anatomic Location	Definition	Average Diameter
Aortic root	Portion of ascending aorta containing aortic valve, annulus, sinuses of Valsalva	37 ± 3 mm
Ascending aorta	Extends from aortic root to right brachiocephalic artery origin	31 ± 4 mm
Arch	Extends from right brachiocephalic artery to ligamentum arteriosum attachment	26 ± 4 mm
Descending aorta	Extends from ligamentum arteriosum to aortic hiatus at the diaphragm	24 ± 3 mm

Table 135.2   Possible Causes of Thoracic Aorta Aneurysm

ASVD*	Aortic Dissection	Infectious Aortitis	Non-Infectious Aortitis	Congenital	Other
		Streptococcus sp.	Rheumatoid arthritis	Bicuspid aortic valve	XRT[¥]
		Staphylococcus sp.	Ankylosing spondylitis	Marfan syndrome	Trauma
		Gonorrhea	Giant cell arteritis	Ehlers-Danlos syndrome	Aortic cannulation site
		Syphilis	Takayasu arteritis	Medial degeneration	Scleroderma
		Salmonella sp.	Relapsing polychondritis		Psoriasis
		M. tuberculosis			SLE[j]
		Rheumatic fever			Ulcerative colitis
					Reiter syndrome

*ASVD, atherosclerotic vascular disease
[¥]XRT, radiation therapy
[j]SLE, systemic lupus erythematosus

Clinical Findings

Most patients with TAAs are asymptomatic. Symptoms usually result from compression of adjacent mediastinal structures and may include SVC syndrome; stridor or dyspnea; dysphagia; and hoarseness from recurrent laryngeal nerve compression. Twenty-five percent of patients may complain of substernal chest, shoulder, or back pain.

Imaging

Chest Radiography

- Contour abnormality and tortuosity of aorta (**Figs. 135.1A, 135.2A, 135.3A, 135.5A, 135.5B**)
- Widened superior mediastinum or elevation of aortic-pulmonary stripe (**Figs. 135.5A, 135.5B**)
- Mediastinal mass, varying size and shape, continuous with, or in close proximity to, thoracic aorta (**Figs. 135.1A, 135.2A, 135.3A**)
- Ascending aorta/proximal arch aneurysms: project anteriorly and rightward (**Fig. 135.2A**)
- Distal arch/descending aorta aneurysms: project posteriorly and leftward (**Figs. 135.3A, 135.5A, 135.5B**)
- Curvilinear peripheral calcifications
- Extrinsic compression of trachea, bronchi, esophagus
- Complications related to rupture (see below)

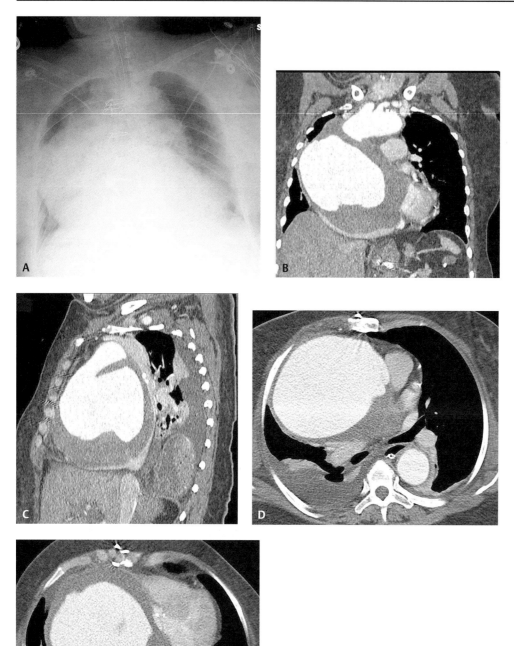

Fig. 135.2 AP chest radiograph **(A)** of a 69-year-old woman admitted to the CCU with chest pain and heart failure shows a large convex right-sided mediastinal mass silhouetting the entire right heart and normal mediastinal lines and stripes. MDCTA coronal **(B)**, sagittal **(C)**, and axial **(D,E)** images confirm the mediastinal mass is a massive ascending aorta aneurysm occupying most of the right thorax. Note its relationship to the arch and great vessels, the mass effect on the right heart, and the abundant mural thrombus.

MDCTA

Comprehensive evaluation of TAA morphology, extent, presence of thrombus, great vessels and mediastinal relationships, and complications such as dissection and rupture

- Abnormal aortic dilatation (**Fig. 135.1B, 135.1C, 135.2D, 135.2E, 135.3B, 135.4A, 135.4B**)
- Intramural circumferential or crescent thrombus (**Fig. 135.1B, 135.1C, 135.2D, 135.2E, 135.3B, 135.4A, 135.4B**)

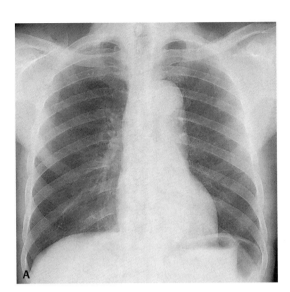 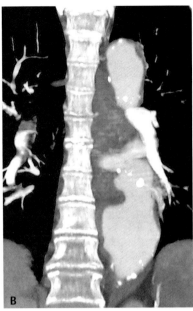

Fig. 135.3 Screening PA chest X-ray **(A)** of a 70-year-old asymptomatic man with hypertension shows an abnormal contour to the descending thoracic aorta projecting leftward and silhouetting the left paraspinal line. MDCTA coronal image **(B)** reveals a distal TAA with irregular mural thrombus and peripheral calcifications.

- High-attenuation thickened aortic wall; aortitis
- Complications (see below)
- 2-D and 3-D reformatting techniques: maximum intensity projection (MIP), curved planar reformation (CPR), multiplanar reformation (MPR), and volume-rendered imaging (VR) complement diagnostic interpretation (**Figs. 135.1C, 135.1D, 135.1E, 135.2B, 135.2C, 135.3B, 135.4B, 135.5C**)

Complications

- Hemothorax; hemomediastinum; hemopericardium; and/or contrast extravasation
- High-attenuation "crescent" in mural thrombus of TAA; may represent an acute contained leak or impending rupture
- *Draped aorta sign*—another CT manifestation of contained rupture or leak; posterior wall of aorta is closely apposed to spine
- *Aortobronchial fistula* (90% between descending TAA and consolidated left lung); *aortoesophageal fistula* (hemomediastinum; TAA intimately related to esophagus; rarely, contrast media extravasation into esophagus)

TAA Mimics

Normal variants that can mimic TAA include:

- Prominent ductus diverticulum (see Case 101)
- Aortic spindle (see Case 101)
- Aortic nipple (**Fig. 135.6**)

Prognosis

- Mean growth rate TAA: 0.1 cm/year (rate greater for descending as opposed to ascending TAA)
- Risk of rupture increases with increasing size
  - 2% for aneurysms <5 cm
  - 3% for aneurysms 5 to 5.9 cm
  - 7% for aneurysms ≥6 cm

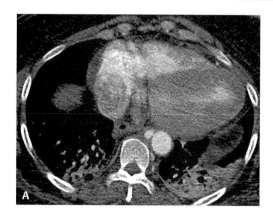

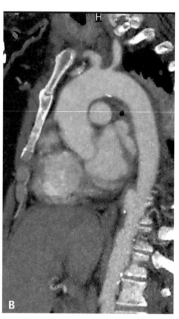

Fig. 135.4   MDCTA axial **(A)** and sagittal oblique **(B)** images of two different patients with IVDA and MRSA sepsis show saccular aneurysms of the descending aorta manifest as focal contour abnormalities with a well-defined neck and variable degrees of mural thrombus.

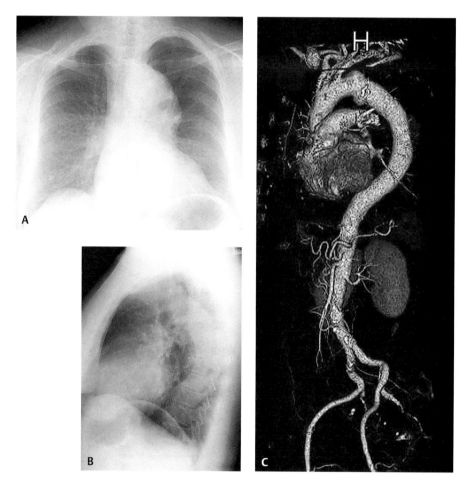

Fig. 135.5   66-year-old woman with poorly controlled hypertension and TAA. PA **(A)** and lateral **(B)** chest radiographs show a widened mediastinum and focal abnormal contour of the transverse aorta. The TAA and its great vessel relationships are nicely depicted on the 3-D volume-rendered CTA **(C)**. (*See color insert following page 108.*)

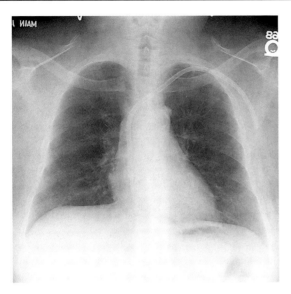

Fig. 135.6 PA chest radiograph of a woman with SVC stenosis from long-standing hemodialysis and resultant recruitment of mediastinal blood flow via the left second superior intercostal vein. This small focal protuberance along the superomedial or inferolateral aorta (aka aortic nipple) should not be confused with TAA. *(Image courtesy of James Messmer, MD, VCU Medical Center, Richmond, Virginia.)*

- Elective TAA repair has lower mortality rate (9%) than does emergent repair (22%)
- One of the greatest risks in elective repair is spinal cord ischemia and paralysis from injury to the artery of Adamkiewicz (i.e., usually arises from thoracic aorta between T8 and L1). Reattachment of large intercostal or lumbar arteries during graft replacement may reduce postoperative paraplegia to 16%.

Management

- TAAs are considered for repair when:
  - Symptomatic
  - Ascending TAA ≥5.5 cm in diameter
  - Descending TAA ≥6.5 cm in diameter
  - Annual TAA growth rate >1 cm
  - TAA ≥5.0 cm (Marfan syndrome)
- Ascending aorta or arch aneurysms: surgical replacement with synthetic conduit; aortic valve replacement in selected cases (see Case 192)
- Descending aorta aneurysms: surgical replacement with synthetic conduit or endovascular stenting (see Case 192)
- Reporting the relationship between the TAA and the great vessel branches is necessary in planning endovascular stent deployment (see Case 192)

PEARLS

- *Bicuspid aortic valve*: independent risk factor for TAA; unrelated to aortic stenosis.
- *Annuloaortic ectasia*: characterized by dilatation of sinuses of Valsalva and effacement of sinotubular junction, producing "pear-shaped" ascending aorta that tapers to a normal arch, most commonly associated with Marfan syndrome. Other causes include Ehlers-Danlos syndrome, osteogenesis imperfecta, and homocystinuria. One-third of cases are idiopathic.
- *Syphilitic aortitis:* most commonly affects ascending aorta (36% of cases), followed by the arch (34%), proximal descending aorta (25%), and distal descending aorta (5%). Syphilitic aneurysms have high rate of rupture; responsible for patient death in 40% of cases.
- Previous *aortic dissection* with persistent false lumen may produce aneurysmal dilatation of false lumen. Such pseudoaneurysms are contained only by the outer media and adventitia and may progressively enlarge over time and rupture.
- Abdominal aortic aneurysm (AAA) occurs in 28% of patients with TAA; necessary to include entire thoracoabdominal aorta in initial MDCTA evaluation of patients with TAAs.

- *Ectasia*: also defined as dilatation of a vessel, but commonly used by radiologists to describe age-related tortuosity of the aorta. This descriptor should be *avoided* because one cannot typically distinguish a tortuous aorta from TAA on conventional radiography alone. If chest radiography reveals an enlarged aortic silhouette, exercise a low threshold for obtaining further imaging in the appropriate clinical setting.

Suggested Reading

1. Agarwal PP, Chughtai A, Matzinger FRK, Kazerooni EA. Multidetector CT of thoracic aortic aneurysms. Radiographics 2009;29(2):537–552

2. Coady MA, Rizzo JA, Hammond GL, Kopf GS, Elefteriades JA. Surgical intervention criteria for thoracic aortic aneurysms: a study of growth rates and complications. Ann Thorac Surg 1999;67(6):1922–1926, discussion 1953–1958

3. Coady MA, Rizzo JA, Hammond GL, et al. What is the appropriate size criterion for resection of thoracic aortic aneurysms? J Thorac Cardiovasc Surg 1997;113(3):476–491, discussion 489–491

4. Dapunt OE, Galla JD, Sadeghi AM, et al. The natural history of thoracic aortic aneurysms. J Thorac Cardiovasc Surg 1994;107(5):1323–1332, discussion 1332–1333

5. Halliday KE, al-Kutoubi A. Draped aorta: CT sign of contained leak of aortic aneurysms. Radiology 1996;199(1): 41–43

CASE 136

■ Clinical Presentation

66-year-old woman with poorly controlled hypertension presented to the Emergency Department with sudden, sharp, tearing intractable chest pain

■ Radiologic Findings

MDCTA axial (**Figs. 136.1A, 136.1B, 136.1C**), coronal MIP (**Fig. 136.1D**), and sagittal MIP (**Fig. 136.1E**) images demonstrate an intimomedial flap limited to a significantly dilated ascending aorta and aortic root. Note the atheromatous changes in the thoracic aorta, its branch vessels, and the left main origin as well as left anterior descending coronary artery.

■ Diagnosis

Acute Dissection of the Thoracic Aorta (Type A)

■ Differential Diagnosis

- Other Causes of Acute Coronary Syndrome

■ Discussion

Background

Aortic dissection (AD) is the *most common* acute emergency condition of the aorta and is often fatal. The reported incidence is 2,000 new cases per year (USA). AD occurs two to three times more often than a ruptured abdominal aortic aneurysm, and it is two to three times more common in men. One-half of aortic dissections in women under 40 years of age occur during pregnancy. Patient outcome and survival are determined by the type and extent of AD and the presence of associated complications. There are two systems of classification (**Fig. 136.2**). The *DeBakey system* is based on the extent of the dissection, and the *Stanford system* classifies dissections by their proximal extent. *DeBakey type I* dissections (29–34%) involve the ascending aorta and extend around the arch and continue distally (**Figs. 136.2, 136.3A, 136.3B, 136.3C**). *DeBakey type II* dissections (12–21%) involve the ascending aorta only (**Figs. 136.1A,136.1B, 136.1C, 136.1D, 136.1E, 136.2**). *DeBakey type III* dissections (>50%) begin beyond the thoracic aorta branch vessels and continue down the descending aorta (*IIIA*), often below the diaphragm into the abdominal aorta (*IIIB*), and sometimes as far distally as the femoral arteries (**Figs. 136.2, Fig. 136.4A, 136.4B, 136.4C, 136.4D, 136.4E, 136.4F**). *Stanford type A* dissections (70%) involve the ascending aorta, regardless of where the entry tear begins and how far distally the dissection extends, and are equivalent to *DeBakey type I* and *type II* ADs (**Figs. 136.1A, 136.1B, 136.1C, 136.1D, 136.1E, 136.2**). *Stanford type B* dissections (20–30%) begin after the arch vessels and are equivalent to *DeBakey type III* (**Figs. 136.2, Fig. 136.4A, 136.4B, 136.4C, 136.4D, 136.4E, 136.4F**). An AD <2 weeks old is considered acute, whereas one >2 weeks old is considered chronic.

663

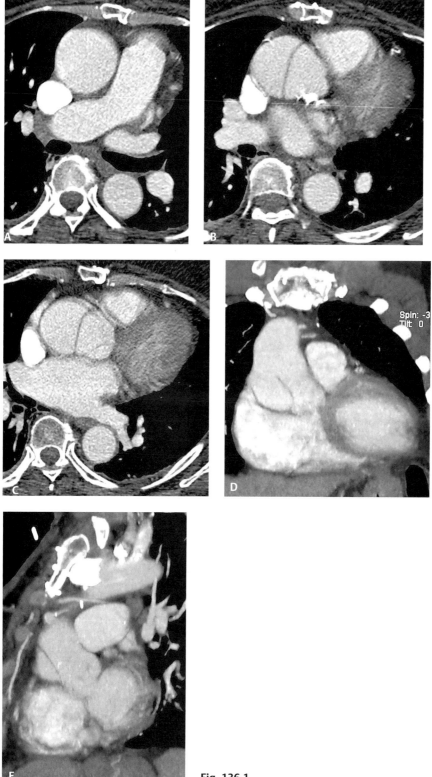

Fig. 136.1

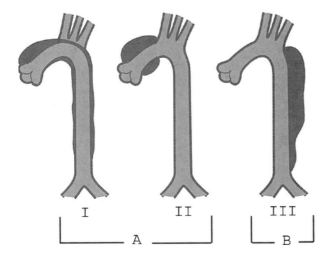

Fig. 136.2 Artist's illustration depicting the three major types of aortic dissection. Stanford type A is equivalent to DeBakey type I and/or II. Stanford B is equivalent to DeBakey type III.

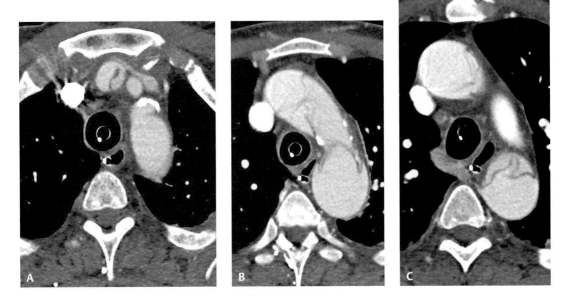

Fig. 136.3 MDCTA axial images show a type I (type A) AD of ascending and descending thoracic aorta **(B,C)** with extension into the brachiocephalic artery **(A)**. Note the displaced intimal calcifications in the ascending aorta.

Etiology

Spontaneous separation of the aortic intima and adventitia allows circulating blood to gain access to and split the media of the aortic wall, creating a false lumen. This false lumen typically has pressures greater than or equal to that of the true lumen. The pressure difference, loss in transmural pressure across the intimomedial flap, and reduced elastic recoil in its thin outer wall due to elastin deficiency, result in expansion of the false lumen and compression-obstruction of the true lumen. These same factors predispose the false lumen to rupture.

Clinical Findings

AD occurs most often in hypertensive patients and those with Marfan syndrome. Other risk factors include congenital bicuspid aortic valve, aortic valvular stenosis, coarctation of the aorta, pregnancy, Ehlers-Danlos syndrome, Turner syndrome, Behçet disease, aortitis (systemic lupus erythematosus), crack cocaine abuse, infection, and cardiac surgery. Classically, patients present with an acute onset of tearing central chest pain radiating to the back. Deficits of major arterial pulses occur in two-thirds of patients and are more common

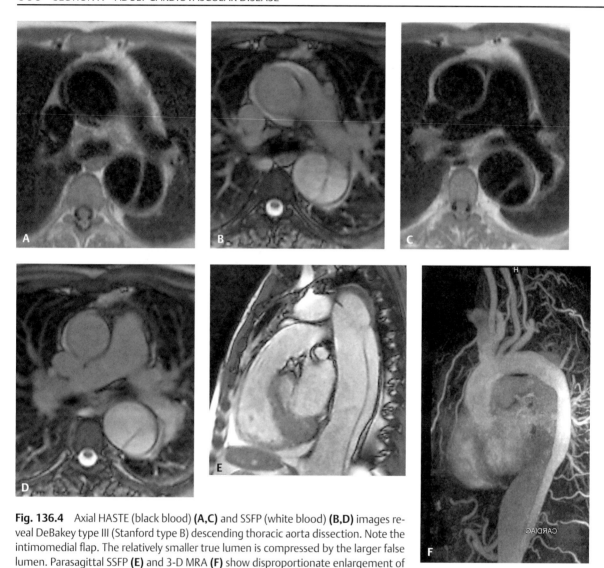

Fig. 136.4 Axial HASTE (black blood) **(A,C)** and SSFP (white blood) **(B,D)** images reveal DeBakey type III (Stanford type B) descending thoracic aorta dissection. Note the intimomedial flap. The relatively smaller true lumen is compressed by the larger false lumen. Parasagittal SSFP **(E)** and 3-D MRA **(F)** show disproportionate enlargement of the false lumen and the relationship of the AD to the branch vessels.

with type A dissection. Up to 20% of patients may present with syncope, which may be the result of hypotension from cardiac tamponade or obstruction of cerebral vessels. Aortic regurgitation with a diastolic murmur is heard in two-thirds of patients with proximal dissections and may be complicated by heart failure.

Complications

Complications include retrograde dissection (e.g., aortic regurgitation, coronary artery occlusion with myocardial ischemia-infarction, rupture into the pericardial sac [**Fig. 136.5A**] or pleural space [**Fig. 136.5B**]), major branch vessel involvement and or occlusion (**Fig. 136.5C**), limb and organ ischemia, aorta rupture, and saccular aneurysm formation. Main abdominal arterial branch involvement occurs in 27% of cases.

Imaging Findings

Chest Radiography

- Normal in 10–40% of patients
- Widening of superior mediastinum and aorta (most common) (**Fig. 136.6**)

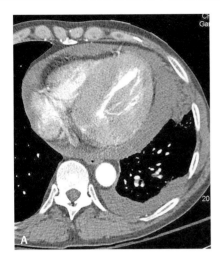
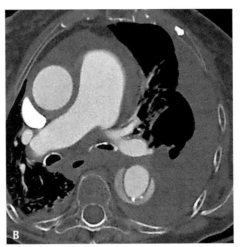
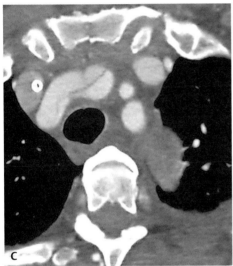

Fig. 136.5 Complications of AD in three different patients. Axial MDCTA **(A)** shows hemopericardium and left hemothorax complicating Type A dissection (outside field of view). Axial MDCTA **(B)** reveals Type B AD complicated by left hemothorax and hemomediastinum. Note the classic *beak sign* of the false lumen and the displaced intimal calcifications. Axial MDCTA **(C)** demonstrates a Type A AD with extension into the brachiocephalic artery. Note the contrast differential between the high-attenuation true lumen and low-attenuation false lumen.

- Change in contour of cardiac or aortic silhouette (**Fig. 136.6**)
- Double contour to aortic arch
- Central displacement of calcified plaque from outer aortic contour >10 mm
- Disparity in size between ascending and descending aorta
- ± left effusion

MDCTA/MRI

- Classic intimomedial flap (70%) (**Figs. 136.1, 136.3, 136.4**)
- Circumferential intimal flap; due to dissection of entire lumen (**Fig. 136.7A**)
- Narrow true lumen with filiform shape (**Figs. 136.3B, 136.3C**)
- Intimomedial intussusception; "windsock" appearance; true lumen internal; false lumen external
- Calcified false lumen; chronic AD with mural calcifications of false lumen
- *Mercedes-Benz sign*: rare configuration of intimal flaps; three-channel dissection; results from secondary dissection within one of the channels (**Fig. 136.7B**)
- Additional false lumen features
  - Larger cross-sectional area than true lumen (**Figs. 136.4, 136.5B, 136.5C**)
  - *Cobweb sign*: slender linear areas of low attenuation due to residual ribbons of media incompletely sheared away (**Figs. 136.3B, 136.3C**)
  - *Beak sign:* wedge of hematoma that creates a space for propagation of false lumen (**Fig. 136.5B**)

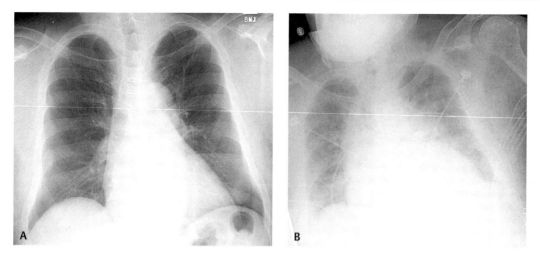

Fig. 136.6 Baseline PA chest radiograph **(A)** of a 60-year-old man with hypertension shows an enlarged heart and surgical changes from remote CABG. AP portable chest X-ray **(B)** 12 months later, when he presented with severe chest pain and hypotension, shows a widened mediastinum; markedly enlarged cardiomediastinal silhouette; change in contour of the ascending and descending aorta; and pulmonary edema. MDCTA (not illustrated) demonstrated a Type A AD with hemopericardium.

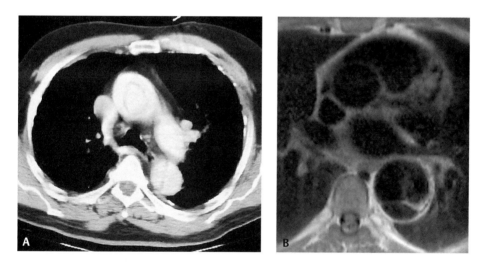

Fig. 136.7 Atypical presentations of AD in two different patients. Contrast-enhanced CT **(A)** shows a circumferential intimomedial flap of the ascending aorta and a classic intimomedial flap in the descending aorta. Asbestos-related pleural plaques are an incidental finding. Axial HASTE MRI **(B)** reveals a three-channel descending thoracic aorta AD due to secondary dissection within one of the channels.

- True lumen: in continuity with undissected aorta; false lumen may thrombose
- Secondary findings of AD
  - Internal displacement of calcifications (**Figs. 136.3B, 136.5B**)
  - Delayed or diminished enhancement of false lumen (**Figs. 136.3A, 136.3C, 136.4F, 136.5B, 136.5C**)

Management

- Type A: Typically requires urgent surgical intervention (see Case 192)
- Type B: Medical management of hypertension unless there are complications related to the AD (**Table 136.1**)

Table 136.1   Indications for Surgical Intervention or Stent Deployment: Type B Aortic Dissection

Aorta rupture

Hemodynamic instability

Descending aorta diameter >6.0 cm

Poor perfusion of thoracoabdominal aorta

Mesenteric, renal, extremity ischemia (expanding false lumen, compressing and compromising true lumen)

Pseudocoarctation syndrome

Distal embolization

Prognosis

Type A

- Left untreated, often rapidly fatal; death rate 1% per hour for the first 48 hours; 75% of untreated patients die within two weeks
- Long-term survival of treated patients: 60% at 5 years and 40% at 10 years
- Operative mortality <10%

Type B

- Medical treatment results in an 80–90% 30-day survival
- Untreated type B dissections: 40% mortality rate
- Surgical repair may be complicated by paraplegia

PEARLS

- Most common risk factor for AD is hypertension (60–90%).
- Arteries supplied exclusively by false lumen are rarely compromised.
- AD may be associated with branch vessel obstruction.
- *Static obstruction*: intimal flap enters branch vessel origin without re-entry point.
  - Increased pressure or thrombus formation in false lumen results in focal stenosis and end-organ ischemia.
  - Treated with intravascular stent deployment.

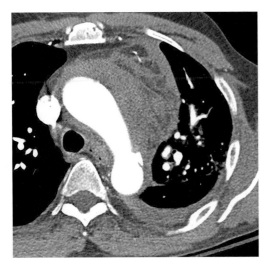

Fig. 136.8   Axial MDCTA image shows a penetrating ulcer in the proximal descending thoracic aorta projecting beyond the aortic lumen and complicated by extensive hemomediastinum and left hemothorax.

- *Dynamic obstruction:* affects vessels arising from true lumen; intimal flap spares branch vessel but prolapses over and covers its origin.
  - ○ Creates pressure deficit in true lumen and resultant ischemia.
  - ○ Treated with intimal flap fenestration to decrease false lumen pressures.
- Recognition and differentiation of penetrating ulcers (PUs) from AD is important. In comparison with *type A* or *B* AD, patients with PU are older (mean age 77 years); have larger aortic diameters (mean 6.5 cm); have ulcers primarily in descending aorta (87%); and more often have ulcers associated with prior diagnosed or managed abdominal aortic aneurysms (AAA) (40%). Risk for rupture is higher among patients with PU (40%) than patients with *type A* or *type B* AD (**Fig. 136.8**). Surgical management is advocated for ascending aorta PUs and for descending aorta PUs characterized by early clinical or radiologic signs of deterioration.

Suggested Reading

1. Castañer E, Andreu M, Gallardo X, Mata JM, Cabezuelo MA, Pallardó Y. CT in nontraumatic acute thoracic aortic disease: typical and atypical features and complications. Radiographics 2003;23(Spec No):S93–S110

2. Coady MA, Rizzo JA, Hammond GL, Pierce JG, Kopf GS, Elefteriades JA. Penetrating ulcer of the thoracic aorta: what is it? How do we recognize it? How do we manage it? J Vasc Surg 1998;27(6):1006–1015, discussion 1015–1016

3. Liu Q, Lu JP, Wang F, Wang L, Tian JM. Three-dimensional contrast-enhanced MR angiography of aortic dissection: a pictorial essay. Radiographics 2007;27(5):1311–1321

4. McMahon MA, Squirrell CA. Multidetector CT of aortic dissection: a pictorial review. Radiographics 2010;30(2):445–460

CASE 137

■ Clinical Presentation

75-year-old woman presented to the Emergency Department with chest pain over the previous several hours with an abrupt increase in severity and intensity just prior to CT imaging

■ Radiologic Findings

Unenhanced chest CT images (**Figs. 137.1A, 137.2A, 137.3A, 137.4A, 137.5A**) demonstrate aneurysmal dilatation of the ascending aorta (5.6 cm) relative to the descending aorta with an associated eccentric high-attenuation intramural fluid collection. An intimomedial flap is suggested in the ascending aorta (**Figs. 137.2, 137.3**). Displaced intimal calcifications are seen in the descending aorta at 2:00 (**Fig. 137.1**) and 6:00 (**Fig. 137.4**). Note the high-attenuation pericardial effusion (i.e., hemopericardium) (**Figs. 137.4, 137.5**) and the extensive coronary artery calcifications. Contrast-enhanced CT images at approximately the same anatomic levels (**Figs. 137.1B, 137.2B, 137.3B, 137.4B, 137.5B**) depict a smooth, non-enhancing, eccentric region of aortic wall thickening involving the ascending aorta and confirm the presence of a spiraling intimomedial flap. Extensive mural thrombus is present in the descending aorta.

■ Diagnosis

Stanford Type A Intramural Hematoma Complicated by Overt Dissection

■ Differential Diagnosis

- Acute presentation in symptomatic patient
  - None
- Incidental finding in asymptomatic patient
  - Aortitis: normal interspersed segments between involved sites
  - Periaortic Lymphoma: thickened aortic wall with irregular external border
  - Atheroma: irregular intraluminal surface

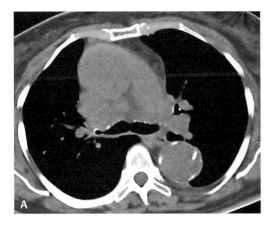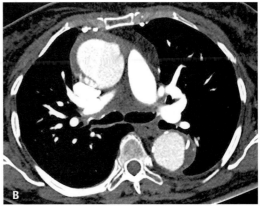

Fig. 137.1

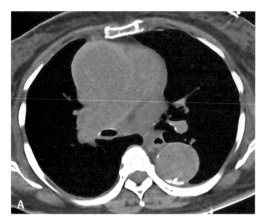 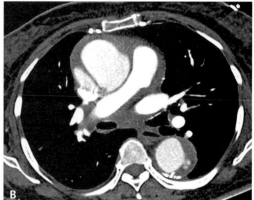

Fig. 137.2

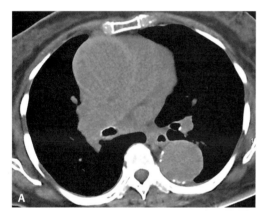 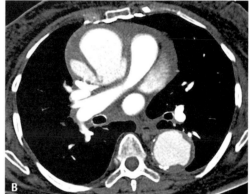

Fig. 137.3

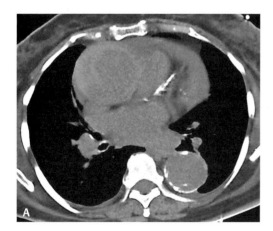 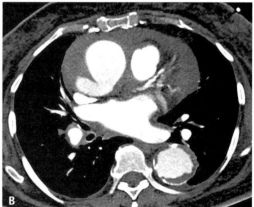

Fig. 137.4

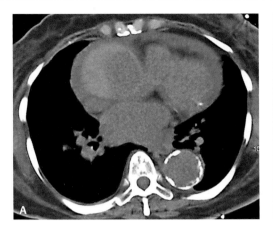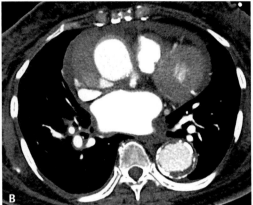

Fig. 137.5

■ Discussion

Background

Aortic intramural hematoma (IMH) is often described as an atypical or "flapless" aortic dissection and is thought to represent either an early-stage limited dissection or thrombosis of the false lumen in dissection. The distinguishing feature is the absence of the intimal disruption that characterizes classic aortic dissection. The Stanford system for classification of typical aortic dissection (AD) is applicable to the classification of IMH. That is, *Stanford type A IMH* involves the ascending aorta, with or without involvement of the descending aorta, and *Stanford type B IMH* involves the descending thoracic aorta, distal to the left subclavian artery origin. However, IMH exhibits a more variable natural history than classic AD, and may be characterized by periods of stabilization, regression, resolution, or progression to overt dissection. *Type A IMH* is more likely to progress to overt dissection than *type B IMH*. This is likely what occurred in this particular case.

Etiology

IMH results from rupture of the vasa vasorum and hemorrhage into the tunica media with resultant weakening of the aortic wall.

Clinical Findings

IMH is found in 5–20% of patients presenting with signs suggestive of acute (AD); 57% are classified as type A and 43% as type B, and 94% of IMHs are non-traumatic. Among IMHs of a traumatic etiology, 75% occur in the setting of a motor vehicle collision. Of affected patients with IMH, 61% are men. The mean age at presentation is 63 years for men and 68 years for woman. IMH and AD have similar predisposing risk factors, the most common being hypertension, as well as clinical signs and symptoms (e.g., chest and/or back pain). Less commonly, patients may experience syncope, hoarseness, anterior spinal syndrome, or acute renal insufficiency. Additional clinical findings include ECG changes, aortic regurgitation, and pericardial and pleural effusion.

Imaging Findings

MDCT (sensitivity/negative predictive value approach 100%)

Unenhanced CT

- Narrow window recommended (200 width; 40 level) for optimal depiction of IMH (**Figs. 137.1A, 137.2A, 137.3A, 137.4A, 137.5A, 137.6A**)
- Enlarged aorta diameter (**Figs. 137.1A, 137.2A, 137.3A, 137.4A, 137.5A, 137.6A**)

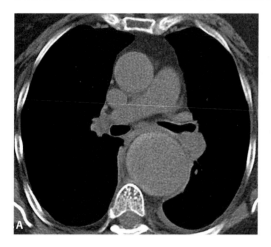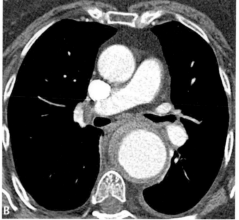

Fig. 137.6 Unenhanced chest CT **(A)** of a 64-year-old woman with severe chest pain and type B IMH shows aneurysmal dilatation of the descending thoracic aorta and a crescentic region of high attenuation involving the aortic wall from 6:00 through 1:00. On the contrast-enhanced CT at the same level **(B)** this intramural fluid collection appears as a non-enhancing, smooth, crescentic region of aortic wall thickening partially encompassing the aortic lumen. Note the absence of an intimomedial flap.

- ± Compression of aortic lumen
- Crescentic, eccentric, high-attenuation region of aortic wall thickening (**Figs. 137.1A, 137.2A, 137.3A, 137.4A, 137.5A, 137.6A**)
- Inward displacement of intimal calcifications
  - IMHs: often appear semicircular or curvilinear
  - ADs: more often appear linear

Contrast-enhanced CT

- Intramural fluid collection appears as a non-enhancing, smooth, crescentic region of aortic wall thickening (**Figs. 137.1B, 137.6B**)
- Intramural fluid collection extends partially or entirely around opacified aortic lumen (Figs. (**Figs. 137.1B, 137.6B**)
- No intimomedial flap, tear, or penetrating ulcer is present (**Fig. 137.6B**)
- Concomitant findings: mediastinal hematoma; pericardial or pleural effusion (**Figs. 137.4B, 137.5B**)

Transesophageal Echocardiography (TEE)

- (Sensitivity 90–100%; specificity 91–100%)
- Focal aortic wall thickening
- Eccentric aortic lumen
- Displaced intimal calcifications
- Hypoechoic areas in aortic wall
- Limited evaluation of the aorta
- False positive or equivocal results: severe atherosclerosis with focal wall thickening

MRI (sensitivity 100%) (Figs. 137.7A, 137.7B, 137.7C, 137.7D, 137.7E, 137.7F)

- Aortic dilatation
- Crescentic intramural fluid collection (**Figs. 137.7A, 137.7B, 137.7C, 137.7D, 137.7E, 137.7F**)
- GRE (white blood sequences)
  - Acute IMH (<7days): increased SI T2WI
  - Subacute/chronic IMH (≥7days): intermediate SI T2WI

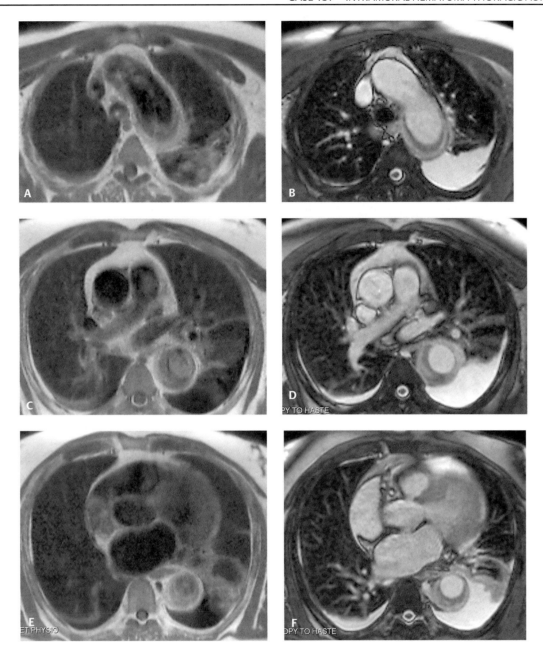

Fig. 137.7 MRI of a 56-year-old hypertensive man presenting to the emergency department with syncope, chest pain, and type B IMH. HASTE (i.e., ultrafast T2-weighted pulse sequence **A, C, F**) shows a dilated distal transverse and descending thoracic aorta with a posteriorly located crescent of high signal intensity in a thickened aortic wall. SSFP sequence **(B,D,F)** reveals similar findings to better advantage. Note the absence of an intimomedial flap and luminal deformity. Bilateral pleural effusions are present.

- Spin-echo (black blood sequences)
  - Acute IMH: intermediate SI T1WI secondary to oxyhemoglobin
  - Subacute/chronic IMH: increased SI T1WI secondary to methemoglobin
- Dynamic phase-contrast images: absence of flow in aortic wall

Angiography (sensitivity 83%)

- Limited usefulness for IMH

Complications

- *New intimal tear* (manifests with formation of ulcer-like projections not present at time of initial diagnosis)
  - Type A IMH >> Type B IMH
  - More commonly occurs in ascending aorta and aortic arch
  - One-third of patients within first three months of follow-up imaging
- *Saccular aneurysm* formation at site of IMH
  - Pseudoaneurysm
  - Most commonly located in distal aortic arch
  - Typically manifest one week to seven months after initial IMH diagnosis
  - Enlarge at average rate of 1.3 cm/year; considerable potential for rupture
- *Fusiform aneurysm* formation at site of IMH
  - True aneurysm
  - More commonly located in descending aorta
- *Progression to overt aortic dissection* (**Figs. 137.1B, 137.2B, 137.3B, 137.4B, 137.5B**)
  - Type A IMH >> Type B IMH
  - Frequency type A IMH: 15–87.5%
  - Imaging predictors of IMH progression to AD requiring surgical management
- Thicker IMH (16 mm vs. 10.5 mm)
- Greater degree of luminal compression (ratio <0.75 of minimum and maximum transverse diameters of aortic lumen at site of maximal IMH thickness)
- Maximal aortic diameter ≥50 mm strongest predictor (PPV 83%, NPV 100%)
- Predictive values of aortic regurgitation, mediastinal hematoma, and pericardial and pleural effusion indeterminate

Management

- Type B IMH: conservative
- Type A IMH: less well established
- Careful monitoring with regular follow-up imaging is mandatory even if the hematoma shows improvement or complete resolution because structural weakening of aorta may result in delayed aneurysm formation or AD
- No established guidelines on optimal frequency and longitudinal duration for surveillance; recommendations include
  - Weekly CT for first month after diagnosis
  - Two or three CT exams during first year after diagnosis

Prognosis

- Morbidity and mortality rate due to IMH: similar to AD
- IMH mortality rate: 21%
- One week after symptoms: IMH attenuation similar to unopacified blood (NCCT)
- Follow-up imaging may reveal decrease in IMH thickness within a few months and complete resolution within a year

PEARLS

- Absence of an intimomedial flap, intimal tear, or penetrating ulcer is a prerequisite for the diagnosis of IMH.
- Radiologist should document maximal aortic diameter, maximal axial thickness of the IMH, and minimum and maximum transverse diameters of aortic lumen at the level of maximal IHM thickness. Data are useful for predicting the outcome of IMH.

Suggested Reading

1. Bluemke DA. Definitive diagnosis of intramural hematoma of the thoracic aorta with MR imaging. Radiology 1997;204(2):319–321

2. Chao CP, Walker TG, Kalva SP. Natural history and CT appearances of aortic intramural hematoma. Radiographics 2009;29(3):791–804

3. Kaji S, Nishigami K, Akasaka T, et al. Prediction of progression or regression of type A aortic intramural hematoma by computed tomography. Circulation 1999;100(19, Suppl):II281–II286

4. Sawhney NS, DeMaria AN, Blanchard DG. Aortic intramural hematoma: an increasingly recognized and potentially fatal entity. Chest 2001;120(4):1340–1346

5. Yoshida S, Akiba H, Tamakawa M, et al. Thoracic involvement of type A aortic dissection and intramural hematoma: diagnostic accuracy—comparison of emergency helical CT and surgical findings. Radiology 2003;228(2):430–435

CASE 138

■ Clinical Presentation

35-year-old woman with dyspnea on exertion

■ Radiologic Findings

PA (**Fig. 138.1**) and lateral (**Fig. 138.2**) chest radiographs demonstrate mild cardiomegaly, an enlarged left atrial appendage (*arrow*) (**Fig. 138.1**), moderate left atrial enlargement (*arrowhead*) with elevation of the left mainstem bronchus (**Fig. 138.2**), and normal pulmonary vascularity. Contrast-enhanced chest CT (mediastinal window) (**Figs. 138.3, 138.4**) shows enlargement of the left atrium and the left atrial appendage (**Fig. 138.3**). Note calcifications of the mitral valve leaflets (**Fig. 138.4**).

■ Diagnosis

Mitral Stenosis

■ Differential Diagnosis

- Left Atrial Enlargement of Other Etiology
  - Myxoma
  - Left Atrial Thrombus

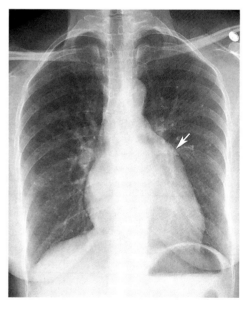

Fig. 138.1

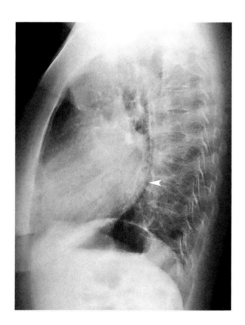

Fig. 138.2

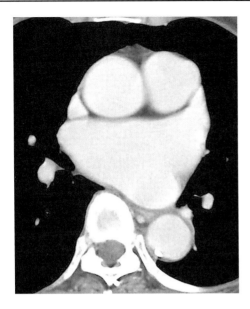

Fig. 138.3

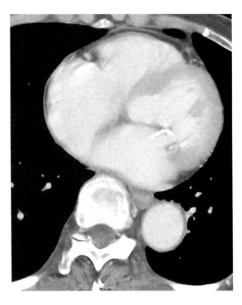

Fig. 138.4

■ Discussion

Background

The mitral valve is characterized by its bicuspid morphology with anterior and posterior leaflets. The anterior mitral valve leaflet is in fibrous continuity with the posterior and left aortic valve leaflets. In normal hemodynamics, diastolic elevation of left atrial pressure forces the mitral valve open and systolic elevation of left ventricular pressure forces it closed. Mitral stenosis refers to valvular obstruction of antegrade blood flow within the left heart and is a lesion of pressure overload. Volume overload follows and results in left atrial enlargement. Rheumatic mitral stenosis almost always has a secondary component of mitral insufficiency.

Etiology

While mitral stenosis may be congenital, it more commonly results from rheumatic heart disease, a complication of rheumatic fever. Rheumatic fever is a systemic inflammatory disorder caused by group A beta hemolytic *Streptococcus*. Approximately 30% of affected patients develop rheumatic heart disease. The mitral valve is most commonly affected (50%), followed by combined involvement of the mitral and aortic valves (20–50%). Tricuspid valve involvement may result in trivalvular disease. The pulmonic valve is rarely affected.

Clinical Findings

Rheumatic fever typically affects patients between the ages of 5 and 15 years. Only 50% of patients with rheumatic mitral stenosis are aware of a past episode of rheumatic fever. Patients remain asymptomatic for at least one decade but eventually develop dyspnea. With sustained volume overload, the left atrium enlarges and atrial fibrillation may ensue. Turbulent flow may result in the formation of left atrial thrombus, particularly within the atrial appendage, and subsequent systemic embolization. Untreated patients develop secondary pulmonary arterial hypertension leading to right ventricular hypertrophy, followed by right ventricular failure with systemic venous hypertension, peripheral edema, hepatic congestion, ascites, and fatigue. A late consequence of untreated mitral stenosis is pulmonary hemosiderosis due to repeated episodes of alveolar hemorrhage.

Imaging Findings

Chest Radiography

- Normal heart size in early disease
- Cardiomegaly secondary to right ventricular failure (late) (**Figs. 138.1, 138.2**)
- Left atrial appendage enlargement (**Figs. 138.1, 138.5**)
- Left atrial enlargement (**Figs. 138.1, 138.2, 138.5**); double contour with the right atrium, elevated left mainstem bronchus; carinal splaying (**Fig. I.2**)
- Pulmonary venous hypertension (**Fig. 138.5**); typically cephalization of blood flow
- Findings of pulmonary arterial hypertension
- Calcified mitral valve (rarely detected on radiography)
- Calcified left atrial wall; calcified left atrial thrombus
- Pulmonary infarction
- Pulmonary hemosiderosis: 2–5 mm densely calcified nodules in mid- and lower lung, more frequently on the right
- *"Double density" sign*: enlarging right side of left atrium pushes into adjacent lung on frontal radiography
- *"Walking man" sign*: posterior displacement of left upper and lower lobe bronchus relative to the right on lateral radiography

MDCT

- Left atrial enlargement (**Figs. 138.3, 138.6A, 138.6B**)
- Mitral valve leaflet calcification (**Fig. 138.4**); valve leaflet fusion, valve may exhibit a funnel morphology
- Transvalvular pressure gradient with mitral valve area of less than 2.3 cm^2
- Visualization of intra-atrial thrombus (may be calcified) (**Fig. 138.6B**) and/or left atrial wall calcification (**Fig. 138.6A**)
- Right ventricular hypertrophy followed by right ventricular failure, right chamber enlargement, and pulmonary venous hypertension
- Assessment of cardiac function and valvular stenosis with or without insufficiency

MRI

- Spin-echo and double inversion recovery techniques: assess atrial volume, identify atrial thrombus, visualize right ventricular hypertrophy or enlargement

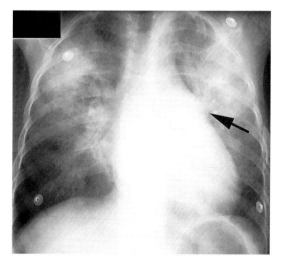

Fig. 138.5 PA chest radiograph of a young man with mitral stenosis and atrial fibrillation demonstrates pulmonary edema with preferential involvement of the upper lobes. Note left atrial appendage enlargement (*arrow*) and cardiomegaly. *(Image courtesy of Diane C. Strollo, MD, University of Pittsburgh Medical Center, Pittsburgh, Pennsylvania.)*

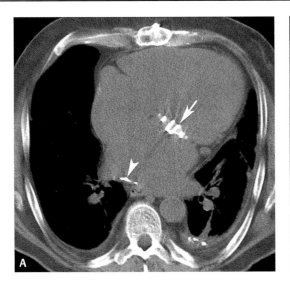 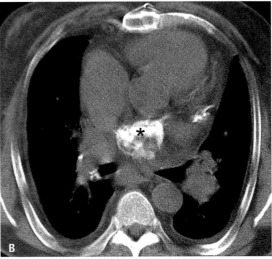

Fig. 138.6   Unenhanced chest CT (mediastinal window) **(A,B)** demonstrates left atrial enlargement **(A)**, a prosthetic mitral valve (*arrow*) **(A)**, left atrial wall calcification (*arrowhead*) **(A)**, and densely calcified left atrial thrombus (*asterisk*) **(B)**. *(Images courtesy of Helen T. Winer-Muram, MD, Indiana University Medical Center, Indianapolis, Indiana.)*

- Gradient-echo techniques
  - High-velocity jet across stenotic mitral valve: diastolic signal void extending from leaflets into left ventricle
  - Assess mitral valve morphology and maximum leaflet separation
- Velocity-encoded cine MRI: mean pressure gradients, blood flow velocity

Angiography

- Left atrial enlargement with normal-to-small left ventricle
- Doming of mitral valve leaflets on left ventriculography
- Mitral stenosis with or without insufficiency on ventriculography

Management

- Mitral valvuloplasty
- Mitral valve commissurotomy
- Mitral valve replacement

Prognosis

- 15–20% five-year survival in untreated patients with resting dyspnea

PEARLS

- Echocardiography is the primary imaging modality for assessment of valvular heart disease.
- Optimal visualization of the mitral valve on CT can be achieved with reformatted images in the two-chamber long axis plane perpendicular to the mitral valve during mid-diastole.

Suggested Reading

1. Chen JJ, Manning MA, Frazier AA, Jeudy J, White CS. CT angiography of the cardiac valves: normal, diseased, and postoperative appearances. Radiographics 2009;29(5):1393–1412

CASE 139

■ Clinical Presentation

Asymptomatic 55-year-old man

■ Radiologic Findings

PA (**Fig. 139.1**) and lateral (**Fig. 139.2**) chest radiographs demonstrate dilatation of the ascending aorta (*arrow*) (**Fig. 139.1**) and dense calcification of the aortic valve (*arrowheads*) (**Fig. 139.2**). The heart size and pulmonary vascularity are normal.

■ Diagnosis

Aortic Stenosis; Bicuspid Aortic Valve

■ Differential Diagnosis

• Hypertension

■ Discussion

Background

The aortic valve has a tricuspid morphology with right, left, and posterior leaflets. In normal hemodynamics, systolic elevation of left ventricular pressure forces the valve open, and diastolic elevation of systemic pressure (relative to left ventricular pressure) forces it closed. Aortic stenosis refers to obstruction of antegrade

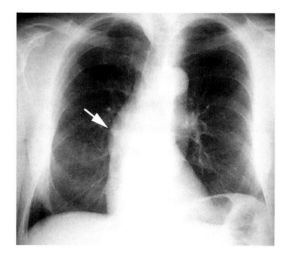

Fig. 139.1

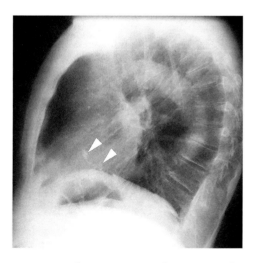

Fig. 139.2 *(Images courtesy of Diane C. Strollo, MD, University of Pittsburgh Medical Center, Pittsburgh, Pennsylvania.)*

682

blood flow between the left ventricle and the systemic circulation and may be valvular, supravalvular, or subvalvular (asymmetric septal hypertrophy). Aortic stenosis is a lesion of pressure overload, but almost always exhibits a component of secondary aortic insufficiency as calcium deposits on the stenotic valve often interfere with normal closure.

Etiology

Congenital aortic stenosis may manifest with a *unicuspid* (patients under 15 years), *bicuspid* (patients 15–65 years), or *tricuspid* (patients over 65 years) aortic valve. However, over 95% of patients with congenital aortic stenosis have unicuspid or bicuspid aortic valves. The latter occur in 1.5% of live births, and aortic stenosis is the most common complication. *Acquired aortic stenosis* may occur as a sequela of rheumatic heart disease or as a degenerative condition in patients over 65 years of age.

Clinical Findings

Patients with aortic stenosis may be entirely asymptomatic and are often diagnosed because of an ejection murmur on auscultation or an abnormal chest radiograph. Asymptomatic patients are usually under the age of 20 years. Approximately 75% of patients with congenital and rheumatic aortic stenosis are men, whereas degenerative aortic stenosis affects men and women equally. Degenerative stenosis is associated with hypertension, smoking, and blood lipid abnormalities. Sustained pressure overload results in left ventricular hypertrophy, increased cardiac work (to generate higher-than-normal systolic pressures), and increased oxygen consumption (to supply an increased left ventricular mass), which produce chest pain. Subsequent left ventricular failure results in dyspnea. Patients with moderate to severe aortic stenosis may not be able to increase their cardiac output in response to exercise-induced peripheral vasodilatation. These patients develop ventricular tachycardia, which may progress to ventricular fibrillation and result in syncope, pre-syncope or sudden death.

Imaging Findings

Chest Radiography

- Normal heart size; left ventricular configuration: spherical ventricular border, concave left mid-heart border, border forming or dilated ascending aorta (**Fig. 139.1, 139.2**)
- Dilatation of ascending aorta (**Fig. 139.1**)
- Calcification of aortic valve leaflets (**Fig. 139.2**)
- Cardiomegaly with left heart failure or associated aortic insufficiency

MDCT

- Post-stenotic dilatation of the ascending aorta (**Fig. 139.3A**)
- Aortic valve thickening and calcifications (**Figs. 139.3B, 139.4**)
- Left ventricular hypertrophy (**Fig. 139.3C**)
- Decreased excursion of valve cusps on cine angiography
- Morphologic assessment of bicuspid aortic stenosis, especially with severe calcification
- Planimetric valve orifice measurements allows evaluation similar to that achieved with echocardiography, and can be used to grade the severity of stenosis as follows:
  - Mild aortic stenosis (>1.5 cm^2)
  - Moderate aortic stenosis (1.0–1.5 cm^2)
  - Severe aortic stenosis (<1.0 cm^2)
  - Critical aortic stenosis (<0.6 cm^2)

MRI

- Spin-echo or double inversion recovery techniques: left ventricular hypertrophy and post-stenotic aortic dilatation
- Gradient echo technique:
  - Thick dark aortic valve leaflets

- ○ Systolic turbulent flow and signal loss distal to aortic valve, signal void post-stenotic jet within signal-enhanced ascending aorta
- ○ Assessment of type of aortic stenosis (valvular, supravalvular, subvalvular) and valve morphology
- Velocity-encoded cine MR: quantification of aortic stenosis; gradient (gradient = 4 × peak velocity^2) mm Hg.

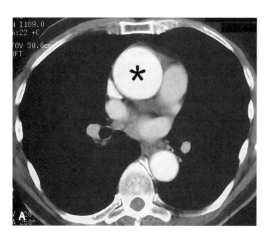
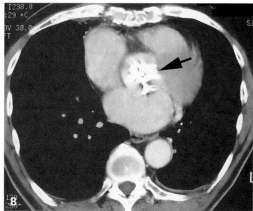
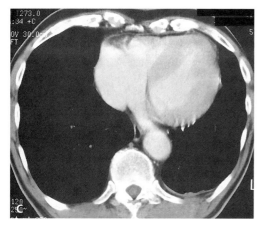

Fig. 139.3 Contrast-enhanced chest CT (mediastinal window) of an asymptomatic middle-aged man with aortic stenosis demonstrates post-stenotic dilatation of the ascending aorta (*asterisk*) **(A)**, dense calcification of the stenotic aortic valve (*arrow*) **(B)**, and left ventricular hypertrophy **(C)**. *(Images courtesy of Diane C. Strollo, MD, University of Pittsburgh Medical Center, Pittsburgh, Pennsylvania.)*

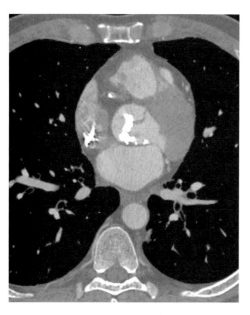

Fig. 139.4 Contrast-enhanced chest CT (mediastinal window) of a 45-year-old man who presented with chest pain demonstrates a densely calcified stenotic bicuspid aortic valve.

Angiography

- Domed thickened aortic valve at systole
- Eccentric contrast jet
- Evaluation of coronary arteries

Management

- Surgical aortic valve replacement
- Percutaneous aortic valve replacement
- Coronary bypass if significant coronary artery stenosis

Prognosis

- Symptomatic untreated patients survive up to five years
- 1–3% surgical mortality from aortic valve replacement

PEARLS

- Echocardiography is the primary modality of choice for assessment of valvular disease.
- MR imaging of the valves can provide qualitative and quantitative assessment of valve disease.

Suggested Reading

1. Chen JJ, Manning MA, Frazier AA, Jeudy J, White CS. CT angiography of the cardiac valves: normal, diseased, and post-operative appearances. Radiographics 2009;29(5):1393–1412

2. Feuchtner GM, Müller S, Bonatti J, et al. Sixty-four slice CT evaluation of aortic stenosis using planimetry of the aortic valve area. AJR Am J Roentgenol 2007;189(1):197–203

3. Liu F, Coursey CA, Grahame-Clarke C, et al. Aortic valve calcification as an incidental finding at CT of the elderly: severity and location as predictors of aortic stenosis. AJR Am J Roentgenol 2006;186(2):342–349

4. Tanaka R, Yoshioka K, Niinuma H, Ohsawa S, Okabayashi H, Ehara S. Diagnostic value of cardiac CT in the evaluation of bicuspid aortic stenosis: comparison with echocardiography and operative findings. AJR Am J Roentgenol 2010;195(4):895–899

CASE 140

■ Clinical Presentation

65-year-old man with nonspecific chest discomfort and a remote myocardial infarction in the left anterior descending vascular territory 6 years prior

■ Radiologic Findings

Coned-down PA (**Fig. 140.1A**) and lateral (**Fig. 140.1B**) chest radiographs demonstrate ovoid, curvilinear, laminated rings of calcification located more than 2 mm within the outer confines of the cardiac silhouette delineating the anterior and apical walls of the left ventricle. These calcifications are seen to better advantage on the accompanying inverted PA (**Fig. 140.1C**) and lateral (**Fig. 140.1D**) images.

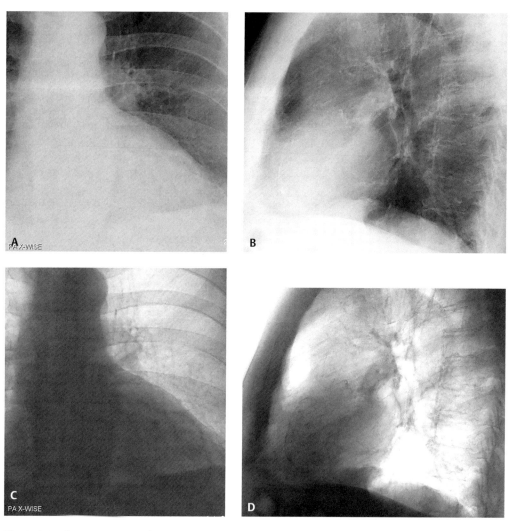

Fig. 140.1 *(Images courtesy of James Messmer, MD, VCU Medical Center, Richmond, Virginia.)*

■ Diagnosis

Calcified Left Ventricular Aneurysm

■ Differential Diagnosis

- Myocardial Calcifications
  - ○ Atherosclerosis in Aorta or Coronary Arteries
  - ○ Aortic or Mitral Valvular or Annular Calcifications
  - ○ Mural Calcifications Post-Infarction
  - ○ Calcified Thrombus
  - ○ Cardiac Fibroma
- Pericardial Calcifications (calcific pericarditis) (see Case 141)
  - ○ Post-Traumatic
  - ○ Post-Infectious
  - ○ Viral Agents
    - – Coxsackievirus
    - – Influenza A and or B
  - ○ *Mycobacterium tuberculosis*
  - ○ Histoplasmosis
  - ○ Systemic Lupus Erythematosus
  - ○ Uremia
  - ○ Rheumatic Heart Disease
- Pericardial Cyst

■ Discussion

Background

Left ventricular aneurysms are a potential complication of myocardial infarction. Such aneurysms are classified as either *true* or *false*. A *true ventricular aneurysm* is a chronic complication of myocardial infarction, usually involves the apical or anterolateral wall (85%), and most often follows the left anterior descending coronary artery (LAD) vascular territory. The aneurysm sac contains endocardium, epicardium, and thinned fibrous scar tissue as a remnant of the left ventricular muscle. *True aneurysms* contained by diseased myocardium can bulge and may be functionally akinetic or dyskinetic. A *false aneurysm* or *pseudoaneurysm* represents pericardium that contains a ruptured left ventricle. Such aneurysms usually involve the inferior and/or posterior ventricular wall. The focal rupture in the myocardial wall creates the neck of the false aneurysm. Because the clinical differentiation between true and false aneurysm is critical, further evaluation with various imaging modalities is often necessary.

Etiology

Left ventricular aneurysms most often develop as sequelae of transmural infarction and may present within 48 hours of the infarction. Past incidence rates of 8–15% following ST segment elevation myocardial infarcts may be decreasing with current improved revascularization techniques. Myocardial calcifications may form as early as six years post-infarction. Other causes of ventricular aneurysm include congenital (Ravitch syndrome), Chagas disease, myocarditis, hibernating myocardium, and sarcoidosis. Trauma is the most common cause of a false aneurysm.

Clinical Findings

A *true aneurysm*, particularly if small, may cause no symptoms. Fifty percent of *true aneurysms* develop mural thrombus that can potentially embolize (**Fig. 140.3**). The bulge in the myocardium subtracts from the stroke volume and the resultant decrease in cardiac output may adversely affect myocardial remodel-

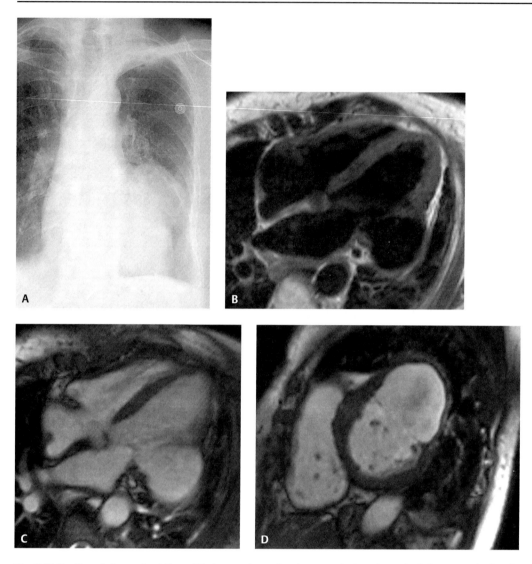

Fig. 140.2 Coned-down chest X-ray **(A)** shows a large, focal, convex bulge along the left ventricular border. Accompanying cardiac MRI four-chamber HASTE **(B)** and SSFP **(C)** and short-axis SSFP **(D)** sequences confirm pseudoaneurysm of the anterior, anterolateral, and posterolateral ventricular wall.

ing. Rupture is an uncommon phenomenon; therefore, surgical resection is necessary only when refractory angina pectoris, heart failure, systemic embolization, or refractory dysrhythmias occur. In contradistinction, *false ventricular aneurysms* have a high risk of rupture and require repair.

Imaging Findings

Chest Radiography

- Localized bulge along left heart border (**Fig. 140.2A**)
- Shelf-like or squared-off appearance to mid-lateral margin of heart border
- Rim or laminated rings of calcification confined to one cardiac chamber, more than 2 mm within the cardiac contour (e.g., remote infarction) (**Figs. 140.1A, 140.1B, 140.1C, 140.1D**)
- Left ventricular enlargement
- Cardiac decompensation

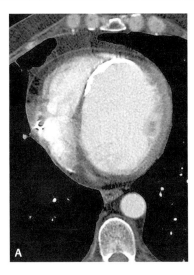
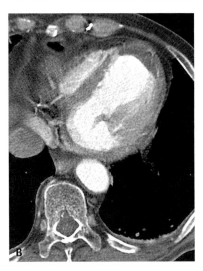

Fig. 140.3   MDCT **(A)** of a 56-year-old man who had myocardial infarction eight years earlier shows a true left ventricular aneurysm. Note the ventricular dilatation and thinning of the inferoseptal wall and associated curvilinear calcifications. MDCT **(B)** of a 69-year-old man with a true left ventricular wall apical aneurysm with muscle thinning and low-attenuation thrombus formation.

MDCT

- Reliable for identifying LV aneurysms and assessing resectability (**Figs. 140.3A, 140.3B**)
- May demonstrate regional wall thinning; mural thrombus; ± calcification (**Figs. 140.3A, 140.3B**)
- Differentiation of *true aneurysm* from *pseudoaneurysm* requires identifying the small ostium connecting aneurysm with LV cavity
- *False aneurysms* are usually substantially larger than *true aneurysms*

Cardiac MRI

- Spin-echo; HASTE (black blood); SSFP (white blood); and cine images may reveal a focal out-pouching in left ventricular wall (**Figs. 140.2B, 140.2C, 140.2D**)
- Delayed hyperenhancement of myocardium consistent with scar
- Adjacent myocardium not part of aneurysm shows no delayed hyperenhancement
- Hypokinesis, akinesis, or dyskinesis of affected myocardial wall on cine images
- Low signal intensity on single-shot inversion recovery with a long inversion time consistent with thrombus
- Signal dropout from associated calcification

Management

- Anticoagulation for systemic embolization prophylaxis
- Ablation for dysrhythmias
- Aneurysmectomy if medical treatment for dysrhythmias, angina, systemic embolization, or heart failure is unsuccessful

Prognosis

- Related to degree of clot burden, dysrhythmias, and/or effect on stroke volume
- Rupture rate, true aneurysm: 4%

PEARLS

- Myocardial calcifications lie ≥2 mm within the external cardiac contour; they are linear or laminated and limited to the left ventricle.
- Pericardial calcifications are usually thin and curvilinear and conform to the pericardium and many times to the atrioventricular groove.
- More shaggy, thick, and amorphous-appearing calcifications are seen with tuberculous pericarditis.

Selected Reading

1. Brown SL, Gropler RJ, Harris KM. Distinguishing left ventricular aneurysm from pseudoaneurysm. A review of the literature. Chest 1997;111(5):1403–1409
2. Burgener FA, Kormano M. Predominantly left ventricular or generalized cardiac enlargement. In: Differential Diagnosis in Conventional Radiology. New York: Thieme; 2007:316
3. Grizzard JD, Judd R, Kim R. Cardiovascular MRI in Practice: A Teaching File Approach. Springer; 2008
4. Webb WR, Higgins CB. Myocardial and pericardial disease. In: Thoracic Imaging: Pulmonary and Cardiovascular Radiology. Philadelphia: Lippincott Williams & Wilkins; 2004:723

CASE 141

■ Clinical Presentation

61-year-old woman with remote history of tuberculosis, but no current respiratory complaints

■ Radiologic Findings

PA (**Fig. 141.1A**) and lateral (**Fig. 141.1B**) chest X-rays reveal thick, chunky, amorphous calcifications over most of the heart's surface (*arrows*) and along the atrioventricular groove. The left chest wall is deformed secondary to remote trauma. Amorphous pleural calcifications are seen in the posterior and lateral left thorax from a remote traumatic hemothorax (calcific pleuritis). Note the asymmetric left apical pleural fibrosis.

■ Diagnosis

Pericardial Calcifications—Secondary to Remote Tuberculous Pericarditis, Non-Constrictive

■ Differential Diagnosis

* Pericardial Calcifications from Other Causes of Remote Pericarditis
* Myocardial Calcifications

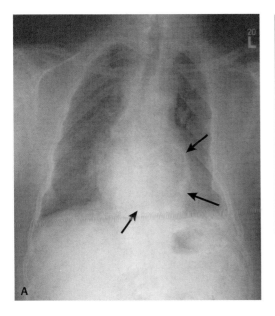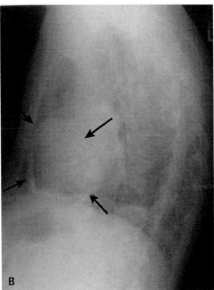

Fig. 141.1

■ Discussion

Background

Normal pericardium is composed of two layers: a tough fibrous *parietal pericardial layer* and a smooth *visceral pericardial layer.* Approximately 20–50 mL of transudative fluid is normally present between these two layers, which minimizes friction during the cardiac cycle. Inflammation of the pericardial layers is called *pericarditis. Acute* and *subacute pericarditis* may be associated with fibrin deposition along these layers and concomitant pericardial effusion. Subsequent organization results in fibrosis, scarring, and sometimes calcification, most often of the parietal pericardium. Thin, linear, "eggshell calcifications" are more often associated with viral and uremic pericarditis. Shaggy, thick, amorphous calcifications are more often associated with tuberculous pericarditis. Calcium deposits tend to be most obvious in the atrioventricular groove, where more fat is usually found. The thickened, fibrotic pericardium may impair normal late diastolic ventricular filling. Approximately 9% of patients with acute pericarditis develop constrictive physiology.

Etiology

Those clinical entities associated with acute pericarditis are likewise responsible for the development of constrictive pericarditis. These most commonly include idiopathic (presumably viral) (e.g., coxsackievirus A and B, adenoviruses), tuberculosis, cardiac surgery–related, and radiation therapy–induced. Less common causes include neoplasia, uremia, various connective tissue disorders (e.g., rheumatoid arthritis, systemic lupus erythematosus, scleroderma), drug-induced (e.g., procainamide, hydralazine), and myocardial infarction.

Clinical Findings

Calcific pericarditis without constriction is often asymptomatic and found incidentally on chest exams. However, it can be associated with *constrictive pericarditis,* in which case patients may present with dyspnea (most common), fatigue, orthopnea, and heart failure. Such patients may also experience lower extremity edema. Unexplained jugular venous distension, pleural effusion, hepatomegaly, and ascites may be evident on physical exam. Kussmaul sign (i.e., elevation of systemic venous pressures with inspiration) is a common but nonspecific finding. Patients with calcified pericarditis and constrictive pericarditis are typically more symptomatic than those without calcified pericarditis.

Imaging Findings

Chest Radiography

- May be normal even with clinical constrictive pericarditis; alternatively may show signs of heart failure
- 20–30% of patients with constrictive pericarditis–pericardial calcifications
  - Pericardial calcification may be present without constrictive physiology
  - Constrictive physiology may be present without pericardial calcification
- Patterns of pericardial calcification
  - Diffuse, thin, eggshell calcifications
  - Thick, irregular, amorphous calcified masses (**Figs. 141.1A, 141.1B**)
- Thicker and more irregular than myocardial calcifications; usually spare cardiac apex and portions of left atrium (contrast with Case 140) (**Figs. 141.1A, 141.1B**)
- Calcifications not restricted to left ventricular surface; more typical of myocardial calcifications (see Case 140) (**Figs. 140.1A, 140.1B, 140.1C, 140.1D**)

MDCT (Constrictive Pericarditis)

- May be normal
- Normal pericardium thickness: 1–2 mm
- Abnormal pericardial thickness: ≥3–4 mm
- CT superior to MRI in detecting pericardial calcification (**Figs. 141.2A, 141.2B**); however, MRI superior to CT in demonstrating associated physiologic abnormalities

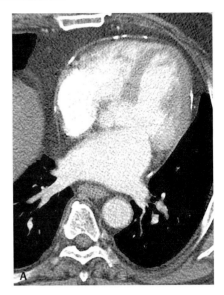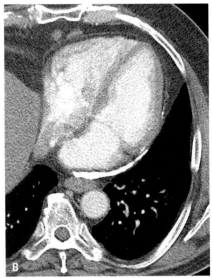

Fig. 141.2 Contrast-enhanced CT (mediastinal window) of a 65-year-old man with dyspnea and constrictive pericarditis shows multi-focal, interrupted, curvilinear pericardial calcifications most pronounced at the left atrial ventricular groove.

- Impaired right ventricular filling may manifest as:
  - Distension of inferior vena cava, hepatic veins, right atrium, coronary sinus
  - Hepatosplenomegaly
  - Ascites
- ± Normal right ventricular size but abnormal tubular morphology (tubularization)

MRI

- Sensitive for imaging pericardium/measuring pericardial thickness (**Figs. 141.3A, 141.3B, 141.3C, 141.3D**)
- Adherence of visceral and parietal pericardium (**Figs. 141.3A, 141.3B**)
- ± Normal right ventricular size but abnormal tubular morphology (tubularization)
- As with CT, may see signs of impaired right ventricular filling
- Real-time imaging provides more "direct method" of visualizing altered physiology
  - Paradoxical septal bounce (*shivering septum sign*)
  - Present in up to 85% of patients with constrictive pericarditis
  - Deep inspiration shows abnormal ventricular interdependence such that augmentation of RV filling results in right-to-left septal displacement; absent in patients with restrictive cardiomyopathy
- Delayed-enhancement imaging: may show focal or diffuse pericardial enhancement; nicely illustrated on PSIR (phase-sensitive inversion recovery) sequences (**Figs. 141.1C, 141.1D**)

Management

- Asymptomatic calcified pericarditis does not require treatment
- Constrictive pericarditis ±calcified pericarditis
  - Surgical pericardiectomy: procedure of choice in select patients
  - Response may be less dramatic in cases where constriction has been present for a prolonged period of time due to development of extensive atrophy and fibrosis

Prognosis

- Untreated constrictive pericarditis can be life threatening
- Symptoms following pericardiectomy commonly improve
  - Evidence of abnormal diastolic filling often remains
  - 60% of patients have complete normalization of cardiac hemodynamic function

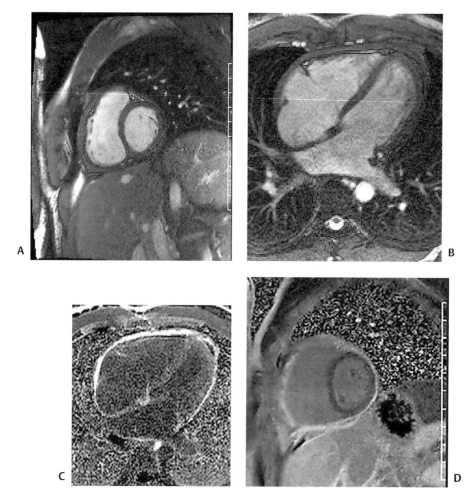

Fig. 141.3 Cardiac MRI of an 18-year-old with dyspnea and constrictive pericarditis. Short-axis SSFP **(A)** and four-chamber SSFP **(B)** images show concentric pericardial thickening, estimated at 7 mm, over the right ventricular free wall. The right ventricle is adherent to the parietal pericardium. Mild right atrial dilatation is seen. Real-time provocative four-chamber and short-axis cine images obtained while the patient took in a deep breath (not illustrated) showed abnormal ventricular coupling manifest by pronounced septal displacement during deep inspiration ("septal bounce"). PSIR four-chamber **(C)** and short-axis **(D)** images demonstrate enhancement of the thickened pericardium.

PEARLS

- Normal pericardial thickness does *not* exclude underlying constrictive pericarditis.
- Thickened pericardium does not indicate a given patient has constrictive pericarditis; imaging finding must be correlated with the clinical signs and symptoms.
- MR is useful in distinguishing constrictive pericarditis from restrictive cardiomyopathy, conditions which have very similar clinical presentations.

Suggested Reading

1. Breen JF. Imaging of the pericardium. J Thorac Imaging 2001;16(1):47–54

2. Francone M, Dymarkowski S, Kalantzi M, Rademakers FE, Bogaert J. Assessment of ventricular coupling with real-time cine MRI and its value to differentiate constrictive pericarditis from restrictive cardiomyopathy. Eur Radiol 2006;16(4):944–951

3. Grizzard JD, Ang GB. Magnetic resonance imaging of pericardial disease and cardiac masses. Cardiol Clin 2007;25(1): 111–140, vi

4. Srichai MB, Axel L. Magnetic resonance imaging in the management of pericardial disease. Curr Treat Options Cardiovasc Med 2005;7(6):449–457

CASE 142

■ Clinical Presentation

40-year-old woman with long-standing uremia presents with increasing shortness of breath

■ Radiologic Findings

PA (**Fig. 142.1A**) chest X-ray reveals an enlarged cardiomediastinal silhouette with an increase in the transverse diameter but no increase in its height, and straightening of the upper mediastinal borders, creating a globular or water bottle morphology (*water bottle sign*). The vascular clarity is slightly diminished and bilateral pleural effusions are present, right greater than left. Lateral (**Fig. 142.1B**) exam also shows globular enlargement of the cardiomediastinal silhouette and separation of the outer retrosternal and inner epicardial fat lines—*fat pad* or *Oreo cookie sign*). This latter sign is seen to better advantage on the coned-down lateral view (**Fig. 142.1C**) (*arrows*).

■ Diagnosis

Pericardial Effusion

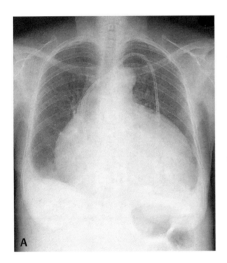
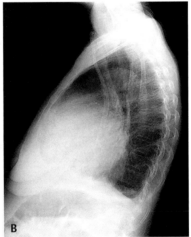
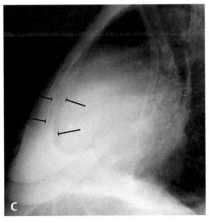

Fig. 142.1

695

■ Differential Diagnosis

- Global Cardiomegaly—Cardiomyopathy

■ Discussion

Background

The pericardium consists of two layers. *Visceral pericardium* is attached to the surface of the heart and the proximal great vessels. *Parietal pericardium* forms the free wall of the pericardial sac. The sac normally contains 20–50 mL of fluid. The *most common* cause of pericardial effusion is myocardial infarction with left ventricular failure. Fifty percent of patients with chronic renal failure develop uremic pericarditis. Coxsackievirus group B, *Staphylococcus*, and *Haemophilus influenzae* are common infectious agents associated with pericardial effusion. Today, tuberculous pericarditis is unusual except in the HIV-AIDS population, in which pericardial effusion of any etiology is a poor prognostic sign.

Etiology

Increased volumes of pericardial fluid and alterations in the composition of normal pericardial fluid may occur in the setting of numerous diseases (**Table 142.1**).

Clinical Findings

Patients may have a relatively large pericardial effusion and experience little or no clinical signs or symptoms, particularly if the fluid has increased slowly over time. This more commonly occurs when the pericardial effusion is the result of neoplasia or a chronic inflammatory disorder (e.g., rheumatoid arthritis). Alternatively, patients with pericardial effusion may experience dyspnea, orthopnea, both pleuritic and non-pleuritic chest pain, cough, syncope or near syncope, fatigue, tachycardia, and low-grade fever. *Tamponade* occurs when the volume of pericardial fluid compromises blood return to the right heart, affecting cardiac output, and is usually caused by serous or bloody fluid.

Imaging Findings

Chest Radiography

- Normal until volume of fluid >250 mL
- Increased transverse dimension of cardiomediastinal silhouette (*water bottle sign*) (80% specific; 46% sensitive) (**Fig. 142.1A**)
- Enlargement of cardiomediastinal silhouette compared with antecedent chest exams (41% specific; 71% sensitive)
- Separation of retrosternal and epicardial fat stripe >2 mm (*fat pad* or *Oreo® cookie sign*) (94% specific; 12% sensitive); seen best with moderate-large pericardial effusions (**Figs. 142.1B, 142.1C**)
- Cardiomegaly with normal pulmonary vascular clarity
- Left pleural effusion (100% specific; 20% sensitive)

Table 142.1 Causes of Pericardial Effusion

Serous	Hemorrhagic	Fibrinous	Chylous
Heart failure	Acute infarction	Infections	Congenital
Hypoalbuminemia	Cardiac surgery	Uremia	SVC obstruction
Irradiation	Trauma	Rheumatoid arthritis	Cardiothoracic surgery
Myxedema	Coagulopathy	Systemic lupus erythematosus	Neoplasia
Drug reactions	Neoplasia	Hypersensitivity reaction	Thoracic duct injuries
	Aortic dissection	HIV-AIDS	

MDCT

- Small effusions first collect dorsal to left ventricle and along left atrium
- Larger effusions collect ventral and lateral to right ventricle
- Even larger effusions may envelop the myocardium (*halo sign*) (**Figs. 142.2A, 142.2B, 142.2C, 142.2D, 142.2E, 142.3**)
- Loculations most often form along right anterolateral pericardium

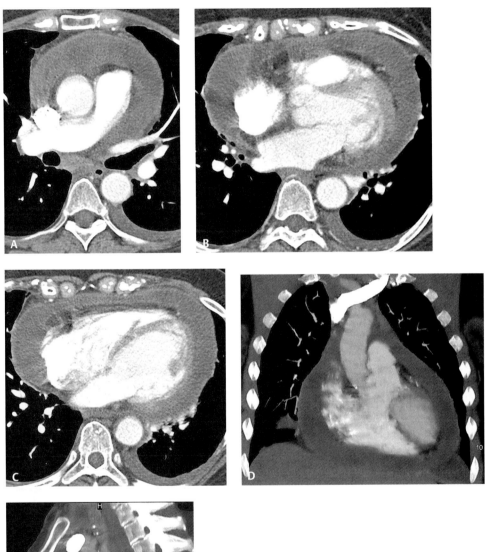

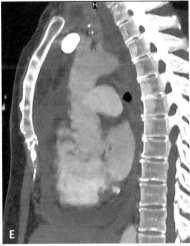

Fig. 142.2 Contrast-enhanced axial CT images (mediastinal window) of a 38-year-old man with chronic renal failure and dyspnea show a large pericardial effusion enveloping the heart (*halo sign*) and extending into the more cephalad pericardial recesses **(A)**. Coronal MIP **(D)** also shows the halo of pericardial fluid engulfing the heart and extending to the origin of the great vessels. Sagittal MIP **(E)** (lateral chest X-ray equivalent) demonstrates the *fat pad* or *Oreo® cookie sign*. Note separation of the lucent outer retrosternal fat stripe from the inner lucent epicardial fat stripe by the intervening layer of pericardial fluid.

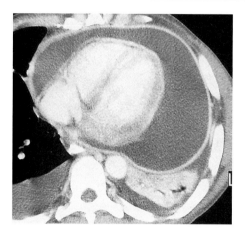

Fig. 142.3 Contrast-enhanced chest CT (mediastinal window) of a 42-year-old man with HIV and dyspnea with a tuberculous pericardial effusion and tamponade shows a massive pericardial fluid collection enveloping the myocardium (*halo sign*) and subtle effacement of the right atrium and right ventricle. Note the thickened and enhancing visceral and parietal pericardium.

- Pericardial thickening, nodularity, enhancement (**Fig. 142.3**)
- Attenuation coefficients rarely helpful in narrowing differential diagnosis; hemopericardium is an exception

MRI

- Similar morphologic features to those depicted on CT
- Transudates: low signal intensity T1WI
- Exudates: higher signal intensity T1WI
- Cine sequences may reveal hemodynamic consequences of pericardial effusion; compression/deformity of right atrium is of hemodynamic significance (**Fig. 142.4**)

Management

- Directed toward underlying cause
- Pericardiocentesis or pericardial window when clinically necessary

Prognosis

- Dependent upon underlying cause

PEARLS

- Echocardiography is the modality of choice for detecting pericardial effusion, although CT and MRI are more sensitive for detection of smaller-volume effusions.
- Reliable distinction between benign and malignant pericardial effusion is not possible on the basis of Hounsfield units alone.

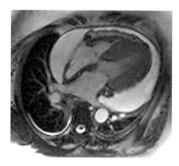

Fig. 142.4 Cardiac MRI (four-chamber SSFP) of a 30-year-old woman with uremia and dyspnea shows a large, simple but hemodynamically significant pericardial effusion of homogeneous signal intensity. Note the effacement of the lateral wall of the right atrium.

Suggested Reading

1. Eisenberg MJ, Dunn MM, Kanth N, Gamsu G, Schiller NB. Diagnostic value of chest radiography for pericardial effusion. J Am Coll Cardiol 1993;22(2):588–593

2. Wang ZJ, Reddy GP, Gotway MB, Yeh BM, Hetts SW, Higgins CB. CT and MR imaging of pericardial disease. Radiographics 2003;23(Spec No):S167–S180

CASE 143

■ Clinical Presentation

72-year-old woman with cough, sinusitis, and renal insufficiency

■ Radiologic Findings

PA chest radiograph (**Fig. 143.1**) demonstrates a right upper lobe mass-like consolidation with associated volume loss. Unenhanced chest CT (lung window) (**Figs. 143.2, 143.3, 143.4**) shows a peripheral wedge-shaped right upper lobe consolidation and multi-focal peripheral subpleural and angiocentric pulmonary masses and nodules.

■ Diagnosis

Wegener Granulomatosis or ANCA-Associated Granulomatous Vasculitis

■ Differential Diagnosis

* Multicentric Primary or Secondary Neoplasia
* Multifocal Pneumonia
* Bland or Septic Emboli, Pulmonary Infarcts
* Other Pulmonary Vasculitis
* Cryptogenic Organizing Pneumonia

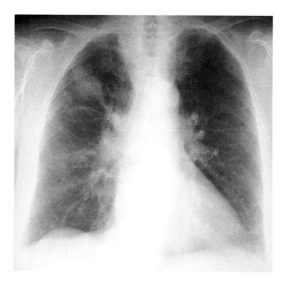

Fig. 143.1

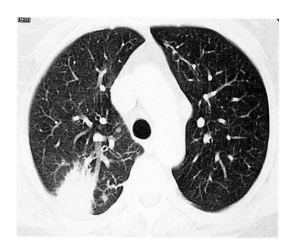

Fig. 143.2

700

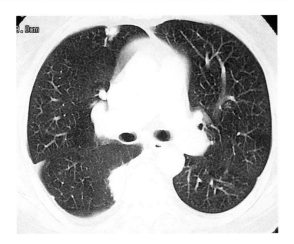

Fig. 143.3

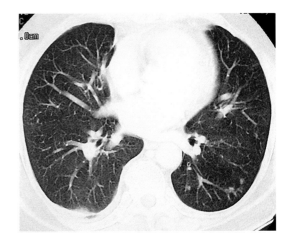

Fig. 143.4

■ Discussion

Background

The pulmonary vasculitides include several disorders characterized by inflammation of the pulmonary blood vessel walls. The term *ANCA-associated granulomatous vasculitis* has been proposed to replace the eponymous term *Wegener granulomatosis*, the most common pulmonary vasculitis. The diagnosis of pulmonary vasculitis requires careful correlation of clinical and imaging findings with the underlying histologic features and the exclusion of infectious granulomatous diseases, many of which often exhibit histologic features of vasculitis.

Etiology

The etiology of pulmonary vasculitis is unknown.

Clinical Findings

ANCA-associated granulomatous vasculitis (Wegener granulomatosis) is a systemic necrotizing vasculitis that commonly affects the lung, with an annual incidence of one case per 100,000 population. Although many organs are affected, *classical Wegener granulomatosis* is characterized by the clinical triad of febrile sinusitis, pulmonary disease, and glomerulonephritis; *limited Wegener granulomatosis* affects primarily the lung. Affected patients are typically adults in the fourth and fifth decades of life, and men are slightly more commonly affected than women. Early symptoms usually relate to upper respiratory tract involvement and include rhinitis, sinusitis, and otitis media. Approximately 60–80% of affected patients develop pulmonary involvement, with cough, dyspnea, hemoptysis, chest pain, and fever. Wegener granulomatosis may produce tracheobronchial stenosis, resulting in stridor, dyspnea, wheezing, and hemoptysis. Renal failure is a late manifestation of the disease. A cytoplasmic pattern of antineutrophil cytoplasmic autoantibody (c-ANCA or proteinase p-ANCA), when confirmed by standard ELISA, has a diagnostic specificity of 99%.

Imaging Findings

Chest Radiography

- Bilateral multi-focal well-defined pulmonary nodules or masses (**Fig. 143.1**)
- Cavitary nodules, masses, or consolidations; typically thick irregular walls, may evolve to thin-walled cavitary lesions (**Fig. 143.5**)
- Multi-focal consolidations (**Fig. 143.1**)

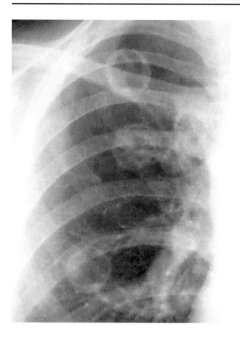

Fig. 143.5 Coned-down PA chest radiograph of a 20-year-old woman with Wegener granulomatosis demonstrates multi-focal cavitary left lung nodules with thin but irregular cavity walls.

- Patchy ground glass opacities
- Visualization of airway stenosis or secondary findings of atelectasis or consolidation
- Rarely lymphadenopathy
- Pleural effusion

MDCT / HRCT

- Multifocal irregular pulmonary nodules, masses, or consolidations (**Figs. 143.2, 143.3, 143.4**)
- Cavitation: typically in nodules over 2.0 cm in diameter; thick irregular cavity walls (**Figs. 143.6, 143.7**)
- Angiocentric (feeding vessels entering the lesions) and subpleural distribution of nodules/masses (**Figs. 143.2, 143.3, 143.4**)
- Peripheral subpleural wedge-shaped nodules or consolidations (**Figs. 143.2, 143.3**)
- *CT halo sign*: ground glass attenuation surrounding pulmonary lesions (**Fig. 143.6**)

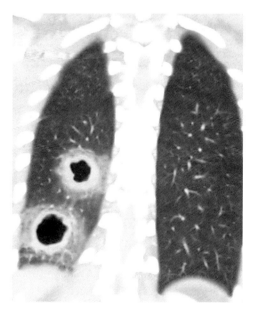

Fig. 143.6 Coronal chest CT (lung window) of a 29-year-old man with Wegener granulomatosis demonstrates two right lower lobe cavitary masses with thick nodular cavity walls and surrounding ground glass attenuation, the *CT halo sign*.

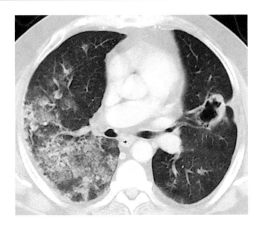

Fig. 143.7   Contrast-enhanced chest CT (lung window) of a 45-year-old man with Wegener granulomatosis who presented with hemoptysis and pulmonary hemorrhage demonstrates a right upper lobe cavitary lesion with thick nodular cavity walls and right lung ground glass opacity and consolidation representing pulmonary hemorrhage. Note trace bilateral pleural effusions.

- Ground glass opacity and consolidation (**Fig. 143.7**)
- Centrilobular nodules and tree-in-bud opacities (10%)
- Focal or diffuse airway stenosis or endoluminal nodules or masses with secondary consolidation or atelectasis
- Pleural effusion in less than 10% of cases (**Fig. 143.7**)

Management

- Combination therapy with cytotoxic drugs (cyclophosphamide, azathioprine) and corticosteroids
  - May be complicated by opportunistic infection
  - May relapse

Prognosis

- 90–95% five-year survival in treated patients
- Poor prognosis in patients with pulmonary hemorrhage and/or renal failure

PEARLS

- Progression of imaging abnormalities or development of air-fluid levels within cavitary lesions in patients with Wegener granulomatosis who are undergoing therapy should suggest superimposed pulmonary infection.
- *Churg-Strauss syndrome* (allergic angiitis and granulomatosis) begins as a prodromal disease characterized by asthma, allergic rhinitis, and peripheral eosinophilia and evolves to a systemic vasculitis. Cardiac involvement is more common than in Wegener granulomatosis, and sinus and renal diseases are less severe. Affected patients are young adults with recurrent consolidations, air space opacities, and/or pulmonary nodules, which may exhibit a peripheral distribution as seen in eosinophilic pneumonia.

Suggested Reading

1. Castañer E, Alguersuari A, Gallardo X, et al. When to suspect pulmonary vasculitis: radiologic and clinical clues. Radiographics 2010;30(1):33–53
2. Chung MP, Yi CA, Lee HY, Han J, Lee KS. Imaging of pulmonary vasculitis. Radiology 2010;255(2):322–341
3. Ananthakrishnan L, Sharma N, Kanne JP. Wegener's granulomatosis in the chest: high-resolution CT findings. AJR Am J Roentgenol 2009;192(3):676–682
4. Travis WD, Colby TV, Koss MN, Rosado-de-Christenson ML, Müller NL, King TE Jr. Pulmonary vasculitis. In: King WD, ed. Atlas of Nontumor Pathology: Non-Neoplastic Disorders of the Lower Respiratory Tract, fasc 2, ser 1. Washington, DC: American Registry of Pathology and Armed Forces Institute of Pathology; 2001:233–264

CASE 144

■ Clinical Presentation

38-year-old woman with weight loss, fever, myalgias, and pulseless left upper extremity

■ Radiologic Findings

Refer to **Figs. 144.1A, 144.1B, 144.1C, 144.1D, 144.1E, 144.1F, 144.1G, 144.1H, 144.1I, 144.1J, 144.1K**. Axial HASTE (black blood) (**Figs. 144.1A, 144.1B, 144.1C, 144.1D, 144.1E**) chest MRI images demonstrate marked narrowing of the left subclavian artery by a thick collar of intermediate signal intensity (**Fig. 144.1A**). Transverse (**Figs. 144.1B, 144.1C**) ascending and proximal descending (**Fig. 144.1D**) and distal thoracic aorta (**Fig. 144.1E**) likewise show a thickened wall of intermediate signal intensity contrasted with the low-signal aortic lumen. Aortic wall thickening is seen to better advantage in the same regions of interest on the post-contrast-enhanced VIBE axial MRI images (**Figs. 144.1F, 144.1G, 144.1H**). Ten-minute-delayed post-contrast sagittal oblique (**Fig. 144.1I**) and four-chamber (**Fig. 144.1J**) images show peripheral enhancement of the thickened aortic wall. 3-D MRA (**Fig. 144.1K**) reveals luminal narrowing of the brachiocephalic and left common carotid artery and near complete occlusion of the left subclavian artery, which fills via the left vertebral artery. Note the small left common carotid artery aneurysm. Left subclavian steal was confirmed on cine VENC sequences (not illustrated)

■ Diagnosis

Takayasu Arteritis

■ Differential Diagnosis

• Large-Vessel Vasculitides of Other Etiologies

■ Discussion

Background

Takayasu arteritis (aka pulseless disease; aortitis syndrome; idiopathic medial aortopathy) is an idiopathic granulomatous inflammation of the large arteries that may affect the aorta, its great vessels, and the pulmonary arteries. Marked intimal proliferation and fibrosis of the media and adventitia eventually lead to stenosis, occlusion, and, occasionally, post-stenotic dilatations and aneurysm formation. The inflammatory process tends to be segmental with a patchy distribution. Four major types have been described (**Table 144.1**).
The *most common* type is type III (65% of patients). The most commonly involved vessels include the left subclavian artery (50%), left common carotid artery (20%), brachiocephalic trunk, renal arteries, celiac trunk, superior mesenteric artery, and pulmonary arteries (50%). Infrequently, the axillary, vertebral, coronary, and iliac arteries are involved.

Etiology

Non-specific, cell-mediated inflammatory process of unknown etiology.

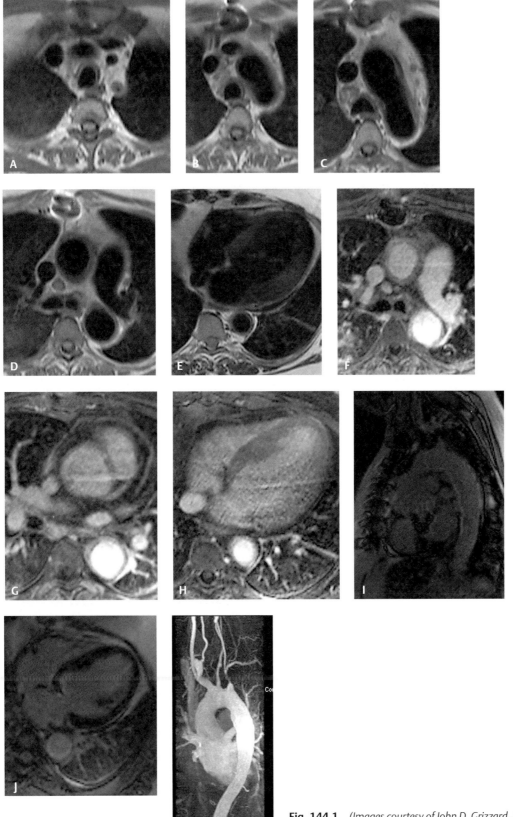

Fig. 144.1 *(Images courtesy of John D. Grizzard, MD, VCU Medical Center, Richmond, Virginia.)*

Table 144.1   Takayasu Arteritis: Classification based on Vessel Involvement

Type	Vessel Involvement
Type I (classic pulseless)	Brachiocephalic artery + carotid arteries + subclavian arteries
Type II	Combination of Type I + III
Type III (atypical coarctation)	Thoracic and abdominal aorta distal to arch and great vessels
Type IV (dilated)	Extensive dilatation of entire aorta and great vessels

Clinical Findings

Takayasu arteritis most commonly occurs in women; the female-to-male ratio is 8:1. Ninety percent of patients are younger than 30–40 years. Clinical manifestations can be divided into two phases: an *early* (prepulseless) *phase*, with systemic symptoms (e.g., low-grade fever, malaise, weight loss, fatigue, tachycardia, pain adjacent to inflamed arteries [carotodynia]); and a *late* (*pulseless* or *occlusive*) *phase*, the most common symptom being related to vascular stenosis with diminished or absent pulses (96% of patients), often associated with limb claudication and blood pressure discrepancies. Not uncommonly, the disease is recurrent, leading to the coexistence of these phases simultaneously.

Imaging Findings

Chest Radiography

- Often normal
- Widened superior mediastinum
- Focal oligemia lung parenchyma
- Premature aortic calcification in younger patient population

MDCT/MRI

- MRI modality of choice: also avoids ionizing radiation exposure in young women

Early Stage

- Vessel wall thickening; crescentic; circumferential; irregular

Late Stage

- Vessel wall thickening; crescentic; circumferential; irregular (**Figs. 144.1A, 144.1B, 144.1C, 144.1D, 144.1E, 144.1F, 144.1G, 144.1H, 144.1I, 144.1J, 144.1K**)
- Luminal changes (**Figs. 144.1A, 144.1B, 144.1C, 144.1D, 144.1E, 144.1F, 144.1G, 144.1H, 144.1I, 144.1J, 144.1K**)
- Luminal narrowing, aneurysmal dilatation, and occlusion (**Figs. 144.1A, 144.1B, 144.1C, 144.1D, 144.1E, 144.1F, 144.1G, 144.1H, 144.1I, 144.1J, 144.1K**)
- Subclavian steal phenomenon may develop (**Fig. 144.1K**)
- Contrast enhancement of thickened vessel walls: some degree of active disease is present (**Figs. 144.1F, 144.1G, 144.1H, 144.1I, 144.1J**)
- MRI—assess pressure differentials across stenotic lesions (VENC sequences)
- Mural calcium deposition in vessel walls in chronic phases; CT better than MRI

PET-FDG

- Useful indicator of vessel wall inflammation
- Intensity of FDG accumulation decreases in response to therapy

Management

- Early corticosteroid therapy: may lead to clinical improvements; subdue active inflammatory phase; control or slow progression of disease
- Methotrexate and intravenous cyclophosphamide: glucocorticoid-resistant arteritis
- Angioplasty: generally contraindicated during acute phase of disease; may be successful once acute phase has abated

Prognosis

- Mortality; usually from vascular complications (e.g., hypertension, stroke, and aortic insufficiency)

PEARLS

- Takayasu arteritis affects almost exclusively patients younger than 40 years, involves primarily the aorta and its great vessels, and generally spares the cranial arteries.
- Takayasu arteritis is the only form of aortitis that produces both stenosis and occlusion of the aorta.
- Unilateral pulmonary artery occlusion can occur in advanced cases; Takayasu arteritis should be considered in cases of chronic pulmonary artery obstruction of unknown origin.

Suggested Reading

1. Castañer E, Alguersuari A, Gallardo X, et al. When to suspect pulmonary vasculitis: radiologic and clinical clues. Radiographics 2010;30(1):33–53
2. Engelke C, Schaefer-Prokop C, Schirg E, Freihorst J, Grubnic S, Prokop M. High-resolution CT and CT angiography of peripheral pulmonary vascular disorders. Radiographics 2002;22(4):739–764

CASE 145

■ Clinical Presentation

89-year-old woman with shortness of breath

■ Radiologic Findings

Contrast-enhanced chest CT (**Figs. 145.1A, 145.1B, 145.1C, 145.1D**) (mediastinal window) through the four chambers of the heart reveals a smooth-bordered fatty attenuation mass within the interatrial septum that straddles the fossa ovalis, resulting in a dumbbell shape. Note the mild deformity of the right and left atrial walls that form a smooth interface with the mass, and the absence of an intracavitary component. Right middle lobe atelectasis, left lower lobe air space disease with associated bronchiectasis, and mitral valve annulus calcification are also present.

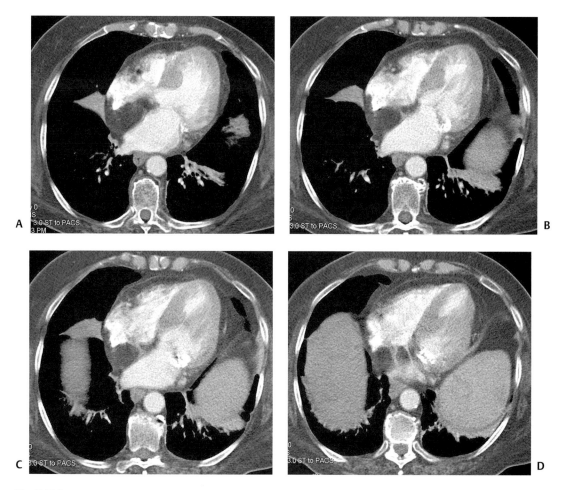

Fig. 145.1

708

■ Diagnosis

Lipomatous Hyperplasia of the Interatrial Septum

■ Differential Diagnosis

Primary Benign Tumors in the Region of the Interatrial Septum

- Myxoma
- Fibroma
- Fibroelastoma

Fat-Containing Cardiac Tumors

- Lipoma
- Liposarcoma

■ Discussion

Background

Lipomatous hyperplasia of the interatrial septum (LHAS) represents benign adipose cell hyperplasia within the interatrial septum of the heart. The prevalence of LHAS is estimated to be 1–8%.

Etiology

Embryologically, the interatrial septum is formed by fusion of the septum primum and the septum secundum. These early outgrowths of tissue from the walls of the immature atria fuse following birth, forming the interatrial septum. In some cases, mesenchymal cells carried along with this immature tissue become trapped within the interatrial septum during the fusion process. These mesenchymal cells later develop into adipocytes when appropriately stimulated.

Clinical Findings

There is an association between LHAS and increasing age as well as obesity. In most patients, LHAS is asymptomatic. However, in some cases LHAS is associated with supraventricular dysrhythmias, syncope, and sudden death. It is postulated that the increased septal fat disrupts normal myocardial fiber organization and subsequent fibrosis impairs contractility and electrical conductance, resulting in dysrhythmias and sudden death.

Imaging Findings

MDCT

- Bilobed fatty expansion of interatrial septum sparing the fossa ovalis (**Figs. 145.1A, 145.1B, 145.1C, 145.1D**)
- No invasion of adjacent vasculature
- No intracavitary extension (**Figs. 145.1A, 145.1B, 145.1C, 145.1D**)
- Flattening of right anterior wall of left atrium (**Figs. 145.1A, 145.1B, 145.1C, 145.1D**)
- Mild deformity of posterior right atrial wall (**Figs. 145.1A, 145.1B, 145.1C, 145.1D**)
- No contrast enhancement (**Figs. 145.1A, 145.1B, 145.1C, 145.1D**)

MRI

- Similar imaging features to CT (**Figs. 145.2A, 145.2B, 145.2C, 145.2D**)
- Bilobed fatty expansion of interatrial septum sparing the fossa ovalis (**Figs. 145.2A, 145.2B, 145.2C, 145.2D**)

- T1WI/T2WI: increased signal intensity consistent with its fatty nature (**Figs. 145.2A, 145.2B, 145.2C, 145.2D**)
- HASTE: increased signal intensity (**Fig. 145.2C**)
- STIR: Fat-suppressed images confirm fatty nature of the lesion
- Perfusion: No hypervascularity
- Delayed-enhanced sequences: No enhancement (**Fig. 145.2D**)

PET

- Marked preferential FDG uptake within the interatrial septum

Management

- Usually no treatment is necessary
- Indications for surgical resection include:
  - SVC obstruction
  - Intractable rhythm disturbances
  - Caution: condition may be an incidental finding in patients referred for cardiac surgery or other cardiac pathology

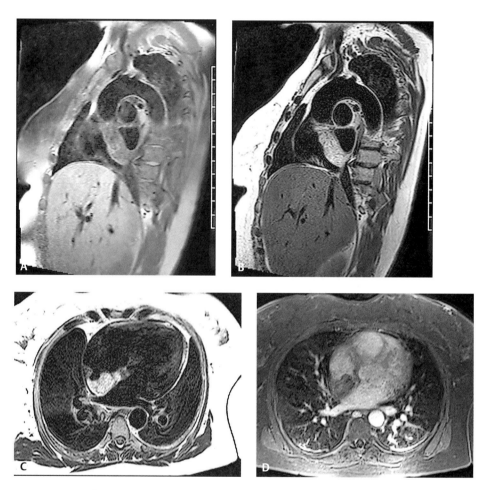

Fig. 145.2   Cardiac MRI of an obese man referred for evaluation of an atrial mass seen on echocardiography. T1- **(A)** and T2- **(B)** weighted modified short-axis images reveal a well-defined, non-invasive fatty mass localized to the interatrial septum without vascular invasion, obstruction, or intracavitary extension. HASTE four-chamber acquisition **(C)** with heavy T2 weighting again confirms the fatty nature of the interatrial lesion. Axial delayed post-Gd-DTPA VIBE **(D)** shows the relationship of the interatrial lesion to the fossa ovalis. Note the lack of contrast enhancement. *(Images courtesy of John D. Grizzard, MD, VCU Medical Center, Richmond, Virginia.)*

Prognosis

- Intra-atrial septal thickness >3 cm is associated with an increased incidence of supraventricular dys-rhythmias

PEARLS

- Non-enhancing, smoothly marginated, homogeneous dumbbell-shaped mass of fat attenuation on CT or MRI within the interatrial septum is highly characteristic of this benign condition and should obviate biopsy or excision.
- Increased FDG uptake on PET imaging is likely related to the presence of brown fat in the septum. Correlation with CT or MRI should be performed to avoid the false-positive diagnosis of malignancy.

Suggested Readings

1. Araoz PA, Mulvagh SL, Tazelaar HD, Julsrud PR, Breen JF. CT and MR imaging of benign primary cardiac neoplasms with echocardiographic correlation. Radiographics 2000;20(5):1303–1319

2. Fan CM, Fischman AJ, Kwek BH, Abbara S, Aquino SL. Lipomatous hypertrophy of the interatrial septum: increased uptake on FDG PET. AJR Am J Roentgenol 2005;184(1):339–342

3. Meaney JF, Kazerooni EA, Jamadar DA, Korobkin M. CT appearance of lipomatous hypertrophy of the interatrial septum. AJR Am J Roentgenol 1997;168(4):1081–1084

4. Salanitri JC, Pereles FS. Cardiac lipoma and lipomatous hypertrophy of the interatrial septum: Cardiac Magnetic Resonance Imaging Findings. J Comput Assist Tomogr 2004;28(6):52–56

CASE 146

■ Clinical Presentation

68-year-old woman experiencing dyspnea when lying flat, intermittent palpitations, and chest pain

■ Radiologic Findings

Cardiac MRI: Axial HASTE (**Fig. 146.1A**) shows a slightly heterogeneous, well-defined right atrial mass adherent to the fossa ovalis slightly higher in signal intensity than normal myocardium. On the T1-weighted short-axis image (**Fig. 146.1B**) the mass is isointense to muscle, whereas on the T2-weighted short-axis acquisition (**Fig. 146.1C**) it is much brighter in signal intensity. Short-axis views show that the mass spans the fossa ovalis between the atrial chambers. STIR sequence (**Fig. 146.1D**) confirms the non-fatty nature of the mass. Short-axis SSFP during diastole (**Fig. 146.1E**) and systole (**Fig. 146.1F**) show the mass prolapsing between the atria during the cardiac cycle, which is better appreciated on GRE cine images (not illustrated). Four-chamber perfusion GRE during passage of gadolinium-DTPA (**Fig. 146.1G**) shows opacification of the atrium but no uptake by the mass itself. Post-Gd-DTPA, four-chamber imaging reveals heterogeneous uptake of contrast by the mass (**Fig. 146.1H**)

■ Diagnosis

Right Atrial Myxoma

■ Differential Diagnosis

* Other Primary Cardiac Tumors
* Secondary Cardiac Tumors
* Atrial Thrombus

■ Discussion

Background

Secondary cardiac masses are 20–40 times more common than *primary cardiac masses.* Whereas most *secondary cardiac masses* are malignant, most primary *cardiac masses* are benign. *Myxoma* is the most common primary benign cardiac mass. Approximately 90% of myxomas are solitary pedunculated masses, but as many as 5% may present as multiple masses. These relatively gelatinous tumors most often arise in close proximity to the fossa ovalis. Nearly 75–85% originate in the left atrium, up to 25% occur in the right atrium and/or extend through the fossa ovalis (**Figs. 146.1A, 146.1B, 146.1C, 146.1D, 146.1E, 146.1F, 146.1G, 146.1H**), and approximately 5% arise within the ventricles. Multiple myxomas may be associated with various syndromes, including Carney syndrome (e.g., atrial myxomas, melanotic schwannomas, Cushing syndrome, multiple cerebral fusiform aneurysms, and breast fibroadenomas).

Etiology

Most cases of atrial myxoma are *sporadic.* Approximately 10% of myxomas may be inherited in an autosomal dominant manner. Multiple tumors occur in approximately 50% of familial cases and in these latter cases are more frequently located in the ventricle.

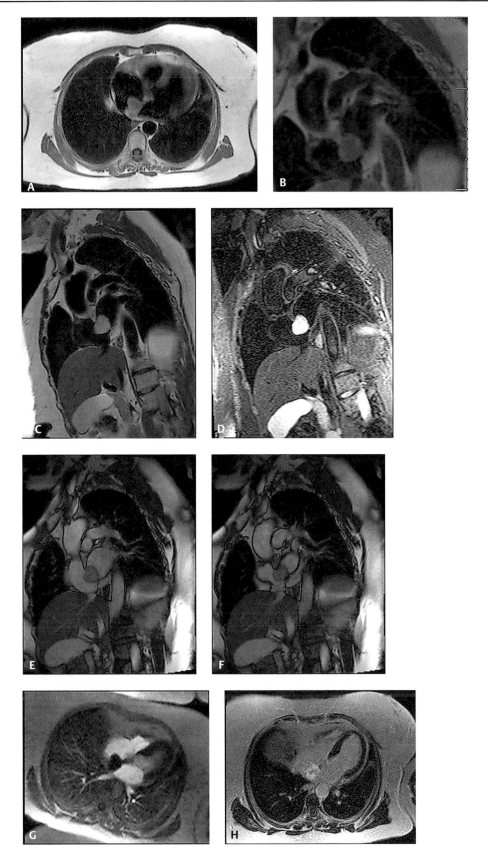

Fig. 146.1   *(Images courtesy of John D. Grizzard, MD, VCU Medical Center, Richmond, Virginia.)*

Clinical Findings

Approximately 75% of *sporadic myxomas* occur in females. However, the female sexual predilection is less pronounced in *familial atrial myxomas*. The mean age at presentation for *sporadic* cases is 56 years, whereas the mean age for *familial myxoma* is 25 years. Most patients with *sporadic myxomas* are symptomatic and most commonly present with dyspnea. In approximately 20% of cases, the myxoma does not cause symptoms and is incidentally discovered. Symptoms are produced by mechanical cardiac chamber or valvular obstruction or tumor embolization. Tumor embolism occurs in 30–40% of patients. The site of embolism depends upon whether the myxoma is located in the left or right atrium. The symptoms and signs of *left atrial myxomas* often mimic mitral stenosis. *Right atrial myxomas* grow to approximately twice the size of typical *left atrial myxomas* before becoming symptomatic, and are sometimes associated with tricuspid stenosis and atrial fibrillation. Symptoms may be precipitated by a change of body position and may include orthopnea, difficulty breathing when asleep, chest pain, syncope or near syncope, and palpitations. Constitutional symptoms are observed in 50% of patients and include fever, weight loss, arthralgias, and Raynaud phenomenon. Hemoptysis due to pulmonary edema or infarction is seen in up to 15% of patients. Abnormal heart sounds, including a "tumor plop" may be heard during auscultation when the tumor moves as the patient changes position.

Imaging Findings

Chest Radiography

- Enlarged left atrial appendage and enlarged left atrium; mimicking mitral stenosis (see Case 138)
- Enlarged pulmonary veins and cephalization of blood flow; mimicking mitral stenosis (see Case 138)
- ± Unusual intracardiac tumor calcification

Transthoracic Echocardiography (TTE)

- Assess tumor location, size, attachment, and mobility
- Doppler can show hemodynamic consequences of atrial myxoma—consistent with resultant mitral stenosis or regurgitation

Transesophageal echocardiography (TEE)

- Better resolution and specificity, and 100% sensitivity compared with TTE
- Better visualization of tumor morphology and size, and the presence of a stalk

MDCT

May be useful in differentiating *atrial myxoma* from *intracardiac thrombus.*

Atrial Myxoma

- Attenuation: 43 ± 14 HU (**Fig. 146.2**)
- Larger than thrombus: 33 ± 16 mm (**Fig. 146.2**)
- Unenhanced scans: lower in attenuation than atrial blood
- Contrast-enhanced scans: heterogeneous mass (reflecting hemorrhage, necrosis, cyst formation, fibrosis, calcification) (**Fig. 146.2**)
- Location: in or near fossa ovalis (**Fig. 146.2**)
- Shape: smooth to lobular, often with polypoid projections (**Fig. 146.2**)
- Mobility: cine sequences may demonstrate prolapse across fossa ovalis or into ventricular cavity depending on length of the peduncle
- May demonstrate calcification(s)

Intracardiac Thrombus

- Attenuation: 57 ± 30 HU
- Smaller than myxomas: 21 ± 7 mm
- Homogeneous more commonly but may appear heterogeneous

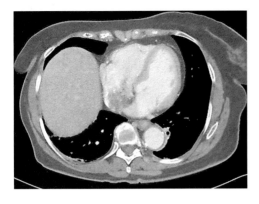

Fig. 146.2 Contrast-enhanced axial chest CT of a 78-year-old woman with palpitations shows a right atrial myxoma. A 3.0 cm heterogeneous lobulated mass is seen attached to the fossa ovalis and effaces the interatrial septum.

- Location: posterior or lateral wall of atrium; atrial appendage
- Shape: flat, smooth, lobulated, or pedunculated
- May demonstrate calcification(s)

MRI

- Site of attachment better visualized, with a post-surgical correlation of 83%
- Cine MR gradient echo (GRE) images can demonstrate mobility of the tumor
- Useful in differentiating *atrial myxoma* from *intracardiac thrombus.*

Atrial Myxoma

- HASTE: heterogeneous mass; signal intensity slightly higher than normal myocardium(**Fig. 146.1A**)
- T1WI: mass iso-intense relative to myocardium (**Fig. 146.1B**)
- T2WI: mass increased SI relative to myocardium (**Fig. 146.1C**)
- STIR: mass demonstrates no fat suppression (**Fig. 146.1D**)
- SSFP cine sequence: increased SI (T2/T1 ratio) secondary to gelatinous composition of tumor with a high fluid-like content (relative T2 weighting) (**Figs. 146.1E, 146.1F**)
- Cine images: pedunculated mass may prolapse across fossa ovalis (**Figs. 146.1E, 146.1F**) or atrial-ventricular valve
- Perfusion GRE: no uptake of Gd-DTPA by the mass (**Fig. 146.1G**)
- Post-Gd-DTPA: heterogeneous enhancement of mass possible (**Fig. 146.1H**)

Intracardiac Thrombus

- Location: usually atrial appendage; broad-based; irregular contour; may appear layered
- Thrombus adherent to cardiac chamber walls is akinetic on cine acquisitions
- SSFP sequence: intermediate/decreased SI relative to normal myocardium (**Figs. 146.3A, 146.3B**)
- Post-Gd-DTPA: no to mild heterogeneous enhancement
- Signal intensity characteristics vary depending on acuteness or chronicity on the thrombus: (**Table 146.1**)

Management

- Surgical resection of the myxoma is the treatment of choice
- Damaged valves may require annuloplasty or prosthetic replacement

Prognosis

- Surgery for sporadic atrial myxoma is usually curative
  - Long-term prognosis excellent
  - Recurrence rate: 1–5%
  - Recurrence after four years is uncommon

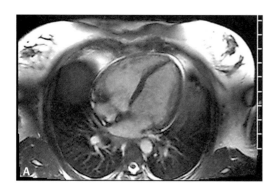
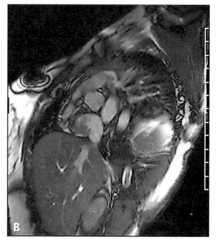

Fig. 146.3   Four-chamber **(A)** and short-axis **(B)** SSFP cardiac MRI acquisitions of a 28-year-old woman with right atrial thrombus adherent to the posterolateral wall of the right atrium. The atrial thrombus manifests as an irregular lobulated mass of intermediate to diminished signal intensity relative to the myocardium.

Table 146.1   MRI Signal Intensity Characteristics of Intracardiac Thrombus

	T1	Proton Density	T2	GRE	HASTE
Acute thrombus	Intermediate	Intermediate	Intermediate/ increased	Intermediate	Intermediate
Chronic thrombus	Intermediate	Intermediate/ decreased	Intermediate/ decreased	Decreased/ markedly decreased	

- Recurrence rate for familial atrial myxoma: 20%
- Untreated myxoma can be complicated by systemic embolization
- Sudden death may occur in up to 15% of patients with untreated atrial myxoma
  ○ Secondary to coronary or systemic embolization
  ○ Obstruction of blood flow at the mitral or tricuspid valve

PEARLS

- MRI is more sensitive than echosonography or CT for differentiating atrial myxoma from atrial thrombus. Thrombus is usually situated in the posterior atrial wall and has a layered appearance. The presence of a stalk and mobility favor atrial myxoma.
- On CT, atrial myxomas and thrombi can sometimes be differentiated by their distinguishing features of size, origin, shape, mobility, and prolapse. Attenuation coefficients and or the presence of calcification are not useful discriminating features.

Suggested Reading

1. Araoz PA, Mulvagh SL, Tazelaar HD, Julsrud PR, Breen JF. CT and MR imaging of benign primary cardiac neoplasms with echocardiographic correlation. Radiographics 2000;20(5):1303–1319

2. Grebenc ML, Rosado-de-Christenson ML, Green CE, Burke AP, Galvin JR. Cardiac myxoma: imaging features in 83 patients. Radiographics 2002;22(3):673–689

3. Grizzard JD, Judd RM, Kim RJ. Cardiovascular MRI in Practice: A Teaching File Approach. London: Springer-Verlag, Limited; 2008:262–263

4. Scheffel H, Baumueller S, Stolzmann P, et al. Atrial myxomas and thrombi: comparison of imaging features on CT. AJR Am J Roentgenol 2009;192(3):639–645

CASE 147

■ Clinical Presentation

19-year-old man with known sickle cell anemia and new onset of cough, fever, and chest pain

■ Radiologic Findings

PA (**Fig. 147.1**) and lateral (**Fig. 147.2**) chest radiographs demonstrate moderate cardiomegaly, low lung volumes, and bilateral basilar linear opacities. Note characteristic H-shaped endplate vertebral deformities in the thoracic spine (**Fig. 147.2**).

■ Diagnosis

Sickle Cell Disease: Acute Chest Syndrome

■ Differential Diagnosis

*   Bacterial Pneumonia
*   Pulmonary Embolism/Infarction

■ Discussion

Background

Sickle cell anemia is a hemolytic anemia that results from the production of abnormal hemoglobin molecules, which deform the red blood cells and impair their transit through vascular channels. Resultant vascular occlusion produces tissue ischemia and infarction. Acute chest syndrome is the second leading cause of hospitalization in patients with sickle cell anemia.

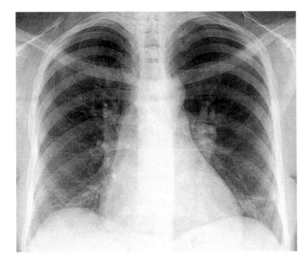

Fig. 147.1

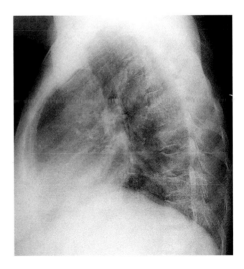

Fig. 147.2

717

Etiology

The cause of acute chest syndrome is poorly understood. It may follow bacterial or viral pneumonia in up to 40% of cases. Because patients admitted for pain crisis may subsequently develop acute chest syndrome, osseous infarction with fat embolism has been proposed as a possible etiology. While pulmonary vascular occlusion is probably a component of acute chest syndrome, it may be the initiating insult in some cases. Acute chest syndrome may follow general anesthesia in up to 10% of affected patients.

Clinical Findings

Acute chest syndrome occurs more frequently in children than in adults, and 50% of children with sickle cell anemia will experience at least one episode during their lifetime. Patients present acutely with fever, chest pain, cough, and dyspnea and may progress to respiratory failure and death. The majority of affected patients (70%) are hypoxemic.

Imaging Findings

Chest Radiography

- Bilateral patchy air space disease (**Figs. 147.1, 147.2, 147.3A**) and consolidation (**Fig. 147.4**) with a predilection for the middle and lower lobes
- Pleural effusions
- Visualization of osseous findings of sickle cell anemia, such as medullary humeral head infarcts and H-shaped thoracic vertebrae (**Fig. 147.2**)

MDCT/HRCT

- Air space disease (**Fig. 147.3B**); consolidation
- Areas of vascular attenuation attributed to hypoperfusion
- Late focal or diffuse pulmonary fibrosis
- Pleural effusions (**Fig. 147.3B**)

Management

- Hydration/transfusion
- Supplemental oxygen; mechanical ventilation and extracorporeal membrane oxygenation in severe cases
- Analgesia
- Antibiotic therapy for underlying or suspected infection

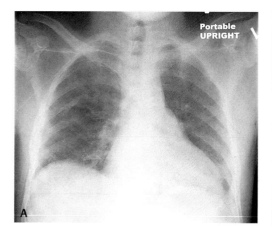 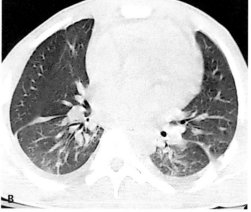

Fig. 147.3 PA chest radiograph **(A)** of a 22-year-old man with sickle cell disease and chest pain shows low lung volumes, cardiomegaly, and mild basilar linear opacities. Unenhanced chest CT (lung window) **(B)** shows mild basilar ground glass opacities, basilar subsegmental atelectasis, and small bilateral pleural effusions.

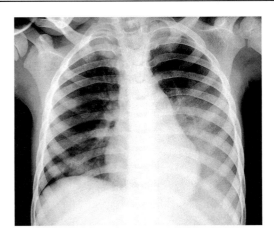

Fig. 147.4   PA chest radiograph of a child with sickle cell disease and acute chest syndrome demonstrates a left lower lobe consolidation. *(Image courtesy of Gael J. Lonergan, MD, Austin, Texas.)*

Prognosis

- Usually response to therapy and hospital discharge within one week
- Leading cause of death in patients with sickle cell anemia; mortality rate higher in adults (4.3%) than in children (1.8%)
- Death from acute episode
- Death from chronic pulmonary disease (pulmonary fibrosis, pulmonary hypertension) secondary to repeated episodes

PEARLS

- Chest radiographs may be initially normal in patients with acute pain crises who later develop acute chest syndrome.
- Bacterial/viral pneumonia must be excluded in all patients with suspected acute chest syndrome.

Suggested Reading

1. Lonergan GJ, Cline DB, Abbondanzo SL. Sickle cell anemia. Radiographics 2001;21(4):971–994

CASE 148

■ Clinical Presentation

37-year-old man with long-standing history of alcohol abuse and liver disease admitted with an acute episode of gastrointestinal bleeding and progressive dyspnea

■ Radiologic Findings

PA (**Fig. 148.1A**) and lateral (**Fig. 148.1B**) chest radiograph with accompanying PA view coned to the lung bases (**Fig. 148.1C**) demonstrates abnormal peripheral basilar reticular opacities. There is no evidence of heart failure or pleural effusion. Chest CT (lung window) (**Figs. 148.1D, 148.1E, 148.1F, 148.1G, 148.1H**) shows the reticular opacities representing multiple dilated distal pulmonary arteries that do not taper normally and extend to the pleural surface (*long arrows*) and juxtapleural telangiectasia (*short arrows*).

■ Diagnosis

Hepatopulmonary Syndrome

■ Differential Diagnosis

None

■ Discussion

Background

Hepatopulmonary syndrome (HPS) is defined by the triad of liver disease, increased alveolar-arterial oxygen gradient ≥15 mm Hg while breathing room air, and intrapulmonary vascular dilatations. HPS develops in 15–20% of patients with cirrhosis. There are two types based on pulmonary angiography. *Type I* is the most common (86%) and manifests as distal vascular dilatation with juxtapleural telangiectasia. *Type II* (14%) is characterized by the formation of small, discrete peripheral arteriovenous malformations.

Etiology

It is postulated that HPS is due to increased hepatic production or decreased hepatic clearance of vasodilators, particularly nitric oxide, by the impaired liver. This results in precapillary pulmonary artery dilatation, the formation of direct arteriovenous communications, and dilated pleural vessels. The vascular dilatation causes over-perfusion of the lung relative to its ventilation, leading to ventilation-perfusion mismatch and hypoxemia.

Clinical Findings

HPS manifests clinically as progressive dyspnea, cyanosis, spider nevi, and digital clubbing in a patient with cirrhosis. Patients may also complain of platypnea and have orthodeoxia. Pulmonary artery pressures are usually normal or reduced.

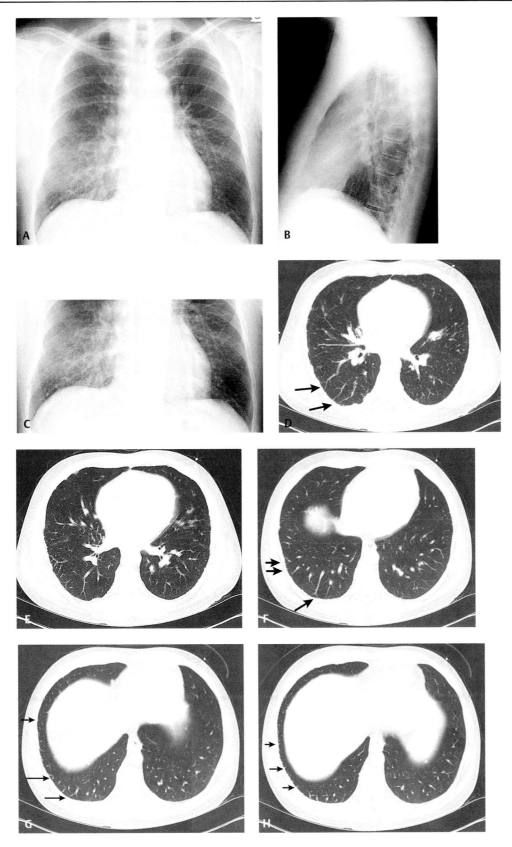

Fig. 148.1

Imaging Findings

Chest Radiography

- Normal; most common
- Basilar, medium-size nodular or reticular opacities (**Figs. 148.1A, 148.1C**)

Echosonography

- Bubble test is useful
  - Intravenous microbubbles (>10 mm diameter) from agitated normal saline normally obstructed by pulmonary capillaries (normally <8–15 mm) rapidly transit the lung and appear in the left atrium within seven heart beats

Nuclear Scintigraphy

- Intravenous technetium-99m (^{99m}Tc)–labeled macroaggregated albumin may transit the lungs and appear in the brain, liver, and spleen
- Distinction must be made from an underlying intracardiac right-to-left shunt

Arteriography

- Type I
  - Distal peripheral arterial dilatation
  - "Spidery" appearance of lower lobe peripheral juxtapleural vessels
- Type II
  - Small, discrete lower lobe pulmonary arteriovenous fistulae

MDCT/HRCT

- Type I
  - Dilatation of distal peripheral lower lobe pulmonary arteries that do not taper normally and extend out to the pleural surface (**Figs. 148.1D, 148.1F, 148.1G, 148.2**)
  - Increased number of visible peripheral pulmonary artery branches (**Figs. 148.1D, 148.1E, 148.1F, 148.1G, 148.1H, 148.2**)
  - Juxtapleural telangiectasia (**Figs. 148.1F, 148.1G**)
  - Increased lower lobe segmental arterial diameter compared with adjacent bronchi
- Type II
  - Nodular dilatation of peripheral pulmonary vessels, which are connected to a feeding artery and a draining vein
- Intrathoracic portosystemic collateral vessels (e.g., coronary vein into esophageal or paraesophageal varices and cardiophrenic varices)
- Cirrhosis, hepatosplenomegaly, varices, ascites

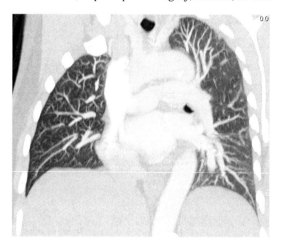

Fig. 148.2 Sagittal oblique MIP chest CT (lung window) illustrates dilatation of the distal peripheral basilar pulmonary arteries. Note the lower lobe vessels do not taper appropriately and extend out to the diaphragmatic pleural surface.

Management

- Currently no effective medical therapies; garlic powder and iloprost (Ventavis/Ilomedine; Schering AG) inhalation may be associated with some clinical improvement in the pre- and post-transplant period
- Somatostatin (vasodilation inhibitor): modest benefit in some patients
- Inhaled nitric oxide synthesis inhibitors; may be an option in the future
- Mainstay of therapy: supplemental oxygen
  - Patients with PaO_2 <55 mm Hg, or PaO_2 >55 mm Hg with polycythemia, cor pulmonale, or cognitive impairment, should receive 100% oxygen
  - If PaO_2 increases to >150 mm Hg and hypoxia is corrected, oxygen therapy should be continued (i.e., type I)
  - If hypoxia is not corrected, or PaO_2 <150 mm Hg after receiving 100% oxygen, pulmonary angiography should be considered for potential embolotherapy (i.e., type II)
- HPS may regress after liver transplantation or if underlying liver disease improves

Prognosis

- Poor without treatment
- Preoperative PaO_2 ≤50 mm Hg alone or in combination with an isotopic shunt fraction ≥20% are the strongest predictors of postoperative mortality
- Liver transplantation is the most effective therapy, correcting the syndrome in more than 80% of patients within 15 months of transplantation

PEARLS

- Do not confuse *hepatopulmonary syndrome* (shunting and V/Q mismatch due to vascular dilatation and arteriovenous malformations) with *portopulmonary hypertension* (development of pulmonary hypertension in a cirrhotic patient with portal hypertension).
- HPS is characterized by the triad of liver disease, increased A-a gradient, and intrapulmonary vascular dilatations. The liver dysfunction may not be severe.

Suggested Reading

1. Fallon MB. Mechanisms of pulmonary vascular complications of liver disease: hepatopulmonary syndrome. J Clin Gastroenterol 2005;39(4, Suppl 2):S138–S142
2. Kim YK, Kim Y, Shim SS. Thoracic complications of liver cirrhosis: radiologic findings. Radiographics 2009;29(3): 825–837
3. Rodríguez-Roisin R, Krowka MJ. Hepatopulmonary syndrome—a liver-induced lung vascular disorder. N Engl J Med 2008;358(22):2378–2387

CASE 149

■ Clinical Presentation

66-year-old man who had undergone a remote coronary artery bypass was readmitted with chest pain and had a new pulmonary artery catheter placed

■ Radiologic Findings

Coned-down AP chest radiograph (**Fig. 149.1A**) demonstrates a pulmonary artery (Swan-Ganz) catheter extending into the right lower lobe pulmonary artery; its tip projects beyond the right mid-clavicular line and is surrounded by focal indistinct ground glass opacity. Follow-up coned-down PA chest radiograph one week later (**Fig. 149.1B**) shows a new nodular opacity at the site of the previous catheter tip. Contrast-enhanced chest CT (**Fig. 149.1C**) reveals a focal collection of contrast enhancement (pseudoaneurysm) in the right lower lobe surrounded by parenchymal consolidation. Coned-down AP radiograph (**Fig. 149.1D**) obtained during pulmonary angiography illustrates a pseudoaneurysm in a right lower lobe pulmonary artery conforming to the previously demonstrated abnormality on chest radiography and chest CT.

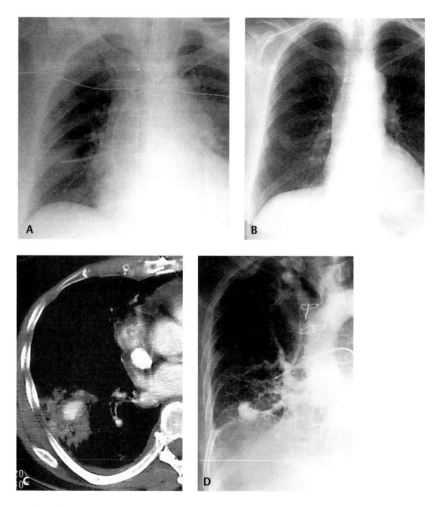

Fig. 149.1

724

■ Diagnosis

Pulmonary Artery Catheter-Related Vascular Pseudoaneurysm; Right Lower Lobe Pulmonary Artery

■ Differential Diagnosis

- Acute Invasive Aspergillosis (nodule with *halo sign*)

■ Discussion

Background

Pulmonary artery aneurysms and pseudoaneurysms are uncommon and may be related to previous trauma, including iatrogenic events from improper placement of Swan-Ganz catheters. Other causes include blunt trauma, Behçet disease, infection (mycotic pseudoaneurysm), and Hughes-Stovin syndrome (recurrent thrombophlebitis, pulmonary artery formation and rupture).

Pulmonary artery (Swan-Ganz) catheters are used to monitor the hemodynamic status of critically ill patients and enable clinicians to differentiate cardiogenic edema, noncardiogenic edema, and septicemia. Catheters may be introduced via an internal jugular, subclavian, or, less often, femoral venous approach, and are then "floated" beyond the pulmonic valve into the right or left main pulmonary artery. A balloon is located at the catheter tip, and when it is inflated (i.e., "wedged"), the resulting pulmonary artery wedge pressure (PAWP) serves as an indirect measurement of left atrial and left end-diastolic volume. Over-distension of the balloon tip may cause pseudoaneurysm formation or rupture of the affected pulmonary artery. The overall complication rate associated with placement of Swan-Ganz catheters is 17%. The incidence of associated pulmonary artery rupture ranges from 0.05% to 0.4% of cases and is related to inflation in a peripheral pulmonary artery, hyperinflation of the catheter's balloon tip, or vigorous flushing through the catheter. Recognized risk factors include age greater than 60 years, female gender, anti-coagulant therapy, pulmonary artery hypertension, and chronic steroid use. Right lower lobe and middle lobe pulmonary artery branches are most often affected. Associated consolidation on imaging studies conforms to parenchymal hemorrhage. If the initial arterial disruption is contained by a hematoma within the lung parenchyma, a pseudoaneurysm forms. A nodular opacity corresponding to pseudoaneurysm formation typically appears one to three weeks following pulmonary artery catheter placement.

Clinical Findings

Affected patients may be asymptomatic or complain of hemoptysis. Recognition of a new focal opacity on serial chest radiography may lead to the diagnosis. Comparison with prior imaging studies is important, with attention to the previous location of pulmonary artery catheters. Rupture of a pulmonary artery may be associated with localized hematoma formation, but disruption of larger vessels may lead to exsanguination.

Imaging Findings

Chest Radiography

- Well-defined, persistent pulmonary nodule/mass adjacent to catheter tip or at site of previous catheter tip (**Fig. 149.1B**)
- Nodule may appear elliptical with its long axis paralleling the pulmonary vasculature
- Ground glass opacity in the vicinity of the malpositioned catheter tip (**Fig. 149.1A**)
- Pleural effusion may be present

MDCT

- Pulmonary artery pseudoaneurysm: enhancing focal mass; may be associated with thrombus or ground glass opacity (**Fig. 149.1C**)
- Ipsilateral effusion
- Coronal and sagittal reformations may aid in elucidating the vascular nature of the focal mass or nodular opacity

Angiography

- Focal area of abnormal contrast at site of previous catheter tip (**Fig. 149.1D**)

Management

- Place affected lung in dependent position; protects contralateral lung if bleeding ensues
- Affected lung placed in nondependent position after placement of double-lumen endotracheal (ET) tube; reduction of pulmonary artery pressure
- Localization of source of bleeding (e.g., CT, pulmonary angiography)
- Embolization of affected vessel
- Occasionally direct repair of injured vessel, temporary ligation of involved artery, and/or resection of affected lung segment

Prognosis

- Pulmonary artery catheter-induced pulmonary artery pseudoaneurysms: 45–65% mortality rate
- Survival dependent on clinical discovery/treatment before pseudoaneurysm rupture

PEARLS

- Contrast-enhanced chest CT imaging is the modality of choice for diagnosing pulmonary artery pseudoaneurysm; pulmonary angiography may be considered as an alternative and can used to direct embolization therapy.

Suggested Reading

1. Poplausky MR, Rozenblit G, Rundback JH, Crea G, Maddineni S, Leonardo R. Swan-Ganz catheter-induced pulmonary artery pseudoaneurysm formation: three case reports and a review of the literature. Chest 2001;120(6): 2105–2111

2. Tseng M, Sadler D, Wong J, et al. Radiologic placement of central venous catheters: rates of success and immediate complications in 3412 cases. Can Assoc Radiol J 2001;52(6):379–384

3. Hunter TB, Taljanovic MS, Tsau PH, Berger WG, Standen JR. Medical devices of the chest. Radiographics 2004;24(6): 1725–1746

4. Ferretti GR, Thony F, Link KM, et al. False aneurysm of the pulmonary artery induced by a Swan-Ganz catheter: clinical presentation and radiologic management. AJR Am J Roentgenol 1996;167(4):941–945

CASE 150

■ Clinical Presentation

76-year-old woman status 11 days post median sternotomy and coronary artery revascularization, complaining of pain and the sensation of movement in her anterior chest wall, especially with coughing

■ Radiologic Findings

Initial postoperative coned-down inverted chest radiograph (**Fig. 150.1A**) shows normal midline alignment of the sternal cerclage wires. Follow-up coned-down inverted chest radiograph on postoperative day 11 (**Fig. 150.1B**) reveals approximately 2.0 cm lateral displacement of the sixth cerclage wire (*annotations*).

■ Diagnosis

Sternal Wound Dehiscence

■ Differential Diagnosis

Sternal Wound Dehiscence with Mediastinitis

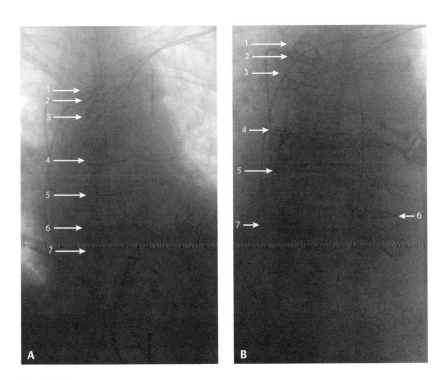

Fig. 150.1

■ Discussion

Background

Median sternotomy is the preferred surgical approach to expose the mediastinum, pericardium, heart, and great vessels. Surgical complications occur in 5% of patients and include wound dehiscence, mediastinitis, and sternal osteomyelitis. *Deep sternal wound* infections arise from hematogenous seeding of the wound, or from direct extension of an adjacent infection. *Staphylococcal* species are responsible in most cases. *Dehiscence* usually develops within the first 7–10 days following surgery. *Risk factors* include hypertension, tobacco abuse, insulin-dependent diabetes, obesity, intra-aortic balloon pump, immunosuppression, prolonged bypass time and/or prolonged mechanical ventilation, female gender, re-operation, and harvest of both internal mammary arteries.

Clinical Findings

Signs and symptoms include wound pain with or without drainage, sternal instability, palpable sternal clicking with deep breathing or coughing, fever, and leukocytosis. Normal postoperative sternotomy incision pain usually subsides over the first month.

Imaging Findings

Chest Radiography

- Mid-sternal stripe of lucency on frontal exams: originally believed to be indicative of sternal dehiscence, now recognized as normal postoperative finding until sternal halves reunite (**Fig. 150.2**)
- Sternal wires displaced to one side or the other as they tend to pull through the sternum, rather than break (**Fig. 150.2**)
- Sternal wire displacement (i.e., offset of one or more wires relative to the others in the vertical axis) (**Fig. 150.1**)
- Sternal wire rotation (i.e., alteration in the axis of a wire compared with its original orientation)
- Sternal wire disruption (i.e., fracture or unraveling of a wire) (**Fig. 150.3**)

MDCT

- Normal postoperative findings for the first two or three weeks include parasternal soft-tissue edema, localized hematoma, sternal nonunion, and minimal pericardial thickening
- Most small collections of parasternal air resorb within the first seven postoperative days

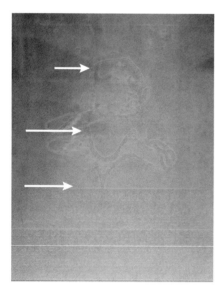

Fig. 150.2 Coned-down AP chest X-ray of 39-year-old man five days following a median sternotomy and aortic valve replacement shows a 2–4 mm wide mid-sternal stripe of lucency between the recently bisected sternal halves (*arrows*). This normal postoperative finding should not be misinterpreted as sternal dehiscence.

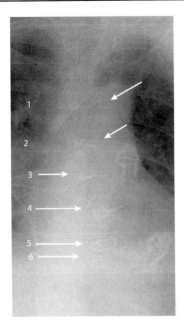

Fig. 150.3 Coned-down AP chest exam of a 63-year-old man six days following median sternotomy and CABG with complaints of "clicking" on deep inspiration reveals fracture of the first wire with lateral displacement of the left half 2 cm and progressive left lateral displacement of wires 2, 3, 4, and fracture of wire 2 (*see annotations*).

- Sternal wires displaced to one side or the other as they pull through the sternum (**Figs. 150.4A, 150.4B, 150.4C, 150.4D, 150.4E, 150.4F**)
- Identifiable *presternal complications*: draining sinus tracts and abscesses (**Figs. 150.4A, 150.4B, 150.4C, 150.4D, 150.4E, 150.4F**)
- Identifiable *retrosternal complications*: hematoma, abscess, draining sinus tracts, mediastinitis, pericardial effusion, and empyema (**Figs. 150.4A, 150.4B, 150.4C, 150.4D, 150.4E, 150.4F**)
- CT findings of *mediastinitis* include: small air bubbles or an air-fluid level in a mediastinal collection
- Limited value in evaluation of sternal osteomyelitis; tagged WBC scan better

Management

- Wide debridement of devitalized infected soft tissue and bone
- Culture-specific antibiotics
- Flap closure (e.g., muscle, musculocutaneous, omentum) for best wound healing

Prognosis

- Mortality rate <10% with appropriate early and aggressive treatment

PEARLS

- Shift in sternal wire(s) positioning on serial postoperative radiographs is best appreciated when the current exam is compared with the first postoperative exam.
- Radiographic abnormalities precede clinical diagnosis in more than two-thirds of patients.
- Sternal wire breaks alone are not an indicator of sternal dehiscence, and single breaks are usually of no clinical significance.
- "Mid-sternal stripe" is a normal 2–4 mm radiographic gap seen in 30–60% of postoperative chest radiographs; no clinical significance.
- First rib fractures are seen on 6% of chest X-rays after routine median sternotomy.

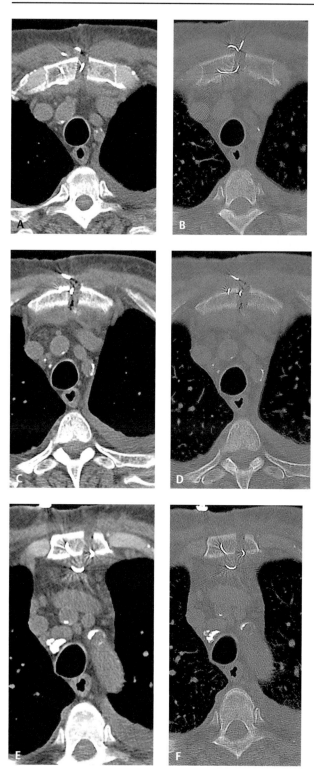

Fig. 150.4 CT of a 65-year-old man status post median sternotomy and CABG complicated by sternal dehiscence and deep wound infection. Axial unenhanced CT images (mediastinal window, **A**, **C**, **E**; accompanying bone window, **B**, **D**, **F**) show separation of the two sternal halves with fragmentation of cerclage wires, several of which are no longer anchored in the bone. Abnormal soft tissue is seen between the sternal halves and an air-containing sinus tract communicates with the retrosternal compartment and pre-sternal soft tissues **(C,D)**.

Suggested Reading

1. Boiselle PM, Mansilla AV. A closer look at the midsternal stripe sign. AJR Am J Roentgenol 2002;178(4): 945–948

2. Boiselle PM, Mansilla AV, Fisher MS, McLoud TC. Wandering wires: frequency of sternal wire abnormalities in patients with sternal dehiscence. AJR Am J Roentgenol 1999;173(3):777–780

3. Boiselle PM, Mansilla AV, White CS, Fisher MS. Sternal dehiscence in patients with and without mediastinitis. J Thorac Imaging 2001;16(2):106–110

4. Restrepo CS, Martinez S, Lemos DF, et al. Imaging appearances of the sternum and sternoclavicular joints. Radiographics 2009;29(3):839–859

CASE 151

■ Clinical Presentation

26-year-old man with non-ischemic cardiomyopathy and progressive decline in cardiac function

■ Radiologic Findings

Baseline AP chest radiograph (**Fig. 151.1A**) shows global enlargement of the cardiac silhouette and decreased vascular clarity from mild pulmonary edema. Note the left subclavian approach transvenous right ventricular ICD. Chest radiograph two days later after medical therapy failure reveals placement of an intra-aortic balloon pump (**Fig. 151.1B**). Note the radio-opaque metallic marker of the device confirming appropriate positioning in the proximal descending thoracic aorta (*arrow*). The edema has improved. Chest radiograph obtained three days later shows placement of a left ventricle assist device (LVAD) (**Fig. 151.1C**). The inflow housing, outflow housing, and conduit can be seen. The sternum is still open. Note the lap sponges at the pericarinal level.

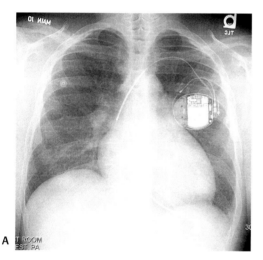

A

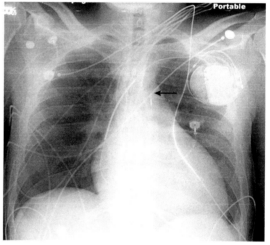

B

C

Fig. 151.1

732

■ Diagnosis

Circulatory Assist Devices: Intra-Aortic Balloon Pump, Left Ventricular Assist Device

Differential Diagnosis

None

■ Discussion

Background

Circulatory assist devices were initially used to support patients in hemodynamic collapse. Today, these devices are used for a wide range of clinical conditions ranging from prophylactic insertion for invasive procedures to cardiogenic shock and cardiopulmonary arrest. The two most commonly employed devices are the intra-aortic balloon counterpulsation pump and the left ventricular assist device.

Intra-Aortic Balloon Pump (IABP)

The IABP remains the most commonly used mechanical circulatory assist device. Its primary purpose is to increase myocardial oxygen supply while reducing its demand. Secondary purposes include improving cardiac output and ejection fraction; increasing coronary perfusion pressure and systemic perfusion; and reducing heart rate, pulmonary capillary wedge pressure, and systemic vascular resistance. Early indications for use included cardiac surgery, left ventricular failure, unstable angina, and failure to come off cardiopulmonary bypass. Prophylactic applications include stabilizing both cardiac and non-cardiac surgical patients. More recent applications include supporting cardiac patients during coronary angiography and percutaneous transluminal angioplasty, drug-induced cardiac failure, myocardial contusion, or septic shock, and as a bridge to transplant.

Left Ventricular Assist Device (LVAD)

The LVAD is a mechanical circulatory assist device used to partially or completely replace the function of the failing heart. Indications for short-term use include cardiogenic shock or post-cardiopulmonary bypass (CPB) low-output syndrome. Long-term use is reserved for patients with end-stage heart failure who are not candidates for heart transplant (destination therapy) and as a bridge to eventual transplantation. The pumps used in the LVAD are divided into two main types: (1) the pulsatile pump, a positive displacement pump that mimics the natural pulsatile action of the heart and requires an air vent tube; and (2) the continuous-flow pump, which uses either a centrifugal or axial flow pump and contains a central rotor that rotates in response to an electric current applied to permanent magnets.

Clinical Findings

IABP

The 8.5–9.5F vascular catheter is introduced percutaneously via the femoral or axillary artery or directly into the descending thoracic aorta at thoracotomy. It is advanced retrograde just distal to the left subclavian artery. A 26–28 mm inflatable balloon is mounted on this vascular catheter. Helium gas is pumped from the bedside console to the balloon. The balloon inflates with the onset of diastole and deflates during isometric contraction or early systole and is phasically pulsed in counterpulsation to the patient's cardiac cycle. Total or regional blood flow is improved during balloon inflation, as is collateral coronary artery circulation.

LVAD

A pre-procedural TEE is performed to assess for the presence of a patent foramen ovale, aortic insufficiency, left ventricular thrombus, and right ventricular function. LVAD placement requires a median sternotomy with the midline incision continued into the upper abdomen halfway between the xiphoid process and umbilicus. A subrectus pocket is created in the left upper quadrant for the LVAD itself. A left ventricular apical cannulation site for the inflow housing and conduit is created slightly lateral to the left anterior descending coronary artery and is secured by circumferential sutures, vascular pledgets, and an inner felt strip. An arteriotomy is made in the ascending aorta for the outflow housing and conduit. The air vent drivelines exit via a percutaneous tunnel in the right upper quadrant. Comparing patients treated with LVAD versus inotropic therapy while awaiting transplantation indicates that patients treated with LVAD have improved clinical and metabolic function at the time of transplant, with better blood pressure control and better serum sodium and creatinine levels. LVAD patients also tend to do better clinically following transplantation than patients treated with only inotropes. In one retrospective study, after transplant, 58% of inotropic patients experienced renal failure and 32% experienced right heart failure versus incidence rates of 17% and 6% in the LVAD patients, respectively.

Complications

IABP

Vascular complications are common and most often related to femoral or iliac injury. The most common vascular complication is limb ischemia (14–45%). Iatrogenic injury of the thoracic aorta is less common but is often fatal. Patients with extensive atherosclerotic disease are at increased risk. If the catheter is advanced too distal (e.g., aortic root), it may obstruct blood flow to the aortic arch and its trifurcated vessels (**Fig. 151.2**). The latter may be associated with acute cerebral vascular accident. If the catheter is not advanced far enough, counterpulsation is less effective and renal insufficiency may occur when the balloon occludes the renal arteries (**Figs. 151.3A, 151.3B**).

LVAD

The *most common complications* include bleeding, infection, and mechanical failure. The flowing of blood over non-biologic surfaces predisposes patients to thrombosis, necessitating anticoagulation, with its complications. Infection can be caused by a variety of organisms including Gram-positive bacteria (e.g., *Staphylococcus* sp., *Enterococccus* sp.), Gram-negative bacteria (e.g., *Pseudomonas aeruginosa*, *Enterobacter* sp., *Klebsiella* sp.); and various fungi (e.g., *Candida albicans*). Mechanical failure is more of a problem for patients with destination therapy, as the device must be replaced every two or three years.

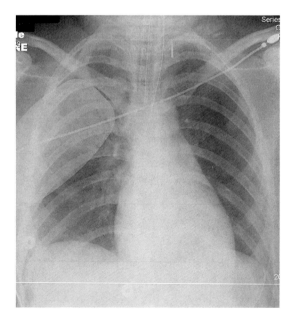

Fig. 151.2 AP chest radiograph of a 16-year-old with cardiogenic shock following a drug overdose reveals a malpositioned IABP. The metallic marker indicates the device is positioned far too high, overlying the expected location of the left common carotid artery.

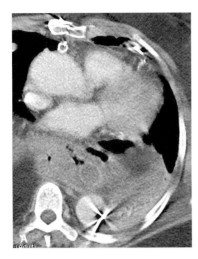 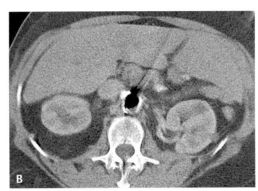

Fig. 151.3 Contrast-enhanced CT (mediastinal window) through the lower thorax **(A)** and upper abdomen **(B)** of a 65-year-old man with distal esophageal cancer status post recent coronary bypass with post-bypass low-output syndrome and errant IABP placement. The IABP is positioned far too low. The metallic marker of the device is seen during systole in the distal thoracic aorta **(A)**. The inflated balloon during diastole is seen at the level of the left renal artery **(B)**.

Imaging Findings

Chest Radiography

IABP

- Catheter tip is visible as an opaque 3 × 4 mm rectangle (**Figs. 151.1B, 151.2**)
- Tip should be positioned in proximal descending thoracic aorta, 2.0 cm below left subclavian artery and superior contour of transverse aorta (**Figs. 151.1B, 151.2**)
- If catheter is advanced into aortic arch, the opaque rectangular tip is foreshortened or appears as a radio-opaque ring
- Complicating dissection should be suspected when there is loss of definition of the descending thoracic aorta shadow

MDCT

- Catheter tip is visible as a high-attenuation 3 × 4 mm rectangular metallic density in the aortic lumen (**Fig. 151.3A**)
- Catheter tip/balloon positioning relative to branch vessels (**Figs. 151.3A, 151.3B**)
- Balloon may be visible depending on counterpulsation cycle
  - Collapsed and not perceptible: systole (**Fig. 151.3A**)
  - Distended and gas filled: diastole (**Fig. 151.3B**)

LVAD

Chest Radiography

- Post median sternotomy changes (**Figs. 151.1C, 151.4A, 151.4B**)
- Various components of LVAD device can be identified
  - Pump: prosthetic left ventricle in subrectus pocket (**Figs. 151.4A, 151.4B**)
  - Left ventricular apex inflow valve housing and conduit (**Figs. 151.4A, 151.4B**)
  - Ascending aorta outflow valve housing and conduit (**Figs. 151.4A, 151.4B**)
  - Air vent drive line cable—exits right upper quadrant, courses to system controller and external battery pack
- Blood-filled outflow conduit can obscure right heart border and simulate middle lobe air space disease (**Fig. 151.1C, 151.4A**)

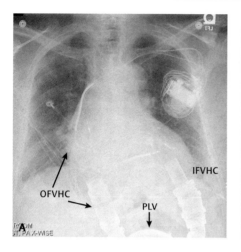 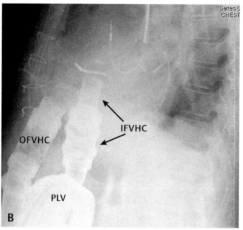

Fig. 151.4 PA **(A)** and coned-down lateral **(B)** chest radiographs of a 63-year-old man following recent uncomplicated LVAD placement show postoperative changes reflective of the recent median sternotomy, left subclavian approach transvenous biventricular ICD, and residual foci of pneumomediastinum **(B)**. The various components of the LVAD can be identified: *IFVHC*, inflow valve housing and conduit; *OFVHC*, outflow valve housing and conduit; *PLV*, prosthetic left ventricle. Note the partial silhouette of the right heart border by the outflow conduit, simulating middle lobe disease.

MDCT

- Similar findings to those identified on conventional radiography (**Figs. 151.5A, 151.5B, 151.5C, 151.5D, 151.5E**)
- Various components of LVAD identified to better advantage (**Figs. 151.5A, 151.5B, 151.5C, 151.5D, 151.5E**)
- Assess for LVAD-related complications:
  ○ Inflow-conduit: improper seating LV cavity; periconduit thrombus or fluid collections
  ○ Outflow-conduit: kinking-best appreciated on MPR or 3-D-VRT reconstructions; periconduit thrombus or fluid collections
  ○ Pump: subrectus or properitoneal pocket fluid collections
  ○ Power cord: abnormal fluid collections/phlegmon; hematoma

Prognosis

IABP

- Early perioperative mortality rate for cardiac failure requiring IABP is as high as 52%. Preoperative serum creatinine level, left ventricular ejection fraction, perioperative myocardial infarction, timing of balloon pump insertion, and indication for operation are independent predictors of early death.
- Hospital survivors have a relatively good long-term prognosis

LVAD

- Extends not only the quantity of life, but also the quality of life
- In small number of cases, LVAD combined with drug therapy has enabled the heart to recover sufficiently and the device to be explanted

PEARLS

- IABP
  ○ Relative contraindications to use include severe aortic valvular insufficiency, known aortic dissection, and severe peripheral vascular disease.
  ○ Catheters positioned too high or too low should be promptly corrected.
  ○ Vascular perforations may require surgical repair or covered endovascular stents.

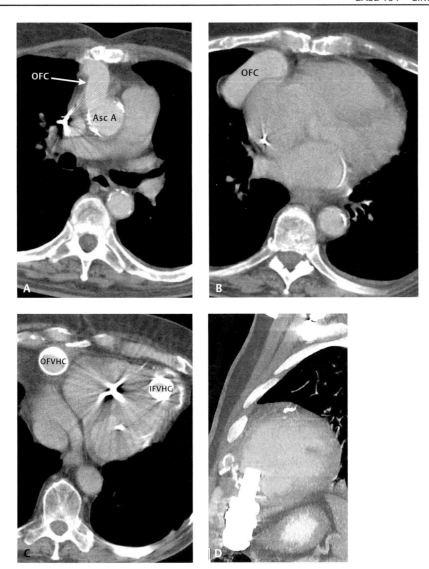

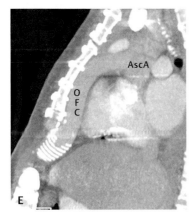

Fig. 151.5 Contrast-enhanced chest CT (mediastinal window) of a 62-year-old man with ischemic cardiomyopathy and end-stage heart failure and LVAD placement. The course of the outflow conduit and its anastomosis with the ascending aorta is delineated **(A,E)**. Note the relationship of the outflow conduit with the right atrium **(B)**, explaining the silhouette sign frequently seen on radiography. The left ventricular apical inflow valve housing and conduit are also seen **(C,D)**. Note the high-attenuation circumferential reinforcing vascular pledgets and felt strip **(C)**. *Asc A*, ascending aorta; *IFVHC*, inflow valve housing and conduit; *OFC*, outflow conduit; *OFVHC*, outflow valve housing and conduit.

- LVAD
    - Ventricular assist devices are designed to assist either the left (LVAD) or right (RVAD) ventricle or both ventricles simultaneously (BiVAD).
    - Device selection depends primarily on the underlying heart disease and the pulmonary arterial resistance.

Suggested Reading

1. Carr CM, Jacob J, Park SJ, et al. CT of left ventricular assist devices. RadioGraphics 2010;(30):429–444

2. Hirsch DJ, Cooper JR Jr. Cardiac failure and left ventricular assist devices. Anesthesiol Clin North America 2003;21(3): 625–638 Review

3. Okuda M. A multidisciplinary overview of cardiogenic shock. Shock 2006;25(6):557–570

4. Pal JD, Piacentino V, Cuevas AD, et al. Impact of left ventricular assist device bridging on posttransplant outcomes. Ann Thorac Surg 2009;88(5):1457–1461, discussion 1461

5. Santa-Cruz RA, Cohen MG, Ohman EM. Aortic counterpulsation: a review of the hemodynamic effects and indications for use. Catheter Cardiovasc Interv 2006;67(1):68–77 Review

6. Trost JC, Hillis LD. Intra-aortic balloon counterpulsation. Am J Cardiol 2006;97(9):1391–1398 Review

CASE 152

■ Clinical Presentation

23-year-old man with non-ischemic cardiomyopathy and end-stage biventricular heart failure who has just undergone a sternal splitting thoracotomy and cardiac surgery as a bridge to orthotopic heart transplant

■ Radiologic Findings

AP chest radiographs without (**Fig. 152.1A**) and with accompanying annotations (**Fig. 152.1B**) demonstrate the normal postoperative appearance of a total artificial heart (TAH) implantation. Both native ventricles have been removed, as have all four native cardiac valves. The mechanical cardiac valves of the TAH are delineated (**Fig. 152.1B**). The air-containing diaphragms related to the artificial right and left ventricles of this pneumatic pulsatile device should not be confused with myocardial chamber air, pneumopericardium, or pneumomediastinum, and are an expected postoperative finding. The left ventricle pneumatic drive line is seen exiting through a port in the left upper quadrant and connects to a bedside console. Two mediastinal and bilateral pleural drains are present. Note the pre-existing ICD leads have been amputated. AV, mechanical aortic valve; MV, mechanical mitral valve; PV, mechanical pulmonic valve; TV, mechanical tricuspid valve.

■ Diagnosis

Total Artificial Heart (TAH) Implantation

■ Differential Diagnosis

None

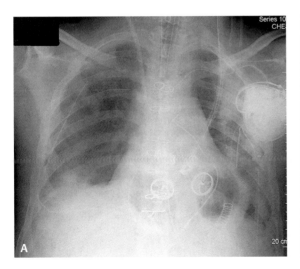
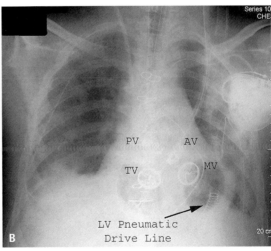

Fig. 152.1

■ Discussion

Background

The total artificial heart (TAH) is presently used in the United States as a bridge for patients with end-stage bi-ventricular heart failure awaiting heart transplantation. This mechanical device is a biventricular orthotopic pneumatic pulsatile pump with two separate artificial ventricles that replace the patient's native ventricles. Each artificial semi-rigid polyurethane ventricle contains a seamless blood-contacting diaphragm, two inter-mediate diaphragms, an air diaphragm, and inflow and outflow mechanical valves. A flexible polyurethane-lined inflow connector is sewn to each atrial cuff of the recipient heart. Dacron graft outflow conduits are sewn to the patient's native aorta and pulmonary artery, respectively. Wire-reinforced conduits covered with Dacron in the transabdominal wall pathways connect to longer drive lines and to an external console that controls the mechanical heart. The external console consists of two pneumatic drivers, one primary and one backup; transport batteries; air tanks; and an alarm and computer monitoring system. Heart rate, percentage of the cardiac cycle occupied by systole, and left and right driving pressures are manually controlled. The TAH is capable of pumping up to 9.5 L of blood per minute. A neopericardium created by Gore-Tex (W. L. Gore & Associates, Flagstaff, AZ) is placed about the TAH to diminish the formation of adhesions between the device and native pericardium and to expedite explantation when an orthotopic human heart becomes available.

Etiology

Worldwide, approximately 3,500 heart transplants are performed every year. Unfortunately, approximately 800,000 people have an irreversible Class IV heart defect (i.e., symptoms occur at rest, and any physical activity brings on discomfort) and therefore need a new organ. This disparity between the supply of available organs for transplant and the demand for such has spurred considerable research into the use of non-human hearts since 1993. The TAH design used and implanted in the United States today is the modern version of the original Jarvik-7 artificial heart first implanted into Barney Clark in 1982. The TAH is primarily used as a bridge to a heart transplant for transplant-eligible patients dying from end-stage biventricular failure.

Clinical Findings

The TAH replaces the patient's diseased ventricles. The device reproduces the same blood flow path as the normal heart. The stroke volume of the device is 70 mL and it weighs roughly 160 g. The TAH decreases the central venous pressure and increases the cardiac index, cardiac output, and end-organ perfusion, thereby increasing organ recovery. The pneumatic drive lines connected to the bedside console may serve as a potential portal of entry for bacteria, increasing the risk for infection for the duration of the device's implantation. To reduce the risk of stroke from blood clots forming on the mechanical parts of the TAH, patients must be anticoagulated.

Imaging Findings

Chest Radiography

- Sternal splitting thoracotomy (**Figs. 152.1A, 152.1B**)
- Sternotomy may be left open in cases of peri-operative bleeding; closed at a later time
- ICD or pacer leads amputated; generator often left in place (**Figs. 152.1A, 152.1B**)
- 1–3 mediastinal drains may be present (**Figs. 152.1A, 152.1B**)
- Unilateral or bilateral pleural drains may be present (**Figs. 152.1A, 152.1B**)
- Two pneumatic drive lines, one for each artificial ventricle, exit through a subcutaneous port in the left upper quadrant (**Figs. 152.1A, 152.1B**)
- Artificial ventricles are not radiographically conspicuous
- Four artificial mechanical valves can be identified (**Figs. 152.1A, 152.1B**)
- Air-containing diaphragms for the artificial ventricles should not be misinterpreted as myocardial air, pneumopericardium, or pneumomediastinum (**Figs. 152.1A, 152.1B**)

MDCT

- Demonstrates various components of the mechanical device (**Figs. 152.2A, 152.2B, 152.2C**)
- Contour abnormalities at the anastomosis between synthetic outflow conduits and native pulmonary artery and native aorta; should not be confused with pseudoaneurysms (**Figs. 152.2A, 152.2B, 152.2C**)

- Neopericardium appears as a high-attenuation curvilinear structure about the implant (**Figs. 152.2B, 152.2C**)
- Tissue expanders are sometimes placed between the artificial left ventricle and neopericardium to minimize adhesion formation and ease explantation

Complications Associated with TAH Implantation

- Infection (72%)
- Bleeding (42%) (**Figs. 152.3, 152.4A, 152.4B**)
  - Mediastinal bleeding
  - Tamponade
- Respiratory dysfunction (30%)
- Liver dysfunction (36%)
- Neurologic (25%)
  - Stroke/transient ischemic attacks
  - Anoxic encephalopathy
  - Metabolic encephalopathy/syncope
- Renal dysfunction (26%)
- Device malfunction (19%)
- Peripheral thromboembolism (11%)

Prognosis

- TAH: highest bridge-to-human heart transplant rate of any heart device
- 79% of TAH recipients successfully transplanted (46% for controls not receiving TAH)

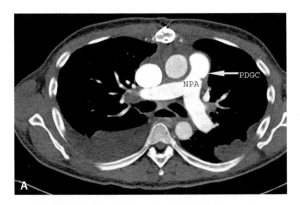

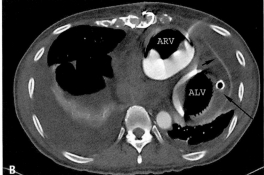

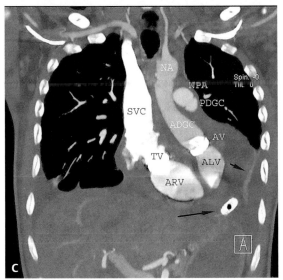

Fig. 152.2 Contrast-enhanced axial **(A,B)** and coronal **(C)** CT (mediastinal window) of a 49-year-old man with TAH shows the normal post-surgical appearance of the native arterial and Dacron synthetic graft conduit (PDGC) anastomoses. The artificial ventricular chambers and the neopericardium (*short black arrow*) can be seen. The left ventricular pneumatic drive line is seen in the left upper quadrant (*long black arrow*). Note the loculated left pleural effusion and the dependent layering right effusion. *ALV*, artificial left ventricle; *ARV*, artificial right ventricle; *ADGC*. aorta Dacron synthetic graft conduit; *NA*, native aorta; *NPA*, native pulmonary artery; *PDGC*, pulmonary artery Dacron synthetic graft conduit.

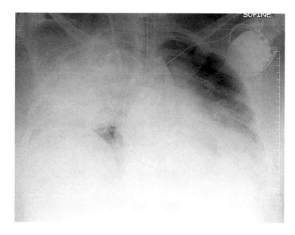

Fig. 152.3 AP chest radiograph of a 60-year-old man with acute right hemothorax occurring on the first postoperative day following TAH implantation. The hemothorax was successfully evacuated.

- Overall survival rate at one year: 70% among patients receiving TAH (31% for controls)
- One-year and five-year survival rates after heart transplant among these patients: 86% and 64%, respectively

PEARLS _____

- All central venous catheters should terminate in a location far removed from the artificial mechanical tricuspid valve; catheter entanglement can cause device failure.
- Radiologists should scrutinize all suture lines on postoperative CT scans in patients with suspected postoperative bleeding or hypotension as this may be a site of suture line dehiscence and bleeding that can be easily repaired (**Figs. 152.4A, 152.4B**).

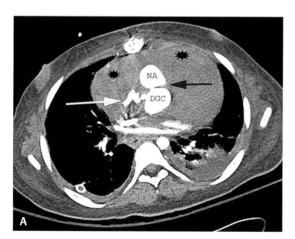
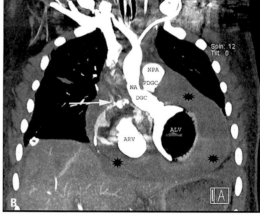

Fig. 152.4 Contrast-enhanced axial **(A)** and coronal MIP **(B)** chest CT (mediastinal window) of 19-year-old man two weeks post TAH implantation with hypotension demonstrates a serpiginous jet of contrast extravasation from the synthetic-to-native aorta conduit anastomosis (*white arrow*). Note the large volume of mixed-attenuation hemopericardium. *ALV*, artificial left ventricle; *ARV*, artificial right ventricle; *DGC*, aorta Dacron graft conduit; *NA*, native aorta; *NPA*, native pulmonary artery; *PDGC*, pulmonary artery Dacron graft conduit; *black arrow*, Dacron graft conduit-to-native aorta anastomosis; *asterisk*, hemopericardium. Re-exploration revealed a suture line dehiscence that was successfully repaired

Suggested Reading

1. Copeland JG, Smith RG, Arabia FA, et al; CardioWest Total Artificial Heart Investigators. Cardiac replacement with a total artificial heart as a bridge to transplantation. N Engl J Med 2004;351(9):859–867

2. http://www.syncardia.com/dldir1/8263_C026.pdf (accessed October 10, 2009)

3. Roussel JC, Sénage T, Baron O, et al. CardioWest (Jarvik) total artificial heart: a single-center experience with 42 patients. Ann Thorac Surg 2009;87(1):124–129, discussion 130

Section XI

Abnormalities of the Mediastinum

OVERVIEW OF ABNORMALITIES OF THE MEDIASTINUM

The mediastinum is defined as the space between the lungs and pleural surfaces. It contains the heart, great vessels, thymus, trachea, esophagus, nerves, lymph nodes, and other soft tissues. A variety of disease processes may arise in the mediastinum, including neoplastic, developmental, infectious, and inflammatory conditions. Evaluation of the mediastinum on radiography requires knowledge of the normal mediastinal interfaces so that deviations from normal can be detected in a timely fashion and evaluated with advanced cross-sectional imaging techniques.

Radiographic evaluation of mediastinal contour abnormalities often includes localization of the lesion in a specific mediastinal compartment for the purposes of differential diagnosis. Once the affected mediastinal compartment is identified, a focused differential diagnosis can be provided. Most mediastinal abnormalities are further evaluated with CT. Contrast administration can be helpful as approximately 10% of mediastinal contour abnormalities are related to vascular lesions and anomalies. In addition, contrast administration often helps in the assessment of the mediastinal lesion being evaluated and its relationship to the adjacent tissues, including the vascular structures. Magnetic resonance imaging is also useful for evaluating the mediastinum but is not as frequently used as CT. MR imaging also allows evaluation of the cardiovascular structures of the mediastinum in patients who cannot tolerate intravenous contrast. In addition, MR can be superior to CT in detecting locally invasive processes.

Mediastinal abnormalities generally consist of neoplasms, developmental lesions, glandular enlargement, vascular lesions, herniations, and other miscellaneous conditions. Many of the mediastinal abnormalities seen in clinical practice relate to mediastinal lymphadenopathies caused either by advanced primary lung cancer, metastatic disease to the mediastinum, or lymphoma. Although lymphadenopathy may also be a feature of infectious/inflammatory processes, the presence of significant lymphadenopathy usually prompts exclusion of malignancy. Benign and malignant primary neoplasms also affect the mediastinum and usually arise from the thymus or from neurogenic structures. Developmental lesions are usually congenital cysts characterized by their unilocular appearance and their fluid content. It should be noted that many mediastinal neoplasms can undergo cystic degeneration. Thus, cystic lesions should be assessed for the presence of associated soft-tissue elements and/or lymphadenopathy to exclude the possibility of a cystic neoplasm. Lesions resulting from glandular enlargement are usually related to the thyroid and the thymus. Imaging diagnosis usually relies on identifying typical features of the gland in question or an anatomic connection with the gland. Two types of vascular lesions affect the mediastinum: those containing blood and those containing lymph. Thus, contrast administration is very useful for evaluation of the former lesions—aneurysms, varices, hemangiomas—while the latter may mimic cystic neoplasms or developmental cystic lesions. Finally, intrathoracic herniations of various abdominal organs and tissues may produce a mediastinal mass that can be assessed and characterized on imaging.

The radiologist plays an important role in the assessment of patients with mediastinal abnormalities. Careful analysis of imaging studies together with knowledge of the clinical history can allow the formulation of a focused differential diagnosis. In addition, knowledge of the appropriate management of various lesions allows the radiologist to play an important role in determining the next step in the evaluation of the affected patient. Recognition of pathognomonic conditions, differentiation between neoplastic and non-neoplastic processes, and distinction between surgical and non-surgical lesions are ways in which the radiologist positively contributes to optimal patient management.

CASE 153

■ Clinical Presentation

Asymptomatic 68-year-old man

■ Radiologic Findings

PA (**Fig. 153.1**) and lateral (**Fig. 153.2**) chest radiographs demonstrate a well-defined left anterior mediastinal mass (*arrows*). Contrast-enhanced chest CT (mediastinal window) (**Figs. 153.3, 153.4**) shows a well-circumscribed ovoid homogeneous soft-tissue mass located in the left lobe of the thymus. A tissue plane separates the mass from the adjacent great vessels.

■ Diagnosis

Thymoma; Encapsulated

■ Differential Diagnosis

- Thymoma, Invasive
- Thymic Carcinoid
- Thymic Carcinoma
- Lymphoma

■ Discussion

Background

Thymoma is an epithelial neoplasm of the thymus. It represents the most common primary neoplasm of the thymus and the most common primary neoplasm of the anterior mediastinum. The recent classification of thymoma by the World Health Organization is based on epithelial cell morphology and lymphocyte-to-epithelial

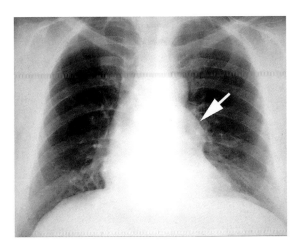

Fig. 153.1

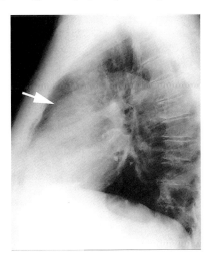

Fig. 153.2

747

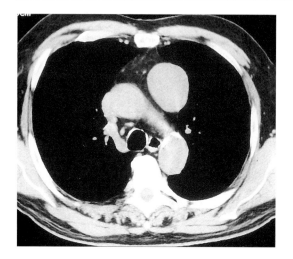

Fig. 153.3

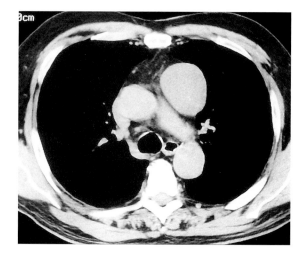

Fig. 153.4

cell ratios. It groups thymomas into types A, AB, B1, B2, and B3, which have been further characterized as *low-risk* (A, AB, B1) and *high-risk* (B2, B3) thymomas. Thymomas may also be classified as *encapsulated* or *invasive*.

Etiology

The etiology of thymoma is unknown. Thymoma is associated with systemic and autoimmune disorders (parathymic syndromes) such as myasthenia gravis, hypogammaglobulinemia, and pure red cell aplasia as well as a variety of non-thymic neoplasms.

Clinical Findings

Patients with thymoma are typically adult men and women who usually present after the age of 40 years (in the fifth and sixth decades of life), although all age groups are affected. While many patients with thymoma are asymptomatic, approximately one-third present with chest pain, cough, dyspnea, and/or symptoms related to local invasion by the tumor (including superior vena cava syndrome). Approximately 15% of patients with myasthenia gravis have thymoma, and up to 50% of patients with thymoma develop myasthenia gravis. Other parathymic syndromes include pure red cell aplasia, polymyositis, systemic lupus erythematosus, rheumatoid arthritis, thyroiditis, and acquired hypogammaglobulinemia.

Imaging Findings

Chest Radiography

- Well-marginated smooth or lobular, typically unilateral, anterior mediastinal nodule or mass; variable size (**Figs. 153.1, 153.2**)
- Located anywhere from thoracic inlet to the cardiophrenic angle; rarely in the neck
- Irregular borders against the lung; ipsilateral diaphragmatic elevation and/or associated pleural nodules/ masses suggest local invasion
- Normal chest radiography in occult thymoma (up to 25%)

MDCT

- Well-defined prevascular (typically unilateral) anterior mediastinal (in anatomic location of thymus) soft-tissue mass of variable size
  - Homogeneous with uniform contrast enhancement (**Figs. 153.3, 153.4, 153.5**)
  - Heterogeneous (**Fig. 153.6**)
    - Low attenuation from cystic change, hemorrhage, necrosis

- – Predominantly cystic (mural soft-tissue nodules)
- – Calcification; peripheral curvilinear, punctate, coarse (**Fig. 153.6**)
- Lobular (**Figs. 153.5, 153.6, 153.7**) or smooth (**Figs. 153.3, 153.4**) contours
- Absent tissue planes described in both encapsulated (**Fig. 153.6**) and invasive thymomas (**Fig. 153.7**)
- Visualization of direct signs of invasion (fat, cardiovascular structures, lung) or pleural implantation (**Fig. 153.7**); may progress to circumferential pleural thickening
- Vascular encasement, irregular contour of vascular lumen, endoluminal tumor in invasive thymoma

MRI

- T1-weighted images: intermediate signal intensity similar to skeletal muscle
- T2-weighted images: high signal intensity; cystic areas with high signal intensity
- Homogeneous/heterogeneous signal intensity; visualization of intrinsic fibrous septa
- Visualization of tumor capsule (low signal intensity, ≤2 mm)
- Smooth contours, round shapes, and capsule visualization suggestive of low-risk thymomas

PET-CT

- No significant difference in SUV between low-risk and high-risk thymomas; differentiation from thymic carcinoma
- Detection of metastatic disease

Staging (Masaoka-Koga System)

- *Stage I*—grossly and microscopically encapsulated thymoma
- *Stage IIa*—microscopic capsular invasion
- *Stage IIb*—macroscopic invasion through the capsule
- *Stage III*—macroscopic invasion of neighboring organs
- *Stage IVa*—pleural or pericardial dissemination
- *Stage IVb*—lymphatic or hematogenous metastases

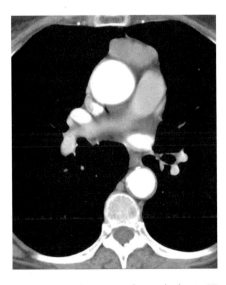

Fig. 153.5 Contrast-enhanced chest CT (mediastinal window) of an asymptomatic 35-year-old woman with an encapsulated thymoma shows a homogeneous small lobular anterior mediastinal soft-tissue nodule and preservation of tissue planes against adjacent vascular structures.

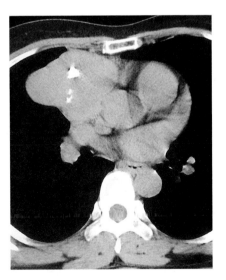

Fig. 153.6 Contrast-enhanced chest CT (mediastinal window) of an asymptomatic 48-year-old woman with an incidentally discovered thymoma shows a large lobular right anterior mediastinal mass with multifocal central calcifications. Note that this encapsulated thymoma exhibits focal obliteration of adjacent tissue planes.

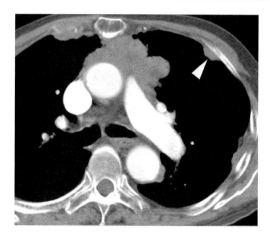

Fig. 153.7 Contrast-enhanced chest CT (mediastinal window) of a 45-year-old man with invasive thymoma demonstrates a poly-lobular thymic soft-tissue mass. Note absence of tissue planes between the mass and the thoracic great vessels and multi-focal bilateral pleural tumor implants (*arrowhead*).

Management

- Complete surgical excision
- Adjuvant radiation for resected thymomas with positive surgical margins and incompletely resected thymomas
- Preoperative chemotherapy for stage III disease
- Adjuvant therapy for local disease control or palliation in patients with stage IV disease
- Chemotherapy for stage IV disease, and for incompletely resected/unresectable thymomas
- Annual imaging follow-up of all treated patients

Prognosis

- Encapsulated and minimally invasive (adjacent fat) thymoma: 95–100% five-year survival; small percentage of local recurrences
- Invasive thymoma (pericardium, lung, cardiovascular structures): 50–60% five-year survival, worse with pleural/pericardial tumor dissemination
- Reported recurrences 10–20 years after initially successful treatment

PEARLS

- The term *thymoma* is reserved for primary epithelial thymic neoplasms without overt atypia of the epithelial component.
- Although *invasive thymomas* may be regarded as malignant lesions, they are histologically indistinguishable from *encapsulated thymomas*.
- Obliteration of adjacent tissue planes on cross-sectional imaging is not diagnostic of local invasion; identification of intact tissue planes does *not* exclude local invasion.

Suggested Reading

1. Marom EM. Imaging thymoma. J Thorac Oncol 2010;**5**(10, Suppl 4):S296–S303

2. Nasseri F, Eftekhari F. Clinical and radiologic review of the normal and abnormal thymus: pearls and pitfalls. Radiographics 2010;30(2):413–428

3. Nishino M, Ashiku SK, Kocher ON, Thurer RL, Boiselle PM, Hatabu H. The thymus: a comprehensive review. Radiographics 2006;26(2):335–348

4. Rosado-de-Christenson ML, Strollo DC, Marom EM. Imaging of thymic epithelial neoplasms. Hematol Oncol Clin North Am 2008;22(3):409–431

5. Travis WD, Brambilla E, Müller-Hermelink HK, et al. Tumours of the thymus. In: Travis WD, Brambilla E, Müller-Hermelink HK, et al., eds. World Health Organization Classification of Tumours. Pathology and Genetics of Tumours of the Lung, Pleura, Thymus and Heart. Lyon: IARC Press; 2004:145–248

CASE 154

■ Clinical Presentation

45-year-old man with Cushing syndrome

■ Radiologic Findings

PA (**Fig. 154.1**) and lateral (**Fig. 154.2**) chest radiographs demonstrate a large, well-defined anterior mediastinal mass that extends predominantly to the left. Note the significant mass effect on the anterior trachea (**Fig. 154.2**). Contrast-enhanced chest CT (mediastinal window) (**Figs. 154.3, 154.4**) demonstrates a large, lobular, slightly heterogeneous anterior mediastinal mass with marked mass effect on the great vessels and the airways.

■ Diagnosis

Thymic Carcinoid

■ Differential Diagnosis

- Thymoma
- Thymic Carcinoma
- Lymphoma
- Seminoma

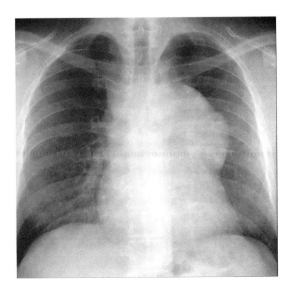

Fig. 154.1

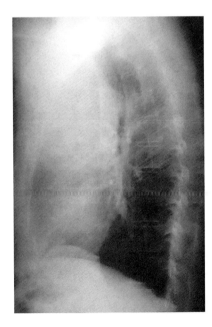

Fig. 154.2

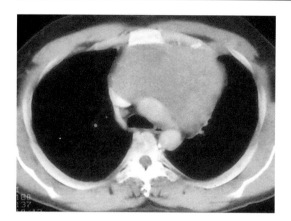

Fig. 154.3

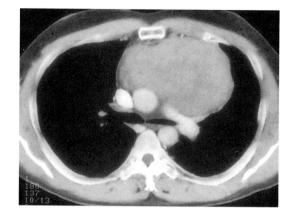

Fig. 154.4

■ Discussion

Background

Thymic carcinoid is a rare primary malignant neuroendocrine thymic neoplasm.

Etiology

The etiology of thymic carcinoid is unknown. It is histologically indistinguishable from bronchial carcinoid, but exhibits a higher frequency of atypical histology and a more aggressive behavior. This neoplasm may be functionally active and may produce a clinical hormone syndrome.

Clinical Findings

Thymic carcinoid affects men more commonly than women (3:1 male-to-female ratio) over a wide age range, with a mean age of 43 years. Most patients are symptomatic at presentation, with cough, dyspnea, chest pain, and/or symptoms related to invasion of adjacent structures. Approximately 50% of thymic carcinoids are functionally active and may initially manifest with Cushing syndrome or in association with the syndrome of multiple endocrine neoplasia (MEN).

Imaging Findings

Chest Radiography

- Large spherical, lobular, anterior mediastinal soft-tissue mass (indistinguishable from thymoma) (**Figs. 154.1, 154.2**)
- Typically well-defined borders on radiography, even with local invasion (**Figs. 154.1, 154.2**)

MDCT

- Typically large homogeneous or heterogeneous (necrosis) anterior mediastinal mass (indistinguishable from thymoma) (**Figs. 154.3, 154.4, 154.5**)
- Lymphadenopathy
- Invasion of adjacent structures, pleural effusion/tumor implants, distant metastases

Scintigraphy

- Evaluation of patients with clinical evidence of ectopic ACTH production
- Uptake of octreotide: In-111-diethylenetriaminepentaacetic acid (DTPA)-D-Phe[1] in occult thymic carcinoids (non-specific finding; uptake in other primary and metastatic thymic neoplasms) (**Fig. 154.5A**)

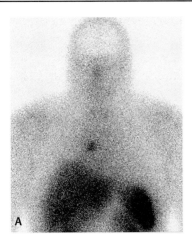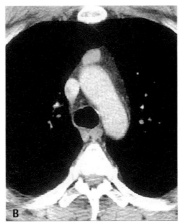

Fig. 154.5 Octreotide scintigraphy **(A)** of a middle-aged man who presented with Cushing syndrome demonstrates focal abnormal mediastinal uptake. Contrast-enhanced chest CT (mediastinal window) **(B)** demonstrates an ovoid soft-tissue nodule in the right lobe of the thymus, which corresponds to the area of abnormal uptake and represents an occult thymic carcinoid.

Management

- Aggressive surgical excision
- Adjuvant radiation therapy and chemotherapy

Prognosis

- Frequent disease progression, recurrence, and/or metastases
- Poor prognosis: 31% five-year survival
- Aggressive behavior and worse prognosis in patients with MEN syndrome or clinical Cushing syndrome

PEARLS

- Thymic carcinoid exhibits a high incidence of local recurrence, and follow-up imaging is often performed.
- Thymic carcinoid may be indistinguishable from thymoma. The presence of a clinical hormone syndrome suggests the diagnosis; visualization of lymphadenopathy suggests thymic/anterior mediastinal malignancy (carcinoid, carcinoma, lymphoma).
- Thymic carcinoma (WHO Type C thymoma) exhibits cytologic atypia and histologic features analogous to carcinomas of other organs and lacks immature lymphocytes characteristically found in thymomas. Radiologically, it manifests as a large anterior mediastinal mass (**Fig. 154.6**) with frequent central necrosis, calcification, local invasion, lymphadenopathy, and distant metastases.

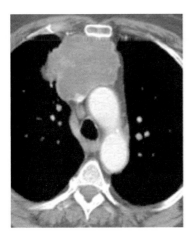

Fig. 154.6 Contrast-enhanced chest CT (mediastinal window) of a 64-year-old woman with chest pain and thymic carcinoma demonstrates a lobular right anterior mediastinal soft-tissue mass with central low attenuation representing necrosis and local invasion of the adjacent superior vena cava.

Suggested Reading

1. Jung K-J, Lee KS, Han J, Kim J, Kim TS, Kim EA. Malignant thymic epithelial tumors: CT-pathologic correlation. AJR Am J Roentgenol 2001;176(2):433–439

2. Nasseri F, Eftekhari F. Clinical and radiologic review of the normal and abnormal thymus: pearls and pitfalls. Radiographics 2010;30(2):413–428

3. Rosado de Christenson ML, Abbott GF, Kirejczyk WM, Galvin JR, Travis WD. Thoracic carcinoids: radiologic-pathologic correlation. Radiographics 1999;19(3):707–736

4. Rosado-de-Christenson ML, Strollo DC, Marom EM. Imaging of thymic epithelial neoplasms. Hematol Oncol Clin North Am 2008;22(3):409–431

5. Travis WD, Brambilla E, Müller-Hermelink HK, et al. Tumours of the thymus. In Travis WD, Brambilla E, Müller-Hermelink HK, et al., eds. World Health Organization Classification of Tumours. Pathology and Genetics of Tumours of the Lung, Pleura, Thymus and Heart. Lyon: IARC Press; 2004:145–248

CASE 155

■ Clinical Presentation

Asymptomatic 12-year-old boy

■ Radiologic Findings

PA (**Fig. 155.1**) and lateral (**Fig. 155.2**) chest radiographs demonstrate a right anterior-inferior mediastinal mass that conforms to the shape of the heart and mimics cardiomegaly. Note the lesion is not visible on the lateral chest radiograph (**Fig. 155.2**). Unenhanced chest CT (mediastinal window) (**Fig. 155.3**) shows a well-defined right juxtacardiac mass composed of soft-tissue elements intermixed with areas of fat. Note mild mass effect on the heart and visualization of intact adjacent subepicardial fat.

■ Diagnosis

Thymolipoma

■ Differential Diagnosis

- Morgagni Hernia
- Lipoma/Liposarcoma
- Mature Teratoma

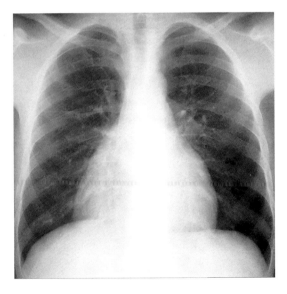

Fig. 155.1

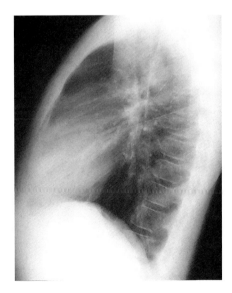

Fig. 155.2

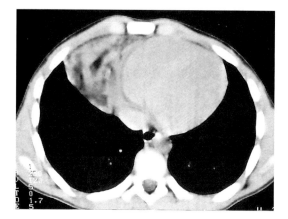

Fig. 155.3

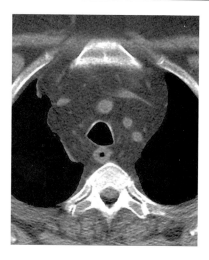

Fig. 155.4 Unenhanced chest CT (mediastinal window) of an obese 40-year-old man with mediastinal lipomatosis demonstrates fat attenuation tissue surrounding normal mediastinal structures without resultant mass effect.

■ Discussion

Background

Thymolipoma is a rare benign primary thymic neoplasm. Thymolipomas are characterized by their soft consistency and preferential growth in the inferior portion of the anterior mediastinum. These lesions may reach very large sizes in spite of minimal symptoms.

Etiology

The etiology of thymolipoma is unknown.

Clinical Findings

Patients with thymolipoma are usually young adults in the third decade of life, and men and women are equally affected. Patients may be entirely asymptomatic. Symptomatic patients present with complaints related to mass effect by large lesions and may complain of cough, dyspnea, and/or chest pain.

Imaging Features

Chest Radiography

- Well-defined unilateral or bilateral anterior inferior mediastinal mass (**Fig. 155.1**)
- Conforms to the shape of adjacent structures; may mimic cardiomegaly or diaphragmatic elevation (**Fig. 155.1**)
- Positional changes in shape due to soft consistency

MDCT

- Anatomic connection with the thymus
- Admixture of linear, whorled, or rounded soft-tissue elements with fat attenuation (**Fig. 155.3**)
- Less commonly, predominant fat attenuation lesion with small internal soft-tissue foci

MRI

- T1WI: high-signal-intensity areas intermixed with intermediate-signal-intensity foci (roughly isointense to muscle)
- Documentation of anatomic connection with the thymus and absence of local invasion

Management

- Surgical excision
- Observation of patients who are not surgical candidates

Prognosis

- Excellent
- No reports of malignant transformation

PEARLS _____

- Diagnosis of thymolipoma should be considered in any asymptomatic patient with an anterior-inferior mediastinal mass that conforms to the shape of adjacent structures and produces little mass effect. The demonstration of fat and soft-tissue elements within the lesion and an anatomic connection to the thymus strongly supports the diagnosis.
- Differential diagnosis of fat-containing soft-tissue mediastinal masses includes:
    - **Mediastinal lipomatosis**—deposition of non-neoplastic unencapsulated mature adipose tissue in the superior mediastinum, pleuropericardial angles, and paravertebral regions in association with obesity or endogenous/exogenous hypercortisolism; characteristic imaging findings of mediastinal enlargement produced by homogeneous fat attenuation/signal tissue without mass effect (**Fig. 155.4**).
    - **Mediastinal lipoma**—rare mesenchymal mediastinal neoplasm composed of encapsulated adipose tissue, vascular structures, and fibrous septa which typically affects asymptomatic adults evaluated because of an abnormal chest radiograph (although large tumors may produce symptoms of compression); CT/MR demonstrates a non-invasive mass of predominant fat attenuation with small internal soft-tissue foci (**Fig. 155.5**).
    - **Mediastinal liposarcoma**—rare mesenchymal malignant neoplasm of variable degrees of differentiation and histologic makeup that typically affects older individuals, who present with dyspnea, chest pain, cough, or constitutional complaints; imaging features correlate with the histologic composition of the tumor and range from masses of predominant fat attenuation/signal (**Fig. 155.6**) to soft-tissue masses with minimal or absent foci of fat attenuation/signal; soft-tissue components are often dominant, and mass effect is typical.

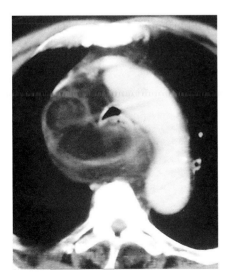

Fig. 155.5 Contrast-enhanced chest CT (mediastinal window) of an asymptomatic man with a mediastinal lipoma demonstrates a middle mediastinal mass of predominant fat attenuation with internal soft-tissue elements, which produce mass effect on the airway and the vascular structures.

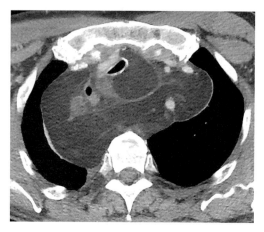

Fig. 155.6 Contrast-enhanced chest CT (mediastinal window) of an elderly man with weight loss, dysphagia, and mediastinal liposarcoma demonstrates a large middle/posterior (and para-vertebral) mediastinal mass of predominant fat attenuation with multi-focal soft-tissue components and marked mass effect on the esophagus and trachea.

○ **Morgagni hernia**—developmental abnormality characterized by a defect in the anteromedial diaphragm through which abdominal contents (including omental fat) may herniate (**Fig. 155.7**). Affected patients are typically asymptomatic but may also present with non-specific abdominal and thoracic complaints. Imaging typically demonstrates a right cardiophrenic angle mass. CT/MR demonstrates fat corresponding to omental herniation and may show bowel loops within the mass, serpiginous omental vessels, and discontinuity of the adjacent diaphragm (**Fig. 155.7**).

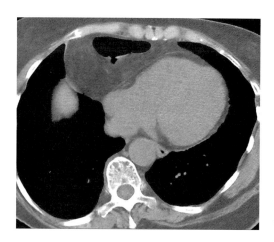

Fig. 155.7 Unenhanced chest CT (mediastinal window) of an asymptomatic 54-year-old woman with a Morgagni hernia reveals a right cardiophrenic angle mass of predominant fat attenuation with an internal air-filled bowel loop.

Suggested Reading

1. Nasseri F, Eftekhari F. Clinical and radiologic review of the normal and abnormal thymus: pearls and pitfalls. Radiographics 2010;30(2):413–428

2. Nishino M, Ashiku SK, Kocher ON, Thurer RL, Boiselle PM, Hatabu H. The thymus: a comprehensive review. Radiographics 2006;26(2):335–348

3. Eisenstat R, Bruce D, Williams LE, Katz DS. Primary liposarcoma of the mediastinum with coexistent mediastinal lipomatosis. AJR Am J Roentgenol 2000;174(2):572–573

4. Rosado-de-Christenson ML, Pugatch RD, Moran CA, Galobardes J. Thymolipoma: analysis of 27 cases. Radiology 1994;193(1):121–126

CASE 156

■ Clinical Presentation

Asymptomatic 42-year-old woman status post chemotherapy for malignancy

■ Radiologic Findings

Contrast-enhanced chest CT (mediastinal window) (**Fig. 156.1**) demonstrates diffuse enlargement of a homogeneous thymus without mass effect, local invasion, or lymphadenopathy. Contrast-enhanced chest CT (mediastinal window) (**Fig. 156.2**) performed after corticosteroid therapy demonstrates prompt reduction in the size of the thymus and a normal anterior mediastinum.

■ Diagnosis

Thymic Hyperplasia

■ Differential Diagnosis

*   Thymoma
*   Lymphoma

■ DISCUSSION

Background

Thymic hyperplasia is an uncommon condition that results in a global increase in the size and weight of the thymus (based on the expected size of the thymus for the individual's age). The condition is also known as "true" thymic hyperplasia and as "rebound" thymic hyperplasia; the latter term is used specifically when hyperplasia follows chemotherapy, steroid therapy, or recovery from a severe systemic insult. Rebound thymic hyperplasia is typically defined as a 50% increase in thymic volume over baseline.

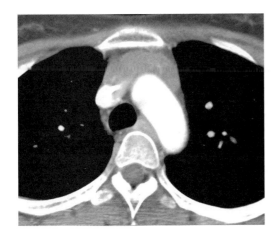

Fig. 156.1

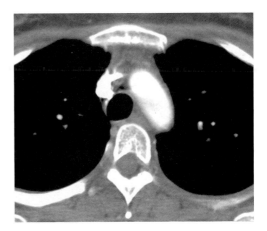

Fig. 156.2

Etiology

True thymic hyperplasia may be an isolated finding in infants presenting with respiratory distress and thymic enlargement. It may also occur as a rebound phenomenon secondary to thymic atrophy caused by chemotherapy for malignancy (testicular cancer, breast cancer, lymphoma, and other malignancies). In these cases, thymic enlargement typically occurs between two weeks and 14 months after chemotherapy. It has been postulated that it is caused by chemotherapy-induced gonadal atrophy and a resultant increase in luteinizing hormone secretion. Hyperplasia is also reported after treatment of hypercortisolism (Cushing syndrome) and following conditions of severe stress, including sepsis and burns. Some authors propose high-dose corticosteroid administration, which typically results in a decrease in the size of the hyperplastic thymus.

Clinical Findings

Patients with thymic hyperplasia are typically children, adolescents, and young adults. Affected individuals are usually asymptomatic, but may also present with dyspnea and/or dysphagia.

Imaging Features

Chest Radiography

- Focal or diffuse anterior mediastinal widening
  - Most commonly appreciated in children (**Fig. 156.3**)
  - May not be evident in adults

MDCT

- Diffuse symmetric thymic enlargement based on measured thymic thickness (**Figs. 156.1, 156.4**)
  - *Thymic thickness* refers to the *short-axis* measurement of a thymic lobe; *thymic width* refers to the *long-axis* measurement of a thymic lobe (**Fig. 156.4**)
  - Maximal normal thickness in individuals under 20 years: 1.8 cm
  - Maximal normal thickness in individuals over 20 years: 1.3 cm
- Preservation of normal thymic attenuation

MRI

- Decreased signal intensity on opposed-phase images relative to in-phase images on chemical shift MRI

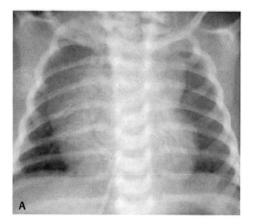 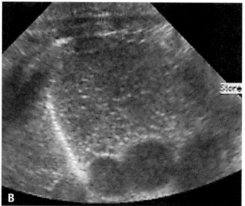

Fig.156.3 AP chest radiograph (**A**) of a term newborn with mild respiratory distress demonstrates a large thymus. Transverse ultrasound through the thymus (**B**) demonstrates normal homogeneous thymic echotexture and no mass effect on the great vessels.

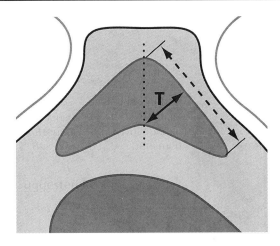

Fig. 156.4 Artist's illustration of the method employed for measuring the thymus on CT. The thickness (*T*) of each lobe is measured perpendicular to the long axis of the lobe.

PET-CT

- FDG uptake reported in patients with thymic hyperplasia; SUV measurements may not allow differentiation between thymic hyperplasia and neoplastic involvement

Management

- Recognition and observation in patients with appropriate history
- Biopsy or excision in patients without associated conditions or airway compression or in cases in which residual or recurrent malignancy must be excluded

Prognosis

- Excellent
- May be a marker of improved survival in some patients with malignancy

PEARLS

- Thymic hyperplasia presents a diagnostic dilemma in patients who are treated for mediastinal lymphoma, as residual or recurrent lymphoma must be excluded.
- True thymic hyperplasia is not to be confused with thymic lymphoid hyperplasia (autoimmune or lymphofollicular thymitis), characterized by secondary lymphoid follicles with germinal centers in an otherwise histologically normal thymus. While affected patients may exhibit thymic enlargement, the thymus is often of normal appearance on imaging studies. This condition is associated with autoimmune disorders such as myasthenia gravis, hyperthyroidism (Graves disease), hypothyroidism, Addison disease, sarcoidosis, pure red cell aplasia, acromegaly and Beckwith-Wiedemann syndrome.

Suggested Reading

1. Ford ME, Stevens R, Rosado-de-Christenson ML, Hall NC, Suster S. Rebound thymic hyperplasia after pneumonectomy and chemotherapy for primary synovial sarcoma. J Thorac Imaging 2008;23(3):178–181

2. Inaoka T, Takahashi K, Mineta M, et al. Thymic hyperplasia and thymus gland tumors: differentiation with chemical shift MR imaging. Radiology 2007;243(3):869–876

3. Nasseri F, Eftekhari F. Clinical and radiologic review of the normal and abnormal thymus: pearls and pitfalls. Radiographics 2010;30(2):413–428

4. Nishino M, Ashiku SK, Kocher ON, Thurer RL, Boiselle PM, Hatabu H. The thymus: a comprehensive review. Radiographics 2006;26(2):335–348

5. Sehbai AS, Tallaksen RJ, Bennett J, Abraham J. Thymic hyperplasia after adjuvant chemotherapy in breast cancer. J Thorac Imaging 2006;21(1):43–46

CASE 157

■ Clinical Presentation

74-year-old woman with cough and chest pain

■ Radiologic Findings

PA (**Fig. 157.1**) and lateral (**Fig. 157.2**) chest radiographs demonstrate a large left anterior mediastinal mass with a thin peripheral rim of curvilinear calcification. Unenhanced chest CT (mediastinal window) (**Figs. 157.3, 157.4**) shows a heterogeneous spherical mass in the left lobe of the thymus. Note the peripheral curvilinear calcification and internal areas of soft tissue, fluid, and fat attenuation.

■ Diagnosis

Mature Teratoma

■ Differential Diagnosis

None

■ Discussion

Background

Germ cell neoplasms typically occur in the gonad but may also affect extragonadal sites, usually the anterior mediastinum (near or within the thymus). Mature teratoma is a benign neoplasm that accounts for approximately 70% of all primary mediastinal germ cell neoplasms.

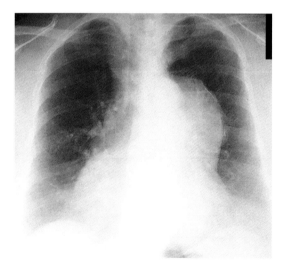

Fig. 157.1

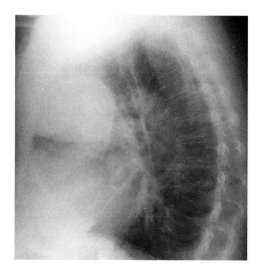

Fig. 157.2

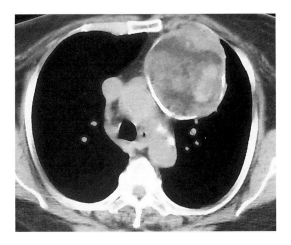

Fig. 157.3

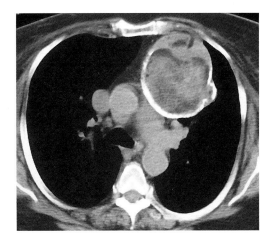

Fig. 157.4

Etiology

The etiology of germ cell neoplasms is poorly understood. It is theorized that extragonadal mature teratomas may arise from primitive germ cells that are "misplaced" along midline structures during their embryologic migration from the yolk sac to the gonad.

Clinical Findings

Patients with mature teratoma are typically children and young adults (usually under 40 years of age). Patients may be asymptomatic or may present with signs and symptoms of compression of adjacent structures, including chest pain, dyspnea, and cough, or because of symptoms related to tumor rupture.

Imaging Findings

Chest Radiography

- Well-defined unilateral anterior mediastinal mass (**Figs. 157.1, 157.2**)
- Calcification in 22% (**Figs. 157.1, 157.2**)
- Mass effect with resultant consolidation/atelectasis
- Occasional pleural effusion (does not necessarily denote tumor rupture)

MDCT

- Well-defined heterogeneous anterior mediastinal mass (**Figs. 157.3, 157.4, 157.5, 157.6**)
- Multilocular cystic mass (85%); fluid attenuation (89%) (**Figs. 157.3, 157.4, 157.5, 157.6**)
- Fat attenuation (76%) (**Figs. 157.3, 157.4, 157.5, 157.6**); fat-fluid levels (11%)
- Calcification (53%) (**Figs. 157.3, 157.4, 157.5**)
- Soft-tissue elements (**Figs. 157.3, 157.4, 157.5, 157.6**)
  - Thin capsule and internal tissue septa
  - Rarely nodular soft tissue in capsule and septa
  - Increased conspicuity of soft-tissue elements after intravenous contrast administration

MRI

- Heterogeneous mediastinal mass
- High signal intensity content on T1WI (corresponding to fat) and variable signal intensity on T2WI; not diagnostic of fat, may be seen in hemorrhagic cysts
- Fat saturation MR imaging such as phase-shift gradient-echo imaging or proton-selective fat saturation imaging for detection of fat and distinction from hemorrhage

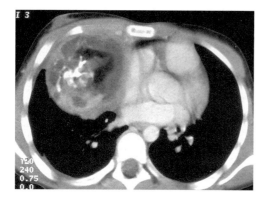

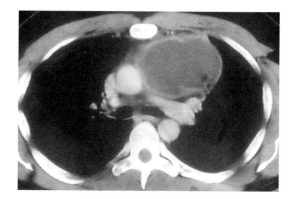

Fig. 157.5 Contrast-enhanced chest CT (mediastinal window) of a 10-year-old girl with chest discomfort and a mediastinal mature teratoma demonstrates a spherical multilocular cystic anterior mediastinal mass with fluid, fat, soft tissue, and calcium attenuation. Note mass effect on the heart and small ipsilateral pleural effusion.

Fig. 157.6 Contrast-enhanced chest CT (mediastinal window) of a young man who presented with chest discomfort demonstrates a large left anterior mediastinal mature teratoma. The lesion is predominantly cystic, exhibits a thin soft-tissue capsule, and contains a small focus of fat attenuation.

Management

- Complete surgical excision

Prognosis

- Excellent in mature teratoma
- Excellent in immature teratoma of infancy and childhood
- Poor in immature teratoma of adulthood and in all teratomas with malignant elements

PEARLS

- Demonstration of fat attenuation within a well-circumscribed cystic mediastinal mass is virtually diagnostic of *mature teratoma* (**Fig. 157.6**).
- While most *mature teratomas* exhibit fat, calcium or both, approximately 15% do not. Thus, *mature teratoma* should be considered in the differential diagnosis of any multilocular cystic anterior mediastinal mass.
- Rupture of a *mature teratoma* may result in increased heterogeneity within the mass, adjacent consolidation/atelectasis, and a higher prevalence of pleural/pericardial effusions.
- *Immature teratoma* consists of more than 10% of immature neuroectodermal and mesenchymal tissues. These neoplasms may be indistinguishable from mature teratoma on imaging studies or may manifest as predominantly solid masses. They often exhibit a highly aggressive behavior in affected adults.
- *Malignant immature teratoma* and *teratoma* with *additional malignant components* may represent malignant degeneration of a former immature or mature teratoma and may contain foci of carcinoma, sarcoma, or other malignant germ cell histologies. While these tumors may exhibit fat and/or calcium attenuation and may mimic mature teratoma on imaging studies, they often display a predominance of enhancing soft-tissue elements, may show extensive areas of necrosis, and may exhibit indistinct margins, obliteration of tissue planes, or frank local invasion.

Suggested Reading

1. Jeung M-Y, Gasser B, Gangi A, et al. Imaging of cystic masses of the mediastinum. Radiographics 2002;22(Spec No): S79–S93

2. Moeller KH, Rosado-de-Christenson ML, Templeton PA. Mediastinal mature teratoma: imaging features. AJR Am J Roentgenol 1997;169(4):985–990

3. Nasseri F, Eftekhari F. Clinical and radiologic review of the normal and abnormal thymus: pearls and pitfalls. Radiographics 2010;30(2):413–428

4. Strollo DC, Rosado-de-Christenson ML. Primary mediastinal malignant germ cell neoplasms: imaging features. Chest Surg Clin N Am 2002;12(4):645–658

5. Ueno T, Tanaka YO, Nagata M, et al. Spectrum of germ cell tumors: from head to toe. Radiographics 2004;24(2): 387–404

CASE 158

■ Clinical Presentation

35-year-old man with facial swelling and flushing

■ Radiologic Findings

PA (**Fig. 158.1**) chest radiograph demonstrates a large, lobular, well-defined anterior mediastinal mass, which extends to both sides of the midline and is associated with elevation of the right hemidiaphragm. Contrast-enhanced chest CT (mediastinal window) (**Figs. 158.2, 158.3**) demonstrates a bulky anterior mediastinal mass of homogeneous soft-tissue attenuation and lobular borders. The mass encases the right brachiocephalic artery, the left common carotid artery, and the bilateral brachiocephalic veins (**Fig. 158.2**) and invades the superior vena cava (**Fig. 158.3**).

■ Diagnosis

Seminoma

■ Differential Diagnosis

- Lymphoma
- Thymoma, invasive

■ Discussion

Background

Seminoma is an uncommon neoplasm that represents approximately 40% of primary mediastinal malignant germ cell neoplasms of a single histology. *Non-seminomatous malignant germ cell neoplasms* (GCNs) are aggressive neoplasms and include embryonal carcinoma, endodermal sinus (yolk sac) tumor, and choriocarcinoma. These lesions typically exhibit more than one germ cell histology and may contain foci of seminoma.

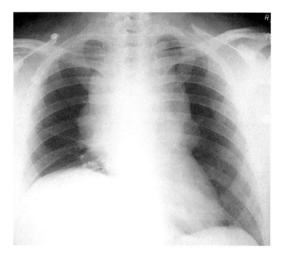

Fig. 158.1

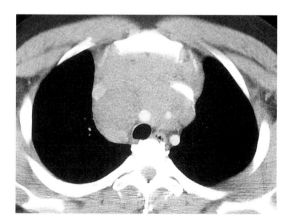

Fig. 158.2

766

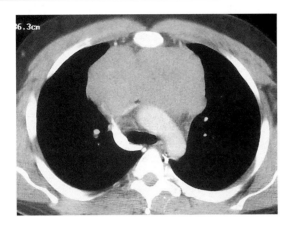

Fig. 158.3

Clinical Findings

Seminoma affects almost exclusively men in the third and fourth decades of life, who typically present with symptoms related to mass effect or local invasion, including chest pain, dyspnea, and superior vena cava syndrome. Up to 30% of affected patients are asymptomatic at presentation. *Non-seminomatous malignant GCN* affects almost exclusively young men who usually present with symptoms of mediastinal compression and/or invasion or with systemic complaints or symptoms related to metastatic disease. Patients may also present with precocious puberty or gynecomastia. Approximately 20% of affected patients have Klinefelter syndrome, and these patients may develop a concurrent hematologic malignancy.

Imaging Findings

Chest Radiography

Seminoma

- Bulky, often well-defined anterior mediastinal mass (**Fig. 158.1**)
- Extends to both sides of midline (**Fig. 158.1**)
- Mass effect

Non-Seminomatous Malignant GCN

- Large, bulky anterior mediastinal mass
- Extends to both sides of midline
- Well- or ill-defined margins
- Mass effect
- Frequent associated pleural effusion

MDCT

Seminoma

- Large, homogeneous soft-tissue mass (**Figs. 158.2, 158.3**)
- Rarely central necrosis or cystic change
- Lymphadenopathy

Non-Seminomatous Malignant GCN

- Large, locally invasive, heterogeneous soft-tissue mass (**Fig. 158.4**)
- Contrast-enhanced studies: central low attenuation (corresponding to necrosis) and peripheral frond-like nodular enhancement (**Fig. 158.4**)

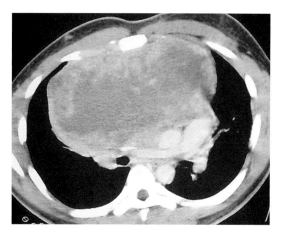

Fig. 158.4 Contrast-enhanced chest CT (mediastinal window) of a 21-year-old man with chest pain, dyspnea, and a non-seminomatous malignant GCN demonstrates a bulky, heterogeneous anterior mediastinal mass with peripheral frond-like contrast enhancement, central irregular low attenuation, and marked mass effect on the adjacent structures.

- Obliteration of adjacent tissue planes or frank local invasion (mediastinum, lung, chest wall) (**Fig. 158.4**)
- Pleural and/or pericardial effusion
- Mediastinal lymphadenopathy

Management

Seminoma

- Radiation therapy
- Cisplatin-based chemotherapy

Non-Seminomatous Malignant GCN

- Chemotherapy
- Surgical excision of residual necrotic and/or viable tumor

Prognosis

Seminoma

- Up to 90% five-year survival

Non-Seminomatous Malignant GCN

- Poor; documented cases of long-term survival

PEARLS

- Evaluation of serologic markers (α-fetoprotein, human chorionic gonadotropin) is useful in the diagnosis of mediastinal malignant GCN and may suggest the histologic types represented.
- Diagnosis of malignant mediastinal GCN will often prompt testicular evaluation to exclude a primary malignancy. However, most testicular GCNs metastatic to the mediastinum exhibit concurrent retroperitoneal lymph node metastases.

Suggested Readings

1. Ravenel JG, Gordon LL, Block MI, Chaudhary U. Primary posterior mediastinal seminoma. AJR Am J Roentgenol 2004;183(6):1835–1837

2. Strollo DC, Rosado-de-Christenson ML. Tumors of the thymus. J Thorac Imaging 1999;14(3):152–171

3. Strollo DC, Rosado-de-Christenson ML. Primary mediastinal malignant germ cell neoplasms: imaging features. Chest Surg Clin N Am 2002;12(4):645–658

CASE 159

■ Clinical Presentation

26-year-old man with chest discomfort

■ Radiologic Findings

PA (**Fig. 159.1**) and lateral (**Fig. 159.2**) chest radiographs demonstrate a large lobular anterior mediastinal mass that extends to both sides of midline, but predominantly to the right. Contrast-enhanced chest CT (mediastinal window) (**Figs. 159.3, 159.4**) reveals a large mediastinal soft-tissue mass of irregular lobular borders, which occupies the anterior mediastinum; encases the left brachiocephalic vein, superior vena cava, and ascending aorta; partially encases the right upper lobe bronchus; and produces an irregular margin with the adjacent right upper lobe. Note associated right paratracheal lymphadenopathy (**Fig. 159.3**).

■ Diagnosis

Hodgkin Lymphoma

■ Differential Diagnosis

- Non-Hodgkin Lymphoma
- Metastatic Mediastinal Lymphadenopathy; Lung Cancer, Extrathoracic Malignancy
- Thymoma, Invasive
- Thymic Malignancy

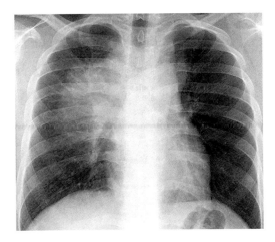

Fig. 159.1

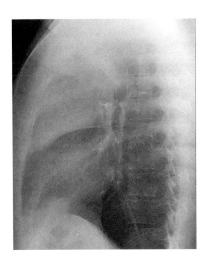

Fig. 159.2

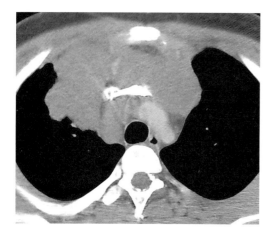

Fig. 159.3

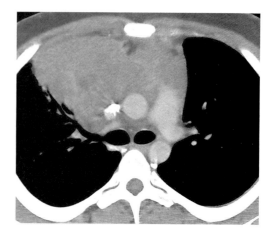

Fig. 159.4

■ Discussion

Background

The lymphomas are a heterogeneous group of malignant neoplasms of the cells of the immune system characterized by proliferation and enlargement of lymph nodes and secondary lymphoid tissues. *Non-Hodgkin lymphoma* is the most frequent lymphoma and accounts for approximately 75% of cases, while *Hodgkin lymphoma* accounts for approximately 25% of lymphomas. However, mediastinal involvement by lymphoma is much more common in patients Hodgkin lymphoma than in those with non-Hodgkin lymphoma. The most common cell type of mediastinal Hodgkin lymphoma is nodular sclerosis. The most common mediastinal non-Hodgkin lymphoma is diffuse large B-cell lymphoma (which, together with follicular lymphoma, accounts for over 50% of all non-Hodgkin lymphomas), although lymphoblastic lymphoma and adult T-cell lymphoma characteristically manifest as large mediastinal masses. The latest WHO classification of lymphoma is complex and consists of over 20 subtypes based on cell of origin (B or T cell), morphologic features, and immunophenotypic characteristics.

Etiology

The etiology of lymphoma is unknown. The increasing incidence of non-Hodgkin lymphoma has been in part attributed to the growing elderly population and the HIV epidemic. Various forms of immunosuppression have been linked to extranodal lymphoma.

Clinical Findings

Hodgkin Lymphoma

Hodgkin lymphoma affects men and women, with a bimodal age distribution characterized by peak incidences in adolescence and young adulthood and a smaller incidence peak after the fifth decade of life. Many patients present with palpable enlarged peripheral lymph nodes, typically in the neck. Chest pain and systemic complaints occur in approximately one-third of affected individuals.

Non-Hodgkin Lymphoma

Non-Hodgkin lymphoma affects patients of both genders and all ages. Most have advanced systemic lymphoma at the time of presentation and are typically symptomatic because of constitutional complaints, palpable lymphadenopathy and/or extranodal disease. Diffuse large B-cell lymphoma (primary mediastinal [thymic] large B-cell lymphoma) typically affects young adults, with a slight female predominance. Affected patients often present with thoracic complaints related to compression and/or invasion of mediastinal structures.

Imaging Features

Chest Radiography

Hodgkin Lymphoma

- Intrathoracic involvement in 75% of cases
- Anterior mediastinal enlargement with "filling" of the retrosternal space on lateral chest radiography (**Figs. 159.1, 159.2**)
- Lobular contours, frequent growth to both sides of the midline, mass effect (**Fig. 159.1**)

Non-Hodgkin Lymphoma

- Intrathoracic involvement in less than half of cases
- Anterior and middle mediastinal enlargement

MDCT

Hodgkin Lymphoma

- Intrathoracic involvement in up to 85% of patients
- Lymphadenopathy affecting contiguous prevascular, paratracheal, and other intrathoracic lymph nodes (**Figs. 159.3, 159.4, 159.5**)
- Nodal coalescence, homogeneous anterior mediastinal soft-tissue mass (**Figs. 159.3, 159.4**)
- Heterogeneity; cystic change, necrosis (**Fig. 159.5**)
- Local invasion of cardiovascular structures, pleura, lung, and/or chest wall (**Fig. 159.5**)
- Rare calcification; usually occurs one year after therapy, affects less than 1% of patients (**Fig. 159.6**), may occur prior to treatment in a small percentage of cases

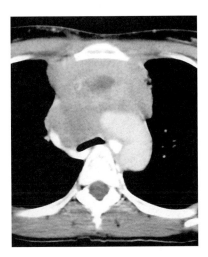

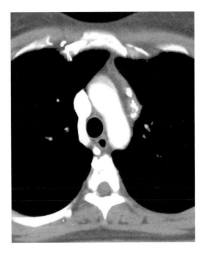

Fig. 159.5 Contrast-enhanced chest CT (mediastinal window) of a young woman with Hodgkin lymphoma who presented with superior vena cava syndrome demonstrates a large heterogeneous prevascular soft-tissue mass, which obstructs the superior vena cava and produces mass effect on the airways and the mediastinal great vessels. The central area of low attenuation likely represents necrosis. Note marked enhancement of the azygos and hemizygos veins.

Fig. 159.6 Contrast-enhanced chest CT (mediastinal window) of a middle-aged woman who is 15 years post successful treatment of Hodgkin lymphoma demonstrates dense mediastinal calcification in areas of prior involvement by lymphoma.

Non-Hodgkin Lymphoma

- Findings indistinguishable from those of Hodgkin lymphoma (**Fig. 159.7**)
- Isolated involvement of mediastinal lymph nodes other than prevascular and paratracheal

MRI

- Increased signal intensity on T2WI in active disease
- Increased signal intensity on T1WI and T2WI in residual fibrous tissue after successful therapy
- Low signal intensity on T2WI in inflammatory and cystic tissue following therapy

PET-CT

- Increased sensitivity and specificity for detection of lymph node and organ involvement when compared with contrast-enhanced CT alone
- Baseline staging and assessment of treatment response; improved sensitivity for extranodal disease
- Correlation of degree of metabolic activity with aggressiveness of lymphoma; low-grade FDG uptake associated with indolent lymphomas

Management

- Radiation, chemotherapy, surgery based on cell type, stage, and metabolic activity
- Palliative treatment for indolent lymphoma

Prognosis

- Use of International Prognostic Index based on age, stage, serum lactate dehydrogenase levels, number of extranodal disease sites, and performance status as predictor of prognosis

PEARLS

- Patients with *Hodgkin lymphoma* often present with palpable peripheral lymphadenopathy. In these cases, the diagnosis is established by lymph node biopsy prior to thoracic imaging. However, up to 10% of affected patients have primary mediastinal Hodgkin lymphoma without superficial lymph node involvement.
- *Mediastinal lymphoma* with nodal coalescence may be indistinguishable from other malignant and locally invasive anterior mediastinal neoplasms. Lymphoma must be considered in the differential diagnosis, particularly when there is imaging evidence of adjacent lymphadenopathy or involvement of multiple lymph node groups (**Figs. 159.3, 159.4, 159.5, 159.7**).

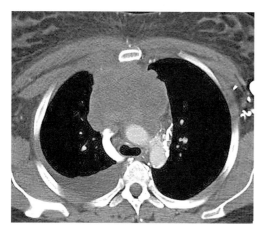

Fig. 159.7 Contrast-enhanced chest CT (mediastinal window) of a 24-year-old woman with weight loss, superior vena cava syndrome, and non-Hodgkin [primary large B-cell] lymphoma demonstrates a large anterior mediastinal mass that completely obstructs the superior vena cava. Note marked enhancement of the azygos venous system as well as mediastinal and chest wall collaterals and moderate right pleural effusion.

- Lymphoma is not a surgical lesion. If lymphoma is suspected, biopsy should be performed for definitive diagnosis.
- *Thoracic Hodgkin lymphoma* may recur in the originally affected mediastinum, in other mediastinal compartments, or in the lung.
- *Mediastinal lymphoma* may manifest with locally invasive disease and superior vena cava syndrome (**Figs. 159.5, 159.7**)
- Advanced lung cancer with mediastinal metastases may manifest as a locally invasive dominant mediastinal mass, particularly in cases of small cell carcinoma.
- Extra-pulmonary malignancies (particularly renal cell, testicular, and head and neck carcinomas) may metastasize to intrathoracic lymph nodes (without concomitant pulmonary metastases) and may manifest as dominant mediastinal abnormalities that mimic lymphoma and metastatic lung cancer (**Fig. 159.8**).

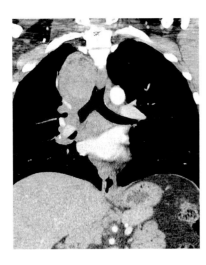

Fig. 159.8   Coronal contrast-enhanced chest CT (mediastinal window) of a 32-year-old woman with metastatic melanoma demonstrates right paratracheal, right hilar, and subcarinal lymphadenopathy.

Suggested Readings

1. Cronin CG, Swords R, Truong MT, et al. Clinical utility of PET/CT in lymphoma. AJR Am J Roentgenol 2010;194(1): W91–W103

2. Paes FM, Kalkanis DG, Sideras PA, Serafini AN. FDG PET/CT of extranodal involvement in non-Hodgkin lymphoma and Hodgkin disease. Radiographics 2010;30(1):269–291

3. Hansell DM, Armstrong P, Lynch DA, et al. Neoplasms of the lungs, airways and pleura. In: Hansell DM, Armstrong P, Lynch DA, McAdams HP, eds. Imaging of Diseases of the Chest, 4th ed. Philadelphia: Elsevier Mosby; 2005:901–1021

4. Strollo DC, Rosado-de-Christenson ML. Tumors of the thymus. J Thorac Imaging 1999;14(3):152–171

CASE 160

■ Clinical Presentation

28-year-old woman with chest pain and dyspnea

■ Radiologic Findings

PA chest radiograph (**Fig. 160.1**) demonstrates decreased right lung volume, right hilar fullness, and paucity of right lower lobe vasculature. Axial and coronal contrast-enhanced chest CT (mediastinal window) (**Figs. 160.2, 160.3**) shows a right hilar soft-tissue mass with multifocal internal calcifications that obliterates the lumen of the right pulmonary artery. Contrast-enhanced chest CT (lung window) (**Fig. 160.4**) reveals attenuation in the caliber of the right lower lobe pulmonary arteries and right lower lobe peripheral ground glass opacity.

■ Diagnosis

Mediastinal Fibrosis

■ Differential Diagnosis

- Lung Cancer
- Lymphoma
- Metastatic Mediastinal Lymphadenopathy
- Other Non-Neoplastic Lymphadenopathies
  - Mycobacterial Infection
  - Fungal Disease
  - Sarcoidosis
  - Silicosis

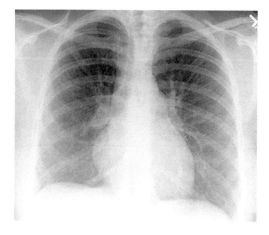

Fig. 160.1

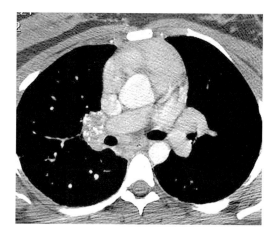

Fig. 160.2

774

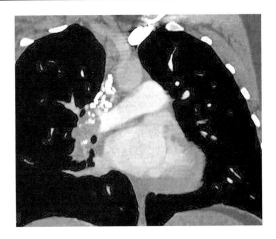

Fig. 160.3

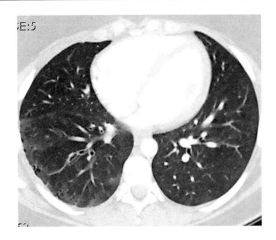

Fig. 160.4

■ Discussion

Background

Mediastinal fibrosis is the proliferation of dense fibrous tissue in the mediastinum with resultant focal or infiltrative masses, which may be locally invasive.

Etiology

Mediastinal fibrosis may be associated with granulomatous infection, typically with *Histoplasma capsulatum* (and rarely with other fungi and *Mycobacterium tuberculosis*). Mediastinal fibrosis also occurs as an idiopathic condition, which may be related to other fibro-inflammatory disorders such as retroperitoneal fibrosis.

Clinical Findings

Mediastinal fibrosis typically affects young patients, but it is reported in all age groups. Affected patients present with signs and symptoms of obstruction of vital mediastinal structures, including the trachea, main bronchi, esophagus, systemic veins, and pulmonary arteries and veins. Symptoms include cough, dyspnea, recurrent infection, hemoptysis, chest pain, and dysphagia.

Imaging Features

Chest Radiography

- Non-specific mediastinal widening often affecting the middle compartment
- Hilar enlargement (**Fig. 160.1**)
- Associated pulmonary granulomas and/or hilar/mediastinal lymph node calcifications (**Fig. 160.1**)

MDCT

- Localized or diffuse, locally invasive soft tissue in the mediastinum/hilum (**Figs. 160.2, 160.3, 160.5, 160.6**)
- May demonstrate intrinsic calcification (**Figs. 160.2, 160.3, 160.5**)
- Location and extent of involvement; exclusion of vascular, airway or esophageal involvement (**Figs. 160.2, 160.3, 160.5, 160.6**)
- Indirect findings:
    ○ Enhanced vascular collaterals, enlargement of uninvolved vessels (**Figs. 160.5, 160.6**)
    ○ Abnormal lung attenuation—wedge-shaped opacities representing infarcts, ground glass opacities, thickening of interlobular septa, post-obstructive pneumonia, and/or atelectasis related to arterial, venous, or bronchial obstruction (**Fig. 160.4**)

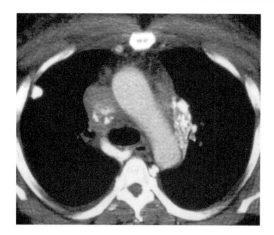

Fig. 160.5 Contrast-enhanced chest CT (mediastinal window) of a middle-aged man with superior vena cava syndrome demonstrates a right paratracheal soft-tissue mass with multi-focal internal calcifications, which obliterates the lumen of the superior vena cava and prominent mediastinal collateral vessels. Note the calcified right upper lobe solitary pulmonary nodule.

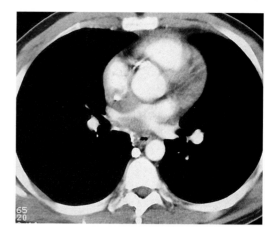

Fig. 160.6 Contrast-enhanced chest CT (mediastinal window) of a 30-year-old man with mediastinal fibrosis and superior vena cava syndrome demonstrates infiltrating middle mediastinal soft tissue that encases and narrows the right superior pulmonary vein.

MRI

- Heterogeneous infiltrative mass of intermediate signal intensity on T1WI
- May demonstrate areas of high and very low signal intensity on both T1WI and T2WI
- Low signal intensity foci on T2WI images corresponding to calcification or fibrosis

Management

- Systemic antifungal agents with reported cases of disease stabilization
- Surgical excision of localized disease; may require vascular/airway reconstruction
- Laser therapy, balloon dilatation, and stenting of obstructed vessels and bronchi; venous bypass grafts for vena cava occlusion

Prognosis

- Mortality of up to 30%; recurrent infection, hemoptysis, cor pulmonale

PEARLS

- Locally invasive mediastinal soft tissue with associated calcification in a young patient from an area where histoplasmosis is endemic suggests the diagnosis of mediastinal fibrosis.
- In the absence of calcification, malignant neoplasia must be considered, and biopsy is indicated.

Suggested Readings

1. Atasoy C, Fitoz S, Erguvan B, Akyar S. Tuberculous fibrosing mediastinitis: CT and MRI findings. J Thorac Imaging 2001;16(3):191–193
2. Rossi SE, McAdams HP, Rosado-de-Christenson ML, Franks TJ, Galvin JR. Fibrosing mediastinitis. Radiographics 2001;21(3):737–757

CASE 161

■ Clinical Presentation

28-year-old man with malaise, fever, night sweats, skin lesions, and palpable supraclavicular lymphadenopathy

■ Radiologic Findings

Contrast-enhanced chest CT (mediastinal window) (**Figs. 161.1, 161.2**) demonstrates multiple borderline enlarged mediastinal and right internal mammary lymph nodes and enlarged right axillary lymph nodes which exhibit intense contrast enhancement.

■ Diagnosis

Multicentric Castleman Disease

■ Differential Diagnosis

* Metastatic Disease
* Lymphoma
* Angioimmunoblastic Lymphadenopathy

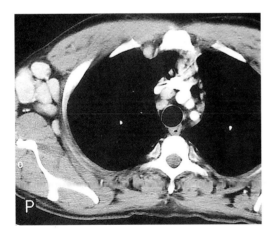

Fig. 161.1

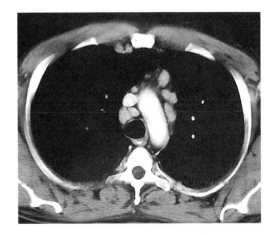

Fig. 161.2 *(Reproduced with permission from Parker MS. Multicentric hyaline-vascular Castleman disease. Clin Radiol 2007; 62:707–710.)*

■ Discussion

Background

Castleman disease, also known as angiofollicular or giant lymph node hyperplasia, is a rare lymphoproliferative disorder characterized by lymph node enlargement with extensive capillary proliferation. Two forms of Castleman disease are recognized, *localized* or *unicentric* (the most common) and *multicentric* or *disseminated*. Three different cell types of Castleman disease are recognized: hyaline-vascular cell, plasma cell, and mixed cellular. Over 90% of cases are of the hyaline-vascular cell type. Although this disorder characteristically affects lymph nodes, pulmonary involvement may also occur.

Etiology

Castleman disease is a disorder of unknown etiology.

Clinical Findings

Localized Castleman disease characteristically affects adults in the third or fourth decade of life. Affected patients are often entirely asymptomatic, but may also present with symptoms of compression or local invasion. Most patients with *multicentric Castleman disease* are symptomatic and present with systemic and constitutional complaints, organomegaly, and frequent palpable lymphadenopathy. Cutaneous lesions may also occur. Multicentric Castleman disease has been described in association with other diseases, including infection with HIV, Kaposi sarcoma, and POEMS syndrome (polyneuropathy, organomegaly, endocrinopathy, monoclonal gammopathy and skin changes). Progression to non-Hodgkin lymphoma has been described in approximately 25% of cases.

Imaging Features

Chest Radiography

- Non-specific mediastinal/hilar enlargement secondary to lymphadenopathy
- Parenchymal abnormalities in cases of multicentric Castleman disease with pulmonary involvement

MDCT

Localized Castleman Disease

- Solitary well-defined mediastinal mass without associated lymphadenopathy
- Dominant mass with associated lymphadenopathy
- Multiple enlarged lymph nodes confined to one mediastinal compartment
- Intense contrast enhancement of soft-tissue masses and affected lymph nodes
- Calcification in 10% of cases

Multicentric Castleman Disease

- Mediastinal/hilar lymphadenopathy
- Supraclavicular/axillary/other intrathoracic lymphadenopathy
- Intense contrast enhancement, particularly with hyaline vascular Castleman disease (**Figs. 161.1, 161.2**)
- Pleural effusion
- Pulmonary involvement by lymphocytic interstitial pneumonia (LIP)
  - ◦ Centrilobular nodules; nodular thickening of bronchovascular bundles
  - ◦ Ground glass opacities
  - ◦ Consolidations

MRI

- Increased signal intensity on T1WI
- Hyperintense on T2WI; visualization of tissue septa
- Contrast enhancement with gadolinium

PET-CT

- Variable FDG uptake; may mimic malignant neoplasm

Management

- Preoperative embolization

Localized Castleman Disease

- Observation and supportive treatment
- Surgical excision

Multicentric Castleman Disease

- Chemotherapy (vinblastine [Velban], etoposide [Eposin]) for acute exacerbations
- Corticosteroids

Prognosis

- Good prognosis for patients with hyaline-vascular localized Castleman disease
- Poor prognosis for patients with multicentric Castleman disease; may progress to lymphoma in approximately 25% of cases

Suggested Readings

1. Guihot A, Couderc L-J, Rivaud E, et al. Thoracic radiographic and CT findings of multicentric Castleman disease in HIV-infected patients. J Thorac Imaging 2007;22(2):207–211

2. Gupta NK, Torigian DA, Gefter WB, et al. Mediastinal Castleman disease mimicking mediastinal pulmonary sequestration. J Thorac Imaging 2005;20(3):229–232

3. Ko S-F, Hsieh M-J, Ng S-H, et al. Imaging spectrum of Castleman's disease. AJR Am J Roentgenol 2004;182(3): 769–775

4. McAdams HP, Rosado-de-Christenson ML, Fishback NF, Templeton PA. Castleman disease of the thorax: radiologic features with clinical and histopathologic correlation. Radiology 1998;209(1):221–228

5. Parker MS. Multicentric hyaline-vascular Castleman's disease. Clin Radiol 2007;62(7):707–710

CASE 162

■ Clinical Presentation

25-year-old woman with cough

■ Radiologic Findings

PA (**Fig. 162.1**) and lateral (**Fig. 162.2**) chest radiographs demonstrate a well-defined middle-posterior mediastinal (subcarinal) mass that projects to the right of the midline on the frontal chest radiograph and projects over the posterior subcarinal region on the lateral chest radiograph. Contrast-enhanced chest CT (mediastinal window) (**Fig. 162.3**) shows a spherical fluid attenuation cystic lesion in the posterior subcarinal region with minimal discontinuous enhancement of a thin cyst wall.

■ Diagnosis

Bronchogenic Cyst

■ Differential Diagnosis

- Other Foregut-Derived Cysts; Esophageal, Gastroenteric
- Pericardial Cyst
- Lymphadenopathy

■ Discussion

Background

Congenital cysts represent approximately 20% of mediastinal masses affecting adults. Bronchogenic cyst is the most common congenital mediastinal cyst and is typically located in the middle-posterior compartment near the carina, but may also affect other mediastinal compartments, the pericardium, diaphragm, pleura, or lung.

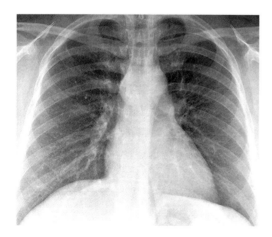

Fig. 162.1

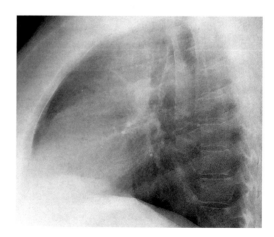

Fig. 162.2

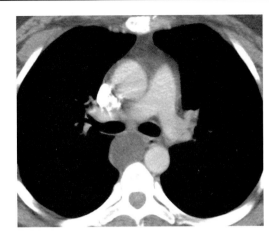

Fig. 162.3

Other foregut-derived congenital cysts include esophageal duplication cysts, which occur in the wall of the esophagus and middle-posterior mediastinum, respectively. Pericardial cysts are typically located in the cardiophrenic angle. Thymic cysts usually affect the anterior mediastinum and often represent acquired lesions.

Etiology

Congenital cysts are typically unilocular thin-walled lesions with a variable fluid content. *Bronchogenic cyst* is thought to result from abnormal budding of the primitive foregut or the developing tracheobronchial tree. The original connection to the foregut is usually obliterated resulting in a blind-ending fluid-filled thin-walled cyst. *Esophageal duplication cysts* may also derive from the primitive foregut as a result of anomalous esophageal development. *Pericardial cysts* are thought to result from disordered formation of the primitive coelomic cavities. While *unilocular thymic cysts* probably represent congenital anomalies related to the fetal thymopharyngeal duct, *multilocular thymic cysts* are generally considered acquired lesions related to trauma (including thoracotomy), thymic neoplasia, and radiation therapy for lymphoma. Multilocular thymic cysts affect approximately 1% of children infected with HIV in association with diffuse infiltrative lymphocytosis syndrome. They are also described in other immune-mediated disorders (e.g., Sjögren syndrome, aplastic anemia, myasthenia gravis).

Clinical Findings

Patients with bronchogenic cyst are typically young children and adults under the age of 40 years. Many are symptomatic and present because of chest pain and/or respiratory complaints related to mass effect on the airways. Patients with esophageal cysts are often asymptomatic adults and children, but some present with symptoms of esophageal/mediastinal mass effect or with local pain related to ectopic gastric mucosa in the cyst wall. Patients with pericardial cysts are invariably asymptomatic and diagnosed incidentally. Patients with thymic cysts are often asymptomatic children and young adults.

Imaging Findings

Radiography

Bronchogenic Cyst

- Well-defined spherical or ovoid middle mediastinal mass (subcarinal, paratracheal) (**Figs. 162.1, 162.2**); characteristic lateral displacement of the superior aspect of the azygoesophageal recess (**Fig. 162.1**)
- May attain large sizes and produce mass effect on adjacent structures

Esophageal Cyst

- Spherical or ovoid middle-posterior mediastinal mass

Pericardial Cyst

- Spherical or ovoid cardiophrenic angle mass; right-sided in 75% of cases

Thymic Cyst

- Well-defined, unilateral anterior mediastinal mass

MDCT

Bronchogenic Cyst

- Well-defined spherical subcarinal or paratracheal mediastinal mass (**Figs. 162.3, 162.4, 162.5**); may affect other mediastinal compartments, lung, diaphragm
- Homogeneous internal attenuation: soft tissue (43%), water (40%) (**Figs. 162.3, 162.4**); no internal enhancement (**Figs. 162.3, 162.4**)
- Thin, smooth wall best seen with contrast-enhanced studies or because of punctate, discontinuous mural calcification (**Fig. 162.4**)
- Rarely: fluid-fluid levels, milk of calcium (**Fig. 162.5**)

Esophageal Cyst

- Relationship to esophagus/esophageal wall (**Fig. 162.6**)
- Otherwise indistinguishable from bronchogenic cyst

Pericardial Cyst

- Smooth spherical/ovoid water attenuation mass at cardiophrenic angle (**Fig. 162.7**)
- Imperceptible non-enhancing cyst wall (**Fig. 162.7**)

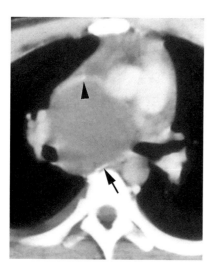

Fig. 162.4 Contrast-enhanced chest CT (mediastinal window) of a young man with a bronchogenic cyst demonstrates a large subcarinal mass of water attenuation with a thin peripheral enhancing wall (*arrow*) and punctate mural calcification (*arrowhead*). Note the small right pleural effusion.

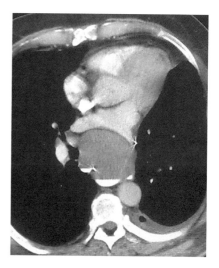

Fig. 162.5 Contrast-enhanced chest CT (mediastinal window) of a 60-year-old man with cough and dyspnea on exertion shows a subcarinal bronchogenic cyst of lobular contours with internal fluid-milk of calcium levels and mass effect on the contrast-filled esophagus and the left atrium. Note left pleural thickening and/or fluid.

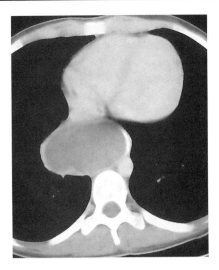

Fig. 162.6 Contrast-enhanced chest CT (mediastinal window) of a 14-year-old girl with dysphagia and an esophageal duplication cyst demonstrates a large ovoid cyst with water attenuation contents. Note the enhancing thin wall, the thin peripheral soft-tissue septa, and the arcuate contour of the contrast-filled esophageal lumen consistent with the mural location of the cyst.

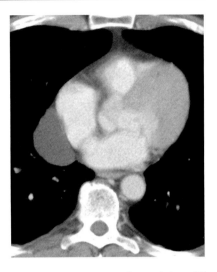

Fig. 162.7 Contrast-enhanced chest CT (mediastinal window) of a 45-year-old woman with an incidentally discovered pericardial cyst demonstrates an ovoid cystic lesion with an imperceptible wall and water attenuation contents adjacent to the right atrium.

Thymic Cyst

- Variable size, unilocular/multilocular cystic lesion with water attenuation contents (**Fig. 162.8**)
- Thin-walled, internal soft-tissue septa (**Fig. 162.8**), soft-tissue components, mural/septal calcifications

MRI

- Intermediate to high signal intensity on T1WI
- High signal intensity on T2WI (**Fig. 162.9**)
- Isointensity with cerebrospinal fluid (**Fig. 162.9**)
- Hemorrhage/infection, high signal intensity on both T1WI and T2WI; fluid-fluid level
- Visualization of thin wall (**Fig. 162.9**) and internal soft-tissue septa when present

Scintigraphy

- Uptake of Tc-99m sodium pertechnetate in ectopic gastric mucosa within esophageal cysts

Management

Bronchogenic/Esophageal Cysts

- Excision
- Aspiration, instillation of sclerosing agents, marsupialization
- Observation of patients who are not surgical candidates

Pericardial Cysts

- Observation

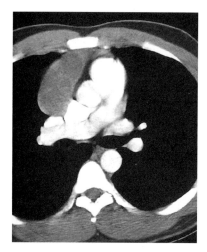

Fig. 162.8 Contrast-enhanced chest CT (mediastinal window) of an asymptomatic 23-year-old man with a thymic cyst demonstrates a multilocular cystic right anterior mediastinal mass in the anatomic location of the thymus. Note the thin enhancing soft-tissue septa that compartmentalize the cyst.

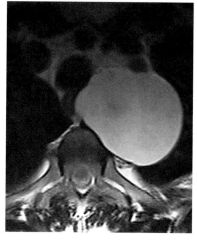

Fig. 162.9 T2-weighted MR of a 30-year-old woman with an incidentally diagnosed bronchogenic cyst demonstrates a spherical left middle-posterior mediastinal cystic mass with a thin low-signal-intensity wall and high-signal-intensity content (isointense with the adjacent cerebrospinal fluid).

Thymic Cysts

- Observation
- Excision for exclusion of cystic neoplasia

Prognosis

- Excellent
- Fluid re-accumulation in aspirated cysts; recurrence of symptoms

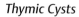

PEARLS

- Diagnosis of *bronchogenic cyst* should be suggested based on location, morphology, and absence of internal enhancement, as attenuation/signal may vary. Visualization of a thin peripheral wall (best seen after intravenous contrast media) and/or fluid-fluid levels strongly supports the diagnosis. MR is helpful in the evaluation of high-attenuation bronchogenic cysts through demonstration of isointensity to cerebrospinal fluid. Bronchogenic cyst is indistinguishable from other foregut cysts; differentiation requires microscopic evaluation of the cyst wall.
- *Thymic cysts* are rare mediastinal lesions. Thus, cystic neoplasia should always be excluded, particularly in the presence of mural nodules and/or lymphadenopathy.
- *Gastroenteric cysts* are rare congenital foregut cysts characterized by their fibrous connection to the vertebrae. They are typically diagnosed in symptomatic infants and manifest as spherical paravertebral soft-tissue masses associated with spinal dysraphism, butterfly or hemivertebrae, and/or scoliosis.

Suggested Readings

1. Choi YW, McAdams HP, Jeon SC, et al. Idiopathic multilocular thymic cyst: CT features with clinical and histopathologic correlation. AJR Am J Roentgenol 2001;177(4):881–885

2. Hansell DM, Armstrong P, Lynch DA, et al. Mediastinal and aortic disease. In: Hansell DM, Armstrong P, Lynch DA, McAdams HP, eds. Imaging of Diseases of the Chest, 4th ed. Philadelphia: Elsevier Mosby; 2005:901–1021

3. Jeung M-Y, Gasser B, Gangi A, et al. Imaging of cystic masses of the mediastinum. Radiographics 2002;22(Spec No): S79–S93

4. McAdams HP, Kirejczyk WM, Rosado-de-Christenson ML, Matsumoto S. Bronchogenic cyst: imaging features with clinical and histopathologic correlation. Radiology 2000;217(2):441–446

CASE 163

■ Clinical Presentation

40-year-old woman with chest discomfort

■ Radiologic Findings

PA (**Fig. 163.1**) and lateral (**Fig. 163.2**) chest radiographs demonstrate a well-defined lobular soft-tissue mass situated predominantly in the right paravertebral region and extending into the middle-posterior mediastinum (**Fig. 163.2**), with associated displacement, pressure erosion, and sclerosis of the adjacent right posterior third rib (*arrow*) (**Fig. 163.1**). Contrast-enhanced chest CT (mediastinal window) (**Fig. 163.3**) shows a heterogeneously enhancing soft-tissue mass, which extends through the neuroforamen into the spinal canal. Contrast-enhanced axial T1WI-MRI (**Fig. 163.4**) reveals heterogeneous enhancement and intraspinal tumor growth (**Fig. 163.4**).

■ Diagnosis

Schwannoma

■ Differential Diagnosis

- Other Neurogenic Neoplasm: Neurofibroma, Ganglioneuroma
- Thoracic Meningocele
- Extramedullary Hematopoiesis

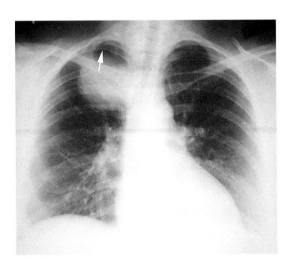

Fig. 163.1

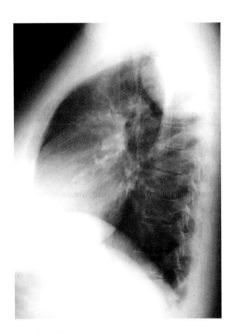

Fig. 163.2

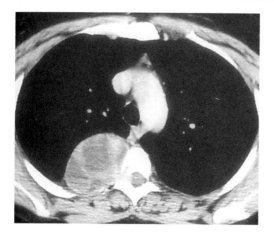

Fig. 163.3

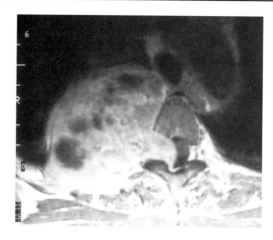

Fig. 163.4

■ Discussion

Background

Neurogenic neoplasms represent approximately 20% of mediastinal masses in adults and approximately 35% in children. They are the most common neoplasms of the paravertebral region (typically located near the neuroforamen), but may arise in other locations. Neoplasms of peripheral nerve origin are typically benign (schwannoma, neurofibroma, plexiform neurofibroma), but malignant peripheral nerve sheath tumors also occur and are more common in patients with NF-1. Schwannoma is the most frequent paravertebral neurogenic neoplasm, followed by neurofibroma. Neoplasms that arise from sympathetic (or parasympathetic) ganglia may be benign (ganglioneuroma) or malignant (ganglioneuroblastoma, neuroblastoma). Malignant sympathetic ganglia neurogenic neoplasms typically affect symptomatic neonates and infants, carry a poor prognosis, and will not be discussed further.

Etiology

The etiology of neurogenic neoplasms is unknown, and most lesions arise spontaneously. Neurofibromatosis-1 (NF-1) is associated with multifocal neurogenic neoplasms and a high risk of malignant transformation.

Clinical Findings

The majority of patients with benign neurogenic neoplasms are asymptomatic. Large lesions may produce symptoms related to mass effect: cough, pain, dyspnea, and/or hoarseness. Approximately 10% exhibit intraspinal growth and may produce symptoms of spinal cord compression. Patients with peripheral nerve neoplasms (schwannoma, neurofibroma, malignant nerve sheath tumor) are typically young adults in the third and fourth decades of life. Patients with sympathetic ganglia neoplasms (ganglioneuroma) are usually older children (over the age of 4 years), adolescents, and young adults. NF-1, the most common neurocutaneous disorder, is an autosomal dominant disease (although approximately 50% of cases occur spontaneously) that manifests with multifocal cutaneous and plexiform neurofibromas, other neurogenic and non-neurogenic neoplasms, skin pigmentation, skeletal defects, and pulmonary fibrosis. Affected patients often exhibit solitary or multiple neurogenic neoplasms of the paravertebral region and other thoracic locations. Patients with NF-1 are at a higher risk of malignant transformation of a neurogenic neoplasm.

Imaging Findings

Chest Radiography

Schwannoma/Neurofibroma

- Well-defined spherical or ovoid smooth or lobular paravertebral soft-tissue mass (**Figs. 163.1, 163.2**)
- Osseous abnormalities in 50% of cases: expansion of neuroforamen, pressure erosion of adjacent vertebrae and ribs, rib deformity (**Fig. 163.1**)

Neurofibromatosis

- Focal or multifocal soft-tissue masses typically adjacent to ribs, in paravertebral regions and in mediastinum
- Rib erosion, separation of adjacent ribs, dysplastic changes (*ribbon rib deformity*); posterior scalloping of vertebral bodies, enlarged neuroforamina
- Short segment acute angulation scoliosis
- Lateral meningocele, right-sided predominance

Malignant Peripheral Nerve Sheath Tumor

- Large, rapidly growing, spherical posterior mediastinal mass

Ganglioneuroma

- Well-defined elongated mass along anterolateral spine
- Vertical orientation, tapered appearance
- Associated benign skeletal erosion/sclerosis

MDCT

- Osseous erosion/deformity, intraspinal extension (**Fig. 163.3**)

Schwannoma/Neurofibroma

- Homogeneous/heterogeneous attenuation, typically lower than that of skeletal muscle
- Heterogeneous enhancement (**Fig. 163.3**)
- Punctate calcification in 10%

Neurofibromatosis

- Focal mass or multi-focal masses affecting multiple thoracic nerves
- Low attenuation, calcification
- Pressure erosion, enlarged neuroforamina
- Lateral thoracic meningocele: homogeneous, spherical, well-defined paraspinal mass of water attenuation with adjacent osseous erosion/sclerosis/neuroforamen enlargement (**Fig. 163.5A**)
- Basal interstitial fibrosis, apical bullae

Malignant Peripheral Nerve Sheath Tumor

- Large round mass (over 5 cm in diameter)
- Large areas of low attenuation, multi-focal calcification
- Mass effect
- Pleural effusion, pleural nodules
- Pulmonary metastases

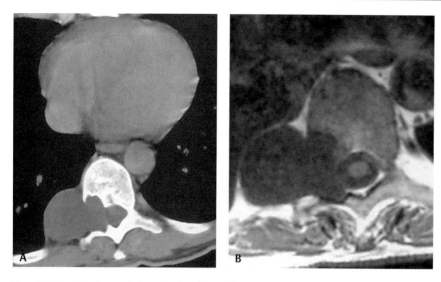

Fig. 163.5   Unenhanced chest CT (mediastinal window) **(A)** of a 45-year-old man with neurofibromatosis-1 demonstrates a low-attenuation spherical right paraspinal mass that extends through the neuroforamen with resultant expansion and adjacent osseous sclerosis and scalloping. Axial T1-weighted MR **(B)** shows the mass exhibits the same signal intensity as that of cerebrospinal fluid.

Ganglioneuroma

- Homogeneous or heterogeneous (**Fig. 163.6**)
- Low to intermediate attenuation (**Fig. 163.6**)
- Punctate to coarse calcification in up to 60% (**Fig. 163.6**)

MRI

- Exclusion of neuroforaminal/intraspinal growth; dumbbell-shaped tumors

Schwannoma/Neurofibroma

- Low to intermediate signal intensity on T1WI
- Intermediate to high signal intensity on T2WI; high-signal-intensity regions related to cystic degeneration (**Fig. 163.4**)

Neurofibromatosis

- Focal or multi-focal neurogenic neoplasms; infiltration of entire nerve trunk in plexiform neurofibromas (the hallmark lesion of NF-1)
- Variable signal intensity on T1WI; peripheral hyperintensity and central hypointensity on T2WI images (*target sign*) (**Fig. 163.7**)
- Lateral thoracic meningocele: low signal intensity on T1WI (**Fig. 163.5B**), high signal intensity on T2WI, parallels cerebrospinal fluid signal; no enhancement

Ganglioneuroma

- Homogeneous intermediate signal intensity on all sequences
- Whorled heterogeneous appearance; curvilinear or nodular low-signal-intensity bands on T1WI and T2WI images

PET-CT

- FDG PET for the diagnosis of malignant peripheral nerve sheath tumors in patients with NF-1; increased specificity for diagnosis with addition of ^{11}C-methionine PET; used to guide biopsy and direct therapy

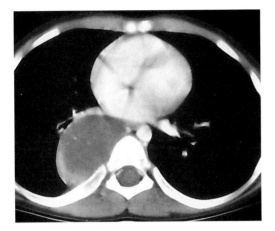

Fig. 163.6 Contrast-enhanced chest CT (mediastinal window) of an asymptomatic 7-year-old boy with a right paravertebral ganglioneuroma demonstrates a heterogeneously enhancing ovoid mass of predominant low attenuation with multi-focal internal punctate calcifications. Note the mass effect on adjacent vessels and bronchi.

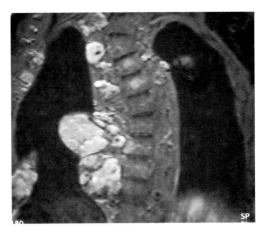

Fig. 163.7 T2-weighted coronal MR of a young woman with neurofibromatosis-1 demonstrates multi-focal paravertebral and chest wall masses of heterogeneous high signal intensity. Note the classic *target sign* appearance exhibited by some of the lesions.

Management

• Surgical excision

Prognosis

• Excellent prognosis for patients with excised benign neurogenic neoplasms
• Excised solitary malignant peripheral nerve sheath tumor: 75% five-year survival
• Patients with neurofibromatosis and malignant peripheral nerve sheath tumor: 15–30% five-year survivals

PEARLS

• Thoracic meningocele (intrathoracic extrusion of meningeal membranes and their fluid content) typically affects patients with neurofibromatosis and manifests on radiography as a well-defined spherical paravertebral mass that may mimic a neurogenic neoplasm. Associated findings include enlargement of an adjacent neuroforamen and pressure erosion/sclerosis of adjacent vertebrae. CT demonstrates osseous "scalloping" and sclerosis and a fluid attenuation lesion (**Fig. 163.5A**). MRI establishes the diagnosis by demonstrating signal intensity that parallels that of adjacent cerebrospinal fluid (**Fig. 163.5B**).

Suqqested Readinq

1. Bredella MA, Torriani M, Hornicek F, et al. Value of PET in the assessment of patients with neurofibromatosis type 1. AJR Am J Roentgenol 2007;189(4):928–935

2. Hansell DM, Armstrong P, Lynch DA, et al. Mediastinal and aortic disease. In: Hansell DM, Armstrong P, Lynch DA, McAdams HP, eds. Imaging of Diseases of the Chest, 4th ed. Philadelphia: Elsevier Mosby; 2005:901–1021

3. Lonergan GJ, Schwab CM, Suarez ES, Carlson CL. Neuroblastoma, ganglioneuroblastoma, and ganglioneuroma: radiologic-pathologic correlation. Radiographics 2002;22(4):911–934

4. Rossi SE, Erasmus JJ, McAdams HP, et al. Thoracic manifestations of neurofibromatosis-I. AJR Am J Roentgenol 1999;173:1631–1638

5. Tanaka O, Kiryu T, Hirose Y, Iwata H, Hoshi H. Neurogenic tumors of the mediastinum and chest wall: MR imaging appearance. J Thorac Imaging 2005;20(4):316–320

CASE 164

■ Clinical Presentation

Elderly woman with respiratory distress and a chronic left neck mass

■ Radiologic Findings

Coned-down PA chest radiograph (**Fig. 164.1**) demonstrates a large, well-defined left-sided mediastinal soft-tissue mass and an associated ipsilateral neck mass. Note marked mass effect on the cervical and intrathoracic portions of the trachea. Contrast-enhanced chest CT (mediastinal window) (**Figs. 164.2, 164.3**) shows a large, heterogeneously enhancing soft-tissue mass that arises from the left lobe of the thyroid gland (**Fig. 164.2**) and extends into the mediastinum (**Fig. 164.3**). Note the large area of central low attenuation surrounded by irregular enhancing soft tissue and significant mass effect on the trachea, esophagus, and mediastinal great vessels.

■ Diagnosis

Mediastinal Goiter

■ Differential Diagnosis

- Thyroid Carcinoma
- Lymphadenopathy; Lymphoma
- Neurogenic Neoplasm

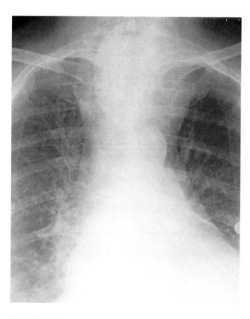

Fig. 164.1

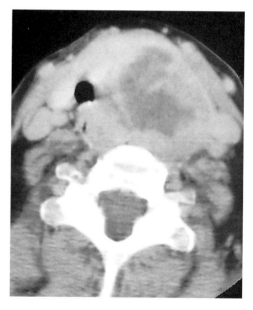

Fig. 164.2

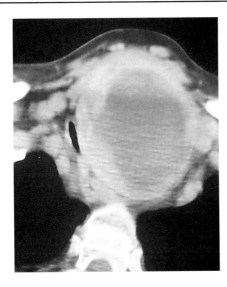

Fig. 164.3

■ Discussion

Background

Mediastinal (intrathoracic, substernal, retrosternal) *goiter* refers to thyroid tissue within the mediastinum. Mediastinal goiter affects approximately 5% of the world population. The term *substernal goiter* is sometimes employed to refer to mediastinal goiters in which over 50% of the mass resides below the thoracic inlet. Approximately 80% of mediastinal goiters arise from the inferior aspect of a thyroid lobe or from the thyroid isthmus and extend into the anterior mediastinum. The rest arise from the posterior aspect of the thyroid, extend into the middle-posterior mediastinum (so-called posterior descending goiters), and are predominantly right-sided.

Etiology

Most mediastinal goiters result from intrathoracic growth of a thyroid goiter, and up to 17% of cervical goiters extend into the thorax. Primary intrathoracic (aberrant or ectopic) goiters are rare (accounting for less than 1% of excised lesions) and are thought to result from abnormal embryologic migration of the thyroid cells.

Clinical Findings

Most affected patients are women in the fifth decade of life. Patients with mediastinal goiter are usually asymptomatic adults with a long history of a thyroid mass. Symptoms of tracheal, esophageal, vascular, or recurrent laryngeal nerve compression may occur, typically dyspnea, wheezing, stridor, dysphagia, and hoarseness.

Imaging Findings

Chest Radiography

- Well-defined smooth or lobular mediastinal soft-tissue mass with frequent mass effect on the airway (**Fig. 164.1**)
  - Associated cervical soft-tissue mass with contralateral airway displacement (**Fig. 164.1**)
  - Isolated mediastinal mass
- Focal or multi-focal calcification
- Right-sided mediastinal mass in most posterior mediastinal goiters, even when originating from the left thyroid lobe

MDCT

- Well-defined high-attenuation soft-tissue mass on unenhanced CT
- Heterogeneous attenuation from focal or multi-focal punctate or coarse calcification or hemorrhage and/or cystic change (**Figs. 164.2, 164.3, 164.4A, 164.4B**)
- Early intense and sustained contrast enhancement; frequent foci of low attenuation (**Figs. 164.4A, 164.4B**)
- Continuity with cervical thyroid (**Figs. 164.2, 164.4A**)

MRI

- Demonstration of continuity with cervical thyroid on sagittal and coronal imaging
- Heterogeneous signal intensity on T1- and T2-weighted images

Scintigraphy

- Uptake of Tc-99m
- Uptake of I-123 and I-131; false positives reported

Management

- Recognition and observation in asymptomatic patients
- Surgical excision in symptomatic patients (tracheal, esophageal, vascular, nerve compression) and in those with malignant transformation

Prognosis

- Favorable prognosis in patients with multinodular goiter
- Guarded prognosis in patients with thyroiditis or malignancy

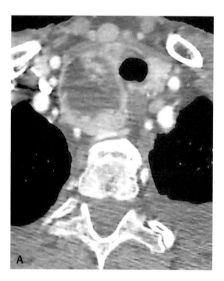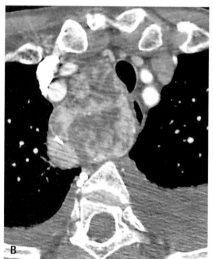

Fig. 164.4   Coned-down contrast-enhanced chest CT (mediastinal window) of an asymptomatic middle-aged woman with a posterior descending goiter demonstrates a heterogeneously enhancing mass with punctate calcifications arising from the posterior aspect of an enlarged heterogeneously enhancing right thyroid lobe and extending into the adjacent mediastinum with mass effect on the trachea and esophagus. Note intense and sustained contrast enhancement of the thyroid and the peripheral aspects of the goiter.

PEARLS

- Presumptive diagnosis of mediastinal goiter can be made in most asymptomatic patients with a known chronic cervical goiter based on clinical presentation and imaging features.
- CT is the imaging modality of choice for the evaluation of mediastinal goiter. While scintigraphy is useful, it may fail to demonstrate features of malignancy, and false positive studies are reported.
- Local invasion and lymphadenopathy should suggest thyroid carcinoma.
- Diagnosis of ectopic mediastinal goiter should be considered in asymptomatic patients with isolated high-attenuation anterior mediastinal masses that exhibit intense and sustained contrast enhancement. The diagnosis may be confirmed with scintigraphy.

Suggested Reading

1. Buckley JA, Stark P. Intrathoracic mediastinal thyroid goiter: imaging manifestations. AJR Am J Roentgenol 1999; 173(2):471–475

2. Hansell DM, Armstrong P, Lynch DA, et al. Mediastinal and aortic disease. In: Hansell DM, Armstrong P, Lynch DA, McAdams HP, eds. Imaging of Diseases of the Chest, 4th ed. Philadelphia: Elsevier Mosby; 2005:901–1021

3. Hopkins CR, Reading CC. Thyroid and parathyroid imaging. Semin Ultrasound CT MR 1995;16(4):279–295

CASE 165

■ Clinical Presentation

24-year-old woman with a palpable neck mass

■ Radiologic Findings

PA chest radiograph (**Fig. 165.1**) demonstrates a well-defined right middle-posterior mediastinal (paratracheal) mass that produces mass effect on the cervical and intrathoracic portions of the trachea. Contrast-enhanced chest CT (mediastinal window) (**Figs. 165.2, 165.3**) shows a multilocular cystic right neck mass of water attenuation contents with thin internal soft-tissue septa (**Fig. 165.2**) that extends into the mediastinum, insinuating between adjacent vascular structures (**Fig. 165.3**), and produces mass effect on the trachea and esophagus (**Fig. 165.3**).

■ Diagnosis

Lymphangioma

■ Differential Diagnosis

- Congenital or Acquired Cyst
  - Bronchogenic Cyst
  - Thyroglossal Cyst
  - Branchial Cleft Cyst
  - Thymic Cyst
- Mature Teratoma

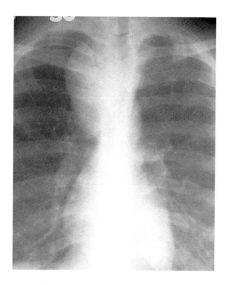

Fig. 165.1

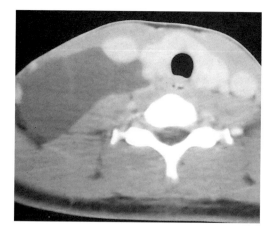

Fig. 165.2

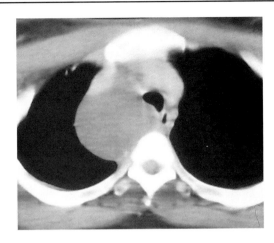

Fig. 165.3

■ Discussion

Background

Lymphangiomas are composed of malformed fluid-filled vascular spaces. Lymphangiomas are classified as cystic hygromas, cavernous lymphangiomas, and capillary lymphangiomas based on the size of the vascular spaces. Recently, lymphangiomas have also been referred to as lymphatic malformations and have been classified as macrocystic (>1 cm cystic spaces) and microcystic (0.5–10 mm cystic spaces) for purposes of minimally invasive management.

Etiology

The etiology of lymphangioma is poorly understood. Developmental, hamartomatous, and neoplastic origins have been postulated.

Clinical Findings

Approximately 90% of patients with lymphangioma are diagnosed in infancy (under the age of 2 years) because of a palpable mass in the neck, head, chest wall, and/or axilla. Approximately 10% of lymphangiomas extend into the mediastinum, and primary mediastinal lymphangiomas are rare. Mediastinal lymphangioma represents up to 4.5% of all mediastinal masses in adults. Affected patients may present with symptoms related to mass effect, including cough, wheezing, and pain. Rarely, mediastinal lymphangiomas result from recurrence of previously excised lymphangiomas. Hemangioma is a related vascular lesion that may coexist with lymphangioma or may occur as an isolated mass.

Imaging Findings

Chest Radiography

- Well-defined mediastinal soft-tissue mass (**Fig. 165.1**)
  - Mediastinal mass with cervical and/or chest wall component (**Fig. 165.1**)
  - Isolated mediastinal mass
- Anterior-superior mediastinum; other compartments also affected
- May produce mass effect on mediastinal structures or cervical trachea (**Fig. 165.1**)

MDCT

- Well-defined mediastinal mass (may exhibit continuity with ipsilateral cervical mass) (**Figs. 165.2, 165.3**)
- Cystic or multilocular (heterogeneous) cystic mass with water attenuation contents and enhancing soft-tissue elements (thin septa, larger soft-tissue components) (**Figs. 165.2, 165.3**)

- Non-enhancing low- (water or soft-tissue) attenuation mass (**Fig. 165.3**)
- May conform to or insinuate around normal structures; may produce mass effect (**Fig. 165.3**)
- Rarely calcification, soft-tissue attenuation, spiculated borders

MRI

- Intermediate to high signal intensity on T1WI
- Heterogeneous high signal intensity on T2WI
  - Low signal intensity on T2WI with hemorrhage or fibrosis
- Enhancing thin tissue septa surrounding intermediate-signal-intensity cystic spaces

Management

- Percutaneous drainage and ablation
- Surgical excision

Prognosis

- Excellent prognosis
- Reports of local recurrence

PEARLS

- *Lymphangioma* should be included in the differential diagnosis of multilocular cystic mediastinal masses affecting young patients, particularly when the lesion exhibits extension into the neck, chest wall, or axilla.
- *Mediastinal hemangioma* is a rare benign vascular mediastinal tumor that is typically diagnosed in asymptomatic young adults and is composed of interconnecting blood-filled endothelial-lined vascular channels with foci of organized thrombus and phleboliths. Radiography demonstrates a well-defined mediastinal soft-tissue mass. CT demonstrates multifocal punctate calcification in 28% of cases (**Fig. 165.4A**), heterogeneous attenuation on unenhanced studies, and intense heterogeneous enhancement that parallels vascular enhancement following contrast (**Fig. 165.4B**).

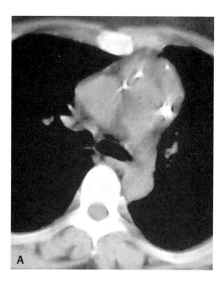 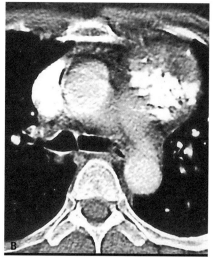

Fig. 165.4 Unenhanced (**A**) and contrast-enhanced chest CT (**B**) (mediastinal window) of an asymptomatic middle-aged woman with a mediastinal hemangioma demonstrates a well-defined heterogeneous mediastinal mass with multifocal punctate calcifications (**B**). Note the intense heterogeneous enhancement after contrast administration, which parallels the attenuation of the pulmonary vessels and the mediastinal veins (**B**).

Suggested Reading

1. Charruau L, Parrens M, Jougon J, et al. Mediastinal lymphangioma in adults: CT and MR imaging features. Eur Radiol 2000;10(8):1310–1314

2. Jeung M-Y, Gasser B, Gangi A, et al. Imaging of cystic masses of the mediastinum. Radiographics 2002;22(Spec No): S79–S93

3. McAdams HP, Rosado-de-Christenson ML, Moran CA. Mediastinal hemangioma: radiographic and CT features in 14 patients. Radiology 1994;193(2):399–402

4. Shaffer K, Rosado-de-Christenson ML, Patz EF Jr, et al. Thoracic lymphangioma in adults: CT and MR imaging features. AJR Am J Roentgenol 1994;162:283–289

5. Shiels WE II. Lymphatic malformation treatment: defining state-of-the-art. Nationwide Children's Hospital, Columbus, OH Issue 33, Fall 2008. www.NationwideChildrens.org/Radiology

CASE 166

■ Clinical Presentation

Asymptomatic elderly man with known cirrhosis and portal hypertension

■ Radiologic Findings

PA (**Fig. 166.1**) and lateral (**Fig. 166.2**) chest radiographs demonstrate a large retrocardiac middle/posterior mediastinal mass, basilar reticular opacities, and elevation of the right hemidiaphragm. Contrast-enhanced chest CT (mediastinal window) (**Figs. 166.3, 166.4**) reveals a complex paraesophageal mass composed of numerous enhancing tortuous serpiginous vascular structures. The degree of contrast enhancement within the lesion parallels that of the adjacent aorta and hemiazygos vein. Note the thickened nodular esophageal wall with minute intensely enhancing foci adjacent to the esophageal lumen and the abdominal ascites.

■ Diagnosis

Paraesophageal and Esophageal Varices

■ Differential Diagnosis

• None

■ Discussion

Background

Paraesophageal and esophageal varices represent dilated extrinsic and intrinsic esophageal veins, respectively. They are supplied by the left gastric vein, which arises at the portal venous confluence and courses through the gastric fundus to drain into the lower esophageal plexus veins, serving as a portosystemic col-

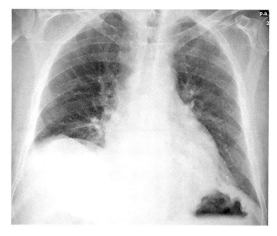

Fig. 166.1

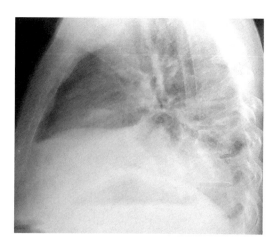

Fig. 166.2

798

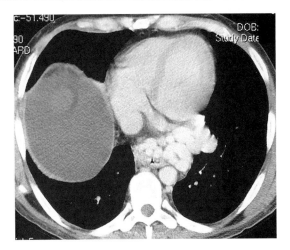

Fig. 166.3

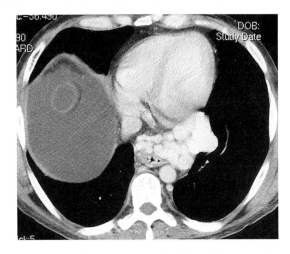

Fig. 166.4   (*Images courtesy of H. Page McAdams, MD, Duke University Medical Center, Durham, North Carolina.*)

lateral pathway in patients with portal hypertension. The posterior branch of the left gastric vein supplies the *paraesophageal varices* and the anterior branch supplies the *gastroesophageal varices*. *Paraesophageal varices* are located outside the esophageal wall, communicate with esophageal varices, and typically drain into the azygos/hemiazygos system, the subclavian/brachiocephalic system, or the inferior vena cava. *Esophageal varices* are located within the wall of the inferior esophagus. These collateral pathways allow decompression of the portal vein into the systemic circulation.

Etiology

Paraesophageal varices result from severe liver disease and portal hypertension (portal venous pressure greater than 10 mm Hg). Two hypotheses are proposed for their pathogenesis: (1) increased sinusoidal pressure (and increased resistance to flow) resulting from collagen deposition in the spaces of Disse and hepatocyte swelling, and (2) endogenous hepatic vasoconstrictors and mesenteric vasodilators that produce increased blood flow and pressure in the portal venous system. It is probable that both mechanisms play a role. Portal venous hypertension results in reversal of flow (away from the liver, or hepatofugal) through intrahepatic arterioportal communications, through the vasa vasora that supply the walls of the portal veins, or at the portal triad through direct blood shunting from the hepatic arteries to the capillaries to the portal vein. The end result is enlargement of portosystemic collateral vessels and the formation of varices.

Clinical Findings

Patients with paraesophageal varices are typically adults with portal hypertension secondary to hepatic cirrhosis and characteristically have a history of alcohol abuse. They may present with fatigue, weight loss, abdominal pain, jaundice, and/or upper gastrointestinal hemorrhage. Physical examination may reveal gynecomastia, digital clubbing, peripheral edema, abdominal ascites, hepatosplenomegaly, and/or enlarged abdominal wall veins. Children may develop portal hypertension secondary to extrahepatic portal venous obstruction.

Imaging Findings

Chest Radiography

- Middle-posterior mediastinal, paraesophageal lobular soft-tissue mass(es) (**Figs. 166.1, 166.2**)
  - Visible in less than 10% of cases
  - Also known as mediastinal pseudotumor
- Obliteration or nodularity of left para-aortic interface

- Lateral displacement of paravertebral stripes
- Lateral displacement or obliteration of azygoesophageal recess
- Splenomegaly

MDCT

- Dilated serpiginous soft-tissue masses closely related to the outer wall of the esophagus; may reach large sizes (**Figs. 166.3, 166.4**)
- Intense contrast enhancement that parallels aortic enhancement (**Figs. 166.3, 166.4**)
- Visualization of vascular communications with the systemic venous circulation (precaval draining vein, preaortic esophageal veins)
- Associated esophageal varices (**Figs. 166.3, 166.4**)
  - Thickened esophageal wall with lobular outer contour
  - Scalloped esophageal lumen with nodular intraluminal protrusions
  - Focal/circumferential mural (nodular) enhancement (similar to that of the thoracic aorta) with associated esophageal wall thickening
- Use of CT angiography with two-dimensional and three-dimensional rendering for anatomic visualization of collateral pathways; evaluation of patients with known cirrhosis/esophageal varices and a mediastinal mass
- Abdominal finding: hepatic cirrhosis; dilated left gastric vein (greater than 5–6 mm in diameter) and/or multiple dilated veins (greater than 4–6 mm in diameter) located between stomach and posterior left hepatic lobe, abdominal ascites (**Figs. 166.3, 166.4**)

MRI

- Use of axial three-dimensional gradient echo MR imaging for depiction of abnormal upper abdominal vascular anatomy
- Use of gadolinium-enhanced three-dimensional MR portal venography

Management

- Sclerotherapy or banding for bleeding esophageal varices

Prognosis

- Poor prognosis in patients with bleeding esophageal varices and paraesophageal varices on CT; prolonged and more frequent sclerotherapy; 20–35% mortality

Suggested Readings

1. Annet L, Peeters F, Horsmans Y, Hermoye L, Starkel P, Van Beers BE. Esophageal varices: evaluation with transesophageal MR imaging—initial experience. Radiology 2006;238(1):167–175

2. Henseler KP, Pozniak MA, Lee FT Jr, Winter TC III. Three-dimensional CT angiography of spontaneous portosystemic shunts. Radiographics 2001;21(3):691–704

3. Kim M-J, Mitchell DG, Ito K. Portosystemic collaterals of the upper abdomen: review of anatomy and demonstration on MR imaging. Abdom Imaging 2000;25(5):462–470

4. Kim YK, Kim Y, Shim SS. Thoracic complications of liver cirrhosis: radiologic findings. Radiographics 2009;29(3): 825–837

CASE 167

■ Clinical Presentation

Middle-aged woman with recurrent epigastric pain

■ Radiologic Findings

PA (**Fig. 167.1**) and lateral (**Fig. 167.2**) chest radiographs demonstrate a moderate-size middle-posterior mediastinal (retrocardiac) mass that contains intrinsic air and fluid and produces lateral displacement of the inferior aspect of the azygoesophageal recess (*arrowhead*). Contrast-enhanced chest CT (mediastinal window) (**Figs. 167.3, 167.4**) shows a moderate hiatus hernia that contains a portion of the stomach and surrounding omental fat.

■ Diagnosis

Hiatus Hernia

■ Differential Diagnosis

• None

■ Discussion

Background

Hiatus hernia results from transient or permanent intrathoracic gastric herniation through an enlarged esophageal hiatus. Herniation of omentum and other portions of the gastrointestinal tract (hollow viscera and solid organs) occasionally occurs. Abdominal fluid may also herniate through the hiatus in patients with

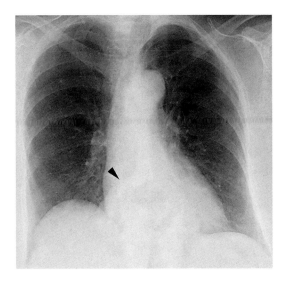

Fig. 167.1

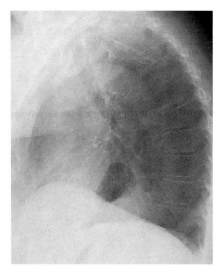

Fig. 167.2

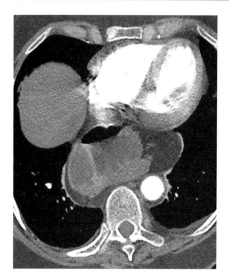

Fig. 167.3

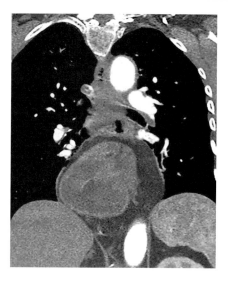

Fig. 167.4

ascites. In paraesophageal hiatus hernia, the gastroesophageal junction remains in its normal location and the herniated stomach migrates above it and resides alongside the esophagus.

Etiology

Hiatus hernia results from acquired widening of the esophageal hiatus related to increased intra-abdominal pressure associated with obesity and pregnancy. Congenital weakness of the esophageal hiatus may play a role in some cases.

Clinical Findings

The prevalence of hiatus hernia increases with age, and most affected patients are older than 60 years. Patients with hiatus hernia are typically asymptomatic middle-aged or elderly individuals who are diagnosed incidentally because of an abnormal chest radiograph. Symptomatic patients complain of burning abdominal pain, most pronounced after meals and in the supine position and typically alleviated by antacids. Upper gastrointestinal bleeding may also occur and may manifest with anemia, frank hematemesis, or melena. Mechanical symptoms, such as early satiety, nausea, and vomiting, may also occur.

Imaging Findings

Chest Radiography

- Retrocardiac middle-posterior mediastinal mass (**Figs. 167.1, 167.2**); typically right lateral displacement of azygoesophageal recess (**Fig. 167.1**)
  - ○ Homogeneous soft-tissue mass
  - ○ Air-filled mass
  - ○ Mass with one or more air-fluid levels (**Figs. 167.1, 167.2**)
- Organo-axial volvulus in cases of significant gastric herniation, with increased risk of incarceration, strangulation, and infarction

MDCT

- Visualization of gastric herniation through esophageal hiatus (**Figs. 167.3, 167.4, 167.5, 167.6**)
- Organo-axial volvulus configuration of the herniated stomach, typically in large herniations (**Fig. 167.5B**)

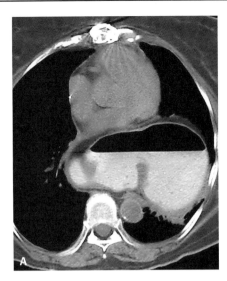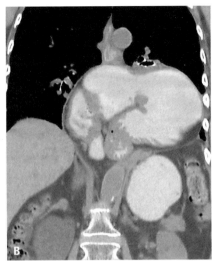

Fig. 167.5   Contrast-enhanced axial **(A)** and coronal **(B)** chest CT (mediastinal window) of an elderly woman with a large hiatus hernia demonstrates herniation of most of the stomach and omental fat through the esophageal hiatus. Note the organo-axial configuration of the stomach **(B)**.

- Visualization of other herniated abdominal organs/structures
- Identification of location of gastroesophageal junction for diagnosis of paraesophageal hernia (**Figs. 167.6A, 167.6B**)

Management

- Recognition and observation
- Antacids in symptomatic patients
- Surgical hernia repair; immediate surgical intervention in cases of strangulation or symptomatic gastric volvulus

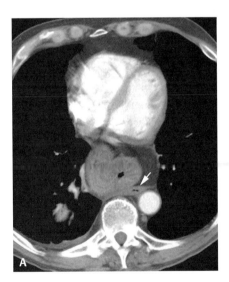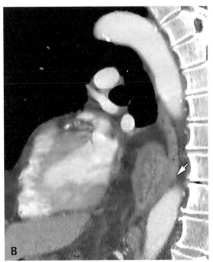

Fig. 167.6   Contrast-enhanced axial **(A)** and sagittal oblique **(B)** chest CT (mediastinal window) of an asymptomatic 67-year-old man with a paraesophageal hiatus hernia demonstrates mediastinal herniation of the stomach and adjacent omental fat. The distal esophagus can be followed to the gastroesophageal junction with the stomach herniating superiorly and alongside the distal esophagus (*arrows*).

Prognosis

- Good

PEARLS

- Asymptomatic organo-axial volvulus may be present in patients with completely intrathoracic stomachs due to large hiatus hernias.
- Acute upper gastrointestinal symptoms in a patient with a known hiatus hernia should prompt exclusion of strangulation or symptomatic gastric volvulus.

PITFALLS

- Large hiatus hernias may lateralize to one side of the hemithorax and may mimic a lung mass or abscess on radiography.

Suggested Reading

1. Barut I, Tarhan OR, Cerci C, Akdeniz Y, Bulbul M. Intestinal obstruction caused by a strangulated Morgagni hernia in an adult patient. J Thorac Imaging 2005;20(3):220–222
2. Hansell DM, Armstrong P, Lynch DA, et al. Mediastinal and aortic disease. In: Hansell DM, Armstrong P, Lynch DA, McAdams HP, eds. Imaging of Diseases of the Chest, 4th ed. Philadelphia: Elsevier Mosby; 2005:901–1021
3. Fraser RS, Müller NL, Colman N, et al. The diaphragm. In: Fraser RS, Müller NL, Colman N, Paré PD, eds. Fraser and Paré's Diagnosis of Diseases of the Chest, 4th ed. Philadelphia: Saunders; 1999:2987–3010

CASE 168

■ Clinical Presentation

35-year-old man with dysphagia, weight loss, and halitosis

■ Radiologic Findings

PA (**Fig. 168.1**) and lateral (**Fig. 168.2**) chest radiographs demonstrate a large, elongate middle-posterior mediastinal mass that extends to the paravertebral region, projects to the right of midline, and produces mass effect on the posterior wall of the trachea (**Fig. 168.2**). Contrast-enhanced chest CT (mediastinal window) (**Figs. 168.3, 168.4**) shows heterogeneous contents and dependent contrast in a dilated esophagus that produces mass effect on the heart and tracheobronchial tree (**Fig. 168.4**).

■ Diagnosis

Achalasia

■ Differential Diagnosis

- Esophageal Dilatation from Progressive Systemic Sclerosis
- Esophageal Dilatation from Acquired Focal Obstruction
  - Carcinoma
  - Metastatic Disease
  - Non-Neoplastic Stenosis

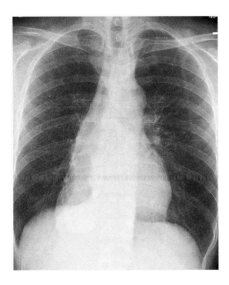

Fig. 168.1

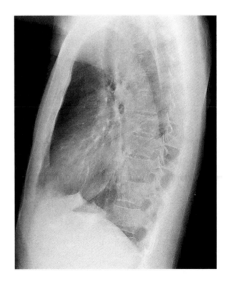

Fig. 168.2

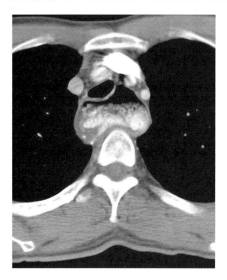

Fig. 168.3

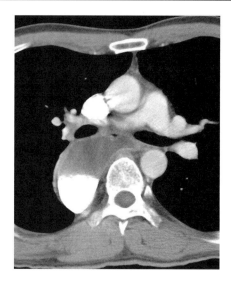

Fig. 168.4

■ Discussion

Background

Achalasia is characterized by absent peristalsis of the esophagus and incomplete relaxation of the lower esophageal sphincter, resulting in marked esophageal dilatation and poor esophageal emptying.

Etiology

In most cases achalasia is a *primary* or *idiopathic* condition that correlates with ganglion cell deficiency in the esophageal myenteric smooth muscle plexus. *Secondary achalasia* (or pseudoachalasia) results from Chagas disease or from malignancy at the gastroesophageal junction. Esophageal dilatation may also result from progressive systemic sclerosis, reflux esophagitis, and mediastinal fibrosis.

Clinical Findings

Patients with *primary achalasia* usually experience an insidious onset of symptoms and typically present between the ages of 30 and 50 years. Symptomatic patients complain of dysphagia, foul breath, regurgitation, chest pain, and symptoms related to aspiration and recurrent pulmonary infection. Patients with *secondary achalasia* (from malignancy) are usually older (over 60 years), have recent onset of dysphagia, and have substantial weight loss.

Imaging Findings

Chest Radiography

- Elongate middle mediastinal mass (dilated esophagus); commonly exhibits an air-fluid level (**Figs. 168.1, 168.2**)
- Marked esophageal dilatation with esophageal displacement to the right of the midline (**Fig. 168.1**)
- Anterior tracheal displacement on lateral chest radiography (**Fig. 168.2**)
- Associated pulmonary consolidation from recurrent aspiration

Barium Esophagogram

- Esophageal dilatation (typically over 4.0 cm in diameter)
- Absent peristalsis

- Smooth narrowing of distal esophagus under 3.5 cm in length (in primary achalasia)
- Failure of lower esophageal sphincter to relax with swallowing

MDCT

- Dilated esophagus with fluid, air-fluid level, internal debris (**Figs. 168.3, 168.4, 168.5**)
- Normal esophageal wall thickness
- Poor visualization of gastric cardia (pseudomass) due to poor esophageal emptying
- Associated pulmonary consolidation, atelectasis, and/or bronchiectasis from mass effect and recurrent aspiration

Management

- Laparoscopic or thoracoscopic esophagogastric myotomy
- Endoscopic injection of botulinum toxin into the lower esophageal sphincter
- Endoscopic balloon dilation of distal esophagus under fluoroscopic guidance; may require repeated treatments; may be complicated by esophageal perforation

Prognosis

- Good

PEARLS

- Some patients with typical imaging findings of achalasia have complete relaxation of the lower esophageal sphincter at manometry during swallowing.
- Approximately 75% of patients with secondary achalasia have carcinoma of the gastric cardia or metastatic disease to this area. These patients may exhibit asymmetric thickening of the distal esophageal wall, a soft-tissue mass at the cardia, and/or mediastinal lymphadenopathy.
- Eccentricity, nodularity, angulation, straightening, and proximal shouldering of the narrowed esophageal segment and a length of narrowing greater than 3.5 cm on barium esophagogram suggest secondary achalasia, and malignancy must be excluded.

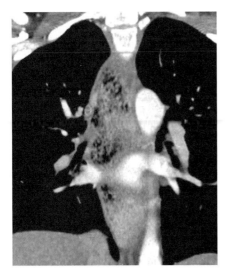

Fig. 168.5 Coronal contrast-enhanced chest CT (mediastinal window) of a 32-year-old woman with primary achalasia demonstrates a large elongate right middle-posterior mediastinal structure corresponding to the debris-filled dilated esophagus.

Suggested Reading

1. Hansell DM, Armstrong P, Lynch DA, et al. Mediastinal and aortic disease. In: Hansell DM, Armstrong P, Lynch DA, McAdams HP, eds. Imaging of Diseases of the Chest, 4th ed. Philadelphia: Elsevier Mosby; 2005:901–1021

2. Mueller CF, Klecker RJ, King MA. Case 3. Achalasia. AJR Am J Roentgenol 2000;175(3):867, 870–871

3. Amaravadi R, Levine MS, Rubesin SE, Laufer I, Redfern RO, Katzka DA. Achalasia with complete relaxation of lower esophageal sphincter: radiographic-manometric correlation. Radiology 2005;235(3):886–891

4. Woodfield CA, Levine MS, Rubesin SE, Langlotz CP, Laufer I. Diagnosis of primary versus secondary achalasia: reassessment of clinical and radiographic criteria. AJR Am J Roentgenol 2000;175(3):727–731

CASE 169

■ Clinical Presentation

25-year-old man with thalassemia major and profound hemolytic anemia

■ Radiologic Findings

PA (**Fig. 169.1**) and lateral (**Fig. 169.2**) chest radiographs demonstrate a well-defined right paravertebral soft-tissue mass (*arrow*) and expansion of osseous medullary spaces. Note the left upper quadrant metallic surgical clips from a prior splenectomy. Contrast-enhanced chest CT (mediastinal window) (**Figs. 169.3, 169.4**) shows an ovoid well-defined right paravertebral soft-tissue mass and a smaller left paravertebral mass. Note expansion and trabeculation of the marrow spaces of adjacent ribs.

■ Diagnosis

Extramedullary Hematopoiesis

■ Differential Diagnosis

- Neurogenic Neoplasm
- Lymphadenopathy

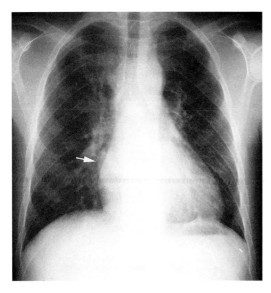

Fig. 169.1

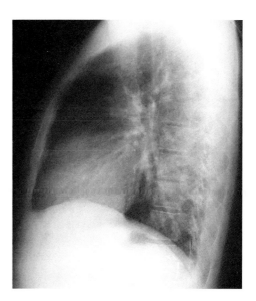

Fig. 169.2

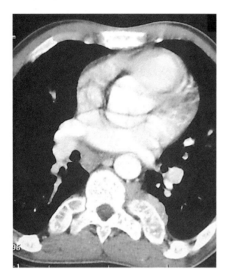

Fig. 169.3

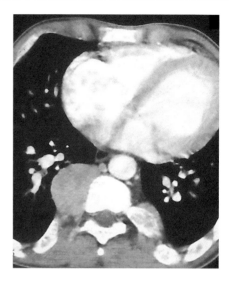

Fig. 169.4

■ Discussion

Background

Extramedullary hematopoiesis (EMH) represents the compensatory formation and maturation of blood elements outside the marrow, most commonly in the liver, spleen, and lymph nodes, but also in the paravertebral region. EMH may also occur in the pulmonary interstitium. It typically results from marrow failure or ineffective production of mature blood elements.

Etiology

The etiology of EMH is incompletely understood. It usually occurs as a response to inadequate erythrocyte production or excessive hemolysis, but it may also represent an abnormal cellular proliferation. It is associated with severe congenital hemolytic anemias (hereditary spherocytosis, thalassemia major), polycythemia vera, lymphoproliferative disorders (myelofibrosis, lymphoma, chronic leukemia), and sickle cell disease. It has also been described in association with hyperparathyroidism and chronic pneumonia. It has been postulated that it may result from paravertebral extrusion of marrow elements through the abnormally thinned cortex of adjacent ribs and vertebrae. An embolic mechanism has also been suggested.

Clinical Findings

Paravertebral EMH does not usually produce symptoms, and affected patients are often diagnosed incidentally because of an abnormal chest radiograph. There are rare reports of associated spontaneous hemothorax and spinal cord compression. Pulmonary EMH may result in cardiopulmonary insufficiency. Patients may also present with symptoms related to one of the associated disease processes.

Imaging Findings

Chest Radiography

- Focal or multi-focal smooth or lobular paravertebral soft-tissue masses
  - Unilateral or bilateral (**Fig. 169.1**)
  - Typically inferior hemithorax between the sixth and twelfth vertebral bodies (**Fig. 169.1**)
  - May affect entire length of thoracic paravertebral region
- Expansion of osseous erythroid bone marrow spaces with coarse trabeculation

MDCT

- Well-defined lobular homogeneous soft-tissue mass(es) (**Figs. 169.3, 169.4**); homogeneous enhancement
- May exhibit internal fat attenuation (**Fig. 169.5**)
- Marrow expansion of adjacent skeletal structures with lacy appearance of ribs and vertebrae (**Figs. 169.3, 169.4**)
- Rarely abnormal interstitial and ground glass pulmonary opacities; pleural effusion

MRI

- Extramedullary mass with slightly higher signal intensity than that of adjacent marrow on T1WI and T2WI
- May involve the intraspinal epidural space

Scintigraphy

- Uptake of Tc-99m-labeled monoclonal antibody
  - High sensitivity
  - Binds to hematopoietic cells beyond promyelocytes
- Uptake of In-111-chloride and Tc-99m-labeled colloids

Management

- Recognition and observation in asymptomatic patients
- Regression with blood transfusion and hydroxyurea
- Splenectomy in cases of spherocytosis
- Steroids and radiation therapy for epidural involvement with spinal cord compression

Prognosis

- Variable prognosis depending on underlying condition
- Durable control of spinal cord compression in patients treated with radiation

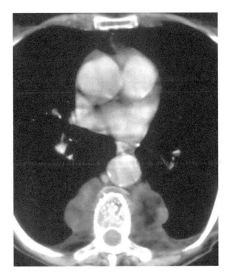

Fig. 169.5 Contrast-enhanced chest CT (mediastinal window) of an elderly woman with chronic anemia and EMH demonstrates bilateral lobular paraspinal soft-tissue masses with central areas of fat attenuation.

Suggested Reading

1. Berkmen YM, Zalta BA. Case 126: extramedullary hematopoiesis. Radiology 2007;245(3):905–908

2. Georgiades CS, Neyman EG, Francis IR, Sneider MB, Fishman EK. Typical and atypical presentations of extramedullary hemopoiesis. AJR Am J Roentgenol 2002;179(5):1239–1243

3. Moellers MO, Bader JB, Alexander C, Samnick S, Kirsch CM. Localization of extramedullary hematopoiesis with Tc-99m-labeled monoclonal antibodies (BW 250/183). Clin Nucl Med 2002;27(5):354–357

CASE 170

■ Clinical Presentation

70-year-old woman evaluated for retropharyngeal abscess and chest pain

■ Radiologic Findings

Contrast-enhanced neck CT (soft-tissue window) (**Fig. 170.1**) demonstrates a complex peripharyngeal fluid collection and a retropharyngeal abscess. Note enhancing borders of the complex fluid collection and air bubbles within the retropharyngeal abscess. Contrast-enhanced chest CT (mediastinal window) (**Fig. 170.2**) shows a mediastinal fluid collection with enhancing borders and intrinsic air bubbles that surrounds the trachea and esophagus and abuts the visualized thoracic great vessels. This process represented mediastinal extension of the retropharyngeal abscess. Note small right pleural effusion.

■ Diagnosis

Mediastinal Abscess

■ Differential Diagnosis

- Tuberculous Mediastinitis
- Infected Neoplasm

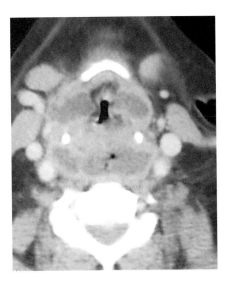

Fig. 170.1

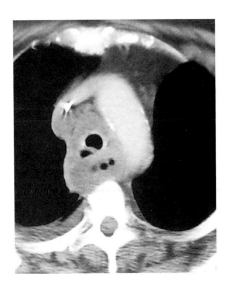

Fig. 170.2 (Images courtesy of Diane C. Strollo, MD, University of Pittsburgh Medical Center, Pittsburgh, Pennsylvania.)

■ Discussion

Background

Acute mediastinal infection is an uncommon but potentially life-threatening inflammatory condition.

Etiology

Most cases of acute mediastinitis (acute mediastinal infection) are the result of surgical intervention or iatrogenic instrumentation. Iatrogenic esophageal perforation during surgery or endoscopy, and accidental perforation from swallowing sharp objects (e.g., fishbone) or forceful vomiting are important etiologies. Postoperative mediastinitis may occur in up to 1% of patients who undergo sternotomy for cardiac surgery. Acute mediastinitis may also result from contiguous or remote spread of infection from an affected organ or site. Other associations are empyema and subphrenic abscess. Pyogenic and tuberculous vertebral infections may cause a paravertebral abscess.

Clinical Findings

Patients with acute mediastinal infection are typically quite ill, present with chest pain, chills, and high fever and may develop septic shock. Patients with esophageal perforation may complain of dysphagia.

Imaging Findings

Chest Radiography

- Focal or diffuse mediastinal widening
- Pneumomediastinum, air in the soft tissues of the neck
- Associated pleural effusion and pulmonary consolidation; pneumothorax, hydropneumothorax

Esophagography

- Identify the of site of perforation

MDCT

- Mediastinal air (bubbly or streaky patterns); often seen in cases of esophageal perforation
- Obliteration of mediastinal tissue planes
- Focal or multifocal abscesses
  - Low-attenuation fluid collections (**Fig. 170.3**), may exhibit enhancing borders (**Figs. 170.2, 170.4**)
  - Intrinsic air, air-fluid levels

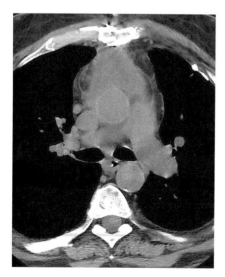

Fig. 170.3 Unenhanced chest CT (mediastinal window) of a 54-year-old man who developed a mediastinal abscess following sternotomy demonstrates a retrosternal low-attenuation fluid collection with higher-attenuation lobular lesion borders. Note the absence of a tissue plane between the fluid collection and the ascending aorta and the induration of the adjacent mediastinal fat.

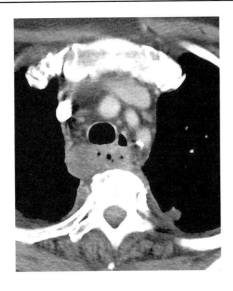

Fig. 170.4 Contrast-enhanced chest CT (mediastinal window) of a 78-year-old woman with pyogenic vertebral osteomyelitis who developed an adjacent mediastinal abscess manifesting as a small fluid collection with intrinsic air-fluid level located posterior to the trachea and the esophagus.

- Extraluminal enteric contrast
- Associated empyema, abscess; adjacent skeletal (spinal) involvement

MRI

- Intermediate signal intensity on T1WI
- High signal intensity on T2WI

Management

- Percutaneous or open drainage
- Antibiotics

Prognosis

- Poor when mediastinitis results from esophageal perforation
- High fatality rate in the presence of sepsis

PEARLS

- Substernal fluid collections and mediastinal gas are normal findings in the two-week period that follows median sternotomy. However, persistence of these findings after postoperative day 14 is highly suggestive of mediastinitis (**Fig. 170.3**).
- Mediastinal pancreatic pseudocysts are rare lesions that affect patients with recurrent pancreatitis, alcohol abuse, or abdominal trauma/surgery. The pseudocyst is a peripancreatic fluid collection surrounded by a fibrous wall that lacks a true epithelial lining. These lesions may communicate with the thorax via the esophageal or aortic hiatus and manifest as a mediastinal mass with associated left or bilateral pleural effusion. CT demonstrates a thin-walled cyst of low attenuation typically located in the middle-posterior mediastinum that often produces mass effect. There is typically an associated pancreatic pseudocyst or peripancreatic fluid collection.

Suggested Readings

1. Hansell DM, Armstrong P, Lynch DA, et al. Mediastinal and aortic disease. In: Hansell DM, Armstrong P, Lynch DA, McAdams HP, eds. Imaging of Diseases of the Chest, 4th ed. Philadelphia: Elsevier Mosby; 2005:901–1021

2. Jeung M-Y, Gasser B, Gangi A, et al. Imaging of cystic masses of the mediastinum. Radiographics 2002;22(Spec No): S79–S93

Section XII

Pleura, Chest Wall, and Diaphragm

OVERVIEW OF PLEURA, CHEST WALL, AND DIAPHRAGM

Diseases that affect the pleura, chest wall, and diaphragm share the property of being extrapulmonary lesions. In many instances, this property will manifest on chest radiography with characteristic findings in terms of location, and at times produce the *incomplete border sign* (see Cases 177 and 182) indicating an extrapulmonary location. Determining the location of an imaging abnormality is the first step in constructing an accurate and meaningful list of differential diagnostic possibilities.

The imaging features of pleural disease are widely varied, ranging from the thin line of a pneumothorax to the exuberant thickening and nodularity that may occur in pleural malignancy. Anatomic features of the pleura influence those imaging manifestations and may cause confusion during image interpretation. The *deep sulcus sign* of pneumothorax in a supine patient, for instance, has its anatomic basis in the deep inferior extension of normal parietal pleura that forms the lateral costodiaphragmatic recess. Malignant tumors can also extend into this potential space (see Cases 175 and 176) and produce characteristic imaging findings that correlate with underlying pleural anatomy.

Some pleural and chest wall lesions have characteristic CT findings, including the shape of loculated pleural effusions and empyema, and the diagnostic fat attenuation detected in chest wall lipomas (see Case 179). The lenticular shape of an empyema with bronchopleural fistula will often lead to a disparity in the length of the associated air-fluid level on orthogonal chest radiographs (see Case 172), in contradistinction to the similarity in length that is often detected in a lung abscess that contains an air-fluid level. These unique imaging features contribute to the range of findings that make the evaluation of pleural and chest wall disease so interesting in daily radiologic practice.

The chest wall may be involved in congenital and developmental conditions, inflammatory and infectious diseases, and soft-tissue and bone tumors. Some of these conditions have characteristic imaging features that allow a confident diagnosis. Others fall within differential diagnostic considerations that can be correlated with demographic and clinical features to narrow the list of possible diagnoses. The radiographic finding of rib destruction in an adult, for example, is most often related to metastatic lesions, but multiple myeloma and chondrosarcoma should also be in the differential diagnosis. Subsequent CT imaging findings might show a characteristic location and cross-sectional features of chondrosarcoma, further narrowing the differential diagnosis (see Case 182).

Knowledge of the characteristic imaging features of pleural and chest wall lesions helps to improve the diagnostic accuracy of imaging interpretation, and results in better patient care.

CASE 171

■ Clinical Presentation

40-year-old man with liver failure, ascites, and absent right-sided breath sounds

■ Radiologic Findings

PA (**Fig. 171.1A**) and lateral (**Fig. 171.1B**) chest radiographs show complete "white-out" of the right hemithorax. No air bronchograms are seen and only the left diaphragm is perceptible on the lateral exam. Note the contralateral displacement of the tracheal air column and mediastinum "away" from the white-out on the PA exam (**Fig. 171.1A**).

■ Diagnosis

Massive Unilateral Pleural Effusion; Hepatic Hydrothorax

■ Differential Diagnosis

- Unilateral Opaque Thorax ("White-out") is quite broad (**Table 171.1**)
- Differential can be narrowed based on location of trachea (**Table 171.2**)
- Other Causes of Unilateral Pleural Effusion (**Table 171.3**)

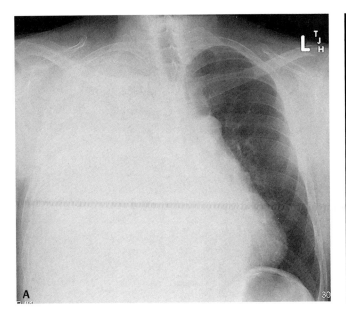 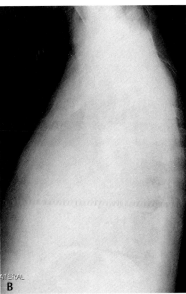

Fig. 171.1

Table 171.1   Unilateral Opaque Thorax ('White-out")

Pleural Disease	Pulmonary Disease	Chest Wall Deformity
Pleural effusion	Total lung collapse	Significant scoliosis
Pleural thickening	Pneumonia	Severe congenital or acquired chest wall deformity
Fibrothorax	Pneumonectomy	Large chest wall hematoma
Diffuse malignant mesothelioma	Pulmonary agenesis	Large chest wall tumor
Metastatic pleural cancer		Diaphragmatic hernia

Table 171.2   Unilateral Opaque Thorax ("White-out") Based on Trachea Location

Pulled "Toward" White-out	Pushed "Away" from White-out	Central Position
Total lung collapse	Pleural effusion	Pleural thickening
Pneumonectomy	Diaphragmatic hernia	Fibrothorax
Pulmonary agenesis	Severe congenital or acquired chest wall deformity	Diffuse malignant mesothelioma
		Metastatic pleural cancer
		Large chest wall hematoma
		Large chest wall tumor

Table 171.3   Unilateral Pleural Effusion Differential Diagnosis

Heart failure

Parapneumonic-empyema

Neoplasia

Pulmonary thromboembolism

Autoimmune-collagen vascular disorders

Trauma

Chylothorax

Subdiaphragmatic diseases and disorders

■ Discussion

Background

Pleural effusion is an abnormal accumulation of fluid in the pleural space and a common manifestation of local and systemic diseases that involve the thorax, affecting an estimated 1.3 million persons each year. The normal pleural cavity contains a small volume of fluid (5–15 mL) that provides a frictionless surface between the visceral and parietal pleura as lung volume changes during respiration. However, between 1 and 2.5 L of pleural fluid is produced each day. Pleural fluid normally forms and flows from capillaries in the parietal pleura into the pleural space and is absorbed through parietal pleural lymphatics. The parietal pleura vasculature drains to the right side of the heart, whereas the visceral pleura vasculature drains to its left side. The formation and absorption of pleural fluid is governed by Starling's equation. That is, the net filtration and resorption of water and its solutes (i.e., pleural fluid) across a semi-permeable membrane (i.e., pleura) are determined by balances between hydrostatic and osmotic pressures. Anything that upsets this balance results in accumulation of pleural fluid: (1) *increased hydrostatic pressure* (e.g., heart failure, constrictive pericarditis); (2) *decreased osmotic pressure* (e.g., cirrhosis, hypoalbuminemia); (3) *decreased pleural space pressure* (e.g., atelectasis); (4) *increased microvasculature permeability* (e.g., neoplasia, inflammatory conditions); (5) *impaired lymphatic drainage* (e.g., neoplasia, fibrosis, radiation therapy); and (6) *increased transportation of fluid from the peritoneal space into the pleural space* (e.g., ascites, nephrotic syndrome).

Etiology

Thoracentesis is usually performed to evaluate pleural effusions of unknown etiology. Fluid is examined grossly and submitted for biochemical analysis, red and white blood cell counts, Gram and acid-fast stains, and cytology. More invasive procedures, including closed, open, or thoracoscopic biopsy, are sometimes necessary to establish a diagnosis. Most effusions are categorized as *transudates* or *exudates* using criteria established by Light. Such categorization is useful in narrowing the differential diagnosis (**Tables 171.4, 171.5**) and dictating patient management. *Exudates* exhibit one or more of the following characteristics: (1) pleural fluid protein/serum protein ratio >0.5; pleural fluid lactic acid dehydrogenase (LDH)/serum LDH ratio >0.6; and (3) pleural fluid LDH ratio greater than two-thirds the normal serum LDH. *Transudates* are characteristically clear, straw-colored, have a low protein concentration, and have few cells. Most *transudates* result from systemic factors that alter pleural fluid formation or absorption (**Table 171.4**). *Exudative* effusions result from diseases that alter the pleural surface and its permeability to protein (**Table 171.5**). Bilateral pleural effusions sometimes have different etiologies (Contarini condition)—for example, an exudative pleural effusion (empyema) in one thorax and a transudative pleural effusion (heart failure) on the other side. Pleural effusions may also be characterized by their composition (e.g., hydrothorax, hemothorax, pyothorax, chylothorax, bilothorax, urinothorax, pyohemochylothorax).

Clinical Findings

The clinical presentation varies depending on the underlying cause of the effusion and how rapidly the pleural fluid accumulated. Some patients are asymptomatic (15%), whereas others present with dull aching chest pain, cough, fever, and dyspnea. Large effusions may displace the mediastinum and cause respiratory distress. Physical exam findings may include decreased or absent breath sounds over the affected thorax and dullness to percussion.

Imaging Findings

Chest Radiography

- Hazy increase in radio-opacity (i.e., ground glass veil) that does not obscure underlying bronchovascular markings on supine chest radiography

Table 171.4   Differential Diagnosis: Transudative Pleural Effusion

Heart failure	Atelectasis	Peritoneal dialysis
Cirrhosis	Myxedema	Urinothorax
Nephrotic syndrome	Pulmonary thromboembolism	

Table 171.5   Differential Diagnosis: Exudative Pleural Effusion

Neoplasia	Infection	Collagen Vascular	Inflammatory	Drug-Related	Other
Primary lung cancer	Parapneumonic	Lupus erythematosus	Asbestos exposure	Lupus-drug induced	Abdominal surgery
Secondary lung neoplasia	Tuberculosis	Rheumatoid arthritis	Post-pericardiotomy syndrome	Amiodarone	Esophageal rupture
Lymphoma	Viral		Pulmonary thromboembolism	Bleomycin	LAM
Mesothelioma	Fungal		Radiation therapy	Bromocriptine	Pancreatitis
Meig syndrome	Parasitic		Trapped lung	Methotrexate	Trauma
	Abdominal abscess		Uremia	Methysergide	Vasculitis
	Hepatitis			Practolol	Yellow-nail syndrome

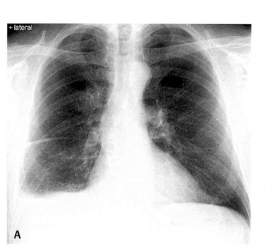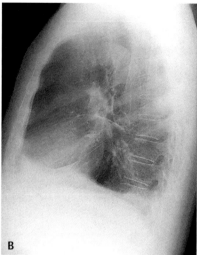

Fig. 171.2 PA **(A)** and lateral **(B)** chest X-rays of a 61-year-old man with primary lung cancer and unilateral right pleural effusion. Note the ill-defined lobulated right suprahilar lung lesion overlying the second anterior medial rib. The effusion forms a meniscus-shaped opacity, blunting the posterolateral sulcus, and extends along the subpulmonic space into the inferior margin of the oblique fissure **(B)**. Similar findings are seen involving the lateral sulcus on the PA view **(A)**. Pleural fluid also extends into the horizontal fissure.

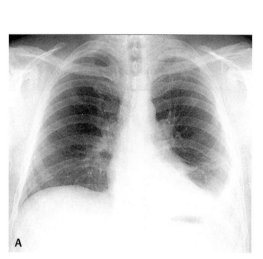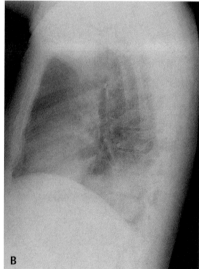

Fig. 171.3 Unilateral left-sided pleural effusion secondary to acute pancreatitis. The effusion forms a smooth meniscus-shaped opacity, the upper border of which curves gently downward from its lateral aspect to the cardiac apex **(A)**. Note blunting of both the posterior and lateral sulcus and the *positive spine sign* **(B)**.

- Radio-opacity involving posterior or lateral costophrenic sulcus with meniscus-shaped upper border (i.e., blunting) on upright radiography (**Figs. 171.2A, 171.2B**)
- Smooth meniscus-shaped opacity, the upper border of which curves gently downward from its lateral aspect to the mid-cardiac region in small to moderate pleural effusions (**Figs. 171.3A, 171.3B**)

Predicting Volume of Pleural Fluid

- Lateral decubitus exam: may demonstrate as little as 5 mL of pleural fluid; also useful in differentiating loculated from mobile pleural fluid collections (**Figs. 171.4A, 171.4B**)
- Posterior costodiaphragmatic sulcus blunting on lateral chest radiography: 20–30 mL

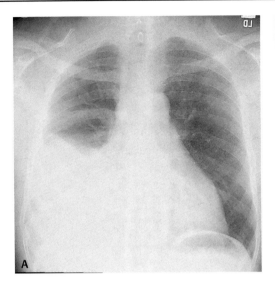
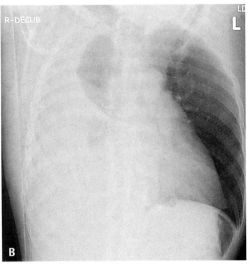

Fig. 171.4 **(A)** PA upright chest X-ray shows a large unilateral right pleural effusion silhouetting the ipsilateral diaphragm and heart border. Right lateral decubitus exam **(B)** confirms the effusion is mobile and layers along the right lateral chest wall.

- Lateral costodiaphragmatic sulcus blunting on frontal chest radiography: 200–300 mL
- Obscuration of ipsilateral hemidiaphragm on frontal radiography: >500 mL (**Fig. 171.4A**)

Subpulmonic Pleural Effusion

- Bilateral subpulmonic effusions unlikely to be recognized; mimics hypoventilation
- Lateral displacement of apex of apparent diaphragm (i.e., pseudodiaphragm) on frontal exams (**Figs. 171.5A, 171.5C, 171.5D**)
- Convex margin of fluid flattens as it contacts oblique fissure and descends abruptly to anterior costophrenic sulcus on lateral radiography; *Rock of Gibraltar sign* (**Fig. 171.5E**)
- ± Small amount of fluid in inferior aspect of oblique fissure on lateral radiography
- Left-sided effusion may be characterized by downward displacement of gastric air bubble from pseudodiaphragm by ≥2.0 cm on upright chest exams (**Figs. 171.5F, 171.5G**)

Interlobar Fluid Collections (Pseudotumor; Vanishing Tumor)

- Most often associated with heart failure; renal failure and hepatic hydrothorax less often (**Figs. 171.6A, 171.6B**)
- Invariably radiographic evidence of concomitant or resolving heart failure
- Homogeneous ovoid opacity oriented along long axis of fissure (**Figs. 171.6A, 171.6B**)
- Evidence of ipsilateral pleural fluid (**Figs. 171.6A, 171.6B**)
- Absence of air bronchograms (**Figs. 171.6A, 171.6B**)
- Morphology changes from one orthogonal view to the next (**Figs. 171.6A, 171.6B**)
- Mobile with decubitus positioning

MDCT

- Sensitive in detection of free pleural fluid
- Layers posteriorly with characteristic meniscoid appearance (**Figs. 171.7A, 171.7B**)
- Attenuation coefficients: 0–20 HU; higher with hemothorax (**Figs. 171.7A, 171.7B, 171.7C, 171.7D**)
- Small effusions may be difficult to differentiate from pleural thickening; fibrosis; dependent atelectasis; decubitus CT imaging aids in differentiation
- Dependent lung may appear to "float" in the fluid of large effusions
- Loculated effusion: sharply marginated lenticular fluid attenuation mass; conforms to concavity of chest wall; forms obtuse margins at its edges; compresses adjacent lung (**Fig. 171.7C**)
- Septations indicative of complicated, organizing effusion (**Fig. 171.7D**)
- Pleural fluid and ascites may occur concurrently; relationship to diaphragm, bare area of liver, and interface with liver and spleen aid in differentiation (**Figs. 171.7A, 171.7B**)

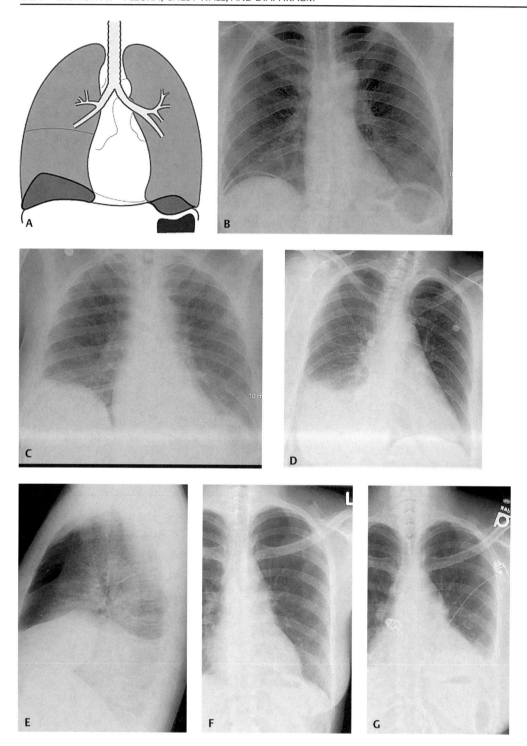

Fig. 171.5 Various depictions of subpulmonic pleural effusion. Artist's illustration (frontal chest X-ray equivalent) **(A)** shows the location and morphology of a subpulmonic effusion. Fluid accumulates in the pleural space between the visceral pleura lining the undersurface of the lower lobe and the parietal pleura covering the ipsilateral diaphragm. Note the preservation of a sharp costophrenic angle and mass effect on the diaphragm. There is characteristic lateral displacement of the apex of the pleural fluid collection (pseudodiaphragm). AP chest exam **(B)** following percutaneous gastrostomy tube placement shows free air beneath the right diaphragm. Note the rounded contour of the right diaphragm. AP chest exam 2 days later **(C)** shows a change in contour of the apparent diaphragm and lateral displacement of its apex from a new subpulmonic effusion. PA **(D)** and lateral **(E)** chest X-rays show a classic right subpulmonic effusion. There is apparent elevation of the diaphragm and lateral displacement of its apex **(D)**. The lateral exam **(E)** reveals a classic *Rock of Gibraltar sign* reflective of subpulmonary fluid between the lung base and diaphragm. Baseline upright PA chest **(F)** and subsequent evolution of a left subpulmonic effusion manifest by downward displacement of the gastric fundus by more than 2.0 cm **(G)**.

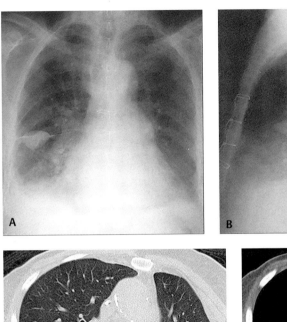

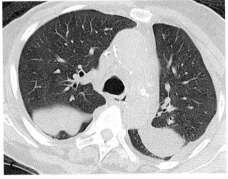

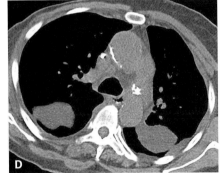

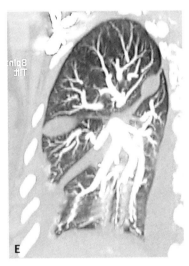

Fig. 171.6   Interlobar fluid collections on radiography and MDCT. PA **(A)** and lateral **(B)** chest radiographs demonstrate a remote median sternotomy. The cardiomediastinal silhouette is enlarged and vascular redistribution is evident. A right-sided pleural effusion is present that partially silhouettes the ipsilateral diaphragm and blunts the posterior and lateral sulcus. An ovoid radio-opacity is present in the right hemithorax. The long axis of this opacity parallels the long axis of the horizontal fissure. The opacity also changes morphology from one orthogonal view to the next, relatively foreshortened on the PA exam **(A)** and becoming more elongated on the lateral exam **(B)**. Both of the latter findings confirm the lesion is pleural-based. Note the absence of air bronchograms. Axial chest CT (lung window, **C**; mediastinal window, **D**) shows homogeneous, ovoid, interfissural fluid collections or pseudotumors in each oblique fissure. Right sagittal MIP CT (lung window) **(E)** of another patient shows interfissural fluid localized in the horizontal and oblique fissure. The oblique fissure appears thickened from fluid.

Ultrasound

- Effusions displace lung away from chest wall; allows visualization of pleural cavity
- Most pleural fluid is anechoic or hypoechoic (e.g., transudate, exudate); may see floating particulate matter
- Septations not apparent on CT are often evident (**Fig. 171.8**); septations, floating particles or layering debris, increased echogenicity more suggestive of exudate
- Collapsed/consolidated lung moves within the effusion during respiration

MRI

- Signal intensity of pleural fluid depends on its biochemical characteristics
- Most cases of non-hemorrhagic or non-chylous effusion:
  - High signal intensity: T2WI (**Fig. 171.9A**)
  - Low signal intensity: T1WI (**Fig. 171.9B**)

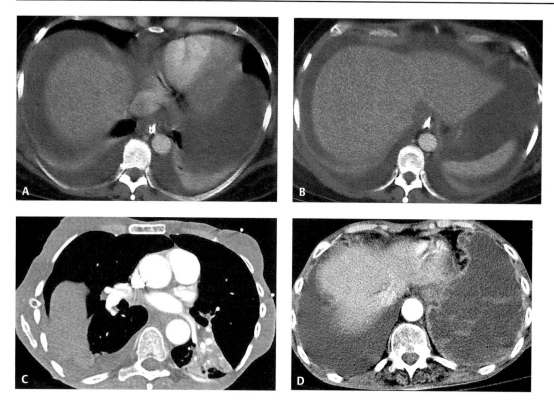

Fig. 171.7 **(A,B)** Contrast-enhanced thoracoabdominal CT images (mediastinal window) show bilateral, dependent layering, low-attenuation pleural effusions and abdominal ascites. Effusions in the costophrenic recess are posterior and medial to the respective diaphragms, displace the crura laterally, and have a fuzzy interface with the liver and spleen. Ascites is located central (medial) to the diaphragm and forms a sharp interface with the anterolateral liver and splenic surface, but is anatomically prevented from extending along the posterior hepatic surface because this region of the liver lacks a peritoneal covering and is directly apposed to the posterior abdominal wall (bare area). Contrast-enhanced CT (mediastinal window) **(C)** shows a loculated high-attenuation (55 HU) right hemothorax. Note the convex lateral border, obtuse margins, and lentiform shape. Contrast-enhanced CT (liver window) **(D)** of a patient with Contarini condition shows a right hydrothorax (8 HU) and a complex, organizing, multi-septated left empyema and parietal pleural enhancement. Septations are often more readily perceived on liver window settings.

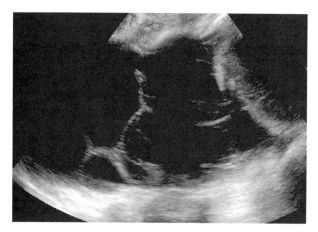

Fig. 171.8 Coronal ultrasound of the right thorax in a young patient with pleural empyema shows unsuspected septations consistent with a complex organized fluid collection. The effusion appeared homogeneous and simple on chest CT (not illustrated).

Management

Transudative Effusion

- Systemic disorder is treated; no further investigation is necessary

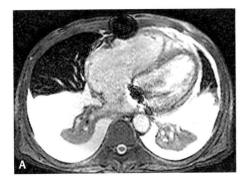 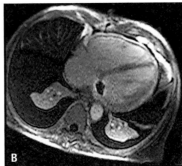

Fig. 171.9 SSFP (T2-weighted) **(A)** and HASTE (T1-weighted) **(B)** axial MRI shows bilateral dependent layering transudative pleural effusions in this patient with mitral regurgitation (note signal dropout from the sternotomy wires and mitral annuloplasty ring). Both atelectatic lower lobes "float" in the pleural fluid.

Exudative Effusion

• Further investigation is warranted to determine its etiology and is then directed toward that disease process

Prognosis

• Dependent upon the underlying disease process

PEARLS

• Heart failure is the most common cause of *transudative* pleural effusion encountered in clinical practice.
• Parapneumonic effusion is the most common cause of *exudative* pleural effusion; neoplasia is the second most common cause.
• *Interlobar pseudotumor*: interlobar accumulation of interfissural fluid that can mimic but should be differentiated from a true lung mass. Although this may occur in any standard or accessory fissure, there is a predilection for it to occur in the horizontal fissure. Remember that these fluid collections are "localized" and not "loculated" within the fissure and will easily layer out on decubitus exams.
• The majority of massive unilateral pleural effusions are malignant (e.g., primary lung cancer, metastatic disease, lymphoma).

Suggested Reading

1. Falaschi F, Battolla L, Mascalchi M, et al. Usefulness of MR signal intensity in distinguishing benign from malignant pleural disease. AJR Am J Roentgenol 1996;166(4):963–968

2. Halvorsen RA, Fedyshin PJ, Korobkin M, Foster WL Jr, Thompson WM. Ascites or pleural effusion? CT differentiation: four useful criteria. Radiographics 1986;6(1):135–149

3. Hierholzer J, Luo L, Bittner RC, et al. MRI and CT in the differential diagnosis of pleural disease. Chest 2000;118(3): 604–609

4. Light RW. Clinical practice. Pleural effusion. N Engl J Med 2002;346(25):1971–1977

5. Travis WD, Colby TV, Koss MN, Rosado-de-Christenson ML, Muller NL, King TE Jr. Pleural disorders. In: King DW, ed. Atlas of Nontumor Pathology: Non-Neoplastic Disorders of the Lower Respiratory Tract, first series, fascicle 2. Washington, DC: American Registry of Pathology; 2002:901–921

CASE 172

■ Clinical Presentation

40-year-old woman with cough and fever

■ Radiologic Findings

Coned-down PA (**Fig. 172.1A**) and lateral (**Fig. 172.1B**) chest radiographs demonstrate a large left pleural effusion with two air-fluid levels. Note the difference in length of the superior air-fluid level on the two orthogonal radiographs (**Figs. 172.1A, 172.1B**). Contrast-enhanced chest CT (mediastinal window) (**Figs. 172.1C, 172.1D**) shows a loculated left pleural effusion with two air-fluid levels (**Fig. 172.1D**) and smooth, mildly thickened enhancing visceral and parietal pleural surfaces (*split pleura sign*) that surround the fluid (**Fig. 172.1D**). Note the mass effect on the adjacent atelectatic left lower lobe (**Fig. 172.1C**).

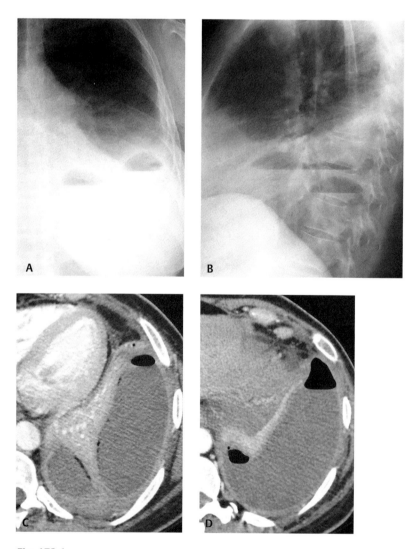

Fig. 172.1

830

■ Diagnosis

Empyema; Bronchopleural Fistula

■ Differential Diagnosis

- Loculated Pleural Effusion—Post Instrumentation
- Malignant Pleural Effusion with Bronchopleural Fistula

■ Discussion

Background

Pleural effusions caused by infection are generally exudative and are classified into three groups, based on pleural fluid analysis. *Simple parapneumonic effusions* are culture and Gram stain negative. *Complicated parapneumonic effusions* are culture and Gram stain negative but have high LDH levels, low pH (<7.2), or low glucose levels (<40 mg/dL). *Empyema* is characteristically purulent on gross inspection, has high neutrophil counts and low pH, and may be culture or Gram stain positive. *Differentiation between parapneumonic pleural effusions and empyemas is based on pleural fluid analysis rather than on imaging features.* Empyema may be associated with bronchopleural fistula when a communication is established between the infected pleural fluid and adjacent airways. Bronchopleural fistula is the most frequent cause of abnormal air collections and air-fluid levels within empyemas. Pleural infection may result in progressive pleural thickening, with formation of an inelastic fibrous membrane that may encase the lung and restrict function (pleural peel).

Etiology

Empyema is most commonly due to pleural extension of infection from adjacent pneumonia, typically caused by Gram-negative bacteria, anaerobic bacteria, *Staphylococcus aureus*, *Streptococcus pneumoniae*, or *Mycobacterium tuberculosis*. Other causes include lung abscess, septic emboli, and subphrenic infection.

Clinical Findings

Affected patients present with fever, chills, cough, and pleuritic chest pain. Physical examination may reveal chest wall erythema and edema. Absence of fever or leukocytosis does not exclude the possibility of empyema. Detection of grossly purulent pleural fluid by thoracentesis is diagnostic.

Imaging Findings

Chest Radiography

- Findings of uncomplicated pleural effusion (see Case 171)
- Ovoid, lenticular, or rounded pleural mass; loculated pleural effusion
- Lesion margins often better defined in one of two orthogonal radiographs, discrepant margin visualization (*incomplete border sign*)
- Bronchopleural fistula
  - Air-fluid level(s) within a pleural mass (loculated empyema) or pleural effusion (**Figs. 172.1A, 172.1B**)
  - Disparity in length of an air-fluid level on paired orthogonal radiographs (**Figs. 172.1A, 172.1B, 172.2**)

MDCT

- Pleural effusion (**Figs. 172.1C, 172.1D, 172.3, 172.5**)
- Focal or multi-focal loculated pleural effusion (**Figs. 172.1C, 172.1D, 172.3, 172.4, 172.5**)
- Loculated pleural fluid forms obtuse angles with adjacent pleura, exhibits a lenticular shape (**Figs. 172.1C, 172.1D, 172.3, 172.4**) and mass effect on adjacent lung (**Figs. 172.1C, 172.3, 172.4**)

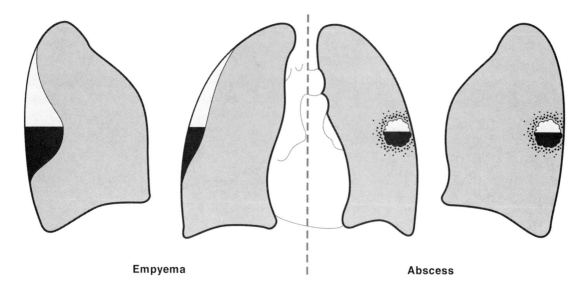

Empyema   **Abscess**

Fig. 172.2 Artist's illustration shows the morphology of empyema with bronchopleural fistula and contrasts it to that of lung abscess. An empyema is an elongate or lenticular fluid collection and, when associated with a bronchopleural fistula, may exhibit discrepant lengths of intrinsic air-fluid levels on orthogonal radiographs. A lung abscess is a spherical lesion that will exhibit no discrepancy in the length of an associated air-fluid level on orthogonal radiographs.

- Uniformly thickened visceral and parietal pleura; exhibits contrast enhancement and surrounds fluid collection; the so-called *split pleura sign* (**Figs. 172.1D, 172.3**)
- Air-fluid level within pleural fluid collection (bronchopleural fistula) (**Figs. 172.1C, 172.1D, 172.4**)

Management

- Prompt closed chest tube drainage
- Antibiotics, empiric initially followed by specific antibiotics based on culture results
- Early administration of fibrinolytic agents through the drainage tube
- Thoracotomy or thoracoscopic lysis of adhesions for patients who fail to respond to antibiotics and closed drainage; open drainage required in up to 30% of patients
- Surgical decortication in late-stage empyema with significantly thickened pleura

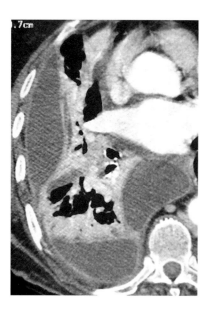

Fig. 172.3 Contrast-enhanced chest CT (mediastinal window) of an 80-year-old woman with empyema demonstrates a multilocular right pleural effusion that produces mass effect on the adjacent lung. The *split pleura sign* is seen in the three areas of loculation.

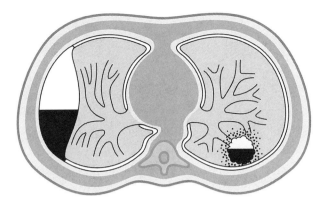

Fig. 172.4 Artist's illustration shows the CT features of empyema and contrasts them with those of lung abscess. An empyema is an elongate pleural collection with borders tapering toward the adjacent pleura and smooth, uniformly thickened walls formed by visceral and parietal pleural surfaces. The pleural collection displaces adjacent parenchymal structures. A lung abscess is spherical in morphology, has thick walls, forms acute borders in relation to the adjacent pleural surface, and does not displace parenchymal structures.

Prognosis

- Good; frequent response to antibiotics and closed chest tube therapy
- Slower recovery for patients requiring open drainage
- Adequate drainage of bronchopleural fistulas imperative to avoid back-spillage into lung and resultant diffuse pneumonitis.
- Variable prognosis depending on patient age, underlying disease, and organism; increased morbidity/ mortality when drainage is inadequate.

PEARLS

- Radiographic evaluation of internal air-fluid levels in thoracic disorders may allow distinction of empyema with bronchopleural fistula from lung abscess:
  - Empyemas exhibit lenticular shapes, disparate lengths of air-fluid levels, and tapering smooth borders (**Figs. 172.1A, 172.1B, 172.2**).
  - Lung abscesses exhibit spherical shapes, air-fluid levels of equal length on orthogonal views, and irregular borders (**Fig. 172.2**).
  - On cross-sectional imaging, empyemas exhibit loculation and lenticular shapes and displace adjacent lung, whereas lung abscesses do not (**Figs. 172.1C, 172.1D, 172.3, 172.4**).
- Post-surgical bronchopleural fistulas develop in 2.5–3% of patients who undergo lobectomy or pneumonectomy, and typically manifest within the first two weeks after surgery. They are usually caused by ne-

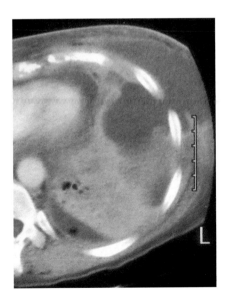

Fig. 172.5 Unenhanced chest CT (lung window) of a 34-year-old immunocompromised woman with empyema necessitatis demonstrates a left anterolateral loculated pleural effusion that extends into the soft tissues of the adjacent chest wall.

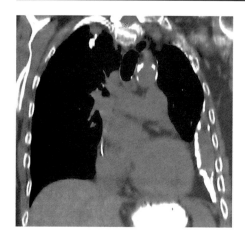

Fig. 172.6 Unenhanced chest CT (mediastinal window, coronal reformation) of an 86-year-old man with calcific fibrothorax related to childhood tuberculosis demonstrates volume loss in the left hemithorax and ipsilateral pleural thickening and calcification that forms a lenticular shape at the site of a previous tuberculous empyema. The patient had decreased left respiratory excursion.

crosis of the bronchial stump or dehiscence of the suture line and most commonly occur following surgery for infectious disease, especially tuberculosis.

- Ultrasonography often reveals septations within empyemas. CT does not reveal such septations directly, but often shows indirect evidence of their presence by demonstrating small air and fluid collections trapped within multiple spaces (**Figs. 172.1C, 172.1D**).
- Empyemas that are untreated or inappropriately treated may drain spontaneously into the subcutaneous tissues of the adjacent chest wall in a process called empyema necessitatis (**Fig. 172.5**).
  ○ This complication is most commonly associated with tuberculosis, actinomycosis, aspergillosis, blastomycosis, and nocardiosis and may result in a palpable mass with associated erythema.
  ○ Prior to the advent of antibiotics, empyema necessitatis was most commonly associated with tuberculosis. Today, it is most often encountered in immunocompromised individuals.
- Tuberculosis is also associated with chronic changes of healed tuberculosis that characteristically manifest as parenchymal scarring and associated pleural thickening, which may be extensive (fibrothorax) and frequently calcifies (**Fig. 172.6**).

Suggested Reading

1. Hansell DM, Lynch DA, McAdams HP, et al. Infections of the lungs and pleura. In: Hansell DM, Lynch DA, McAdams HP, Bankier AA, ed. Imaging of Diseases of the Chest, 5th ed. Philadelphia: Mosby Elsevier; 2010:205–293
2. Stark DD, Federle MP, Goodman PC, Podrasky AE, Webb WR. Differentiating lung abscess and empyema: radiography and computed tomography. AJR Am J Roentgenol 1983;141(1):163–167
3. Travis WD, Colby TV, Koss MN, Rosado-de-Christenson ML, Müller NL, King TE Jr. Pleural disorders. In: King DW, ed. Atlas of Nontumor Pathology: Non-Neoplastic Disorders of the Lower Respiratory Tract. First Series. Fascicle 2. Washington, DC: The American Registry of Pathology; 2002:901–921
4. Silverman SG, Mueller PR, Saini S, et al. Thoracic empyema: management with image-guided catheter drainage. Radiology 1988;169(1):5–9
5. vanSonnenberg E, Nakamoto SK, Mueller PR, et al. CT- and ultrasound-guided catheter drainage of empyemas after chest-tube failure. Radiology 1984;151(2):349–353

CASE 173

■ Clinical Presentation

78-year-old man with a history of colon cancer

■ Radiologic Findings

PA chest radiograph (**Fig. 173.1A**) and coned-down composite views of right lung (**Fig. 173.1B**) demonstrate multi-focal bilateral nodular opacities. Note discrepant visualization of the lesion borders (**Fig. 173.1B**) (ill definition of some lesion borders [*arrowhead*] and sharp margination [*arrow*] of others) consistent with an extrapulmonary location. Unenhanced chest CT (mediastinal window) (**Figs. 173.1C, 173.1D**) shows multi-focal discontinuous areas of pleural thickening along the costal and diaphragmatic pleural surfaces, many of which are adjacent to ribs.

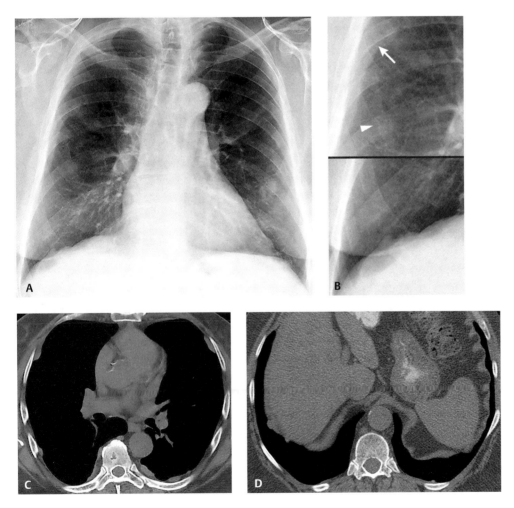

Fig. 173.1

835

■ Diagnosis

Pleural Plaques

■ Differential Diagnosis

None

■ DISCUSSION

Background

Four types of benign asbestos-related pleural disease are recognized: non-calcified pleural plaques, calcified pleural plaques, benign asbestos pleural effusion, and diffuse pleural fibrosis (see Table 125.1). *Pleural plaques* are the macroscopic and radiologic hallmarks of past asbestos exposure and typically develop 15–20 years after initial exposure. Pleural plaques tend to occur adjacent to relatively rigid structures such as the ribs, vertebrae, and the tendinous portion of the diaphragms. Subsequent calcium deposition often occurs in pleural plaques, beginning as fine, punctate flecks that may coalesce over time to form dense streaks or plate-like deposits. *Benign asbestos pleural effusions* are dose-related manifestations of asbestos exposure that may develop within a shorter latency period than that of other asbestos-related pleural diseases (1–20 years). The effusions are typically unilateral, typically exudates, and sometimes hemorrhagic. The diagnosis is established based on a history of exposure and through exclusion of other etiologies, particularly malignancy. *Diffuse pleural thickening* and *diffuse pleural fibrosis* are thought to develop after a previous asbestos-related pleural effusion, involve the visceral pleura, and affect the pleural surface adjacent to the costophrenic angle, a distinguishing feature from pleural plaques.

Etiology

The pathogenesis of pleural plaques is unclear. It has been hypothesized that plaques result from mechanical irritation of the parietal pleura by asbestos fibers. Recent studies suggest that short asbestos fibers (chrysotile) reach the parietal pleura by passage through lymphatic channels, where they cause an inflammatory reaction, whereas larger fibers (amphiboles) are retained in the lung.

Clinical Findings

Patients with pleural plaques are typically asymptomatic and have a history of asbestos exposure. Pleural plaques are invariably found more frequently in men than in women and exhibit increasing incidence and extent with advancing patient age.

Imaging Findings

Chest Radiography

- Bilateral, discontinuous multifocal areas of pleural thickening characteristically distributed on the posterolateral chest wall (ribs 7 to 10), the lateral chest wall (ribs 6 to 9), the domes of the diaphragms, and the mediastinal pleura (**Figs. 173.1A, 173.1B**)
- Characteristic sparing of the pleural surfaces adjacent to the lung apices and costophrenic angles (**Figs. 173.1A, 173.1B, 173.2**)
- Variable calcification (**Fig. 173.2**)
- Characteristic serpentine marginal calcification (so-called holly leaf pattern of calcification) in peripherally calcified plaques imaged *en face* (**Fig. 173.2**)

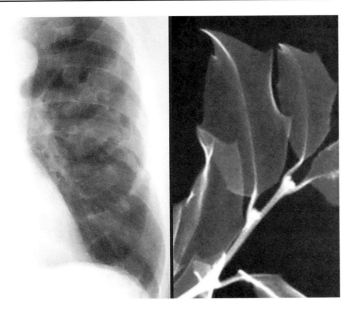

Fig. 173.2 Coned-down PA chest radiograph (*left*) of an 82-year-old man with pleural plaques demonstrate the *holly leaf* appearance of partially calcified plaques when projected *en face*. Note the densely calcified pleural plaques over the central tendinous portion of the left hemidiaphragm. Radiograph of several holly leaves (*right*) shows the scalloped edges resembling the margins of densely calcified pleural plaques when viewed *en face*.

MDCT

- Multifocal discontinuous bilateral pleural nodules; most profuse along paravertebral pleural surfaces and posterolateral chest wall (**Figs. 173.1C, 173.1D, 173.3, 173.4**)
- Pleural plaques along the anterior aspects of the upper ribs on CT, an area poorly visualized on radiography (**Figs. 173.1C, 173.4**)
- More conspicuous calcification of plaques than on radiography

Management

- None

Prognosis

- Good; no proven long-term sequelae
- Conflicting reports regarding likelihood of development of malignant pleural mesothelioma in patients with pleural plaques

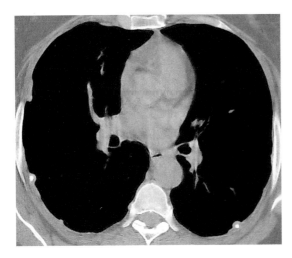

Fig. 173.3 Unenhanced chest CT (mediastinal window) of a 60-year-old man with pleural plaques demonstrates small bilateral multifocal discontinuous pleural nodules, some of which exhibit central calcification.

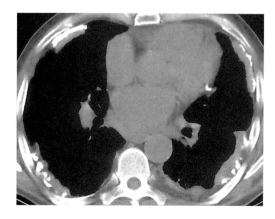

Fig. 173.4 Unenhanced chest CT (mediastinal window) of a 68-year-old man with pleural plaques demonstrates bilateral large, thick, discontinuous foci of pleural thickening with dense calcification extending along multiple ribs.

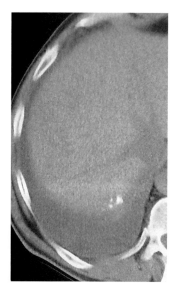

Fig.173.5 Unenhanced chest CT (mediastinal window) of a 63-year-old man with an asbestos-related pleural effusion demonstrates a right-sided pleural effusion and a calcified pleural plaque over the tendinous portion of the right hemidiaphragm.

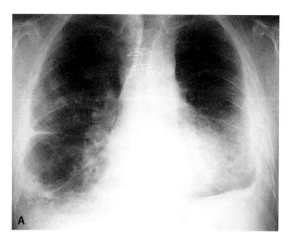
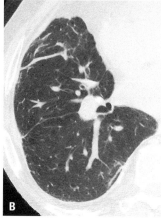

Fig. 173.6 PA chest radiograph (**A**) of a 72-year-old man with dyspnea and asbestosis demonstrates diffuse bilateral smooth pleural thickening that produces blunting of the costophrenic angles. Coned-down HRCT (**B**) shows diffuse continuous bilateral pleural thickening, more pronounced on the left. Note interstitial peripheral parenchymal bands, juxtapleural lines, and architectural distortion (**B**).

PEARLS

- *Asbestos-related pleural effusion* (**Fig. 173.5**) is a diagnosis of exclusion and can only be attributed to asbestos when there is a history of exposure and all other etiologies have been excluded, particularly malignancy.
- *Diffuse pleural fibrosis* typically manifests as diffuse pleural thickening that results in blunting of the costophrenic angles (**Figs. 173.6A, 173.6B**), and may mimic malignant pleural mesothelioma on histologic evaluation.
- *Asbestosis* (**Fig. 173.6B**) (see also Case 125) should *not* be confused with *asbestos-related pleural disease.* The former refers to interstitial lung disease characterized by pulmonary fibrosis resulting from occupational exposure to asbestos. The latter does not affect the lung and typically occurs in asymptomatic individuals.
- *Asbestos-related pleural plaques* do *not* undergo malignant degeneration or transformation into pleural mesothelioma. Plaques are simply a manifestation of having been exposed to asbestos.

Suggested Reading

1. Hansell DM, Lynch DA, McAdams HP, et al. Inhalational lung disease. In: Hansell DM, Lynch DA, McAdams HP, Bankier AA, ed. Imaging of Diseases of the Chest, 5th Edition. Philadelphia: Mosby Elsevier; 2010:451–504

2. Peacock C, Copley SJ, Hansell DM. Asbestos-related benign pleural disease. Clin Radiol 2000;55(6):422–432

3. Cugell DW, Kamp DW. Asbestos and the pleura: a review. Chest 2004;125(3):1103–1117

4. Chapman SJ, Cookson WO, Musk AW, Lee YC. Benign asbestos pleural diseases. Curr Opin Pulm Med 2003;9(4):266–271

5. Travis WD, Colby TV, Koss MN, Rosado-de-Christenson ML, Müller NL, King TE Jr. Pleural disorders. In: King DW, ed. Atlas of Nontumor Pathology: Non-Neoplastic Disorders of the Lower Respiratory Tract. First Series. Fascicle 2. Washington, DC: The American Registry of Pathology; 2002:901–921

CASE 174

■ Clinical Presentation

37-year-old man presents to the Emergency Department with pleuritic chest pain and shortness of breath

■ Radiologic Findings

PA (**Fig. 174.1A**) and lateral (**Fig. 174.1B**) chest X-rays show a right-sided primary spontaneous pneumothorax with near total collapse of the right lung and contralateral mediastinal displacement.

■ Diagnosis

Primary Spontaneous Pneumothorax

■ Differential Diagnosis

- Secondary Spontaneous Pneumothorax
- Traumatic Pneumothorax

■ Discussion

Background

Pneumothorax is the presence of air in the pleural space and is a common form of thoracic disease.

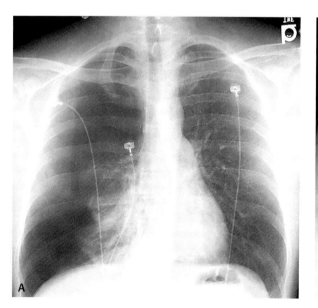
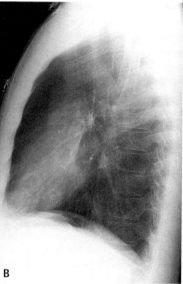

Fig. 174.1

Etiology

Pneumothorax may be classified into one of three major categories: *traumatic,* which can be either *iatrogenic* (following unsuccessful central venous line or pacemaker-ICD placement, CT-guided or transbronchial biopsy, etc.) or *non-iatrogenic* (e.g., following blunt or penetrating chest injuries (see Case 84); *primary spontaneous,* caused by rupture of an air-containing space within (*bleb*) or immediately deep to the pleura (*bulla*) (**Fig. 174.2**); or *secondary spontaneous,* related to underlying lung disease (e.g., emphysema, chronic interstitial fibrosis or cystic lung disease). Pneumothorax may also develop from pneumomediastinum as a result of air tracking from the mediastinal pleura. *Primary spontaneous pneumothorax* occurs most often in men (2–15M: 1F) in the third or fourth decade of life and shows a right-sided predilection and strong association with tobacco abuse. Numerous underlying conditions may be associated with *secondary spontaneous pneumothorax* (**Table 174.1**), the most common of which is COPD. In some cases, the secondary spontaneous pneumothorax is the first clinical manifestation of the underlying disease.

Clinical Findings

Chest pain and/or dyspnea are the classic clinical symptoms of spontaneous pneumothorax. Breath sounds are decreased or absent on auscultation despite normal or increased resonance on percussion.

Imaging Findings

Primary Spontaneous Pneumothorax

Chest Radiography

- Focal areas of apical emphysema or bulla typically not seen
- Visceral pleural reflection
  - Vascular markings do not extend beyond lateral border (**Fig. 174.1A**)
  - Follows contour of the lung (**Fig. 174.1A**)
  - Radiographic density gradient proceeds from "gray" (aerated lung) to"white" (visceral pleural reflection) to "black" (pleural air) (**Fig. 174.1A**)

MDCT

- Focal areas of apical emphysema or bullae identified (>80% of cases) (**Fig. 174.2**)
- Bullae located predominantly in the peripheral upper lobe or apices (**Fig. 174.2**)
- Localized low-attenuation areas ≥3 mm in diameter; ± thin walls (**Fig. 174.2**)

Table 174.1 Conditions Associated with Secondary Spontaneous Pneumothorax

COPD	Connective Tissue Disease	Immunologic Disorders	Neoplasia	Infection	Other
Asthma	Ehlers-Danlos syndrome	Idiopathic pulmonary fibrosis	Mesothelioma	Bacterial pneumonia	Birt-Hogg-Dubé syndrome
Cystic fibrosis	LAM*	Langerhans histiocytosis	Metastatic lung cancer	Fungal pneumonia	Catamenial
Emphysema	Marfan syndrome	Sarcoidosis	Metastatic sarcoma	Hydatid disease	Mitral valve prolapse
	Neurofibromatosis	Wegener granulomatosis	Pleural metastases	PCP	Silicosis
	Tuberous sclerosis		Primary lung cancer		XRT

*LAM, Lymphangioleiomyomatosis

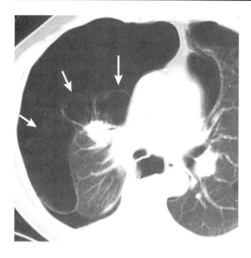

Fig. 174.2 Chest CT (lung window) of a young man presenting with primary spontaneous pneumothorax. Note the extensive upper lobe bulla bilaterally; right greater than left, and the large right pneumothorax. An incidental lung nodule is seen in the partially collapsed upper lobe.

Secondary Spontaneous Pneumothorax

Chest Radiography

- Visceral-parietal pleural separation (**Figs. 174.3A, 174.3D**)
- ± Evidence of underlying condition or predisposing disease (e.g., cystic lung disease, peripheral lung mass, interstitial fibrosis) (**Figs. 174.3A, 174.3D**)

MDCT

- Mirrors conventional radiography findings, albeit more sensitive and specific (**Figs. 174.3B, 174.3C**)

Pseudopneumothorax (skin fold, wrinkle in patient gown or sheet, external dressing)

Chest Radiography

- Typically "black" edge as opposed to "white" visceral pleural reflection, but not always (**Figs. 174.4A, 174.4B, 174.4C, 174.4D**)
- May be linear, curvilinear, multiple; does not usually follow lung contour (**Figs. 174.4A, 174.4B, 174.4C, 174.4D**)
- Vascular markings may or may not project beyond its lateral border (**Figs. 174.4A, 174.4B, 174.4C, 174.4D**)
- Radiographic density gradient proceeds from "gray" (aerated lung) to "black" edge (pseudo-visceral pleural reflection) to "gray" (aerated lung) (**Figs. 174.4A, 174.4B, 174.4C, 174.4D**)

Management

Primary Spontaneous Pneumothorax

- Decompression of affected pleural space
- Blebectomy, bullectomy, or pleurodesis

Secondary Spontaneous Pneumothorax

- Decompression of affected pleural space
- Directed toward underlying condition or predisposing disease process

Prognosis

Primary Spontaneous Pneumothorax

- High recurrence rate in the absence of treatment: 30% ipsilateral; 10% contralateral

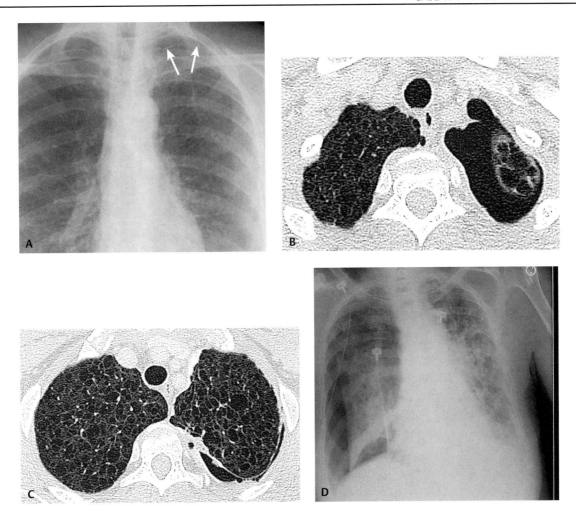

Fig. 174.3 Secondary spontaneous pneumothorax in two different patients. Coned-down AP chest X-ray over the left thorax **(A)** shows an apical pneumothorax *(arrows)* and a background of cystic lung lesions. Accompanying chest CT (lung window) **(B, C)** also reveals the apical, lateral, and posterior pneumothorax. The cystic lesions of lymphangioleiomyomatosis are seen to better advantage. AP portable chest exam **(D)** of a woman with pulmonary fibrosis from advanced sarcoidosis demonstrates a spontaneous right pneumothorax.

Secondary Spontaneous Pneumothorax

- Dependent on underlying condition

PEARLS

- Most air-containing spaces associated with primary spontaneous pneumothorax are bullae.
- Major contributing factor to primary spontaneous pneumothorax is smoking, which increases the likelihood by 22 times in men and by 8 times in women.
- Focal areas of emphysema distend with decrease in atmospheric pressure (e.g., increasing altitude during air flight) and with rapid resurfacing after diving.
- *Catamenial pneumothorax* occurs at the time of menstruation and may be recurrent with the woman's menstrual cycle. Postulated mechanisms include endometrial pleural and diaphragmatic implants (20–60% of patients have pelvic endometriosis) and migration of air from vagina, uterus, and fallopian tubes into peritoneal cavity, across diaphragmatic pores and defects into pleural space.

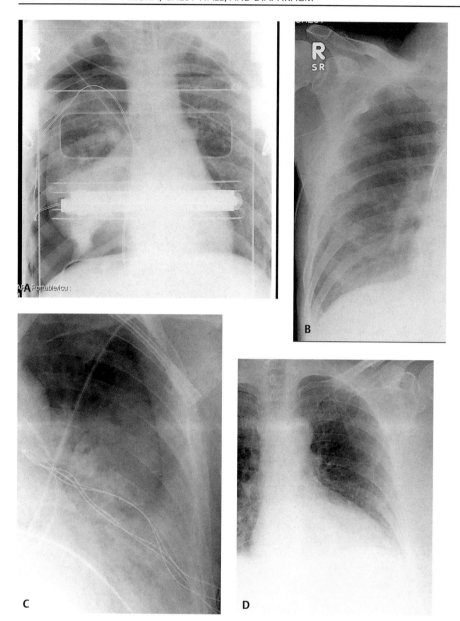

Fig. 174.4 True pneumothorax versus pseudopneumothorax. AP portable chest X-ray **(A)** of a trauma patient with spinal cord injury on a roto-bed and spontaneous right pneumothorax while on positive-pressure ventilation. The visceral pleural reflection follows the contour of the right lung, and vascular markings do not extend beyond the pleural reflection. Note the expected "gray-white-black" gradient. Coned-down chest X-ray over the right thorax reveals **(B)** two skin folds mimicking a pneumothorax. The two curvilinear "black" edges do not conform to the morphology of the lung. The multiplicity of lines also argues against a true pleural reflection. Note the abnormal "gray-black-gray" gradient. Similar findings with a single skin fold are seen on the coned-down chest exam over the left thorax **(C)**. Coned-down chest exam over the left thorax **(D)** of a gown wrinkle mimicking a pneumothorax. Although the "edge" appears white, it does not conform to the lung and vascular markings project beyond its border.

Suggested Reading

1. Alifano M. Catamenial pneumothorax. Curr Opin Pulm Med 2010;16(4):381–386

2. Fraser RS, Müller NL, Colman N, Paré PD. Pneumothorax. In: Fraser and Paré's Diagnosis of Disease of the Chest, 4th ed. New York: WB Saunders Company; 1999:2781–2794

3. Noppen M, De Keukeleire T. Pneumothorax. Respiration 2008;76(2):121–127

4. Wakai A. Spontaneous pneumothorax. Clin Evidence (online) 2008; Mar 10:1505

CASE 175

■ Clinical Presentation

83-year-old man with malaise and right-sided pleuritic chest pain

■ Radiologic Findings

Coned-down PA chest radiograph (**Fig. 175.1A**) demonstrates a moderate right pleural effusion and moderate pleural thickening along the lateral right pleural surface that extends into the interlobar fissure. Coronal T2-weighted MR image (**Fig. 175.1B**) shows circumferential right pleural thickening by high-signal nodular masses. Note extension into the interlobar fissure and right costodiaphragmatic recess, involvement of the mediastinal pleura, and invasion of the diaphragm and mediastinum. Contrast-enhanced chest CT (mediastinal window) (**Figs. 175.1C, 175.1D**) reveals the right pleural effusion; extensive plaque-like and nodular pleural thickening along the costal, diaphragmatic, and mediastinal pleural surfaces; and nodular involvement of the minor fissure.

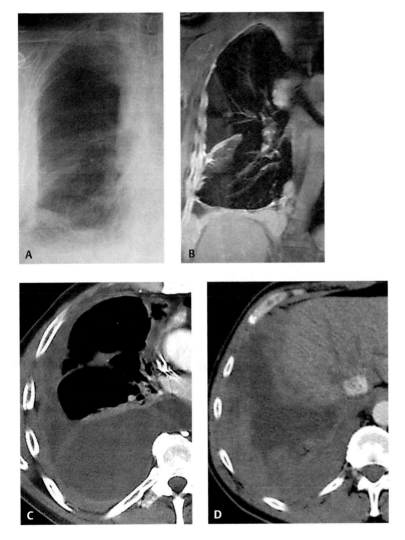

Fig. 175.1

845

■ Diagnosis

Diffuse Malignant Pleural Mesothelioma

■ Differential Diagnosis

- Pleural Effusion of Non-Neoplastic Etiology
- Malignant Pleural Effusion; Pleural Metastases (adenocarcinoma, carcinoma of other cell type, lymphoma)

■ Discussion

Background

Diffuse malignant pleural mesothelioma is a relatively rare pleural malignancy. It is the most common primary pleural neoplasm.

Etiology

The majority of cases of malignant pleural mesothelioma (80–90%) are related to the carcinogenic effects of asbestos, and most lesions occur in individuals with documented occupational or environmental asbestos exposure. Approximately 6% of asbestos workers will develop mesothelioma. While a higher incidence of mesothelioma is observed in patients with continuous exposure to asbestos, intermittent, brief, and indirect exposures have also been implicated in the development of this neoplasm. Occupations with increased exposure to asbestos include construction, shipyard, and insulation work. The latency period between onset of exposure and development of mesothelioma is between 20 and 40 years. Both amphibole and chrysotile asbestos fibers are associated with the development of mesothelioma. Amphiboles are long, needle-like fibers that penetrate deeply into the lung, resist clearance, and are considered more tumorogenic than the serpiginous chrysotile asbestos fibers.

Clinical Findings

Patients with malignant pleural mesothelioma often have an insidious onset of symptoms, commonly dyspnea and chest pain. Affected patients may also present with cough and constitutional symptoms, such as weight loss and fatigue. Most (approximately 75%) affected patients are men, typically between the ages of 40 and 60 years. A history of asbestos exposure is documented in only 40–80% of patients with mesothelioma.

Imaging Features

Chest Radiography

- Unilateral pleural effusion (40%) (**Fig. 175.1A**)
- Unilateral pleural thickening (**Fig. 175.1A**); diffuse, nodular, circumferential, fissural
- Decrease in size of affected hemithorax

MDCT

- Pleural effusion (**Figs. 175.1C, 175.1D, 175.2, 175.3, 175.4A**)
- Plaque-like (**Figs. 175.1C, 175.2, 175.3, 175.4A**) or nodular (**Figs. 175.1D, 175.2, 175.3, 175.4A**) pleural thickening
- Pleural thickening of greater than 1.0 cm (**Figs. 175.1C, 175.1D, 175.2, 175.3, 175.4A**)
- Mediastinal pleural involvement (**Figs. 175.1D, 175.2, 175.3, 175.4A**)
- Lung encasement, extension into interlobar fissures (**Figs. 175.1C, 175.2, 175.3, 175.4A**)
- Invasion of chest wall (**Fig. 175.3**), mediastinum (**Figs. 175.1D, 175.2, 175.3**), diaphragm and/or pericardium
- Concomitant pleural plaques in 25% of cases (**Fig. 175.2**)

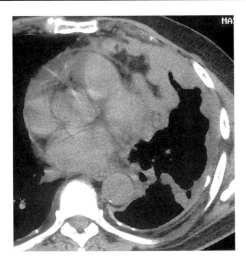

Fig. 175.2 Unenhanced chest CT (mediastinal window) of a 62-year-old man with mesothelioma demonstrates circumferential nodular left pleural thickening with involvement of the major fissure and direct mediastinal invasion. Note decreased size and encasement of the left lung and bilateral calcified pleural plaques. The patient worked in the shipbuilding industry for 35 years and had documented asbestos exposure.

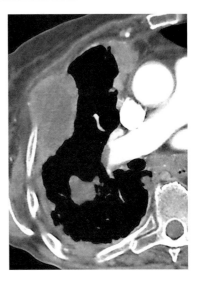

Fig. 175.3 Contrast enhanced chest CT (mediastinal window) reveals circumferential nodular pleural thickening involving the costal and mediastinal pleural surfaces with extension into the interlobar fissure. There is focal invasion of the chest wall anterolaterally and posteriorly and invasion of the anterior mediastinum. Note right hilar and subcarinal lymphadenopathy.

MRI

- Minimally increased signal relative to chest wall muscles on T1WI
- Moderately increased signal relative to muscle on T2WI (**Fig. 175.1B**)
- Improved detection of chest wall, diaphragm, and mediastinum invasion (**Fig. 175.1B**)

PET-CT

- Diffuse uptake of ^{18}FDG in tumor, typically intense (**Fig. 175.4B**)

Management

- Surgery: pleurectomy, extrapleural pneumonectomy for select patients
- Radiation therapy
- Chemotherapy; systemic, intrapleural
- Immunotherapy
- Photodynamic therapy, gene therapy, multimodality therapy

Prognosis

- Poor: 12-month median survival after diagnosis
- Better with early diagnosis and extrapleural pneumonectomy
- Reports of median survival of 18–19 months with radical pleurectomy-decortication and aggressive radiation therapy with or without chemotherapy

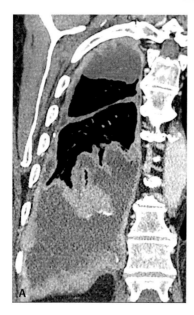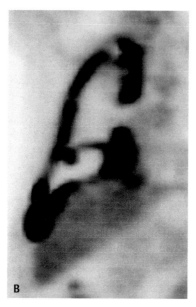

Fig. 175.4 Contrast-enhanced chest CT (coronal reformation) (**A**) shows circumferential nodular pleural thickening involving the costal, mediastinal, and diaphragmatic pleura and extending into the interlobar fissure, with a loculated pleural effusion. PET scan (coronal image) (**B**) demonstrates intense [18]FDG avidity throughout the tumor, demonstrating the circumferential growth pattern of tumor encasing the right lung and extending into the lateral costodiaphragmatic recess.

PEARLS

- Imaging features of mesothelioma cannot be reliably distinguished from those of pleural metastases.
- Clinical staging of mesothelioma relies primarily on CT, but MRI and PET imaging may add important diagnostic and prognostic information.
- Diagnosis is often established through open lung or video-assisted thoracoscopic (VATS) biopsy, whereas fine needle biopsies are usually inadequate.

Suggested Reading

1. Ismail-Khan R, Robinson LA, Williams CC Jr, Garrett CR, Bepler G, Simon GR. Malignant pleural mesothelioma: a comprehensive review. Cancer Contr 2006;13(4):255–263

2. Wang ZJ, Reddy GP, Gotway MB, et al. Malignant pleural mesothelioma: evaluation with CT, MR imaging, and PET. Radiographics 2004;24(1):105–119

3. Antman KH, Pass HI, Schiff PB. Malignant mesothelioma. In: DeVita VT, Hellman S, Rosenberg SA, eds. Cancer: Principles and Practice of Oncology. New York: Lippincott Williams & Wilkins; 2001:1943–1969

4. Sharma A, Fidias P, Hayman LA, Loomis SL, Taber KH, Aquino SL. Patterns of lymphadenopathy in thoracic malignancies. Radiographics 2004;24(2):419–434

5. Miller BH, Rosado-de-Christenson ML, Mason AC, Fleming MV, White CC, Krasna MJ. From the archives of the AFIP. Malignant pleural mesothelioma: radiologic-pathologic correlation. Radiographics 1996;16(3):613–644

CASE 176

■ Clinical Presentation

48-year-old woman with recently diagnosed lung cancer

■ Radiologic Findings

Coned-down PA chest radiograph (**Fig. 176.1A**) demonstrates circumferential nodular right pleural thickening with encasement and loss of volume of the right lung. Note the right upper lobe surgical chain sutures. Unenhanced chest CT (mediastinal window) (**Figs. 176.1B, 176.1C, 176.1D**) shows circumferential nodular pleural thickening that involves the major fissure (**Fig. 176.1C**) and is produced by multi-focal pleural masses of various sizes (**Figs. 176.1B, 176.1C, 176.1D**). Many pleural nodules/masses measure over 1 cm in thickness. Right upper lobe surgical chain sutures (**Fig. 176.1B**) are from prior wedge resection of a primary lung adenocarcinoma.

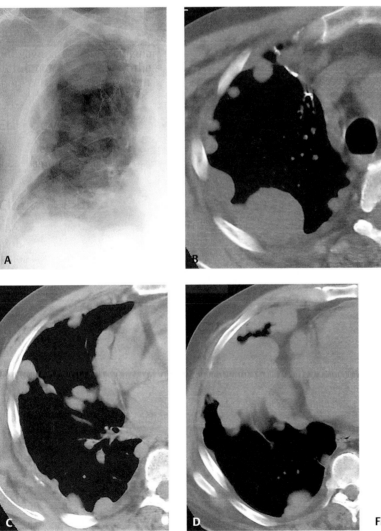

Fig. 176.1

■ Diagnosis

Pleural Metastases; Adenocarcinoma of the Lung

■ Differential Diagnosis

- Pleural Metastases from Extrapulmonary Primary Malignancy
- Diffuse Malignant Pleural Mesothelioma
- Lymphoma
- Invasive Thymoma

■ Discussion

Background

Pleural metastases are the most common pleural malignancy and typically result from primary cancers of the lung, breast, pancreas, stomach, and ovary. However, pleural metastases can originate from primary neoplasms in almost any organ. Malignant pleural effusion is the most common manifestation of metastatic pleural disease and occurs in approximately 60% of patients with pleural metastases. The majority of malignant pleural effusions (75%) occur as a result of lung and breast cancers and lymphoma. Pleural metastases may also manifest as soft-tissue nodules or masses.

Etiology

Pleural metastases may develop from direct pleural invasion by an adjacent peripheral lung cancer. "Drop" metastases may produce circumferential pleural involvement and may develop in patients with invasive thymoma. Metastases may also disseminate to the pleura via hematogeneous and lymphatic routes.

Clinical Findings

Patients with pleural metastases typically have a known primary malignancy. Most present with dyspnea on exertion. Chest pain is relatively uncommon (<25%), in contradistinction to its frequent occurrence in patients with malignant mesothelioma.

Imaging Features

Chest Radiography

- Unilateral or bilateral pleural effusion
- Focal or diffuse pleural thickening (**Fig. 176.1A**)
  - Nodular pleural thickening (**Fig. 176.1A**)
  - Circumferential pleural thickening (**Fig. 176.1A**)
- Pleural effusion and nodular pleural thickening

MDCT/HRCT

- Pleural effusion (**Fig. 176.2**)
- Pleural effusion and nodular pleural thickening/pleural masses (**Figs. 176.2, 176.4**)
- Nodular pleural thickening (**Figs. 176.1B, 176.1C, 176.1D, 176.2, 176.3, 176.4, 176.5**)
  - Circumferential (**Figs. 176.1B, 176.1C, 176.1D, 176.2, 176.4**)
  - Fissural (**Figs. 176.1C, 176.4**)
  - Mediastinal (**Figs. 176.1B, 176.1C, 176.1D, 176.2, 176.4**)
  - Thickening >1.0 cm (**Figs. 176.1B, 176.1C, 176.1D, 176.4, 176.5**)
  - Ossification in osteogenic sarcoma metastases (**Fig. 176.5**)

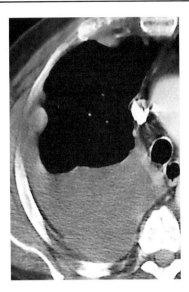

Fig. 176.2 Contrast-enhanced chest CT (mediastinal window) of a 79-year-old man with metastatic melanoma demonstrates a large right pleural effusion. Note multi-focal enhancing soft-tissue nodules along the anterior and lateral pleural surfaces and band-like enhancing soft tissue measuring 1.0 cm in thickness along the right mediastinal pleural surface.

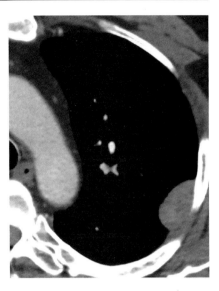

Fig. 176.3 Contrast-enhanced chest CT (mediastinal window) of a 62-year-old woman with metastatic renal cell carcinoma demonstrates a solitary, focal mass along the left lateral pleural surface. The lesion is heterogeneous and exhibits well-defined contours without invasion of adjacent osseous structures. There was no associated pleural effusion.

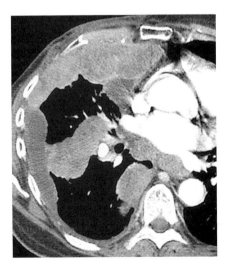

Fig. 176.4 Contrast-enhanced chest CT (mediastinal window) of a 51-year-old woman with metastatic breast cancer shows circumferential marked nodular pleural thickening in the right hemithorax with extension into the interlobar fissure and involvement of the mediastinal pleura. A loculated malignant pleural effusion is demonstrated laterally. Note right hilar and subcarinal metastatic lymphadenopathy.

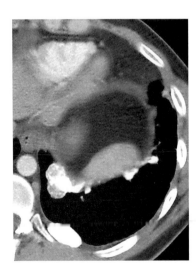

Fig. 176.5 Contrast-enhanced chest CT (mediastinal window) of a 28-year-old man with metastatic osteogenic sarcoma demonstrates ossified nodular pleural metastases along the posterior costal and diaphragmatic pleural surfaces.

Management

- Pleurodesis for control of malignant pleural effusions
- Pleural and systemic chemotherapy
- Radiation therapy

Prognosis

- Poor
- Mean survival for patients with lung cancer and malignant pleural effusion: 2–3 months
- Mean survival for patients with breast cancer and malignant pleural effusion: 7–15 months

PEARLS

- Pleural metastases, invasive thymoma, and lymphoma may be radiologically indistinguishable from diffuse malignant pleural mesothelioma.
- Pleural effusion in the setting of lung cancer does not imply malignancy, as affected patients may develop parapneumonic pleural effusions and pleural effusions unrelated to the primary neoplasm.

Suggested Reading

1. Hansell DM, Lynch DA, McAdams HP, et al. Neoplasms of the lungs, airways, and pleura. In: Hansell DM, Lynch DA, McAdams HP, Bankier AA, ed. Imaging of Diseases of the Chest, 5th ed. Philadelphia: Mosby Elsevier; 2010:787–879

2. Leung AN, Müller NL, Miller RR. CT in differential diagnosis of diffuse pleural disease. AJR Am J Roentgenol 1990;154(3):487–492

3. Aquino SL, Chen MY, Kuo WT, Chiles C. The CT appearance of pleural and extrapleural disease in lymphoma. Clin Radiol 1999;54(10):647–650

CASE 177

■ Clinical Presentation

Asymptomatic 67-year-old man

■ Radiologic Findings

Coned-down PA (**Fig. 177.1A**) and lateral (**Fig. 177.1B**) chest radiographs demonstrate a mass in the posterior right hemithorax. The mass has well-defined lateral and superior borders (**Figs. 177.1A, 177.1B**) and an indistinct inferior border (**Fig. 177.1B**). The lesion's inferior obtuse angles with the adjacent pleura result in incomplete border visualization on the lateral radiograph (*incomplete border sign*). Unenhanced chest CT (mediastinal window) (**Fig. 177.1C**) shows a well-defined homogeneous, lobulated soft-tissue mass that forms obtuse angles with the adjacent pleura. There is no evidence of chest wall involvement.

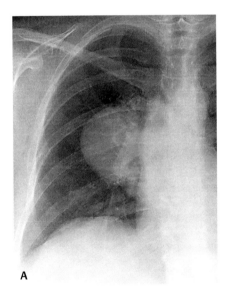

A

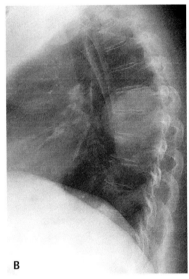

B

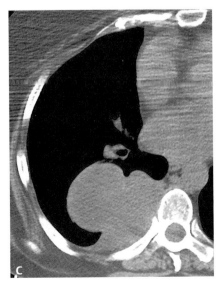

C

Fig. 177.1

■ Diagnosis

Localized Fibrous Tumor of the Pleura

■ Differential Diagnosis

- Other Mesenchymal Pleural Neoplasm
- Chest Wall Neoplasm (schwannoma, neurofibroma)
- Pleural Metastasis

■ Discussion

Background

Localized fibrous tumors of the pleura are rare but represent the second most common primary pleural neoplasm after mesothelioma. They probably arise from submesothelial mesenchymal cells that undergo fibroblastic differentiation. While most are related to the pleura, they have also been described in other intra- and extrathoracic locations. Localized fibrous tumors are not related to mesothelioma or to asbestos exposure.

Etiology

Localized fibrous tumors are neoplasms of unknown etiology.

Clinical Findings

Localized fibrous tumors typically occur in adult men and women in the fifth through eighth decades of life. Many patients (particularly those with small tumors) are asymptomatic and diagnosed incidentally because of an abnormal chest radiograph. Symptoms typically relate to tumor size and include cough, chest pain, and dyspnea. Constitutional symptoms, hypoglycemia, clubbing, and hypertrophic osteoarthropathy rarely occur.

Imaging Features

Chest Radiography

- Well-defined lobular nodules/masses; typically abut the pleura (**Figs. 177.1A, 177.1B**)
- Variable size; approximately one-third occupy half a hemithorax
- May exhibit the *incomplete border sign* (discrepant border visualization on orthogonal radiographs) (**Fig. 177.1B**)
- Approximately 80% extend to or occupy the inferior hemithorax; may mimic diaphragmatic elevation
- Ipsilateral pleural effusion in 20%

MDCT

- Non-invasive lobular soft-tissue mass of variable size; abuts at least one pleural surface (**Figs. 177.1C, 177.2, 177.3, 177.4**)
- Typically exhibit acute angles against adjacent pleura (**Figs. 177.2, 177.3, 177.4**); approximately one-third exhibit at least one obtuse angle (**Fig. 177.1C**)
- Contrast enhancement is typical (**Figs. 177.2, 177.4**)
- Homogeneous attenuation in small lesions; heterogeneous attenuation/enhancement in large lesions (**Figs. 177.2, 177.4**); low-attenuation areas (**Figs. 177.2, 177.4**), calcification and enhancing vessels within lesion
- Ipsilateral pleural effusion in approximately one-third of cases (**Fig. 177.4**)
- May exhibit fissural location (**Fig. 177.3**)
- Malignant tumors may invade the chest wall (**Fig. 177.4**)
- Rare direct visualization of pedicle

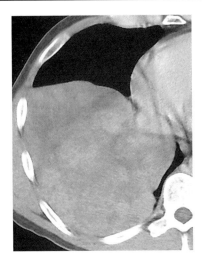

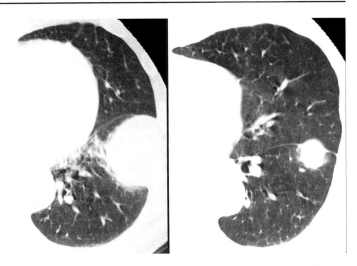

Fig. 177.2 Contrast-enhanced chest CT (mediastinal window) of a 49-year-old man with a large localized fibrous tumor of the pleura shows a large mass in the right inferior hemithorax. The mass exhibits well-defined borders, acute angles with the adjacent pleura, and heterogeneous contrast enhancement with nodular areas of high attenuation surrounded by irregular low-attenuation areas.

Fig. 177.3 Composite chest CT (lung window) of a 58-year-old man with an asymptomatic localized fibrous tumor of the pleura demonstrates a peripheral soft-tissue mass in the mid-left hemithorax that forms acute angles with the adjacent pleural surface (*left*) and extends into the left major fissure (*right*).

MRI

- Well-defined, non-invasive mass of heterogeneous signal
- Low/intermediate signal intensity on both T1WI and T2WI; high signal intensity on T2WI
- Multiplanar imaging helpful in excluding local invasion and establishing intrathoracic location

Management

- Complete surgical excision

Prognosis

- Favorable prognosis with benign course in up to 90% of patients
- Infrequent local recurrence and distant metastases

PEARLS

- Radiographic *incomplete border sign* refers to discrepancy of margin visualization of thoracic lesions and typically implies an extrapulmonary location.
    - It is typically exhibited by lesions that form obtuse borders with the adjacent pleura (**Figs. 177.1A, 177.1B**).
    - Although most thoracic localized fibrous tumors arise from the pleura, they infrequently exhibit the *incomplete border sign* as most of these tumors form acute angles with the adjacent pleura.
- Localized fibrous tumors of the pleura are not related to mesothelioma or asbestos exposure.
    - Benign and malignant variants are described.
    - Prognosis relates more to resectability than to histologic features.

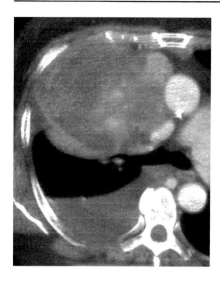

Fig. 177.4 Contrast-enhanced chest CT (mediastinal window) of a 50-year-old man with a malignant localized fibrous tumor of the pleura demonstrates a large heterogeneous soft-tissue mass in the anterior aspect of the right hemithorax that invades the anterior chest wall, produces mass effect on the mediastinum, and exhibits extensive low attenuation with central foci of enhancement. Note the large right-sided pleural effusion.

Suggested Reading

1. Rosado-de-Christenson ML, Abbott GF, McAdams HP, Franks TJ, Galvin JR. From the archives of the AFIP: Localized fibrous tumor of the pleura. Radiographics 2003;23(3):759–783

2. Hansell DM, Lynch DA, McAdams HP, et al. Neoplasms of the lungs, airways, and pleura. In: Hansell DM, Lynch DA, McAdams HP, Bankier AA, ed. Imaging of Diseases of the Chest, 5th ed. Philadelphia: Mosby Elsevier; 2010:787–879

3. England DM, Hochholzer L, McCarthy MJ. Localized benign and malignant fibrous tumors of the pleura. A clinicopathologic review of 223 cases. Am J Surg Pathol 1989;13(8):640–658

4. Magdeleinat P, Alifano M, Petino A, et al. Solitary fibrous tumors of the pleura: clinical characteristics, surgical treatment and outcome. Eur J Cardiothorac Surg 2002;21(6):1087–1093

5. Saifuddin A, Da Costa P, Chalmers AG, Carey BM, Robertson RJ. Primary malignant localized fibrous tumours of the pleura: clinical, radiological and pathological features. Clin Radiol 1992;45(1):13–17

CASE 178

■ Clinical Presentation

47-year-old man with chest pain

■ Radiologic Findings

Coned-down PA (**Fig. 178.1A**) and lateral (**Fig. 178.1B**) chest radiographs demonstrate a left upper lobe mass with associated thickening of the soft tissues of the anterior chest wall (**Fig. 178.1B**). Contrast-enhanced chest CT (mediastinal window) (**Figs. 178.1C, 178.1D**) reveals mass-like consolidation in the medial aspect of the left upper lobe with contiguous involvement of the adjacent anterior mediastinum. Note asymmetric soft-tissue thickening of the adjacent anterior chest wall (**Figs. 178.1C, 178.1D**) that exhibits heterogeneous attenuation (**Fig. 178.1C**) but no osseous destruction.

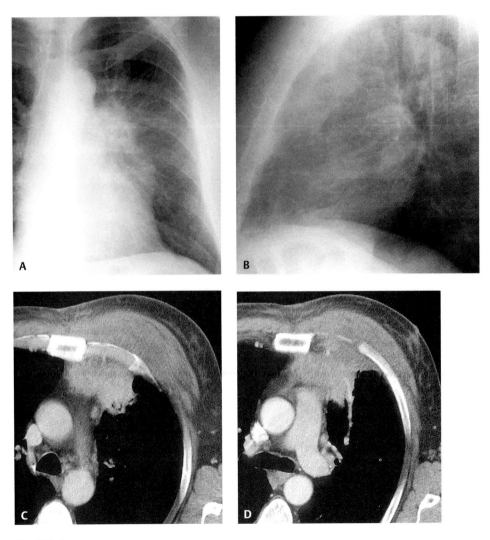

Fig. 178.1

857

■ Diagnosis

Chest Wall Infection (Actinomycosis) with Pulmonary, Mediastinal and Chest Wall Involvement

■ Differential Diagnosis

- Lung Cancer with Adjacent Mediastinal and Chest Wall Involvement
- Pulmonary, Mediastinal, and Chest Wall Involvement by Other Malignancy
- Other Thoracic Infections (aspergillosis, nocardiosis, blastomycosis, tuberculosis, pyogenic infection)

■ Discussion

Background

Actinomycosis is a rare bacterial pneumonia that often extends across anatomic barriers to involve the pleura and chest wall. It typically occurs as a chronic suppurative and granulomatous infection. Spread of infection is related to proteolytic enzymes and fistula formation between involved lung and adjacent tissues. Thoracic infection most commonly occurs through aspiration of contaminated oral secretions. Anaerobic cultures must be obtained for confirmation of the diagnosis; characteristic sulfur granules may be seen.

Etiology

Actinomycosis is caused by infection with organisms in the genus Actinomycetes. The most common pathogen is *Actinomyces israelli*. Less common pathogens include *A. naeslundii, A. viscosus,* and *A. propionica.*

Clinical Findings

Patients with actinomycosis may present with cough, sputum production, and fever and weight loss. Hemoptysis and chest pain occur less frequently. Affected patients often have poor dental hygiene that promotes growth of *Actinomyces* organisms normally present in the oropharynx. The cervicofacial region is most commonly affected. Abdominal infection is usually related to surgery or intestinal trauma, and pelvic disease may be associated with intrauterine devices in women. Cerebral actinomycosis may also occur.

Imaging Features

Chest Radiography

- Peripheral, unilateral patchy consolidation (may be chronic)
- Mass-like consolidation; may mimic lung cancer (**Figs. 178.1A, 178.1B**)
- Multi-focal nodules/masses
- Soft-tissue thickening or mass of adjacent chest wall (**Figs. 178.1A, 178.1B**)
- Wavy periostitis; rarely rib destruction

MDCT

- Mass-like consolidation; homogeneous or heterogeneous with peripheral enhancement and central low attenuation/cavitation (**Figs. 178.1C, 178.1D, 178.3, 178.4**)
- Pleural thickening (**Figs. 178.1C, 178.1D**), pleural effusion
- Hilar/mediastinal lymphadenopathy (**Fig. 178.3**)
- Mediastinal involvement (**Figs. 178.1C, 178.1D**)
- Chest wall soft-tissue mass or thickening (**Figs. 178.1C, 178.1D**)
- Wavy periostitis of adjacent osseous structures; rarely rib destruction

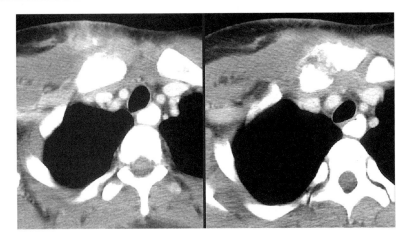

Fig. 178.2 Composite contrast-enhanced chest CT (mediastinal window) of an intravenous drug user with chest wall *Staphylococcus aureus* osteomyelitis demonstrates enhancing soft-tissue infiltration of the subcutaneous fat of the right anterior chest wall, thickening of adjacent muscles, and involvement of the ipsilateral sternoclavicular joint.

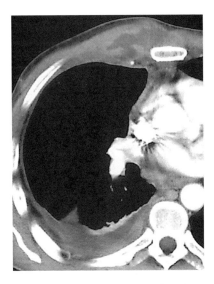

Fig. 178.3 Contrast-enhanced CT (mediastinal window) of a 41-year-old man with tuberculosis demonstrates a heterogeneous irregular mass in the soft tissues of the right anterior chest wall. Note subtle peripheral enhancement and central low attenuation consistent with tissue necrosis. There is right pleural thickening, a small right pleural effusion, and lymphadenopathy in the azygoesophageal recess.

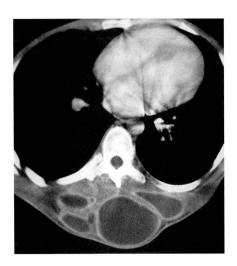

Fig. 178.4 Contrast-enhanced CT (mediastinal window) of a 58-year-old man with coccidioidomycosis demonstrates multiple cystic masses with peripheral enhancement in the soft tissues of the posterior chest wall. The lesions expand and deform the chest wall.

Management

- Prolonged therapy with penicillin: four to six weeks of intravenous penicillin followed by 6–12 months of an oral regimen
- Improved oral hygiene

Prognosis

- Good with antibiotic treatment but slow response; prolonged indolent disease reported
- Cure in 90% of patients treated with penicillin
- Morbidity from central nervous system involvement (i.e., brain abscess, meningitis)

PEARLS

- Thoracic actinomycosis is often difficult to diagnose and can mimic lung cancer and tuberculosis in its clinical presentation and imaging features. The majority of patients undergo surgery for definitive diagnosis.
- Heroin addicts have a striking tendency to develop septic arthritis of the sternoclavicular and sternochondral joints, typically caused by *Staphylococcus aureus* (**Fig. 178.2**) and *Pseudomonas aeruginosa.*
- Tuberculous chest wall abscesses are most frequently found at the margins of the sternum and along rib shafts (**Fig. 178.3**).

Suggested Readings

1. Jeung MY, Gangi A, Gasser B, et al. Imaging of chest wall disorders. Radiographics 1999;19(3):617–637

2. Hansell DM, Lynch DA, McAdams HP, et al. Infections of the lungs and pleura. In: Hansell DM, Lynch DA, McAdams HP, Bankier AA, ed. Imaging of Diseases of the Chest, 5th ed. Philadelphia: Mosby Elsevier; 2010:205–293

3. Mabeza GF, Macfarlane J. Pulmonary actinomycosis. Eur Respir J 2003;21(3):545–551

4. Colmegna I, Rodriguez-Barradas M, Rauch R, Clarridge J, Young EJ. Disseminated *Actinomyces meyeri* infection resembling lung cancer with brain metastases. Am J Med Sci 2003;326(3):152–155

5. Morris BS, Maheshwari M, Chalwa A. Chest wall tuberculosis: a review of CT appearances. Br J Radiol 2004;77(917): 449–457

CASE 179

■ Clinical Presentation

Asymptomatic 91-year-old woman

■ Radiologic Findings

Coned-down PA (**Fig. 179.1A**) and lateral (**Fig. 179.1B**) chest radiographs demonstrate a peripheral opacity in the right superior hemithorax that forms obtuse angles with the adjacent chest wall (**Fig. 179.1A**). There is discrepancy in margin visualization consistent with an extrapulmonary location. Contrast-enhanced chest CT (lung window, **Fig. 179.1C**; mediastinal window, **Fig. 179.1D**) shows a peripheral mass that forms at least one obtuse angle with the adjacent chest wall (**Figs. 179.1C, 179.1D**) and exhibits fat attenuation with scant thin linear soft-tissue elements (**Fig. 179.1D**). The mass is contiguous with subcutaneous fat attenuation tissue.

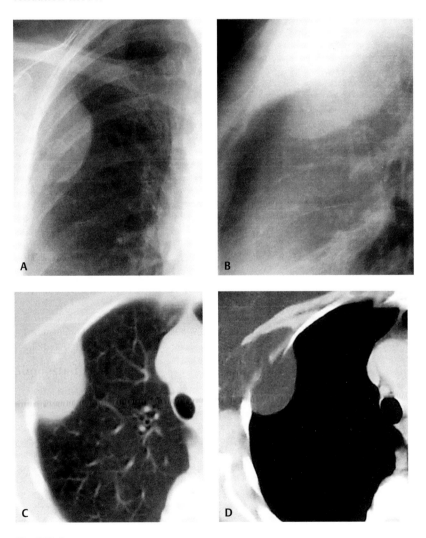

Fig. 179.1

■ Diagnosis

Chest Wall Lipoma

■ Differential Diagnosis

None

■ Discussion

Background

Benign chest wall tumors may originate from blood vessels, nerves, bone, cartilage, or fat. The imaging manifestations of benign and malignant chest wall lesions overlap, but some entities have characteristic imaging features that allow a confident diagnosis. Lipomas represent the most common soft-tissue chest wall tumors. They are well-circumscribed, encapsulated masses of adipose tissue that may lie deep within the chest wall and/or protrude into the thorax, displacing the pleura, mimicking other benign or malignant pleural lesions.

Etiology

The etiology of chest wall lipomas is unknown.

Clinical Findings

Chest wall lipomas are typically incidental findings in asymptomatic patients. They occur most frequently in patients who are 50–70 years of age and are more common in obese individuals.

Imaging Findings

Chest Radiography

- Well-marginated ovoid or lens-shaped chest wall mass (**Figs. 179.1A, 179.1B**)
- Lesions may exhibit the *incomplete border sign* (**Figs. 179.1A, 179.1B**)
- Lesions may change shape with respiration

MDCT

- Chest wall mass with intrathoracic extension and well-defined borders (**Figs. 179.1C, 179.1D**)
- Fat attenuation mass (**Fig. 179.1D**); may contain scant thin linear and punctate soft-tissue elements (**Fig. 179.1D**)
- Occasional punctate calcification
- Completely intrathoracic, subcutaneous, or both (**Figs. 179.1C, 179.1D**)

MRI

- High signal intensity on T1WI
- Decreased signal intensity on T1W1 fat-saturation
- Intermediate signal intensity on T2WI
- Homogenous, smooth-lobulated edged, semicircular, oval, or polygonal-shaped mass

Management

- None
- Surgical excision in selected patients with large lesions

Prognosis

- Excellent

PEARLS

- Predominance of soft-tissue elements in a fatty chest wall lesion should suggest the possibility of *liposarcoma* or *lipoblastoma*. Large lesion size should also prompt exclusion of malignancy.
- *Fibrous dysplasia* is a developmental skeletal anomaly that commonly affects the ribs and may be monostotic (70–80%) or polyostotic.
  - The lesion is related to failure of mesenchymal osteoblasts to achieve normal morphologic differentiation and maturation.
  - Imaging studies typically demonstrate unilateral fusiform rib enlargement and deformity with cortical thickening and increased trabeculation (**Fig. 179.3**).
- *Neurofibromas* are peripheral nerve neoplasms that most commonly affect young adults between the ages of 20 and 30 years.
  - Most patients (60–90%) have type 1 neurofibromatosis (NF1).
  - Neurofibromas may develop along the thoracic spine roots, the paraspinal ganglia of the sympathetic chain, the intercostal nerves, or the peripheral nerves of the chest wall.
  - Neurofibromas arising from intercostal nerves may produce rib erosion, notching, and/or sclerosis (**Fig. 179.4**).
- CT is more cost-effective than radiography for establishing the diagnosis of chest wall *lipoma* and for demonstration of small calcifications and subtle bone destruction. MRI is the preferred modality for delineating intramuscular neurofibromas; for demonstrating soft-tissue, intraspinal, and marrow involvement by neurogenic tumors; and for surgical planning.
- Primary tumors of the diaphragm are uncommon.
  - Lipoma (**Fig. 179.2**) is the most common benign tumor; leiomyoma, hemangioma, and other tumors are rarely encountered.
  - Prominent fat pads and omental fat herniations also occur near the diaphragm.
  - The most common malignant neoplasm of the diaphragm is fibrosarcoma.

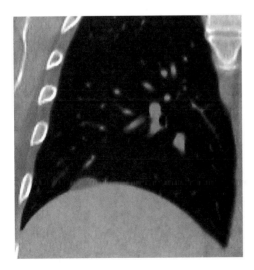

Fig. 179.2 Contrast-enhanced chest CT (mediastinal window, coronal reformation) of a 57-year-old man with a diaphragmatic lipoma shows a well-defined lesion of fat attenuation along the superior surface of the right hemidiaphragm.

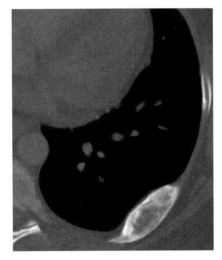

Fig. 179.3 Coned-down chest CT (bone window) of a 42-year-old man with monostotic fibrous dysplasia shows a right rib expansile lesion with intact cortical margins.

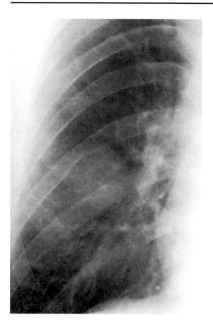

Fig. 179.4 Coned-down PA chest radiograph of a 29-year-old man with neurofibromatosis shows smooth notching and sclerosis of the undersurface of the right eighth posterior rib that conforms to the superior contour of an adjacent nodular opacity with "incomplete" and ill-defined borders.

Suggested Reading

1. Hansell DM, Lynch DA, McAdams HP, et al. Neoplasms of the lungs, airways, and pleura. In: Hansell DM, Lynch DA, McAdams HP, Bankier AA, ed. Imaging of Diseases of the Chest, 5th ed. Philadelphia: Mosby Elsevier; 2010:787–879

2. Tateishi U, Gladish GW, Kusumoto M, et al. Chest wall tumors: radiologic findings and pathologic correlation: part 1. Benign tumors. Radiographics 2003;23(6):1477–1490

3. Kuhlman JE, Bouchardy L, Fishman EK, Zerhouni EA. CT and MR imaging evaluation of chest wall disorders. Radiographics 1994;14(3):571–595

4. Epler GR, McLoud TC, Munn CS, Colby TV. Pleural lipoma. Diagnosis by computed tomography. Chest 1986;90(2): 265–268

CASE 180

■ Clinical Presentation

79-year-old man complains of a "clicking" sensation in his left shoulder with activity and has a palpable infrascapular mass

■ Radiologic Findings

Contrast-enhanced chest CT (mediastinal window) (**Figs. 180.1A, 180.1B, 180.1C, 180.1D**) demonstrates a 6.0 cm left-sided, lenticular, infrascapular mass located medial to the serratus anterior and latissimus dorsi muscles. The attenuation of the mass is similar to adjacent skeletal muscle. More inferiorly, streaks of fat are seen intermingled with the mass.

■ Diagnosis

Elastofibroma Dorsi

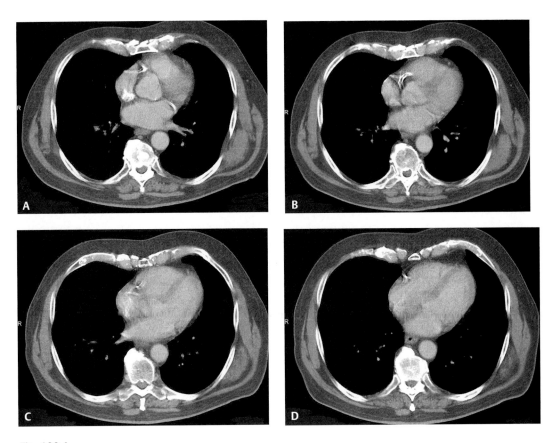

Fig. 180.1

865

■ Differential Diagnosis

Infrascapular Lesion: Decreased to Intermediate Attenuation Similar to Skeletal Muscle

- Extrabdominal Desmoid
- Neurofibroma
- Cicatricial Fibroma
- Malignant Fibrous Histiocytoma
- Sarcoma

■ Discussion

Background

Elastofibroma dorsi (ED) is a slow-growing, benign lesion of unknown cause and is most commonly seen in the periscapular or infrascapular region of the chest wall. Autopsy series report ED 3.0 cm or smaller in 24% of women and 11% of men more than 55 years old. The name reflects its characteristic location at the medial, inferior border of the scapula. ED lesions are periscapular in 99% of cases and bilateral in 10–66% of cases. Synchronous lesions in the infra-olecranon region are common. Other reported locations include the thoracic wall, deltoid muscle, axilla, ischial tuberosity, and greater trochanteric region.

Etiology

Although the etiology is unclear, there is an increased prevalence of ED in manual laborers. Thus, it has been postulated that ED may be reactive in nature and attributable to repetitive mechanical friction of the scapula against the ribs. This theory provides an explanation for the right-sided preponderance. However, up to 32% of cases occur in patients with a family history of ED, suggesting a genetic, nontraumatic origin.

Clinical Findings

Elastofibromas occur most often in elderly women but have been reported in persons aged 6–94 years. Most patients with ED are asymptomatic and small pseudotumors may be overlooked unless the patient is asked to move his or her arm laterally or anteriorly. Only rarely do patients report stiff shoulders, local pain with arm movement, and/or an annoying "click" when using their shoulder.

Imaging Findings

Radiography

- Usually normal

Ultrasonography

One of four ultrasound patterns may be detected:
- Type I (54%): inhomogeneous fasciculated
- Type II (22%): inhomogeneous non-specific
- Type III (15%): hyperechogeneous
- Type IV (9%): hypoechogeneous
- In the absence of a clearly defined cleavage plane, ED is difficult to differentiate from surrounding muscle

MDCT

- Poorly defined, inhomogeneous, unencapsulated, lenticular, soft-tissue mass (**Figs. 180.1A, 180.1B, 180.1C, 180.1D**)
- Attenuation similar to that of skeletal muscle (**Figs. 180.1A, 180.1B, 180.1C, 180.1D**)
- Contains linear streaks of fat attenuation (**Figs. 180.1C, 180.1D**)

MRI

- Similar appearance to CT
- T1/T2-weighted images: signal intensity similar to skeletal muscle with interlaced streaks of fat signal intensity
- Heterogeneous enhancement after gadolinium administration

Management

- Asymptomatic patients: no treatment necessary
- Symptomatic patients:
  - Complete surgical excision is the treatment of choice

Prognosis

- Recurrence after surgery is unusual
- No cases of malignant transformation have been reported

PEARLS

- In most cases, diagnosis can be made on the basis of characteristic CT/MRI imaging findings and typical periscapular or infrascapular anatomic location, avoiding unnecessary biopsy and surgery in asymptomatic patients.
- Elastofibromas are very frequently bilateral. The presence of a similar contralateral periscapular lesion is of great benefit in establishing the correct diagnosis, virtually eliminating malignancy from the differential.

Suggested Reading

1. Battaglia M, Vanel D, Pollastri P, et al. Imaging patterns in elastofibroma dorsi. Eur J Radiol 2009;72(1):16–21 [Epub ahead of print]
2. Kransdorf MJ, Meis JM, Montgomery E. Elastofibroma: MR and CT appearance with radiologic-pathologic correlation. AJR Am J Roentgenol 1992;159(3):575–579
3. Naylor MF, Nascimento AG, Sherrick AD, McLeod RA. Elastofibroma dorsi: radiologic findings in 12 patients. AJR Am J Roentgenol 1996;167(3):683–687

CASE 181

■ Clinical Presentation

17-year-old man with left chest pain and dyspnea

■ Radiologic Findings

Coned-down PA chest radiograph (**Fig. 181.1A**) shows a mass-like opacity in the left hemithorax and a left pleural effusion. Contrast-enhanced chest CT (mediastinal window) (**Figs. 181.1B, 181.1C**) demonstrates a large heterogeneous mass invading the left anterolateral chest wall and destroying the anterolateral aspect of the left sixth rib. The mass contains small areas of indistinct calcification. Note moderate-size left pleural effusion (**Figs. 181.1B, 181.1C**).

■ Diagnosis

Askin Tumor/Primitive Malignant Neuroectodermal Tumor (PNET)

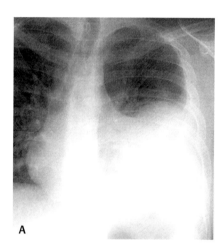
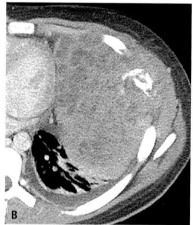
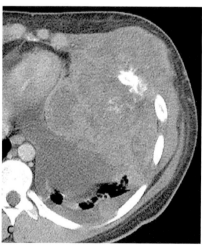

Fig. 181.1

■ Differential Diagnosis

- Metastatic Tumor
- Lymphoma (direct extension)
- Infection (e.g., tuberculosis)

■ Discussion

Background

Primitive neuroectodermal tumors (PNETs), originally known as Askin tumors, are malignant small round cell tumors that typically affect children and adolescents, but may be encountered in adults. They are typically unilateral, aggressive masses that originate in the chest wall, destroy bone, and are typically associated with pleural effusion. Women are affected more commonly than men (3:1). Detection of associated rib destruction establishes the tumor location within the chest wall. In an adult, the most common etiologies of rib destruction are metastatic lesions, multiple myeloma, and chondrosarcoma. In children and adolescents, the most likely neoplasms include Ewing sarcoma, neuroblastoma, lymphoma, and Askin (PNET) tumor.

Etiology

The etiology of Askin tumor is unknown.

Clinical Findings

Askin (PNET) tumor typically manifest as a large, extrapulmonary mass in an adolescent or young adult. Affected patients often complain of localized chest pain.

Imaging Findings

Chest Radiography

- Large, unilateral extrapulmonary chest wall mass (**Fig. 181.1A**)
- Chest wall/pleural location may be difficult to determine (**Fig. 181.1A**)
- Rib destruction
- Ipsilateral pleural effusion: frequent finding (**Fig. 181.1A**)
- Lymphadenopathy

MDCT

- Heterogeneous chest wall mass with intrathoracic extension (**Figs. 181.1B, 181.1C**)
- Rib destruction (**Figs. 181.1B, 181.1C**)
- Pleural effusion (90%) (**Figs. 181.1B, 181.1C**)
- Extension into chest wall, pleura, lung, mediastinum (**Figs. 181.1B, 181.1C**)
- Metastases to hilar/mediastinal lymph nodes

MRI

- Homogeneous and iso- or discretely hypointense in comparison to spinal cord on T1W1
- Heterogeneous and hyperintense on proton density and T2W1
- Stark contrast-enhancement after the administration of paramagnetic contrast agents

Management

- Surgical excision, radiation therapy, chemotherapy

Prognosis

- Overall survival is poor

- *Hodgkin lymphoma* and *non-Hodgkin lymphoma* may occasionally invade the chest wall (**Fig. 181.2**) with or without associated mediastinal or lung involvement.
  - In a minority of patients, the chest wall may be the only site of disease.
  - CT and MR are effective imaging modalities for evaluating tumor extension into chest wall fat or muscle, and for detection of rib destruction.
  - Chest wall involvement by lymphoma may be extensive (**Fig. 181.2**).
- Tumors may arise from any of the various components of the chest wall (muscle, bone, cartilage, fat, fibrous connective tissue, nerves, breast tissue, blood, and lymphatic vessels).
  - Such tumors may displace the adjacent pleura and form obtuse angles at its interface with adjacent pleural surface, and mimic a pleural mass.
- *Fibrosarcoma* and *malignant fibrohistiocytoma* (*MFH*) are the most common malignant tumors that arise in the soft tissues of the chest wall in adults.

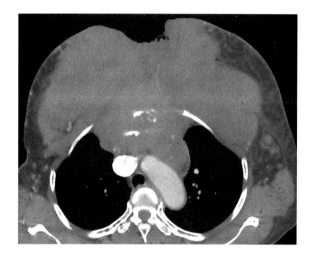

Fig. 181.2 Contrast-enhanced chest CT (mediastinal window) of a 42-year-old man with lymphoma demonstrates a large, lobulated tumor involving the anterior mediastinum and the anterior chest wall. There is osseous destruction of the sternum and ulceration of the anterior skin surface across the midline. Note bilateral internal mammary and left axillary lymphadenopathy.

Suggested Reading

1. Katsenos S, Nikopoloulou M, Kokkonouzis I, Archondakis S. Askin's tumor: a rare chest wall neoplasm. Case report and short review. Thorac Cardiovasc Surg 2008;56(5):308–310

2. Hansell DM, Lynch DA, McAdams HP, et al. Neoplasms of the lungs, airways, and pleura. In: Hansell DM, Lynch DA, McAdams HP, Bankier AA, ed. Imaging of Diseases of the Chest, 5th ed. Philadelphia: Mosby Elsevier; 2010:787–879

3. Takanami I, Imamura T. The treatment of Askin tumor: results of two cases. J Thorac Cardiovasc Surg 2002;123(2): 391–392

4. Sabaté JM, Franquet T, Parellada JA, Monill JM, Oliva E. Malignant neuroectodermal tumour of the chest wall (Askin tumour): CT and MR findings in eight patients. Clin Radiol 1994;49(9):634–638

5. Jeung MY, Gangi A, Gasser B, et al. Imaging of chest wall disorders. Radiographics 1999;19(3):617–637

CASE 182

■ Clinical Presentation

46-year-old man with chest pain and a palpable left anterior chest wall mass

■ Radiologic Findings

Coned-down PA (**Fig. 182.1A**) and lateral (**Fig. 182.1B**) chest radiographs demonstrate a left anterior chest wall mass. The lesion exhibits a well-defined lobulated border with obtuse angles against the adjacent chest wall on the lateral radiograph (**Fig. 182.1B**) and manifests as a left mid-thoracic opacity with poorly defined margins on the frontal radiograph (**Fig. 182.1A**). Unenhanced chest CT (mediastinal window) (**Fig. 182.1C**) shows a heterogeneous left anterior chest wall mass arising at the costochondral-sternal junction with multifocal dense, linear calcifications.

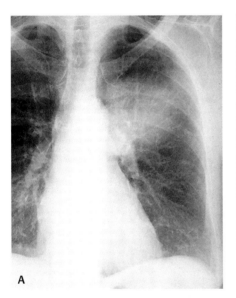
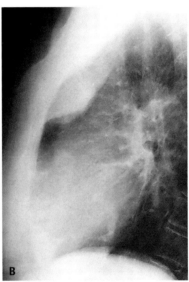
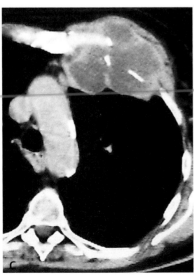

Fig. 182.1

871

■ Diagnosis

Chondrosarcoma

■ Differential Diagnosis

- Metastasis from Primary Chondrosarcoma or Other Primary Malignant Neoplasm
- Primitive Malignant Neuroectodermal Tumor
- Malignant Fibrous Histiocytoma
- Fibrosarcoma; Neurofibrosarcoma

■ Discussion

Background

Chondrosarcomas are malignant neoplasms with cartilaginous differentiation. They represent the most common primary malignant tumor of the chest wall. They typically arise in the anterior chest wall and involve the sternum or costochondral arches. Less frequently they arise in the ribs (17%) and scapulae.

Clinical Findings

Chondrosarcomas occur across a wide age range but typically affect patients between the ages of 30 and 60 years. Most tumors manifest as a palpable chest wall mass that may be painful. The lesion may grow rapidly and cause chest pain. Males are affected slightly more frequently than females (male to female ratio of 1.3:1.0).

Imaging Findings

Chest Radiography

- Large chest wall mass (**Figs. 182.1A, 182.1B**); bone destruction; typically affects sternum, costochondral junction or ribs
- *Incomplete border sign* as in other extrapulmonary masses (see Case 177) (**Figs. 182.1A, 182.1B**)
- Variable intratumoral calcification (rings, arches, flocculent, or stippled)

MDCT

- Well-defined soft-tissue mass (**Fig. 182.1C**)
- Osseous destruction
- Higher sensitivity for detection of tumor calcification, which may be amorphous, popcorn-like, or curvilinear (**Fig. 182.1C**)

MRI

- Lobular chest wall mass
- Heterogeneous signal intensity on T1WI and T2WI images
- Heterogeneous contrast enhancement, especially at the periphery

Management

- Surgical resection
- Chemotherapy and radiation in selected cases

Prognosis

- Five-year survival: >60% (>80% in patients without metastases)
- Poor prognosis associated with incomplete resection, metastases, local recurrence, and patient age over 50 years

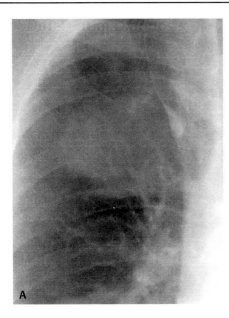
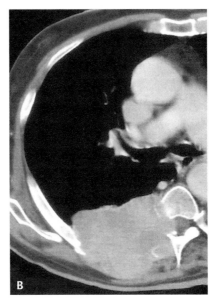

Fig. 182.2 Coned-down PA chest radiograph **(A)** of a 69-year-old man with metastatic hepatocellular carcinoma demonstrates an ill-defined opacity projecting over the right superior hemithorax with associated destruction of the posterior right fifth rib. Note the accessory azygos lobe. Contrast-enhanced chest CT (mediastinal window) **(B)** shows a large soft-tissue mass of the right posterior chest wall with associated rib destruction and invasion of the adjacent soft tissue. Note partial destruction of the adjacent vertebral body and intraspinal tumor growth **(B)**.

PEARLS

- Chest wall metastases represent the most common malignant chest wall neoplasm in adults (**Figs. 182.2A, 182.2B**).
- Chest wall neoplasms that exhibit imaging features of osseous destruction in adults include chest wall metastases (**Figs. 182.2A, 182.2B**), multiple myeloma (**Fig. 182.3**), and neurofibrosarcoma (**Fig. 182.4**).
- CT and MRI have complementary roles in the evaluation of chest wall lesions.
  - CT more readily shows calcifications (**Figs. 182.1C, 182.4**) and bone destruction (**Figs. 182.2B, 182.3, 182.4**), is faster, and is less expensive.
  - MRI may better delineate the extent of tumor invasion and is superior for depicting bone marrow infiltration and the extent of soft-tissue involvement.

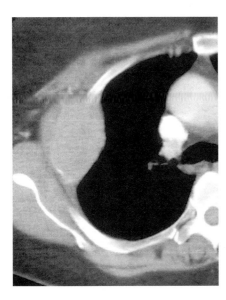

Fig. 182.3 Contrast-enhanced chest CT of a 53-year-old woman with multiple myeloma shows a homogeneous soft-tissue mass in the right lateral chest wall with associated rib destruction, involvement of the chest wall soft tissues, and smooth effacement of the adjacent pleura.

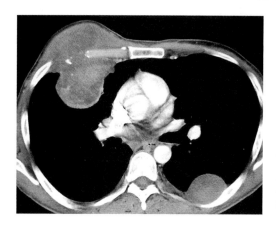

Fig. 182.4 Contrast-enhanced chest CT of a 46-year-old man with neurofibromatosis (NF1) shows a benign neurofibroma manifesting as a well-defined homogeneous soft-tissue mass of the left posterior chest wall with benign pressure erosion on the adjacent rib and a malignant right anterior chest wall neurofibrosarcoma. The neurofibrosarcoma exhibits heterogeneous enhancement, amorphous calcification, extension into the right chest cavity, and invasion of the anterior chest wall soft tissues and osseous structures.

Suggested Reading

1. Müller NL, Silva CIS. Chest wall. In: Silva CIS, Müller NL, Hansell DM, ed. Imaging of the Chest. Philadelphia: Saunders; 2008:1590–1608

2. Tateishi U, Gladish GW, Kusumoto M, et al. Chest wall tumors: radiologic findings and pathologic correlation: part 2. Malignant tumors. Radiographics 2003;23(6):1491–1508

3. Gladish GW, Sabloff BM, Munden RF, Truong MT, Erasmus JJ, Chasen MH. Primary thoracic sarcomas. Radiographics 2002;22(3):621–637

4. Kuhlman JE, Bouchardy L, Fishman EK, Zerhouni EA. CT and MR imaging evaluation of chest wall disorders. Radiographics 1994;14(3):571–595

CASE 183

■ Clinical Presentation

Asymptomatic 35-year-old man

■ Radiologic Findings

PA (**Fig. 183.1A**) and lateral (**Fig. 183.1B**) chest radiographs demonstrate a severe pectus excavatum deformity. Note vertical orientation of the anterior ribs and obscuration of the right cardiac border in the absence of right middle lobe consolidation. Contrast-enhanced chest CT (mediastinal window, **Fig. 183.1C**; lung window, **Fig. 183.1D**) reveals the pectus deformity, with posterior displacement of the sternum and associated leftward displacement of the heart (**Fig. 183.1C**). The illustrated anteroposterior (7.19 cm) and transverse measurements (28.36 cm) (**Fig. 183.1D**) are used to compute the Haller (pectus) index (see below).

■ Diagnosis

Pectus Excavatum

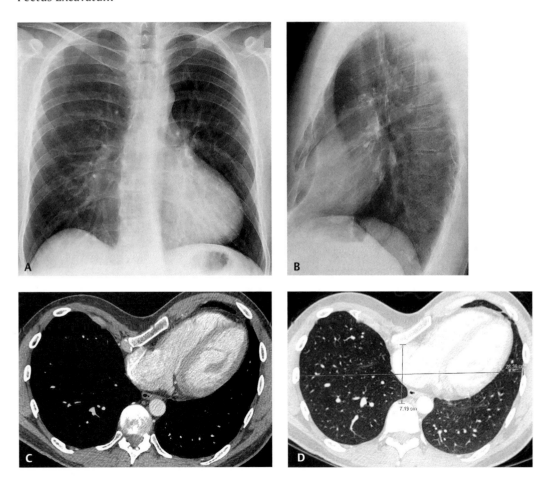

Fig. 183.1

875

■ Differential Diagnosis

None

■ Discussion

Background

Pectus deformities (pectus excavatum and pectus carinatum) are among the most common chest wall anomalies in the general population. There is great variability in the anatomy and morphology of the anterior chest wall of asymptomatic children. Thus, mild asymmetry and mild degrees of pectus deformity are sometimes considered normal variants. Pectus excavatum is also referred to as "funnel chest."

Etiology

Pectus excavatum is thought to result from abnormal growth of the costal cartilages that produces depression of the sternum (typically its inferior portion) often associated with sternal rotation to the right. Typically, there is associated rotation and displacement of the heart and mediastinum to the left. *Pectus carinatum* and localized *pectus excavatum* probably result from sternal growth disturbances with or without associated costal cartilage abnormalities. Severity of pectus excavatum may be determined by computing the Haller index (syn. pectus index), which is defined as the ratio of the transverse diameter (horizontal distance of the inner aspect of the rib cage) and the anteroposterior diameter (shortest distance between the anterior cortex of the vertebrae and the posterior cortex of the sternum at its narrowest point). In the illustrated case (**Fig. 183.1D**), the pectus index is 4 (28/7). A pectus index over 3.25 is one of the parameters used to select candidates for surgical correction of the chest wall deformity. The normal Haller index is about 2.5.

Clinical Findings

Pectus excavatum is found in approximately 0.13–0.4% of the general population and affects males three to four times more frequently than females. While it is usually a sporadic condition, there are reports of an increased familial incidence. Associated conditions include Marfan syndrome, congenital heart disease (2%), and mitral valve prolapse. Most affected patients are asymptomatic. Symptomatic patients complain of dyspnea, chest pain, and palpitations. Severe pectus excavatum deformity may result in exercise-induced cardiopulmonary dysfunction. There is an increased incidence of mild scoliosis (15–22% of cases). There may also be large airway compression, malacia, and a predisposition to atelectasis. Physical examination may reveal a heart murmur related to flow abnormalities from mediastinal distortion. Impaired cardiac function is primarily exercise-induced with decreased stroke volume and respiratory reserve.

Imaging Findings

Chest Radiography

- Mediastinal shift to the left, upturned configuration of cardiac apex, and straightening of left heart border (from mediastinal rotation) on frontal radiographs (**Fig. 183.1A**)
- Posterior depression of inferior sternum with narrow anteroposterior diameter on lateral radiographs (**Fig. 183.1B**)
- Prominent right pulmonary vasculature and poor visualization of right cardiac border, suggesting right middle lobe consolidation/volume loss on frontal radiographs (**Fig. 183.1A**)
- Increased downward sloping of anterior ribs on frontal radiographs (**Fig. 183.1A**)

MDCT

- Location and degree of pectus deformity and its effect on intrathoracic structures (**Fig. 183.1C**)
- Evaluation of mediastinum and airways, and exclusion of pulmonary disease
- Calculation of "pectus index" (i.e., ratio of transverse thoracic diameter to AP diameter at deepest part of pectus deformity) (**Fig. 183.1D**)

- Multiplanar and 3-D volume rendered imaging useful in guiding surgical planning and follow-up results (**Figs. 183.2C, 183.2D**)

Management

- Surgical correction: patients with cardiorespiratory symptoms or for cosmetic reasons
- Resection of costal cartilage with placement of a transverse metallic strut (**Figs. 183.2A, 183.2B, 183.2C, 183.2D**)

Prognosis

- Excellent for asymptomatic patients with mild pectus deformity
- Excellent for surgically treated patients; best results when surgery is performed between ages 4 and 10 years but successful surgery reported in adolescents and adults

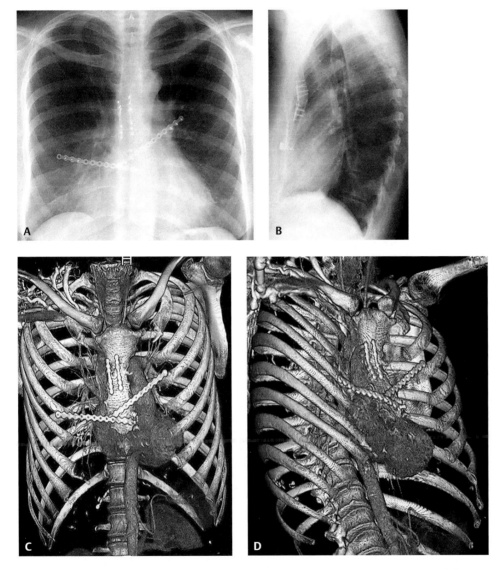

Fig. 183.2   PA **(A)** and lateral **(B)** chest radiographs demonstrate post-surgical changes following corrective surgery for pectus excavatum. Metallic bands and bars extend along and across the sternum, respectively; the bars connect to the anterior aspect of adjacent ribs. The 3-D volume-rendered images show the post-surgical changes to better advantage **(C, D)**. (*See color insert following page 108.*) The pectus index was improved from 3.77 pre-op to 3.0 post-op.

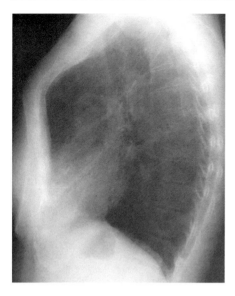

Fig. 183.3 Lateral chest radiograph of an asymptomatic woman with pectus carinatum shows focal sternal deformity with increased anteroposterior thoracic diameter.

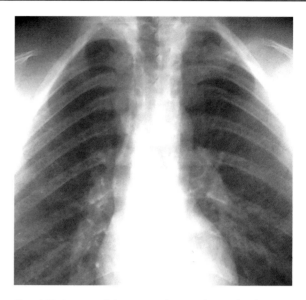

Fig. 183.4 Coned-down PA chest radiograph of an asymptomatic young man with cleidocranial dysostosis shows small rudimentary clavicles bilaterally and a bell-shaped thorax.

PEARLS

- *Pectus carinatum*, or "pigeon breast," is less common than pectus excavatum. It may result from abnormal growth of the costal cartilage or abnormal fusion of the sternal segments and manubrium, with resultant sternal protrusion (**Fig. 183.3**).
- *Cleidocranial dysostosis* is an autosomal dominant disorder of membranous bone in which the outer portions of the clavicles are typically absent.
  - Scapula may be hypoplastic and the glenoid is often small.
  - Thorax may be bell-shaped (**Fig. 183.4**).
- *Poland syndrome* refers to congenital absence or hypoplasia of the pectoralis major muscle.
  - Associated anomalies include malformations of ipsilateral ribs (typically 2–5) and clavicle, and congenital absence of ipsilateral breast tissue (**Figs. 183.5A, 183.5B**).

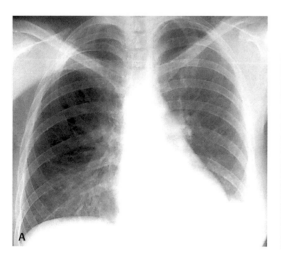
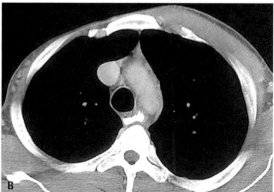

Fig. 183.5 PA chest radiograph **(A)** of an asymptomatic patient with Poland syndrome demonstrates hyperlucency of the right hemithorax secondary to asymmetry of the chest wall soft tissues and absence of the right breast. Contrast-enhanced chest CT (mediastinal window) **(B)** reveals absence of the right pectoralis muscles.

Suggested Reading

1. Müller NL, Silva CIS. Chest wall. In: Silva CIS, Müller NL, Hansell DM, ed. Imaging of the Chest. Philadelphia: Saunders; 2008:1590–1608

2. Haller JA Jr, Kramer SS, Lietman SA. Use of CT scans in selection of patients for pectus excavatum surgery: a preliminary report. J Pediatr Surg 1987;22(10):904–906

3. Grissom LE, Harcke HT. Thoracic deformities and the growing lung. Semin Roentgenol 1998;33(2):199–208

4. Lancaster L, McIlhenny J, Rodgers B, Alford B. Radiographic findings after pectus excavatum repair. Pediatr Radiol 1995;25(6):452–454

5. Takahashi K, Sugimoto H, Ohsawa T. Obliteration of the descending aortic interface in pectus excavatum: correlation with clockwise rotation of the heart. Radiology 1992;182(3):825–828

CASE 184

■ Clinical Presentation

Asymptomatic 53-year-old man with a left posterior mass detected incidentally on chest radiography

■ Radiologic Findings

Coned-down PA (**Fig. 184.1A**) and lateral (**Fig. 184.1B**) chest X-rays show a well-defined mass in the posterior left inferior hemithorax that appears to abut the adjacent diaphragm. Contrast-enhanced chest CT (lung window) (**Fig. 184.1C**) and coronal reformation (**Fig. 184.1D**) demonstrate the well-defined mass abuts, elevates, and deforms the posterior aspect of the left diaphragm and contains the left kidney (**Figs. 184.1C, 184.1D**).

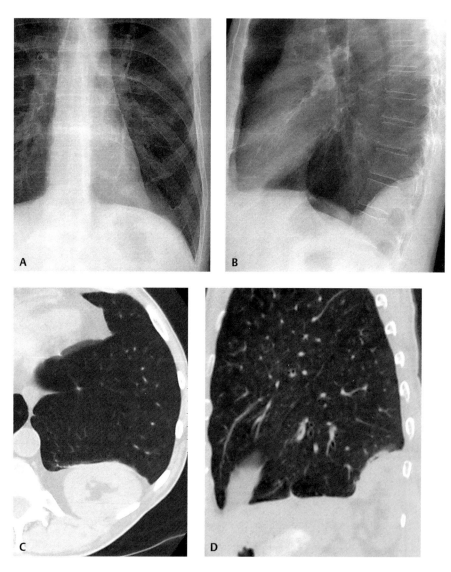

Fig. 184.1

■ Diagnosis

Bochdalek Hernia

■ Differential Diagnosis

None

■ Discussion

Background

Abdominal contents may herniate into the thorax through congenital or acquired diaphragmatic weak areas or through rents caused by trauma. Non-traumatic diaphragmatic herniation occurs most frequently through the esophageal hiatus and is usually related to obesity and/or pregnancy. Less commonly, herniation occurs through the pleuroperitoneal hiatus (Bochdalek hernia) or the parasternal hiatus (Morgagni hernia). *Bochdalek hernias* have been reported to occur more commonly on the left side, although a recent small series described a right-sided predominance (68%) with bilateral involvement in 14% of affected patients. Bochdalek hernias are associated with protrusion of omental or retroperitoneal fat that may be accompanied by abdominal organs, most often the kidney. *Morgagni hernias* are less common and represent 3% of diaphragmatic hernias. They are frequently located lateral to the xiphoid but may be directly posterior to it. The foramina of Morgagni are small triangular diaphragmatic clefts bounded medially by muscle fibers originating from the sternum and laterally by the seventh costal cartilages. Morgagni hernias are typically unilateral and occur more commonly on the right (90%) as the left foramen is protected by the pericardium.

Etiology

Bochdalek hernias are typically acquired lesions of adults and relate to focal weaknesses or defects in the diaphragm near the pleuroperitoneal hiatus.

Clinical Findings

The incidence of Bochdalek hernias in the adult population is approximately 1% and women are more commonly affected. The incidence of Bochdalek hernias increases with age, suggesting that they are acquired lesions. Affected patients are often asymptomatic but may complain of vague symptoms including chest pain, abdominal pain, and rarely bowel obstruction. Large hernias may produce mass effect and pulmonary insufficiency.

Imaging Features

Chest Radiography

- Focal bulge in diaphragm or soft-tissue mass in posterior/posteromedial inferior thorax (**Figs. 184.1A, 184.1B**)
- Opacity may appear less dense than soft tissue (**Fig. 184.1A**)
- May visualize internal air-containing bowel loops

MDCT

- Continuity with diaphragm and abdomen (**Figs. 184.1C, 184.1D**)
- Demonstration of fat attenuation with intrinsic punctate or thin linear soft-tissue foci representing omental vessels (**Fig. 184.2**)
- Herniated viscera, most often the kidney (**Figs. 184.1C, 184.1D**)

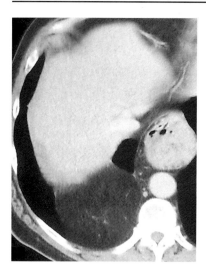

Fig. 184.2 Unenhanced chest CT (mediastinal window) of a 55-year-old man with a Bochdalek hernia reveals herniation of retroperitoneal fat into the right inferior thorax.

Management

• Surgical repair in symptomatic patients

Prognosis

• Good, most patients remain asymptomatic
• Large hernias may contain viscera or bowel that may experience vascular compromise or obstruction

PEARLS

• *Morgagni hernias* manifest as well-defined soft-tissue masses located in the right costophrenic angle in asymptomatic patients (**Figs. 184.3, 184.4, 184.5**). In contrast to *Bochdalek hernias*, a hernia sac is usually present and typically contains omentum (**Figs. 184.3, 184.4**) and/or bowel (**Fig. 184.4**), typically transverse colon. More rarely, the stomach, small bowel, or liver (**Fig. 184.5**) is involved. In some cases, the hernia sac may extend into the pericardium.
• *Congenital Bochdalek hernias* relate to congenital anomalies of the pleuroperitoneal canal, often with partial agenesis of the hemidiaphragm. These lesions are typically left-sided and, when large, are associated with neonatal respiratory distress. Large congenital Bochdalek hernias may contain large amounts of bowel and abdominal viscera and may result in pulmonary hypoplasia.

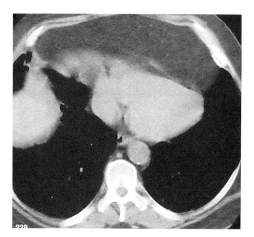

Fig. 184.3 Unenhanced chest CT (mediastinal window) of a 58-year-old man with bilateral Morgagni hernias shows protrusion of omental fat into the anterior thorax.

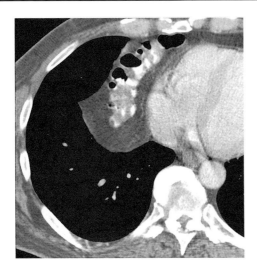

Fig. 184.4 Contrast-enhanced chest CT (mediastinal window) of a 43-year-old man with a Morgagni hernia demonstrates a right costophrenic angle hernia sac that contains air-filled bowel with residual contrast material.

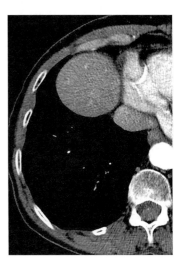

Fig. 184.5 Contrast-enhanced chest CT (mediastinal window) of a 57-year-old man with a Morgagni hernia shows a right costophrenic angle hernia sac that contains liver.

Suggested Reading

1. Hansell DM, Lynch DA, McAdams HP, et al. Congenital anomalies. In: Hansell DM, Lynch DA, McAdams HP, Bankier AA, ed. Imaging of Diseases of the Chest, 5th ed. Philadelphia: Mosby Elsevier; 2010:1065–1119

2. Gaerte SC, Meyer CA, Winer-Muram HT, Tarver RD, Conces DJ Jr. Fat-containing lesions of the chest. Radiographics 2002;22(Spec No):S61–S78

3. Gale ME. Bochdalek hernia: prevalence and CT characteristics. Radiology 1985;156(2):449–452

4. Caskey CI, Zerhouni EA, Fishman EK, Rahmouni AD. Aging of the diaphragm: a CT study. Radiology 1989;171(2):385–389

5. Mullins ME, Stein J, Saini SS, Mueller PR. Prevalence of incidental Bochdalek's hernia in a large adult population. AJR Am J Roentgenol 2001;177(2):363–366

CASE 185

■ Clinical Presentation

45-year-old man 6-weeks status post CABG with complaints of increasing dyspnea on exertion and orthopnea who cannot tolerate lying flat and must sleep with his head elevated on 4–5 pillows

■ Radiologic Findings

Preoperative frontal chest X-ray (**Fig. 185.1A**) shows mild cardiomegaly and a normal relationship of the right and left diaphragms. No underlying lung disease is present. Follow-up postoperative frontal (**Fig. 185.1B**) and lateral (**Fig. 185.1C**) chest radiographs demonstrate marked elevation of the left diaphragm relative to the right. Note the median sternotomy. Subsequent fluoroscopic "sniff test" revealed paradoxical motion of the left diaphragm.

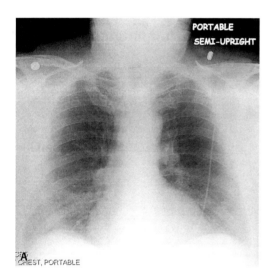
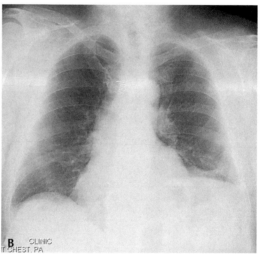
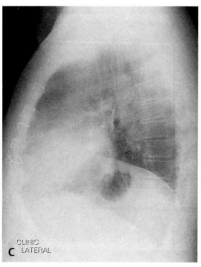

Fig. 185.1

■ Diagnosis

Paralyzed Left Diaphragm

■ Differential Diagnosis

- Eventration of the Diaphragm
  - ○ Congenitally thin muscular portion of diaphragm; appearance increases with age
  - ○ 5R:1L
  - ○ Anteromedial on right; usually involves entire left diaphragm
- Elevation of the Diaphragm
  - ○ Subpulmonic Effusion (see Case 171)
  - ○ Atelectasis
  - ○ Hypoplastic Lung
  - ○ Abdominal Disease (e.g., subphrenic abscess; liver mass; ascites)
  - ○ Idiopathic
- Diaphragmatic Hernia (see Cases 94 and 184)

■ Discussion

Background

The diaphragm is a cone-shaped muscle innervated by the cervical motor neurons of C3–C5 via the phrenic nerves. The diaphragm is the most important muscle of ventilation, the contraction of which creates negative intrathoracic pressure initiating ventilation, expanding the thoracic cavity, and facilitating gas exchange. The diaphragm contributes up to 70% of the total ventilation at rest in both the upright and supine positions. Diaphragmatic paralysis encompasses a spectrum of disease that may involve a single leaflet (unilateral diaphragmatic paralysis) or both leaflets (bilateral diaphragmatic paralysis). Normal ventilation also requires simultaneous contraction of the accessory respiratory muscles (i.e., scalenus muscles, parasternal internal and external intercostal muscles, trapezius, and sternocleidomastoid).

Etiology

Unilateral diaphragmatic paralysis is most often the result of neoplasia (e.g., lymphoma, advanced lung cancer). Other possible causes include non-iatrogenic and iatrogenic trauma, cervical spondylosis, herpes zoster infection, and infrequently sepsis. *Bilateral diaphragmatic paralysis* is usually a sequela of motor neuron disease (e.g., amyotrophic lateral sclerosis), demyelinating disease (e.g., multiple sclerosis), and myopathies (e.g., muscular dystrophy). The incidence of diaphragmatic paresis-paralysis after coronary artery bypass grafting (CABG) ranges from 10% to 60%. Postulated causes include pleurotomy with harvest of the internal mammary artery for grafts (e.g., chest wall and parenchymal trauma, reduced blood flow to ipsilateral intercostal muscles), mechanical injury to the phrenic nerve (i.e., phrenic nerves crosses the internal mammary artery anteriorly (54% of patients) and posteriorly (14% of patients), and the use of cardioplegic solutions.

Clinical Findings

Symptoms depend on whether the diaphragmatic paralysis is unilateral or bilateral, and on the presence of pre-existent lung disease. Patients with *unilateral diaphragmatic paralysis* are often asymptomatic at rest but experience dyspnea with exertion, or dyspnea at rest if they have underlying pre-existent lung disease (e.g., emphysema, pulmonary fibrosis). Patients with *bilateral diaphragmatic paralysis* may present with respiratory failure or dyspnea exacerbated by recumbency. Paradoxical abdominal wall retraction during inspiration may be observed. On PFTs, vital capacity (VC) normally decreases approximately 10% with recumbency. In *unilateral diaphragmatic paralysis* the VC decreases to 20–30% or more of the predicted value, and with *bilateral diaphragmatic paralysis* there is a 50% decrease in VC. Diaphragmatic electromyography (EMG) has a limited role in *unilateral diaphragmatic paralysis* but may reveal a pattern consistent with underlying myopathy or neuropathy. Assessment of transdiaphragmatic pressure differentials (i.e., thin-walled balloon placed transnasally into the distal esophagus to measure pleural pressure changes and a second intra-gastric balloon placed to measure intra-abdominal pressure) can distinguish diaphragmatic paralysis from other causes of respiratory failure.

Imaging Findings

Chest Radiography

Unilateral Diaphragmatic Paralysis

- Unilateral diaphragmatic elevation strongly suggests diagnosis (**Figs. 185.1B, 185.1C**)
- Comparison with serial or remote chest exams helpful in documenting chronicity (**Figs. 185.1A, 185.1B, 185.1C**)
- Lung volume diminished on affected side (**Figs. 185.1B, 185.1C**)
- Ipsilateral basilar atelectatic changes (**Figs. 185.1B, 185.1C**)

Bilateral Diaphragmatic Paralysis

- Often unrecognized or misinterpreted as low lung volumes or hypoventilation

Fluoroscopic "Sniff Test"

- Real-time fluoroscopic study performed to assess diaphragmatic excursion during tidal volume (normal inspiration and expiration) and with exaggerated inspiratory maneuvers designed to isolate diaphragm from accessory respiratory muscles (i.e., through rapid sniffing)
- During inspiration and expiration, normal diaphragm moves down and up, respectively, 2–8 cm
- Rapid repetitive "sniffing" (i.e., as if the patient has a bad runny nose without the benefit of a handkerchief or tissue)
  - Accentuates the difference in a paretic or paralyzed diaphragm, which will exhibit paradoxical motion (i.e., during inspiration, affected diaphragm moves up; and during expiration, affected diaphragm moves down)
  - Must be performed with patient supine or at least semi-recumbent; upright positioning alone has a high false negative rate

Ultrasonography

- Paretic-paralyzed diaphragm exhibits no active caudal excursion with inspiration
- Paradoxical movement with employment of rapid sniffing

MDCT

- Indicated in patients with suspected neoplasia or lymphadenopathy affecting or invading the phrenic nerve

Management

- Most patients: asymptomatic, transient; do not require treatment
- Surgical diaphragmatic plication may benefit symptomatic patients with *unilateral diaphragmatic paralysis*
- *Bilateral diaphragmatic paralysis* depends on the etiology and severity
  - Phrenic nerves intact without myopathy: diaphragmatic pacing (phrenic nerve is electrically stimulated to contract the diaphragm)
  - Phrenic nerves not intact: non-invasive positive-pressure ventilation

Prognosis

- Good in *unilateral diaphragmatic paralysis*, especially in the absence of underlying neurologic or pulmonary disease

- Poor in patients with advanced lung disease, *bilateral diaphragmatic paralysis*, and chronic demyelinating conditions
- Most patients with post–cardiac surgery diaphragmatic paresis-paralysis improve with conservative measures; rarely complicated by hypoventilatory respiratory failure
- Diaphragm function may recover if nerve is not permanently injured; phrenic nerve regeneration occurs at an estimated rate of 1 mm/day
- *Bilateral diaphragmatic paralysis:* may be complicated by increased CO_2 retention, leading to eventual hypercapnic respiratory failure

PEARLS

- "Sniff test"—insensitive with ipsilateral large or subpulmonic pleural effusions.
- Diaphragmatic excursion is paradoxical with diaphragmatic paralysis but not with diaphragmatic eventration.

Suggested Reading

1. Gierada DS, Slone RM, Fleishman MJ. Imaging evaluation of the diaphragm. Chest Surg Clin N Am 1998;8(2): 237–280

2. Kumar N, Folger WN, Bolton CF. Dyspnea as the predominant manifestation of bilateral phrenic neuropathy. Mayo Clin Proc 2004;79(12):1563–1565

3. Qureshi A. Diaphragm paralysis. Semin Respir Crit Care Med 2009;30(3):315–320

4. Ulkü R, Onat S, Balci A, Eren N. Phrenic nerve injury after blunt trauma. Int Surg 2005;90(2):93–95

5. Verhey PT, Gosselin MV, Primack SL, Kraemer AC. Differentiating diaphragmatic paralysis and eventration. Acad Radiol 2007;14(4):420–425

Section XIII

Post-Thoracotomy Chest

CASE 186

■ Clinical Presentation

60-year-old woman status post antecedent left upper lobectomy for adenocarcinoma

■ Radiologic Findings

PA (**Fig. 186.1A**) and lateral (**Fig. 186.1B**) chest X-rays show decreased volume in the left thorax and leftward anterior mediastinal shift. The left diaphragm is elevated and a juxtaphrenic peak is present. The interface between lung and the shifted anterior mediastinum forms an *upper triangle sign* mimicking mediastinal widening (**Fig. 186.1A**) (*white arrows*). The anterior interface of the LLL with the mediastinum correlates with this finding on the lateral exam (**Fig. 186.1B**) (*black arrows*) and should not be confused with a displaced left oblique fissure. Note the absence of a LUL bronchial orifice on the lateral exam (**Fig. 186.1B**)

■ Diagnosis

Left Upper Lobectomy

■ Differential Diagnosis

Left Upper Lobe Collapse (see Case 42)

■ Discussion

Background

The various pulmonary resection techniques include *wedge resection*, excision of tumor confined to one specific area and a small margin of normal lung; *segmentectomy*, exaggerated wedge resection entailing excision of a larger volume of tissue but not the entire lobe; *lobectomy*, excision of entire lobe with or without ac-

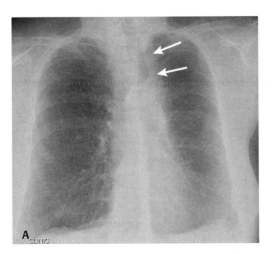 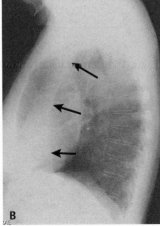

Fig. 186.1 *(Images courtesy of Anthony D. Casssano, MD, VCU Medical Center, Richmond, Virginia.)*

companying lymphadenectomy, typically performed for early stage non–small cell lung cancer (see Section VI); *sleeve lobectomy*, an alternative to pneumonectomy in select cases of cancer involving a lobar orifice and airway reconstruction with end-to-end-anastomosis and wrapping of anastomosis with pleura or other vascularized tissue, for which the most common site is RUL (75%), followed by LUL (16%) and LLL (8%); and *pneumonectomy*, removal of the entire lung (see Case 187). This case will focus on lobectomy. *Lobectomy* can be considered the ultimate form of volume loss. That is, the anatomic and radiologic alterations in pulmonary and extrapulmonary structures closely resemble those of severe lobar collapse (see Section IV). Displacement of mediastinal structures into the post-lobectomy space may mimic lobar collapse. Postoperative pleural effusion or fibrothorax in the post-lobectomy space likewise may simulate lobar collapse on imaging. Reorientation of the left lung after lobectomy is characterized by a pleuromediastinal interface that also simulates lobar collapse. Right-sided lobectomies are characterized by reorientation of the remaining two lobes and apposition of the visceral interlobar pleural surfaces and formation of "neofissures." Neofissures may be difficult to perceive on conventional radiography as they are often not parallel to the X-ray beam axis.

Post-Lobectomy Complications

Early Postoperative Lobectomy Complications

- **Anastomotic dehiscence.** May manifest as an airway complication after sleeve lobectomy (6%) and result in bronchopleural fistula. CT shows a defect in the bronchial wall or extraluminal air about the anastomosis, bronchial irregularity, or narrowing.
- **Bronchopleural fistula.** Dreaded complication with high mortality (see Case 187). Usually develops at the bronchial stump after pneumonectomy or lobectomy.
- **Hemothorax** (see Case 187)
- **Lobar torsion.** Following RUL lobectomy, the RML relocates into the upper thorax. RML torsion may occur if it twists clockwise on its narrow vascular pedicle. The degree of torsion is usually 180°. Torsion of hilar vessels causes impaired circulation and predisposes to hemorrhagic infarction. Affected patients may have bronchorrhea, hemoptysis, shock, and sepsis. Mortality is high if the condition goes unrecognized and the affected lobe is not reduced or excised. Radiography shows rapidly developing consolidation with volume expansion of the affected lobe (**Fig. 186.2A**) and neofissure reorientation. CT findings include amorphous soft-tissue attenuation at the hilum, poor enhancement of torsed lobe with increased volume, ground glass opacity, septal thickening, neofissure reorientation, and tapered obliteration of the affected pulmonary artery and bronchus (**Figs. 186.2B, 186.2C**).
- **Non-obstructive atelectasis.** Results from retained secretions, edema at the anastomosis, interruption of ciliary epithelium and lymphatic vessels, and partial denervation of the reimplanted lobe. This occurs in 5–10% of sleeve resections and more commonly follows those involving the lower lobe. Secondary infection may ensue.
- **Persistent air leak.** Most patients undergoing lobectomy or segmentectomy develop some degree of air leak. This most often occurs in older patients and in those with underlying emphysema or incomplete/absent interlobar fissures and resolves within 24–48 hours. A persistent air leak continues beyond seven days. Imaging studies show persistent pneumothorax, pneumomediastinum, or subcutaneous air.
- **Pneumonia.** Prevalence of post-thoracotomy pneumonia ranges from 2% to 22% and is most common in patients requiring prolonged intubation or having difficulty clearing secretions, and is often the result of aspiration of gastric secretions or secondary bacterial colonization. There is often a time lag between clinical and radiologic presentation. Imaging findings vary from patchy bronchopneumonia to consolidation and necrosis.
- **Pulmonary edema.** Post-thoracotomy edema is life-threatening and usually occurs 2–3 days following pneumonectomy (2.5–5%), lobectomy (<1%), or bilobectomy. Patients experience rapidly progressive dyspnea and hypoxia. Mild forms of hydrostatic edema clear within a few days, whereas more severe cases show rapidly progressive pulmonary edema, consolidation, and ARDS (see Case 187).

Late Postoperative Lobectomy Complications

- **Anastomotic stricture or stenosis.** Most common late complication after sleeve resection (<18% of cases). Imaging reveals narrowing at the surgical anastomosis.
- **Recurrent tumor.** Local tumor recurrence includes ipsilateral mediastinal node metastases, chest wall or parietal pleural implants, and recurrence at the surgical bronchial stump (2.2% of cases). Differentiation from postoperative granulation tissue may require PET imaging.

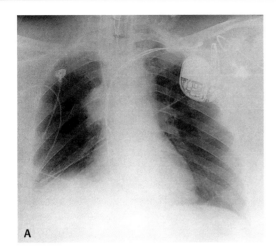
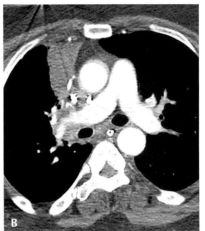
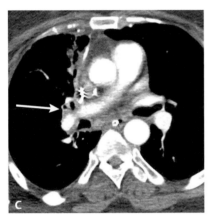

Fig. 186.2   56-year-old man postoperative day 1 following RUL lobectomy with complicating RML torsion. AP chest X-ray **(A)** shows upper lobectomy changes and appropriately positioned tubes and lines, but an unexpected focal mass-like consolidation in the tracheobronchial angle. Contrast-enhanced CT (mediastinal window) **(B,C)** shows focal air space consolidation without enhancement in the medial right upper lobe. Note the kink in the right pulmonary artery and middle lobe bronchus **(C)** (*arrow*). The middle lobe was infarcted at re-exploration.

Normal Postoperative Imaging Findings

Left Upper Lobectomy

Chest Radiography (Figs. 186.1A, 186.1B)

- Decreased volume left thorax ; may mimic LUL collapse (**Figs. 186.1A, 186.1B**)
- Anterior mediastinum displaced leftward; interface between lung and shifted mediastinum creates *upper triangle sign* paralleling infraclavicular tracheal air column; do not confuse with lymphadenopathy (**Fig. 186.1A, 186.1B**)
- ± Ipsilateral juxtaphrenic peak (**Fig. 186.1A**)
- Anterior mediastinal interface with left lower lobe on lateral radiography; do not confuse with displaced left oblique fissure (latter no longer exists) (**Fig. 186.1B**)
- ± Surgical clips and rib distortion

MDCT

- Leftward anterior mediastinal displacement
- Right lung extends across midline anteriorly
- Mild clockwise rotation of aorta; myocardium; increased horizontal orientation left anterior descending coronary artery
- Anteromedial, lateral basal, and posterior basal segments of lower lobe occupy anterior and lateral hemithorax

Left Lower Lobectomy

Chest Radiography

- Decreased volume left thorax; relatively hyperlucent left hemithorax
- Leftward mediastinal displacement
- Pleuromediastinal interface between lung and anterior mediastinum; creates *upper triangle sign* paralleling transverse aorta; do not confuse with lymphadenopathy
- Left hilum appears small and remaining pulmonary arteries displaced caudally
- Pleuromediastinal interface of LUL with mediastinum on lateral radiography

MDCT

- Leftward anterior mediastinal shift; aorta and mediastinum rotate clockwise (**Figs. 186.3A, 186.3B**)
- Right lung extends across midline (**Figs. 186.3A, 186.3B**)
- Left mainstem bronchus displaced posteriorly
- Anterior and apicoposterior segmental bronchi displaced inferiorly and posteriorly
- Lingular bronchus displaced posteriorly and inferiorly; lingula occupies most of lower left thorax (**Figs. 186.3A, 186.3B**)

Right Upper Lobectomy

Chest Radiography

- Decreased volume right thorax (**Figs. 186.4A, 186.4B**)
- Slight shift of trachea and anterior mediastinum rightward (**Figs. 186.4A, 186.4B**)
- RLL overinflates to occupy most of right thorax (**Figs. 186.4A, 186.4B**)
- Proximal right interlobar pulmonary artery displaced superiorly and laterally (**Figs. 186.4A, 186.4B**)
- Right cardiophrenic sulcus blunted by rotation of mediastinal fat (**Figs. 186.4A, 186.4B**)
- Right hemidiaphragm elevated (**Figs. 186.4A, 186.4B**); juxtaphrenic peak may be present
- RML expands to meet RLL superior segment near apex of right thorax; superior aspect of neofissures may be seen on lateral exams

MDCT

- RML and RLL create neofissure by swinging upward to contact each other near apex of right thoracic cavity; extends from apex to hemidiaphragm

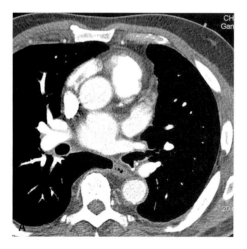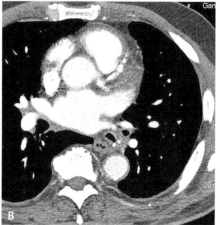

Fig. 186.3   Contrast-enhanced CT (mediastinal window) of a 70-year-old man status post antecedent LLL lobectomy shows mild leftward shift and clockwise rotation of the mediastinum and ipsilateral displacement of the esophagus and azygoesophageal recess **(A,B)**. Right lung extends anteriorly across the midline **(A,B)**. Lingular bronchus is displaced posteriorly and inferiorly **(A)**. Note the surgical sutures at the LLL bronchial stump **(A,B)**.

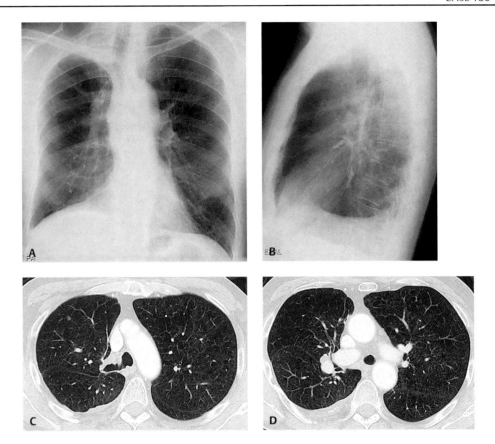

Fig. 186.4 PA **(A)** and lateral **(B)** chest X-rays of a 71-year-old man status post remote right upper lobectomy. The right thorax is smaller than the left and there is cephalad retraction of the right hilum. The trachea is displaced rightward and the right diaphragm is elevated. Ipsilateral apical thickening and obscuration of the posterolateral sulcus and anteromedial sulcus is seen. Note the sutures in the right tracheobronchial angle. CT **(C,D)** (lung window) shows a neofissure between the reoriented RML and RLL lobes. Contrast the orientation of the neofissure with the left oblique fissure.

- RML and RLL are contiguous along lower aspect of oblique fissure, but lower part of oblique fissure shifts anteriorly
- Slight rightward shift and counterclockwise mediastinal rotation
- Left lung extends anteriorly across midline
- Elevation of proximal right interlobar pulmonary artery and ipsilateral diaphragm
- Cranial displacement RLL superior segmental bronchus; obliquely reoriented and anteriorly displaced bronchus intermedius
- Horizontally oriented basilar segmental bronchi arising from RLL bronchus; elevation and lateral displacement of RML bronchus
- Fat displaced into right anterior cardiophrenic sulcus

Right Middle Lobectomy

Chest Radiography

- Decreased volume right thorax
- RUL and RLL expand to contact each other along a curved surface resembling RML collapse; area of contact may appear thick and irregular
- Blunting of cardiophrenic sulcus by mediastinal fat displacement
- Minimal mediastinal shift; anterior ipsilateral elevation of diaphragm

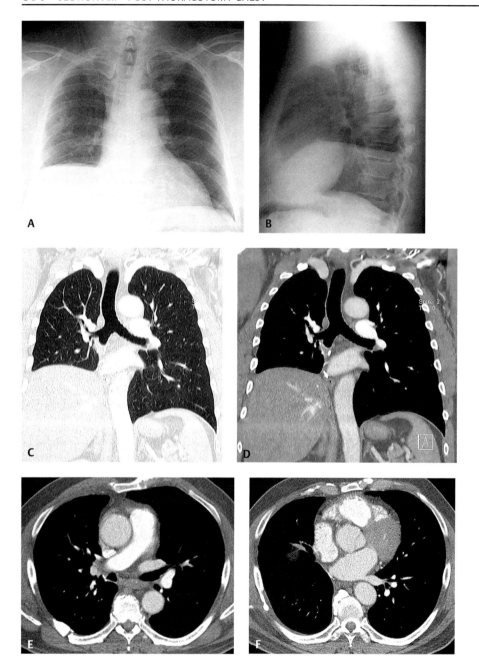

Fig. 186.5 50-year-old man status post antecedent RML-RLL bilobectomy for carcinoid tumor. PA **(A)** and lateral **(B)** chest exams mirror features of combined RML and RLL collapse. Note the relatively small right thorax compared with the left and the ipsilateral mediastinal shift, diaphragmatic elevation, and seventh posterior rib deformity. Coronal **(C,D)** and axial **(E,F)** CT show similar findings. Note the bronchial stump and suture lines across the bronchus intermedius and expected location of the right inferior pulmonary vein. *(Images courtesy of Anthony D. Casssano, MD, VCU Medical Center, Richmond, Virginia.)*

MDCT

- Obliquely oriented neofissure in anteroinferior right thorax; broad-based band posteriorly; more sharply defined and thinner inferiorly
- Blunting of right cardiophrenic sulcus from changes in myocardium orientation and pericardial fat redistribution

Right Lower Lobectomy

Chest Radiography

- Marked volume loss in right thorax; rightward mediastinal shift; creates *upper triangle sign* paralleling infraclavicular tracheal air column; do not confuse with lymphadenopathy
- Right hilum small
- Right diaphragm elevated
- Portion of neofissure separating RML in anterior lung base from RUL in posterior lung base may be seen on lateral exams

MDCT

- Counterclockwise rotation and shift of mediastinum to right
- Hyperexpanded left lung extends across midline anteriorly
- Resected right inferior pulmonary vein
- Posterior and inferior displacement of RUL bronchus and its branches
- Inferior and lateral displacement of RML bronchus
- RML and RUL neofissure may be perceptible as it curves posteriorly and inferiorly toward the posterior costophrenic sulcus

PEARLS

- Anatomic and radiologic alterations in pulmonary and extrapulmonary structures following lobectomy resemble those of severe lobar collapse. Displacement of mediastinal structures into the post-lobectomy space may mimic lobar collapse. Detection of surgical sutures and rib deformity is helpful in differentiation but may be inconspicuous with the ever-increasing use of less invasive resection techniques.
- Following RUL and RML bilobectomy, the airway is reconstructed with anastomosis of the RLL bronchus proximally to the RMSB.
- After LLL lobectomy and lingular segmentectomy, the airway is reconstructed with anastomosis of the upper divisional bronchus of the LUL proximally to the LMSB.
- RML-RLL bilobectomy post-operative changes simulate features of concomitant RML and RLL collapse on imaging studies (**Figs. 186.5A, 186.5B, 186.5C, 186.5D, 186.5E, 186.5F**).

Suggested Reading

1. Holbert JM, Chasen MH, Libshitz HI, Mountain CF. The postlobectomy chest: anatomic considerations. Radiographics 1987;7(5):889–911

2. Kim EA, Lee KS, Shim YM, et al. Radiographic and CT findings in complications following pulmonary resection. Radiographics 2002;22(1):67–86

3. Pinstein ML, Winer-Muram H, Eastridge C, Scott R. Middle lobe torsion following right upper lobectomy. Radiology 1985;155(3):580

4. Seo JB, Lee KS, Choo SW, Shim YM, Primack SL. Neofissure after lobectomy of the right lung: radiographic and CT findings. Radiology 1996;201(2):475–479

CASE 187

■ Clinical Presentation

57-year-old man status post right pneumonectomy for adenocarcinoma

■ Radiologic Findings

First postoperative chest exam (**Fig. 187.1A**) following right pneumonectomy shows an air-containing pleural space, slight ipsilateral mediastinal shift and diaphragmatic elevation, and mild vascular congestion of the contralateral lung. The right sixth posterior rib has been partially resected and the chest tube is in place. Minimal subcutaneous air is present. Frontal chest exams on postoperative day 1 (**Fig. 187.1B**), day 3 (**Fig. 187.1C**), and day 5 (**Fig. 187.1D**) demonstrate gradual but progressive filling of pneumonectomy space with fluid and decreasing volume of air. Note the progressive ipsilateral mediastinal shift, diaphragmatic elevation, and overinflation of the left lung. By post-op day 15 (**Fig. 187.1E**) 90% of the pneumonectomy space is fluid-filled. Three months later (**Fig. 187.1F**) the space is completely obliterated. The mediastinum remains displaced appropriately toward the ipsilateral thorax.

■ Diagnosis

Post-Pneumonectomy; Normal Postoperative Sequence

■ Differential Diagnosis

None

■ Discussion

Background

Pneumonectomy is the treatment of choice for lung cancer, advanced medically refractory infection, and complicated bronchiectasis. Radiologists must be cognizant of the normal postoperative appearance of the post-pneumonectomy chest to avoid misinterpreting expected findings with true complications. Pulmonary resection techniques include *intrapleural pneumonectomy*, resection of the involved lung and surrounding visceral pleura (most common); *extrapleural pneumonectomy*, en bloc resection of the ipsilateral lung, parietal and mediastinal pleura, pericardium, and diaphragm; *intrapericardial pneumonectomy*, which entails opening the pericardium and dividing vessels involved by tumor within the pericardial sac; and *sleeve pneumonectomy*, resection of tumor involving the tracheobronchial angle, carina, or lower trachea and the ipsilateral lung with anastomosis of proximal contralateral mainstem bronchus to the lower trachea.

Normal Post-Pneumonectomy Radiography Changes

The initial postoperative chest radiograph should demonstrate an air-containing ipsilateral pleural space, slight ipsilateral mediastinal shift and diaphragmatic elevation, and mild vascular congestion of the contralateral lung (**Fig. 187.1A**). Thereafter, the normal pneumonectomy space begins to fill with serosanguineous fluid at a rate of about two ribs per day (**Fig. 187.1B, 187.1C, 187.1D**), although the left thorax tends to fill more rapidly than the right. By the end of the second postoperative week, 80–90% of the pneumonectomy space should be obliterated (**Fig. 187.1E**), and complete obliteration is typically seen by 2–4 months (**Fig.**

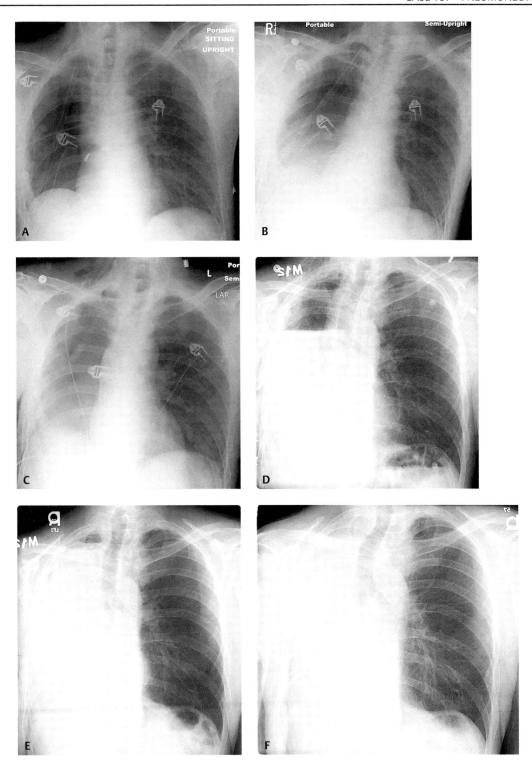

Fig. 187.1

187.1F). The post-pneumonectomy space is usually obliterated by a combination of fluid, ipsilateral diaphragmatic elevation and mediastinal shift, and overexpansion of the contralateral lung. Ipsilateral mediastinal shift is the most reliable radiologic sign of a normal postoperative course.

Post-Pneumonectomy Complications

Complications occur in 20–60% of patients following pneumonectomy. Complications may occur early in the postoperative course or at a later time.

Early Postoperative Complications

- **Hemothorax.** Most commonly results from inadequate hemostasis of a bronchial artery or systemic vessels in the chest wall. Other causes include ligature slippage from a pulmonary vessel and iatrogenic vascular injury. Mortality rate is <0.1%. On radiography, hemothorax presents as a rapidly enlarging pleural effusion. CT features include heterogeneous or high-attenuation pleural effusion or a fluid-hematocrit level.
- **Chylothorax.** Injury to the thoracic duct or one of its branches results in the accumulation of chyle in the pleural space. Potential sites of injury include inferior right paravertebral region during extrapleural pneumonectomy; pericarinal and subaortic region during radical lymphadenectomy; and pulmonary ligaments during intrapleural pneumonectomy.
- **Pulmonary edema.** Life-threatening complication with a prevalence of 2.5–5% and mortality rate of 80–100%. Occurs more commonly following right pneumonectomy. Predisposing factors include large perioperative volume loading, transfusion of fresh frozen plasma, dysrhythmia, and marked postoperative diuresis. Diagnosis requires exclusion of aspiration, acute PTE, pneumonia, and other causes of ARDS. Imaging features mirror those of rapidly progressive pulmonary edema and ARDS.
- **Bronchopleural fistula.** Potentially life-threatening complication with a prevalence of 2–13% and associated mortality of 30–70%. Occurs more commonly following right pneumonectomy. Predisposing factors include active preoperative lung or pleural infection, trauma, preoperative radiation therapy, faulty closure of bronchial stump, and postoperative mechanical ventilation. Imaging features include failure of post-pneumonectomy space to fill with fluid; persistent or progressive ipsilateral pneumothorax; ≥2.0 cm drop in the air-fluid level (decrease <1.5 cm can be ignored unless associated with contralateral mediastinal shift); persistent or progressive pneumomediastinum or subcutaneous air; sudden onset of pneumothorax or reappearance of air in a previously opaque pneumonectomy space; new foci of consolidation in contralateral lung (i.e., transbronchial contamination); and communication or tract from an airway or the lung to the pleural cavity (**Fig. 187.2**).
- **Empyema.** Uncommon but potentially fatal complication with an incidence of 2–16%. Mortality rate ranges between 16% and 71%. Early postoperative empyema is usually related to residual pleural infection. Predisposing factors include completion pneumonectomy (following antecedent lobectomy), right pneumonectomy, preoperative radiation therapy, infected pleural cavity, mediastinal lymphadenectomy, long bronchial stumps, and postoperative ventilatory support. CT is more sensitive than radiography. Imaging features include over-expansion rather than contraction of the pneumonectomy space; excessive rapid filling of the pneumonectomy space (must exclude bleeding and chyle leak); contralateral mediastinal displacement; drop in the air-fluid level or reappearance of air in a previously opaque pneumonectomy space; mass effect on, straightening of, or reversal of inward convexity of mediastinal pleura in the pneumonectomy space; and irregular pleural thickening.
- **ARDS.** Incidence of 5% but a mortality rate of 80%. Radiographic features include rapid evolution of diffuse ground glass or consolidation in the contralateral lung. CT manifestations include ground glass or consolidation with an anteroposterior gradient and interlobular septal thickening.
- **Pneumonia.** Incidence is 2–15% with a mortality rate of 25%. Potential causes include aspiration of gastric secretions, bacterial colonization, and transbronchial contamination via bronchopleural fistula. Imaging features often lag behind the clinical presentation but include foci of ground glass to frank areas of consolidation, necrotizing pneumonia, and abscess formation.
- **Cardiac herniation.** Rare complication in which the heart or a portion of it herniates through the pericardial defect created to access the hilar vessels. The associated mortality rate is 40–50%. This complication usually presents within the first 24 hours following surgery and manifests with sudden hypotension, cyanosis, and hemodynamic collapse. On imaging, right-sided herniation is characterized by shift or rotation of the cardiac apex into the right thorax (**Fig. 187.3**), whereas left-sided herniation presents as hemisphere-shaped left heart border with an incisura between the great vessels and the lateral herniated heart border. Treatment requires immediate surgical reduction.

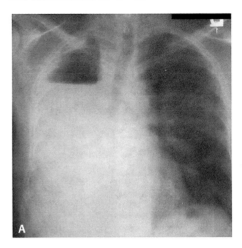

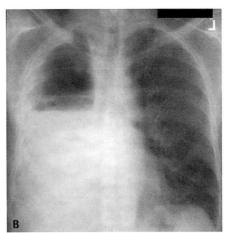

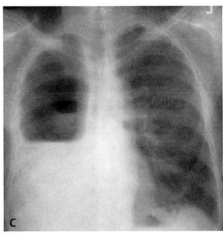

Fig. 187.2 Serial postoperative chest exams of a 62-year-old man after right pneumonectomy. Postoperative day 21 **(A)** chest X-ray shows 80% opacification of the pneumonectomy space and expected ipsilateral mediastinal shift. Postoperative day 23 **(B)** shows a marked drop in the air-fluid level and bubbles of air layering below it. The mediastinum is now midline. Chest radiograph on postoperative day 25 **(C)** shows a further drop in the air-fluid level. Surgical re-exploration revealed a bronchopleural fistula and bronchial stump dehiscence.

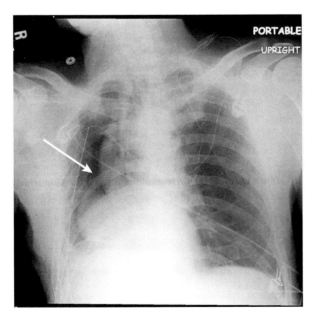

Fig. 187.3 First postoperative chest radiograph of a 59-year-old man who underwent right radical carinal pneumonectomy with mediastinal lymphadenectomy for squamous cell carcinoma and experienced immediate postoperative hypotension and cardiac herniation. The cardiac silhouette is dextroposed, far from the midline, laterally displacing the ipsilateral apically directed thoracostomy tube. Note the characteristic "notch" (*arrow*) between the unusually rounded right heart border and the great vessels. (From Kiev J, Parker MS, Zhao S, Kasirajan V. Cardiac herniation following intra-pericardial pneumonectomy. Am Surg 2007;73(9):906–908. Reprinted with permission.)

Late Postoperative Complications

- **Post-pneumonectomy syndrome.** Delayed complication typically seen in infants, young children, young adults, and women within a year of right pneumonectomy. As the contralateral lung over-expands, it displaces the mediastinum not only rightward but posteriorly, rotating the heart along its main axis counterclockwise. Affected patients present with exertional dyspnea, stridor, and recurrent pneumonia. Imaging studies demonstrate rightward and posterior displacement of the trachea and mediastinum; and stretching, compressing, and narrowing of the left mainstem bronchus between the pulmonary artery anteriorly and the aorta and thoracic spine posteriorly. Surgical implantation of tissue expanders in the post-pneumonectomy space has been advocated as a means of both prevention in children and treatment in young adults.

- **Esophagopleural fistula.** Occurs in 0.2–1.0% of patients and usually presents within two years after the cessation of neoadjuvant therapy. Potential causes include direct esophageal injury at the time of surgery, chronic infection-inflammation, and tumor recurrence. Imaging findings mirror those of bronchopleural fistula. MDCT may directly demonstrate the fistulous communication.

- **Late-onset bronchopleural fistula (BPF).** Approximately 50% of post-pneumonectomy BPFs occur in the first postoperative week and the remainder later. The latter group is usually the result of infection or recurrent tumor. The imaging features are similar to those of BPF seen in the early postoperative period.

- **Late-onset empyema.** Empyema may occur as early as one day following pneumonectomy or weeks, months, or years later. Persistence of fluid in the pneumonectomy space is a potential precursor for late-onset empyema. Imaging features mirror those of empyema discussed earlier.

- **Radiation-induced pericarditis and pleuritis.** Radiation-induced pericarditis has a prevalence of 2–6% and usually manifests six to nine months following completion of therapy. MR is best suited to assess for constrictive physiology and hemodynamic effects. Radiation-induced pleural effusion usually occurs within six months of ceasing therapy and must be differentiated from malignant pleural disease or effusion secondary to constrictive pericarditis.

- **Radiation pneumonitis.** Mediastinal radiation therapy is associated with radiation pneumonitis in 6% of patients and usually occurs 4–12 weeks after completion of therapy. Fibrotic changes evolve over 6–24 months and remain stable after two years. Imaging features include ground glass and consolidation (acute phase) and cicatrization atelectasis, traction bronchiectasis, and bronchiolectasis (late phase).

- **Recurrent and/or metastatic tumor.** Recurrence rate at the bronchial stump is 2.2–37% for all resected tumors. Most recurrences present within two years following the pneumonectomy. Recurrence can be difficult to appreciate on chest radiography because of the changes created by the pneumonectomy and/or concomitant radiation therapy. CT may reveal a new soft-tissue mass at or near the bronchial stump, lymphadenopathy, pleural implants, new lung nodules, and extrathoracic disease (e.g., adrenal gland, liver, bones). PET imaging is very useful in this population.

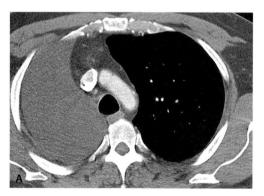 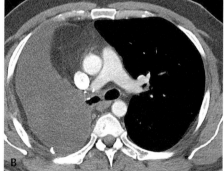

Fig. 187.4 Contrast-enhanced chest CT of a 67-year-old man two years following right pneumonectomy shows a persistent fluid-filled post-pneumonectomy space and expected ipsilateral mediastinal shift and over-expansion of the contralateral lung.

PEARLS

- Radiologists should monitor early serial postoperative chest radiographs for changes in the air-fluid level in the pneumonectomy space; increased air and decreased fluid are cardinal imaging signs of bronchopleural fistula.
- Post-pneumonectomy space remains fluid-filled and marginated by thickened parietal pleura in two-thirds of patients (**Fig. 187.4**); the space becomes obliterated by fibrous tissue and displacement of mediastinal structures in the remaining one-third.
- Persistence of fluid in the pneumonectomy space is a potential precursor for late-onset empyema.

Suggested Reading

1. Chae EJ, Seo JB, Kim SY, et al. Radiographic and CT findings of thoracic complications after pneumonectomy. Radiographics 2006;26(5):1449–1468

2. Fraser RS, Müller NL, Colman N, Paré PD. Complications of therapeutic, biopsy, and monitoring procedures. In: Fraser and Paré's Diagnosis of Diseases of the Chest, 4th ed. Philadelphia: WB Saunders Company; 1999:2665

3. Kiev J, Parker MS, Zhao S, Kasirajan V. Cardiac Herniation following intra-pericardial pneumonectomy. Am Surg 2007;73(9):906–908

4. Kim EA, Lee KS, Shim YM, et al. Radiographic and CT findings in complications following pulmonary resection. Radiographics 2002;22(1):67–86

5. Tsukada G, Stark P. Postpneumonectomy complications. AJR Am J Roentgenol 1997;169(5):1363–1370

CASE 188

■ Clinical Presentation

57-year old man with shortness of breath

■ Radiologic Findings

PA chest radiograph (**Fig. 188.1A**) demonstrates pulmonary hyperinflation with diaphragmatic flattening and increased lucency with giant bullae in both lungs. Compressive changes are noted in the right lower lobe with crowding of bronchovascular structures. Unenhanced chest CT (**Fig. 188.1B**) shows giant bullae in both lungs, right larger than left, with leftward shift of the mediastinal structures. PA chest radiograph following lung volume reduction surgery (**Fig. 188.1C**) demonstrates reduction in overall lung volumes, increased upward convexity of the left hemidiaphragm, and improved aeration in the lung parenchyma bilaterally. A subpulmonic effusion obscures the right lateral sulcus and displaces the apex of the diaphragm laterally.

■ Diagnosis

Lung Volume Reduction Surgery (LVRS) for Giant Bullous Emphysema

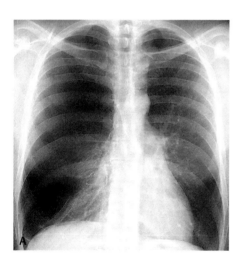
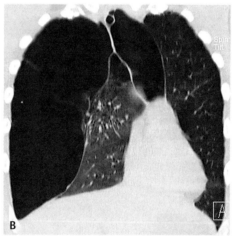
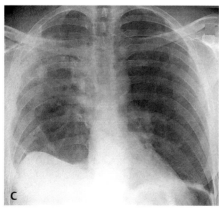

Fig. 188.1 *(Images courtesy of Anthony D. Cassano, MD, Department of Thoracic Surgery, VCU Medical Center, Richmond, Virginia.)*

■ Differential Diagnosis

None

■ Discussion

Background

Lung volume reduction surgery (LVRS) is performed as a palliative technique to restore lung mechanics in patients with severe emphysema who do not respond to medical management. Targeted areas of severely emphysematous lung are resected with the goal of reducing the overall lung volume and improving respiratory mechanics. By removing areas of overinflated, less functional, emphysematous lung, adjacent normal lung is able to decompress, with improved elastic recoil, and the ipsilateral diaphragm becomes less flattened and more convex, thus increasing its surface area and extent of apposition to the lung base. This combination of changes improves lung mechanics, with immediate symptomatic and functional improvements experienced by patients who undergo LVRS. Patient selection involves evaluation of the degree and extent of emphysema and its distribution within the lungs. The best results are derived from patients whose emphysema is heterogeneous in distribution, with upper lobe predominance of disease being the most likely to be associated with improved lung function. Patients whose emphysema is homogeneous in distribution are less likely to experience improved lung function following LVRS. The presence of extensive pleural disease, bronchiectasis, pulmonary artery hypertension, and coronary artery/ischemic heart disease may further limit patient selection for LVRS.

Clinical Findings

Candidates for LVRS have severe emphysema and have not responded to medical therapy. Poor outcomes have been associated with (1) patients with severe COPD and very low FEV_1; (2) patients with uniform distribution of panacinar emphysema; and (3) those patients with severely reduced gas diffusing capacity (DLCO).

Imaging Findings

Chest Radiography

- Hyperinflation, hyperlucency, bullous changes, and regional areas of compressive atelectasis on preoperative radiographs (**Fig. 188.1A**)
- Decreased lung volume, increased upward convexity of the diaphragms, and improved aeration of lung parenchyma following LVRS (**Fig. 188.1C**)

MDCT/HRCT

Preoperative CT

- Emphysema, bullous changes, giant bullae (**Fig. 188.1B**)
- Flattened diaphragm (**Fig. 188.1B**)

Postoperative CT

- Post-surgical changes at site of previous emphysematous/bullous changes
- Improved aeration of decompressed lung parenchyma
- Increased upward convexity of ipsilateral hemidiaphragm

Prognosis

- Immediate symptomatic and functional improvement; stable two years after LVRS
- No difference in overall survival between patients randomized to LVRS and those receiving medical therapy

PEARLS

- Bronchoscopic lung volume reduction (BLVT) entails bronchoscopic placement of one-way intrabronchial valves and is a less invasive technique being utilized to reduce lung volumes by targeting emphysematous areas of lung parenchyma.
  - Technique may be suitable for patients with severe emphysema who are not candidates for LVRS.
  - Early experience suggests collateral ventilation prevents significant atelectasis of occluded segments in many individuals; but some clinical benefit has been reported.

Suggested Reading

1. Hansell DM, Lynch DA, McAdams HP, et al. Diseases of the airways. In: Hansell DM, Lynch DA, McAdams HP, Bankier AA, ed. Imaging of Diseases of the Chest, 5th ed. Philadelphia: Mosby Elsevier; 2010:715–785

2. Cooper JD, Patterson GA. Lung volume reduction surgery for severe emphysema. Semin Thorac Cardiovasc Surg 1996;8(1):52–60

3. Fishman A, Martinez F, Naunheim K, et al; National Emphysema Treatment Trial Research Group. A randomized trial comparing lung-volume-reduction surgery with medical therapy for severe emphysema. N Engl J Med 2003;348(21):2059–2073

4. Takasugi JE, Wood DE, Godwin JD, Richardson ML, Benditt JO, Albert RK. Lung-volume reduction surgery for diffuse emphysema: radiologic assessment of changes in thoracic dimensions. J Thorac Imaging 1998;13(1):36–41

5. Quint LE, Bland PH, Walker JM, et al. Diaphragmatic shape change after lung volume reduction surgery. J Thorac Imaging 2001;16(3):149–155

CASE 189

■ Clinical Presentation

42-year-old man status post Eloesser pleurocutaneous window for chronic empyema

■ Radiologic Findings

PA chest radiograph (**Fig. 189.1A**) reveals partial surgical resection of the right eighth and ninth posterolateral ribs. A large air-filled cavity occupies the lower right thorax, communicating with the chest wall and outside environment. Contrast-enhanced coronal (**Fig. 189.1B**) (bone window) and axial (**Fig. 189.1C**) (mediastinal window) chest CT demonstrates the pleurocutaneous window to better advantage. The overlying ribs and associated intercostal muscles have been resected. Note the continuous epithelial lined parietal pleural surface of the permanent cavity.

■ Diagnosis

Eloesser Pleurocutaneous Window for Chronic Empyema

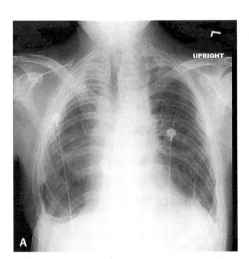

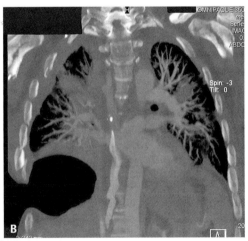

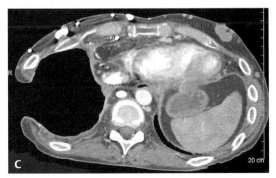

Fig. 189.1

907

■ Differential Diagnosis

None

■ Discussion

Background

Twenty to 60% of all cases of pneumonia are associated with parapneumonic effusions (PPE). PPE accounts for about one-third of all pleural effusions and is the *most common* cause of exudative effusion. Untreated or inadequately treated PPE may progress to *empyema thoracis*, which, by definition, is pus in the pleural space. If not drained, the effusion may become organized as fibroblasts grow into the pleural fluid from both the visceral and parietal pleura. This produces a thick inelastic pleural peel which prevents the lung from expanding, entrapping the lung. The key to successful treatment is evacuation of the infected pleural space and elimination of the dead space in the pleural cavity. However, the underlying pleural infection cannot be eradicated unless this peel is removed. Treatment options include:

- Empyemectomy-decortication and open drainage
- Pleurocutaneous window (Eloesser flap)
- Muscle flap closure without pleural drainage

Clinical Findings

Empyemectomy-decortication and *open drainage* are indicated for late Stage II (fibropurulent) or Stage III (chronic organizing) PPE with inadequate pleural drainage after tube thoracostomy and intrapleural fibrinolytic therapy. Decortication is preferred over open drainage. *Pleurocutaneous window (Eloesser flap)* is indicated for refractory pleural effusions (e.g., empyema, malignant effusions, esophagopleural fistulas) and creates permanent open access to the pleural space. *Muscle flap closure without pleural drainage* provides well-vascularized muscle tissue to close a bronchopleural fistula and obliterate the empyema cavity.

Imaging Findings

Stage III Empyema

- Pleural rind or peel with or without calcific pleuritis (**Fig. 189.3**)
- Entrapment of the adjacent lung
- Rib approximation and contraction of affected hemithorax
- Chest wall invasion or violation (**Figs. 189.3, 189.4**)

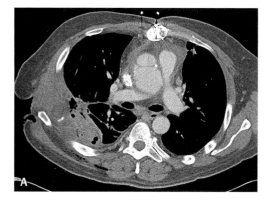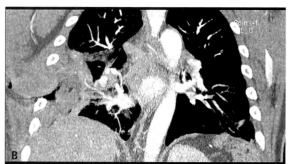

Fig. 189.2 Contrast-enhanced axial (**A**) and coronal (**B**) (mediastinal windows) chest CT reveal expected postoperative imaging findings of a muscle flap closure procedure. The serratus anterior muscle has been brought into the chest through a lateral thoracotomy to obliterate the empyema cavity.

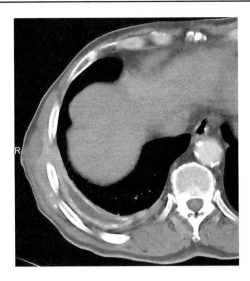

Fig. 189.3 Contrast-enhanced chest CT with Stage III PPE characterized by a pleural peel with calcific pleuritis. The infection has extended into the chest wall, as manifested by inflammatory changes and punctate calcifications in the adjacent serratus anterior and latissimus dorsi muscles and subcutaneous tissues. Note the ipsilateral rib approximation.

Pleurocutaneous Window (Eloesser flap) (Figs. 189.1A-189.1C)

- Surgical resection of at least two posterolateral ribs and associated intercostal muscles
- Large air-filled cavity occupying the lower thorax that communicates with chest wall and outside environment
- Continuous epithelial lined parietal pleural surface of the permanent cavity
- Packing material (e.g., sponges, gauzes) may mimic abscess

Muscle Flap Closure without Pleural Drainage (Figs. 189.2A, 189.2B)

- Lateral thoracotomy
- Partial resection of at least two posterolateral ribs
- Chest wall muscle mobilization in pleural cavity may mimic abscess

Management

- Decortication (preferred over open drainage)
  - Formal thoracotomy
  - All fibrous tissue removed from pleural surfaces
  - All pus evacuated from pleural space
- Open drainage
  - Indicated for those patients too ill to tolerate decortication
  - Segments of one to three ribs overlying the lower part of the empyema cavity are resected, and one or more short large-bore tubes are inserted into the cavity
  - Cavity is irrigated daily with antiseptic solution, and drainage from the tubes is collected in a colostomy bag
- Pleurocutaneous window (Eloesser flap) (**Figs. 189.1A, 189.1B, 189.1C**)
  - Mid-axillary line horizontal incision
  - At least two ribs and intervening intercostal muscles are removed
  - Skin is circumferentially sewn directly to the parietal pleura, creating a continuous epithelial surface and ensuring dependent drainage without the need for tubes
- Muscle flap closure without pleural drainage (**Fig. 189.2**)
  - Latissimus dorsi muscle
    - Ideal bulk, pedicle length, and arc of rotation to fill most thoracic defects
    - May be used as a turn-over flap or advanced directly into the wound
    - Usually provides enough muscle bulk to obliterate an empyema cavity

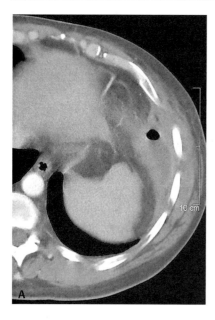 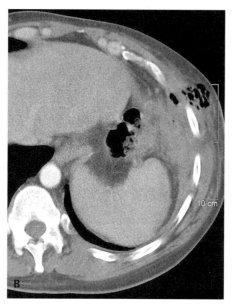

Fig. 189.4 Contrast-enhanced chest CT with complicated PPE, bronchopleural, and empyema necessitatis. The loculated pleural fluid infection has breached the chest wall and extends into the adjacent musculature and subcutaneous tissues. Note the intrathoracic and extrathoracic locules of air and the associated inflammatory changes.

- ○ Serratus anterior muscle (**Fig. 189.2**)
  - – Second most common muscle used to fill an empyema cavity
  - – Muscle is thin enough to fill a small space and can be passed through a lateral thoracotomy incision; can be brought into the chest with the latissimus dorsi muscle on a common pedicle
- ○ Pectoralis major muscle
  - – May be used as either a turn-over flap or placed directly in the wound
  - – Intrathoracic placement requires creation of a window by partial rib resection of the second or third rib to afford maximal length
- ○ Omentum
  - – May be used if empyema space is not large or a well-vascularized reinforcement of a bronchopleural fistula is required
  - – Advantages include its long reach, excellent vasculature, and relative distance from the infectious process

Prognosis

- Overall mortality from empyema is approximately 20%; advanced multilocular empyema can have a mortality of up to 50%
- Empyema may be complicated by
  - ○ Necrosis of visceral pleura, parietal pleural, and/or chest wall
  - ○ Bronchopleural or esophageal fistula
  - ○ Osteomyelitis of the ribs or spine
  - ○ Metastatic hematogenous systemic dissemination (e.g., brain abscess[es])
- Median time for healing treated by open-drainage procedures is 142 days

Suggested Reading

1. Athanassiadi K, Gerazounis M, Kalantzi N. Treatment of post-pneumonic empyema thoracis. Thorac Cardiovasc Surg 2003;51(6):338–341
2. Miller JI Jr. The history of surgery of empyema, thoracoplasty, Eloesser flap, and muscle flap transposition. Chest Surg Clin N Am 2000;10(1):45–53, viii
3. Qureshi NR, Gleeson FV. Imaging of pleural disease. Clin Chest Med 2006;27(2):193–213

CASE 190

■ Clinical Presentation

49-year old man with severe bullous emphysema before and after bilateral lung transplantation

■ Radiologic Findings

PA chest radiograph (**Fig. 190.1A**) demonstrates hyperinflation of the lungs with flattening of both diaphragms, and severe bullous emphysematous changes bilaterally. Post-surgical changes in the lungs and sternum were related to prior thoracotomy for resection of bullae. Unenhanced chest CT (lung window) (**Fig. 190.1B**) shows bullous emphysematous changes with giant bullae bilaterally. PA chest radiograph (**Fig. 190.1C**) following bilateral lung transplants reveals reduced lung volumes, normal bronchovascular structures, and improved configuration of both diaphragms. Unenhanced chest CT (lung window) (**Fig. 190.1D**) after bilateral lung transplantation demonstrates normal lung parenchyma bilaterally.

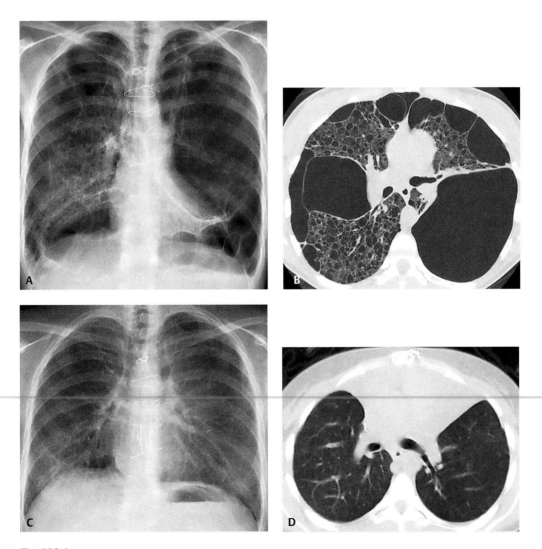

Fig. 190.1

■ Diagnosis

Bilateral Lung Transplantation

■ Differential Diagnosis

None

■ Discussion

Background

In recent decades, single and double lung transplantation have been established as successful treatments for advanced lung disease. Nearly 3,000 lung transplants were performed worldwide in 2009, according to the registry of the International Society for Heart and Lung Transplantation (www.ishlt.org). The most common indications for lung transplantation are emphysema/COPD, idiopathic pulmonary fibrosis (IPF), cystic fibrosis, α-1 anti-protease deficiency, and pulmonary arterial hypertension. *Single lung transplantation* has advantages in terms of extending treatment to more patients, since one donor may supply lung transplants for two individuals. But certain conditions require *double (bilateral) lung transplantation.* Patients with cystic fibrosis or severe bronchiectasis are at risk for suppurative lung infection in both native lungs, and thus double lung transplantation has been the preferred technique for those individuals. In recent years, *single lobe transplants* have been obtained from living donors.

The morbidity and mortality associated with lung transplantation has decreased in recent decades, largely due to advances in surgical techniques. Bronchial connections may be established as end-to-end or telescoping anastomoses. The telescoping technique usually avoids the need for omental or intercostal muscle wrapping at the anastomotic site.

Complications of lung transplantation may be categorized as early or late. The *early complications* include primary graft dysfunction (e.g., ischemic/reperfusion injury or edema), vascular complications, acute rejection, infections, and airway complications (**Fig. 190.2**). *Late complications* include opportunistic infections, bronchiolitis obliterans syndrome (BOS), and post-transplantation lymphoproliferative disorders (PTLD) (see Case 191).

Reperfusion edema occurs in most transplanted lungs. *Airway complications* occur in less than 15% of patients and may consist of partial or complete dehiscence or anastomotic stenosis. *Vascular anastomotic stenosis* or *occlusion* may also occur. *Pulmonary infection* occurs more frequently in lung transplants than in other solid organ transplants; *Pseudomonas aeruginosa* (**Fig. 190.5**), cytomegalovirus (CMV) (**Fig. 190.4**), and *Aspergillus* are the most common infectious agents. *Acute rejection* manifests on imaging studies as air space, nodular, or interstitial opacities and pleural effusion (**Fig. 190.3**). *Chronic rejection* manifests as bronchiolitis obliterans syndrome (BOS) with mosaic attenuation on inspiratory CT, and air trapping on expiratory CT (**Fig. 190.6**).

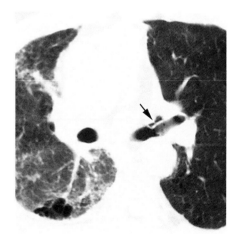

Fig. 190.2 Unenhanced chest CT (lung window) of a patient with anastomotic dehiscence after left lung transplantation shows a club-shaped band of abnormal air (*arrow*) extending along the inner aspect of the left mainstem bronchial anastomosis.

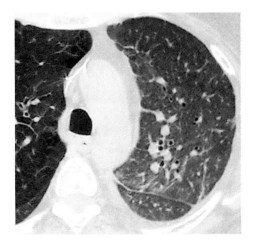

Fig. 190.3 Unenhanced chest CT (lung window) of a patient with acute rejection following left lung transplantation reveals diffuse ground glass opacity in the transplanted left lung, with interlobular septal thickening and pleural effusion.

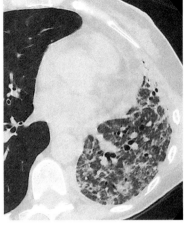

Fig. 190.4 Unenhanced chest CT (lung window) of a patient with CMV infection following left lung transplantation demonstrates diffuse ground glass opacity in the transplanted left lung with patchy areas of consolidation and centrilobular nodules.

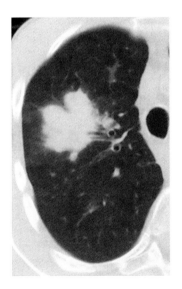

Fig. 190.5 Unenhanced chest CT (lung window) of a patient with *Pseudomonas aeruginosa* infection one month after bilateral lung transplantation demonstrates a large focal mass-like region of consolidation in the right upper lobe with an air bronchogram along its hilar aspect.

Imaging Findings

Chest Radiography

Anastomotic Dehiscence

- Extrapulmonary peribronchial air
- Pneumothorax with persistent air leak

Acute Rejection

- Interstitial pulmonary edema (perihilar, lower lobes)
- Kerley B-lines
- Normal heart size
- Pleural effusions

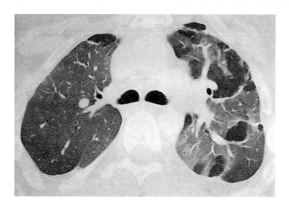

Fig. 190.6 Unenhanced chest CT (lung window; expiration sequence) of a patient with bronchiolitis obliterans syndrome developing one year after bilateral lung transplantation shows bilateral areas of air trapping manifesting as sharply outlined areas of low attenuation that became exaggerated on expiratory imaging.

MDCT/HRCT

Acute Rejection

- Ground glass opacities (**Fig. 190.3**)
- Consolidation
- Interlobular septal thickening (**Fig. 190.3**)
- Pleural effusion (**Fig. 190.3**)

Chronic Rejection

- Mosaic attenuation (inspiratory CT)
- Air trapping (expiratory CT) (**Fig. 190.6**)

Infection

- Ground glass opacities (**Fig. 190.4**)
- Consolidation (**Fig. 190.5**)
- Centrilobular nodules and tree-in-bud opacities
- Typical and atypical findings may occur

Airway Complications

- Extrapulmonary peribronchial air at anastomosis (**Fig. 190.2**)

Management

- Treatment of respective infection
- Adjustment of immune suppression as necessary

Prognosis

- One-year survival: 70%
- Two-year survival: 55%
- Five-year survival: 43%

PEARLS

- CT is the modality of choice for follow-up imaging after lung transplantation. Use of expiratory CT imaging is mandatory for detection of constrictive bronchiolitis in patients suspected of having bronchiolitis obliterans syndrome.

- Bronchiolitis obliterans syndrome is a manifestation of chronic immunologic rejection and the most important cause of long-term graft failure and death. Risk factors include repeated episodes of acute rejection, CMV and RSV infection, GERD, and aspiration.

Suggested Reading

1. Hansell DM, Lynch DA, McAdams HP, et al. The immunocompromised patient. In: Hansell DM, Lynch DA, McAdams HP, et al, eds. Imaging of Diseases of the Chest, 5th ed. Philadelphia: Mosby Elsevier; 2010:295–384

2. Krishnam MS, Suh RD, Tomasian A, et al. Postoperative complications of lung transplantation: radiologic findings along a time continuum. Radiographics 2007;27(4):957–974

3. Ko JP, Shepard JA, Sproule MW, et al. CT manifestations of respiratory syncytial virus infection in lung transplant recipients. J Comput Assist Tomogr 2000;24(2):235–241

4. Murray JG, McAdams HP, Erasmus JJ, Patz EF Jr, Tapson V. Complications of lung transplantation: radiologic findings. AJR Am J Roentgenol 1996;166(6):1405–1411

5. Collins J, Kuhlman JE, Love RB. Acute, life-threatening complications of lung transplantation. Radiographics 1998; 18(1):21–43, discussion 43–47

CASE 191

■ Clinical Presentation

54-year old man with fatigue developing nine months after renal transplantation

■ Radiologic Findings

Unenhanced composite chest CT (lung window) (**Fig. 191.1**) demonstrates multi-focal nodules and masses that are peribronchovascular (*left image*) and subpleural (*middle and right images*) in distribution.

■ Diagnosis

Post-Transplant Lymphoproliferative Disease (PTLD)

■ Differential Diagnosis

- Bacterial or Fungal Pneumonia
- Cryptogenic Organizing Pneumonia (COP)
- Lung Cancer

■ Discussion

Background

All organ transplant recipients are at increased risk for development of a malignancy, at a rate four times that of the general population. This increased risk is attributed to the powerful immunosuppressive regimens used in transplantation, the associated chronic stimulation of the immune system, and increased activity of oncogenic viruses (e.g., Epstein-Barr virus, HPV, and HHV-8) in the transplant population. The risk increases

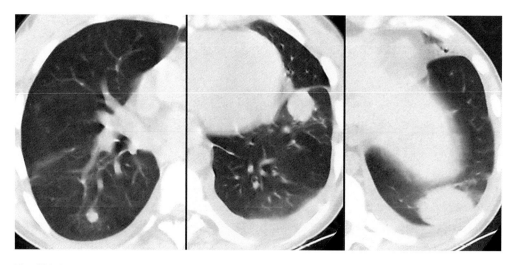

Fig. 191.1

with increasing severity and/or duration of immune suppression. The two most common malignancies that occur following transplantation are post-transplant lymphoproliferative disease or disorder (PTLD) and skin malignancies other than melanoma. Other malignancies that involve the thorax as primary or secondary tumors with increased frequency in the post-transplant population include lung cancer, Kaposi sarcoma, and head and neck tumors. The incidence of PTLD ranges from 1% to 20% and is highest in lung and small bowel transplant recipients. The risk for developing PTLD lasts indefinitely after transplantation but is most common in the first year. In addition to occurring in lung transplant recipients, PTLD may manifest in the lungs of recipients of other solid organ transplants and bone marrow transplants. PTLD also may affect the thymus, pericardium, esophagus, abdominal organs, tonsils, and lymph nodes.

Etiology

Most PTLDs are derived from recipient cells and contain Epstein-Barr virus.

Clinical Findings

The clinical manifestations of PTLD are varied. Patients may present with fever, night sweats, weight loss, and a mononucleosis-like illness; others may complain of symptoms related to mass effects. Some patients will be asymptomatic and the disease may be detected on routine imaging surveillance studies.

Imaging Findings

Chest Radiography

- Solitary (uncommon) or multiple pulmonary nodules
- Consolidation, focal or multi-focal (8%)
- Hilar and mediastinal lymphadenopathy
- Pleural effusion

MDCT/HRCT

- Nodules, peribronchovascular or subpleural in distribution (**Figs. 191.1, 191.2**)
- Multi-focal consolidation
- Hilar and mediastinal lymphadenopathy (**Fig. 191.3**)

PET

- May reveal extranodal sites of disease

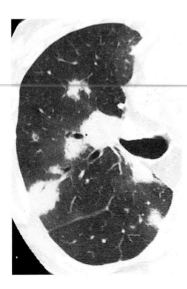

Fig. 191.2 Unenhanced chest CT (lung window) of a 57-year-old woman with PTLD following lung transplantation demonstrates multi-focal irregular nodular opacities that are predominantly peribronchovascular and subpleural in distribution, and right hilar lymphadenopathy.

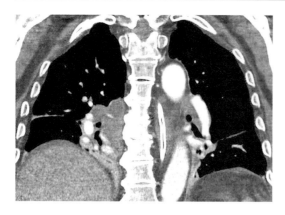

Fig. 191.3 Contrast-enhanced chest CT (mediastinal window; coronal reformation) of a 44-year-old man with PTLD six months after renal transplantation demonstrates bilateral hilar, mediastinal, and paravertebral lymphadenopathy.

Management

- Reduction of immune suppression
- Chemotherapy and radiation for aggressive disease

Prognosis

- 30–60% mortality reported
- Dependent on histopathology and the number of sites involved

PEARLS

- CT detection of a combination of nodules and/or consolidation and lymphadenopathy is highly suggestive of PTLD.

Suggested Reading

1. Gottschalk S, Rooney CM, Heslop HE. Post-transplant lymphoproliferative disorders. Annu Rev Med 2005;56: 29–44

2. Hansell DM, Lynch DA, McAdams HP, et al. The immunocompromised patient. In: Hansell DM, Lynch DA, McAdams HP, Bankier AA, eds. Imaging of Diseases of the Chest, 5th ed. Philadelphia: Mosby Elsevier; 2010:295–384

3. Müller NL, Silva CIS. Immunocompromised host. In: Silva CIS, Müller NL, Hansell DM, eds. Imaging of the Chest. Philadelphia: Saunders; 454–467

4. Collins J, Müller NL, Leung AN, et al. Epstein-Barr-virus-associated lymphoproliferative disease of the lung: CT and histologic findings. Radiology 1998;208(3):749–759

5. Dodd GD III, Ledesma-Medina J, Baron RL, Fuhrman CR. Posttransplant lymphoproliferative disorder: intrathoracic manifestations. Radiology 1992;184(1):65–69

CASE 192

■ Clinical Presentation

Series of five unrelated patients who share in common the surgical placement of synthetic interposition grafts or the deployment of endovascular stent grafts

■ Radiologic Findings

Unenhanced (**Fig. 192.1A**) and contrast-enhanced (**Fig. 192.1B**) axial and sagittal oblique CTAs (**Fig. 192.1C**) of a 70-year-old woman following total ascending aorta and aortic arch replacement with "elephant trunk" reconstruction and interposition graft and a trifurcated Gelweave (Vascutek, Inchinnan, Scotland) 12/8/8

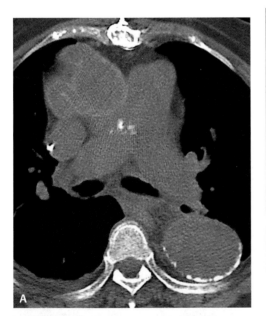
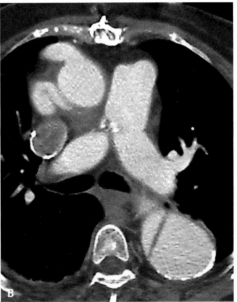
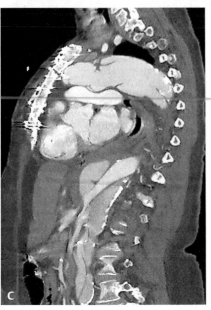

Fig. 192.1 (*Images courtesy of Jennifer Hubert, MD, VCU Medical Center, Richmond, Virginia.*)

919

branch vessel graft with subclavian artery reimplantation show a dissecting descending thoracic-abdominal aortic aneurysm and intimomedial flap. Sagittal oblique CTA (**Fig. 192.2**) of a 62-year-old man with ATAI treated with an endoluminal stent-graft demonstrates coverage of the post-traumatic pseudoaneurysm (*arrow*) but occlusion of the left subclavian artery origin. Coronal CTA (**Fig. 192.3**) of a 46-year-old man with ATAI treated with endoluminal stent-graft shows the stent-graft *en face* and covering the left subclavian artery origin. An Amplatzer occlusion device (AGA Medical Corp., Plymouth, MN) is seen in the proximal subclavian artery (*arrow*). A left-carotid-to-subclavian arterial bypass graft was performed the day before (not illustrated). Arterial phase axial CT (**Fig. 192.4A**) of a 63-year-old man with endovascular stent deployment for treatment of a descending aortic aneurysm shows an intramural-extra-stent collection of blood consistent with "type II endoleak" (*arrow*). Delayed axial (**Fig. 192.4B**) and coronal CTA (**Fig. 192.4C**) images reveal that the endoleak source emanates from the seventh, eighth, and ninth intercostal arteries (*arrows*). Sagittal oblique CTA (**Fig. 192.5**) of a 52-year-old man with ATAI treated with endoluminal stent-graft 12 months earlier and now complicated by a "type III endoleak." Although there is coverage of the post-traumatic pseudoaneurysm, contrast media can be identified both medially (*arrow*) and laterally between adjacent contiguous stent-grafts.

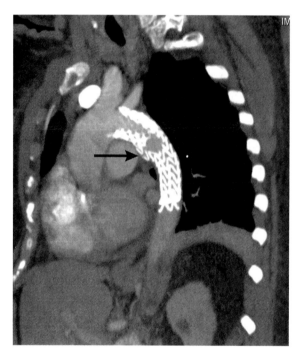

Fig. 192.2

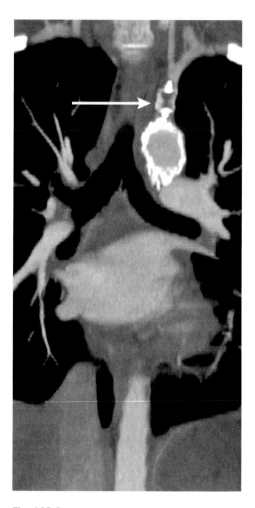

Fig. 192.3

■ Diagnosis

Synthetic Interposition Grafts and Endovascular Stents

■ Differential Diagnosis

None

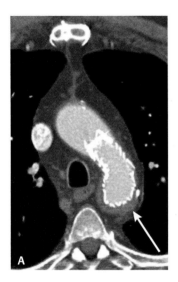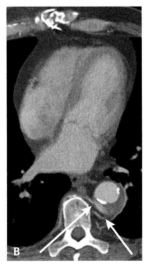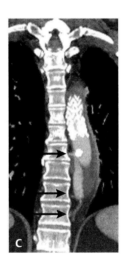

Fig. 192.4

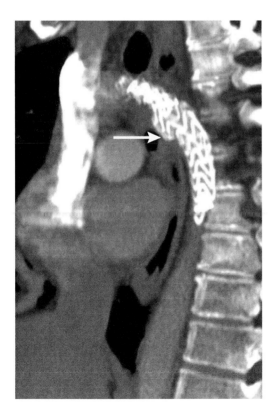

Fig. 192.5

■ Discussion

Background

Synthetic Interposition Grafts

Two common techniques of *aortic root graft repair* are the *interposition graft* and *inclusion graft*. An *interposition graft* entirely replaces the diseased segment of aorta, which is resected and removed. All vascular branches, including the coronary arteries, are reimplanted. Radio-opaque vascular pledgets and rings are used to reinforce the various anastomoses and cannulation sites (**Fig. 192.6**). An *inclusion graft* is inserted directly into the aortic lumen, leaving a potential space between the native aorta and graft. This potential perigraft space may continue to have persistent slow blood flow of little clinical consequence or eventually thrombose. Complex, *extensive thoracic aortic aneurysms* are difficult and challenging to manage. A single operative procedure replacing the ascending aorta, arch, and descending thoracic aorta subjects the patient to a prolonged procedure, multiple incisions, longer cross-clamp times, and increased blood loss. In the past, difficulty establishing proximal control of the aorta during staged repairs was often complicated by excessive and sometimes catastrophic bleeding. In 1983, the *elephant trunk* two-stage technique for reconstructing the diseased aorta was introduced. *Stage I* involves graft replacement of the ascending aorta and aortic arch with or without separate valve replacement. The distal portion of the graft is inverted and its folded edge is sutured to the descending aorta just distal to the left subclavian artery and the outer "windsock" portion or "elephant trunk" is left "hanging" in the descending aorta (**Figs. 192.1C, 192.7A**). *Stage II* is performed at a later date, during which time this portion of the graft is retrieved and the distal anastomosis completed (**Fig. 192.7B**). The technique obviates cross-clamping of the proximal aorta, reducing bleeding and other complications.

Complications

Postoperative complications include graft dehiscence and infection. Suture line surgical dehiscence may lead to pseudoaneurysm formation.

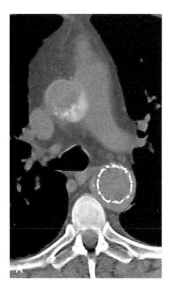 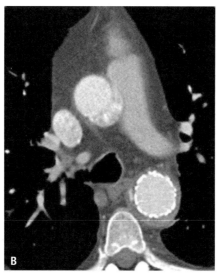

Fig. 192.6 CT of an elderly woman following ascending aorta replacement with an *interposition graft* and deployment of an *endovascular stent-graft* in the descending aorta. (**A**) The synthetic graft appears as a curvilinear high-attenuation crescent and the reinforcing vascular pledgets as an amorphous high-attenuation collection posteromedial to the ascending aorta on the unenhanced scan. (**B**) This latter collection appears more ominous on the contrast-enhanced scan and could easily be misinterpreted as a pseudoaneurysm. Note the hematoma outside the stent-graft lumen consistent with an endoleak.

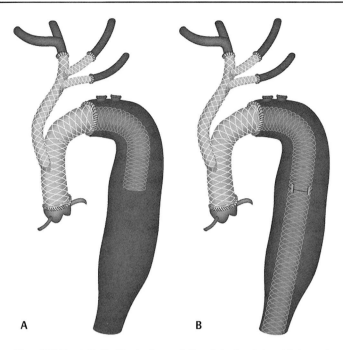

A   B

Fig. 192.7 Artist's illustration of the "elephant trunk" two-staged reconstruction of the diseased thoracic aorta. (**A**) *Stage I* involves replacement of the ascending aorta and, in this case, placement of a Gelweave 12/8/8 trifurcated branch vessel graft with reimplantation of the subclavian artery, similar to the patient in **Figs. 192.1A, 192.1B, 192.1C.** Note the debranching sites of the native branch vessels off the native arch. An additional graft has been sewn into the aorta, and this tubular "elephant trunk" graft hangs in the descending aorta. (**B**) In *stage II* the "elephant trunk" is retrieved and the distal anastomosis is completed. The native aorta is then wrapped around the repair.

Endoluminal Stent-Grafts

Endoluminal stent-grafts have emerged as an alternative to traditional surgical repair of acute and chronic type B aortic dissection (see Case 136), atherosclerotic aneurysms of the thoracic aorta (see Case 135), and post-traumatic aortic pseudoaneurysms (see Case 100). Conventional open surgical therapy has a mortality rate between 3% and 26%, but as high as 75% for emergency repairs. These high rates are partially due to co-morbidities, such as pulmonary and renal insufficiency, coronary artery disease, hypertension and diabetes in elderly patients, and the frequency of coexisting serious non-aortic injuries in trauma patients. The minimally invasive alternative endoluminal stent-graft is associated with an overall 30-day mortality rate of 6%; 3% in those patients undergoing elective treatment and 13% in those undergoing emergent treatment. Additionally, the rates of spinal cord paralysis in conventional open surgical repair range from 1.5% to 19%. Because of the absence of aortic cross-clamping and reperfusion, endoluminal repair of the aorta may have a much lower incidence of spinal cord ischemia. In fact, Piffaretti et al. reported no cases of paraplegia or paralysis in their series of patients treated with endoluminal stent-graft placements. The success of stent-graft treatment is based on the ability of the stent to bridge the pseudoaneurysm and isolate it from the circulation by forming a tight seal between the graft and the aortic wall at both the proximal- and distal-most aspects of the pseudoaneurysm. Because most ATAIs occur at the isthmus just beyond the left subclavian artery takeoff, the origin of this great vessel must often be covered by the stent-graft to obtain a tight proximal seal (**Fig. 192.2**). This often necessitates a pre-procedural left-carotid-to-subclavian arterial bypass graft or surgical transposition of the left subclavian artery to the left carotid artery. The uncovered orifice of the left subclavian artery is then often occluded with either embolization coils or an Amplatzer vascular occluder to reduce the risk of thromboembolism with resultant upper limb claudication (**Fig. 192.3**). The longitudinal flexibility of the stent-graft design and its ability to adequately conform to the curvature of the distal arch and proximal descending aorta and form a tight seal may predispose the stent-graft to leakage. Such endoleaks after thoracic endoluminal therapy are a serious complication and represent one of the limitations of this surgical alternative.

Complications

Endoleaks

Endoleaks are characterized by blood flow outside the stent-graft lumen but within the aneurysm or pseudo-aneurysm. Lifelong imaging surveillance (e.g., CTA, MRA, DSA, and US) of patients treated with endoluminal stent-grafts is necessary to detect endoleaks and assess their long-term durability. CTA is most commonly used for this purpose. A classification system has been developed which organizes endoleaks into one of five categories based on the source of blood flow (**Fig. 192.8**). The radiologist must be cognizant that it is the *source* of blood flow into the endoleak that defines the specific type of endoleak, which subsequently affects patient management.

- *Type I endoleaks* are "attachment site leaks" and are further classified based upon whether the endoleak is proximal (*Type IA*) (**Fig. 192.8B**) or distal (*Type IB*) (**Fig. 192.8C**). The separation between stent-graft and native aortic wall allows direct communication between the aneurysm or pseudoaneurysm and systemic arterial circulation.
- *Type II endoleaks* represent a "collateral vessel leak." There is retrograde blood flow through aortic branch vessels into the aneurysm or pseudoaneurysm (**Fig. 192.8D**). As with Type I endoleaks, there is direct communication from the systemic arterial circulation to the aneurysm or pseudoaneurysm.
- *Type III endoleaks* represent "structural failures in stent-graft integrity." These include stent-graft fractures, holes that form in the device fabric, and junctional separations between multiple devices. Repetitive stresses placed on grafts from arterial pulsations may be responsible (**Fig. 192.8E**). Type III endoleaks are the most dangerous type.
- *Type IV endoleaks* are caused by "stent-graft porosity" (**Fig. 192.8F**). These leaks are uncommon but are most often seen at implantation and manifest as a "blush" on the immediate post-implantation angiogram, when patients are fully anticoagulated.
- *Type V endoleaks* are also referred to as "endotension" and are characterized by expansion of the aneurysm or pseudoaneurysm without an obvious identifiable leak. The exact cause is unknown, but may be related to radiologically occult Type I, II, or III endoleaks.

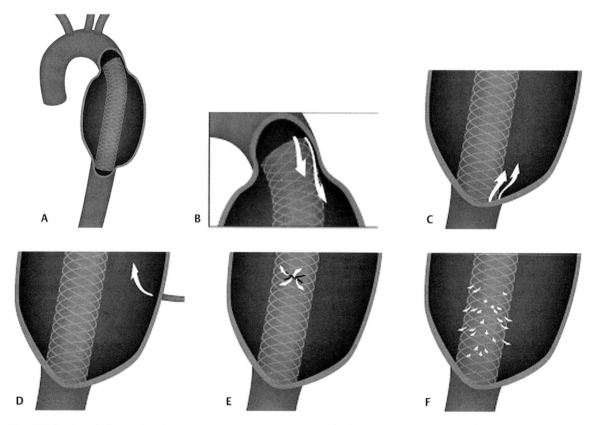

Fig. 192.8 Artist's illustration depicting an endovascular stent and the four types of radiologically demonstrable endoleaks that may complicate endoluminal stent-graft placements. See text for further discussion.

Imaging Findings

- Felt rings and pledgets are often used to reinforce anastomoses and cannula sites and can mimic pseudoaneurysms on contrast-enhanced scans; easily identified because of their high attenuation on unenhanced scans (**Figs. 192.6A, 192.6B**)
- Tissue grafts are indistinguishable from native aortic tissue on contrast-enhanced CT; synthetic grafts have a higher attenuation than native aorta and are easily differentiated on unenhanced scans (**Figs. 192.6A, 192.6B**)
- Normal postoperative appearance of "elephant trunk" reconstruction and interposition grafts can mimic a pseudoaneurysm or dissection with intimomedial flap on enhanced CT; knowledge of the imaging features associated with this procedure and unenhanced CT are necessary for differentiation (**Figs. 192.1A, 192.1B, 192.1C, 192.7A, 192.7B**)
- CTA/MRI-MRA is useful in demonstrating and classifying the type and nature of endoleak complications following stent-graft placements (**Figs. 192.4A, 192.4B, 192.4C, 192.5, 192.8**); both arterial phase and 60-second delayed CTA images through the thoracic aorta stent-graft are often necessary to optimally demonstrate endoleaks
- Visualize "inflow" (*Type Ia*) or "outflow" (*Type Ib*) endoleaks (**Fig. 192.8B, 192.8C**)
- Visualize vessels communicating with endoleak cavity: *Type II* (**Figs. 192.4A, 192.4B, 192.4C, 192.8D**)
- *Type III* endoleaks usually manifest as a contrast collection around the graft but spare the aneurysm sac peripherally (**Figs. 192.5, 192.8E**)

Management

- Aortic grafts may be composed of biologic tissue (porcine) or synthetic
- Type of surgical repair used based on extent of disease, integrity of native aortic tissue, presence or absence of concomitant aortic valvular and coronary artery disease, surgeon preference and experience, need for long-term anticoagulation, and antecedent aortic surgery
- *Type I* and *type III endoleaks*—repaired immediately
  - *Type I*—secure attachment sites with angioplasty balloons, stents, stent-graft extensions, or embolization coils
  - *Type III*—cover defect with stent-graft extension
- *Type II endoleak*—controversial; some surgeons conservatively follow this endoleak as long as aneurysm size does not increase; up to 40% spontaneously thrombose; other surgeons prefer surgical repair
- *Type IV endoleaks*—self-limited, require no treatment, and resolve spontaneously
- *Type V endoleaks*—typically require conversion to an open vascular repair

PEARLS

- Normal postoperative appearance of the thoracic aorta can mimic disease; knowledge and understanding of the surgical procedure performed are both critical for accurate diagnostic interpretation of these studies.

Suggested Reading

1. Agarwal PP, Chughtai A, Matzinger FRK, Kazerooni EA. Multidetector CT of thoracic aortic aneurysms. Radiographics 2009;29(2):537–552

2. Piffaretti G, Tozzi M, Lomazzi C, Rivolta N, Caronno R, Castelli P. Complications after endovascular stent-grafting of thoracic aortic diseases. J Cardiothorac Surg 2006;1:26

3. Riley P, Rooney S, Bonser R, Guest P. Imaging the post-operative thoracic aorta: normal anatomy and pitfalls. Br J Radiol 2001;74(888):1150–1158

4. Safi HJ, Miller CC III, Estrera AL, et al. Staged repair of extensive aortic aneurysms: morbidity and mortality in the elephant trunk technique. Circulation 2001;104(24):2938–2942

5. Sundaram B, Quint LE, Patel HJ, Deeb GM. CT findings following thoracic aortic surgery. Radiographics 2007;27(6):1583–1594

CASE 193

■ Clinical Presentation

49-year-old man diagnosed with esophageal cancer six months earlier and treated with surgery

■ Radiologic Findings

PA (**Fig. 193.1A**) and lateral (**Fig. 193.1B**) chest X-rays demonstrate evidence of a right thoracotomy with associated rib deformity. Surgical clips are seen in the right tracheobronchial angle, perihilar region, and left upper quadrant. There is a partial silhouette of the right interlobar artery, dorsal spine, and cardiophrenic angle by a curvilinear opacity extending from the cardiophrenic angle to the clavicle. Contrast-enhanced axial (**Figs. 193.1C, 193.1D, 193.1E**) and coronal (**Figs. 193.1F, 193.1G, 193.1H**) CT (mediastinal window) shows postoperative changes of an Ivor Lewis intrathoracic esophagectomy and esophagogastric anastomosis. The neoesophagus or gastric tube has been placed in the right paravertebral space.

■ Discussion

Background

Esophageal cancer is the third most common gastrointestinal malignancy and one of the most prevalent cancers in the world. Surgery is the mainstay of treatment for patients with early-stage disease. Locally advanced disease in non-surgical patients is managed with chemotherapy and radiation therapy. Esophageal resection with various forms of reconstruction benefits many patients with esophageal cancer suffering from dysphagia.

Esophageal resection can be performed using either a transthoracic or transhiatal technique.

Transthoracic Esophagectomy

- **Ivor Lewis procedure.** The most commonly performed procedure for treatment of mid- and distal esophageal cancers. An initial laparotomy to mobilize the stomach is followed by a right thoracotomy. The esophagus is excised en bloc and the thoracic duct is ligated. Lymph nodes along the celiac trunk, splenic and common hepatic arteries, and periesophageal, aortopulmonary and subcarina are dissected. A high cervical intrathoracic anastomosis, above the azygos vein, is created between the proximal esophageal remnant and stomach, forming the neoesophagus (**Figs. 193.1A, 193.1B, 193.1C, 193.1D, 193.1E, 193.1F, 193.1G, 193.1H, 193.2A, 193.2B**). The neoesophagus is most commonly positioned in the posterior mediastinum prevertebral space, but may also be placed in the right paravertebral or anterior mediastinal substernal space. Pyloromyotomy or pyloroplasty is performed to prevent post-vagotomy gastric outlet obstruction from pylorospasm (**Fig. 193.2A**).
- **McKeown procedure.** This procedure involves a midline laparotomy, anterolateral thoracotomy, and cervicotomy. Stomach mobilization, lymphadenectomy, and esophageal resection are performed in a manner similar to the Ivor Lewis. The primary difference is that the cervical esophagogastric anastomosis is created in the neck as opposed to the thorax, reducing the potential for sepsis from anastomotic dehiscence.
- **Left thoracoabdominal thoracotomy.** This approach is optimal for lower esophageal and gastric cardia cancer because it provides simultaneous exposure of the upper abdomen and posterior mediastinum through a single incision. Extensive lymphadenectomy can be performed and concomitant left lung lesions resected. The lower esophagus is resected and the stomach mobilized. The esophagogastric anastomosis is performed behind the transverse aorta.

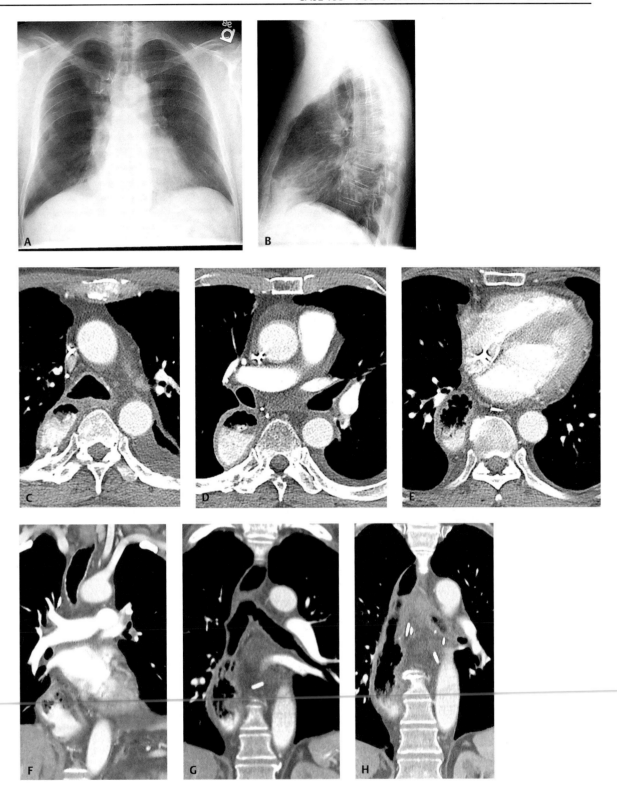

Fig. 193.1

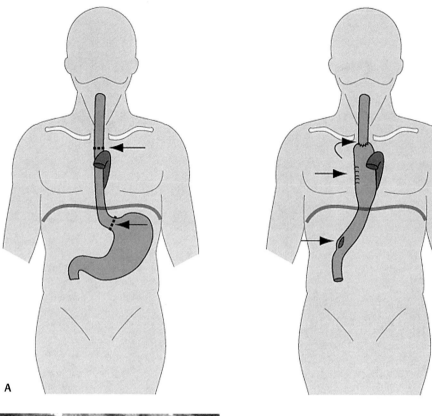

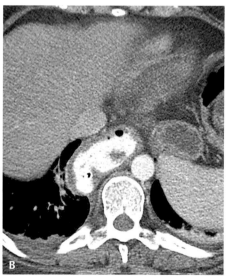

Fig. 193.2 Artist's illustration of the Ivor Lewis transthoracic esophagectomy **(A)**. Laparotomy is performed to mobilize the stomach, perform a pyloromyotomy (*lower arrow, second figure*), and dissect regional lymph nodes. Subsequently, a right thoracotomy is performed to remove the esophagus and dissect those regional nodes (*arrows, first figure*). The neoesophagus is created by joining the esophageal remnant and stomach high in the thorax (*upper arrows, second figure*). Contrast-enhanced chest CT **(B)** of an Ivor Lewis esophagectomy shows the mobilized neoesophagus positioned as is seen most commonly, in the prevertebral posterior mediastinal space.

Trans-hiatal Esophagectomy without Thoracotomy

This procedure is performed for resection of distal esophageal or gastric cardiac neoplasms. Two incisions are made. First, a cervicotomy paralleling the sternocleidomastoid muscle provides access to the proximal esophagus. Second, a supraumbilical-to-xiphoid incision provides access to the distal esophagus. Combined but "blinded" circumferential dissection and mobilization of the intrathoracic esophagus and lymphadenectomy are performed as the surgeon places his or her hand through both the cervical and abdominal incisions. The cervical esophagus is divided, and the stomach with the attached esophagus is removed through the supraumbilical incision. The esophagus is resected. A partial proximal gastrectomy and pyloromyotomy are performed and the cervical esophagogastric anastomosis created (**Fig. 193.3**). Since a formal thoracotomy is avoided, peri-operative respiratory problems are less of an issue and anastomotic leaks are more easily managed.

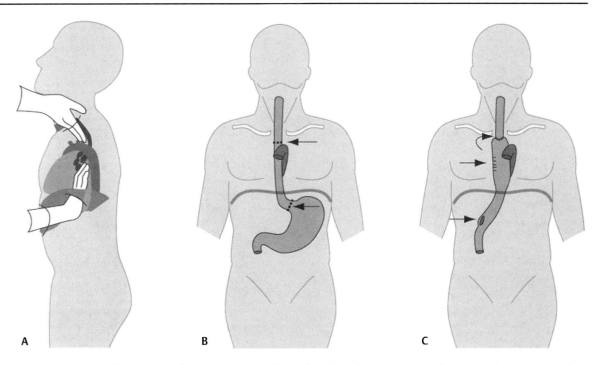

Fig. 193.3 Artist's illustration of the various stages of trans-hiatal esophagectomy. Initially, a cervical incision is made to access the proximal esophagus and a supraumbilical incision to access the distal esophagus. The surgeon then places the hands through the upper and lower incisions and "blindly" dissects and mobilizes the intrathoracic esophagus **(A)**. The cervical esophagus is resected via the cervicotomy and the stomach with attached esophagus removed through the lower incision **(B**, *upper and lower arrows*). A partial gastrectomy and pyloromyotomy are performed and the stomach is mobilized back through the hiatus and drawn into the upper thorax, where the cervical esophagogastric anastomosis is completed **(C**, *arrows*). This procedure avoids the need for a formal thoracotomy.

Bypass Surgery

Bypass provides an alternative conduit for food passage and is most often used in those cases in which the esophagus is completely obstructed by tumor or is dysfunctional because of dysmotility disorders or severe stricture. Various segments of the normal gastrointestinal tract have been mobilized and interposed to serve as this new conduit, including the stomach, jejunum, and colon (**Figs. 193.4A, 193.4B, 193.4C, 193.4D, 193.4E, 193.4F**). The stomach is the most commonly used conduit because it has a reliable blood supply and can be easily mobilized up into the chest as high as the hypopharynx if necessary. The substernal anterior mediastinal route is chosen for most such conduits (**Figs. 193.4A, 193.4B, 193.4C, 193.4D, 193.4E, 193.4F**), but the posterior mediastinum and subcutaneous route can also be used. In cases of antecedent gastric surgery or underlying gastric disease, the colon is the second most often used conduit (**Figs. 193.4A, 193.4B, 193.4C, 193.4D, 193.4E, 193.4F**). Colonic interposition has a reduced prevalence of reflux esophagitis and anastomotic stricture formation. The jejunum is more often used as a free graft to replace the cervical esophagus (i.e., pharyngojejunoesophagostomy) (**Figs. 193.4E, 193.4F**).

Procedure-Specific Limitations

Ivor Lewis Esophagectomy

- Difficult procedure in patients with antecedent right thoracotomy
- Respiratory insufficiency from thoracotomy or prolonged mechanical ventilation

McKeown Esophagectomy

- Radical lymphadenectomy technically more difficult to perform

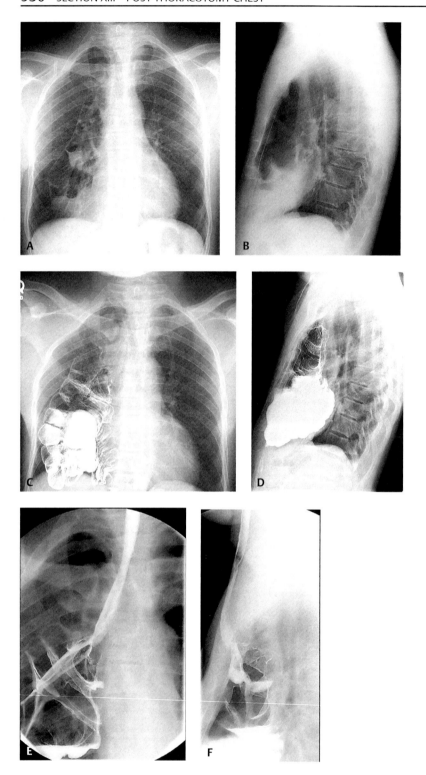

Fig. 193.4 Complex esophageal reconstruction and laryngectomy following remote lye ingestion. PA **(A)** and lateral **(B)** chest radiographs demonstrate a right-sided, substernal-anterior mediastinal mixed-density tubular structure extending from the right tracheobronchial angle to the hiatus. Accompanying PA **(C)** and lateral **(D)** chest radiographs following barium esophagography show this corresponds with an interposed colonic conduit (i.e., colonic interposition) with prolonged stasis and delayed emptying. Note the absent subglottic tracheal air column from the laryngectomy. AP **(E)** and lateral **(F)** fluoroscopic images acquired during barium esophagography show an anteriorly positioned interposed loop of jejunum that anastomoses with the pharynx proximally and the colonic interposition distally. A stricture is present at the distal anastomosis. *(Images courtesy of Roger Tutton, MD, VCU Medical Center, Richmond, Virginia.)*

Transhiatal Esophagectomy without Thoracotomy

- Relative contraindications include antecedent thoracic or mediastinal surgery or radiation therapy; past esophageal perforation
- Absolute contraindications include mediastinal, vascular, or airway invasion
- Limited tumor visualization during procedure
- Only limited lymphadenectomy can be performed

Complications of Esophageal Resection and Reconstruction (up to 60% of cases)

Intraoperative Complications

- Hemorrhage
- Tracheal or mainstem bronchial injury
  - Usually involves membranous airway
  - May be complicated by fistula, respiratory compromise, recurrent pneumonia, or empyema and necessitate stenting or surgical repair
- Recurrent laryngeal nerve injury
  - Prevalence as high as 24% with trans-hiatal esophagectomy
  - Impairs patients' ability to cough, predisposing to aspiration pneumonia

Postoperative Complications

- Lung/pleura (e.g., atelectasis, aspiration, pneumonia, effusion, empyema, ARDS)
- Anastomotic leak, complicated by fistula (esophagobronchial, esophagopleural, esophagocutaneous) (**Fig. 193.5**) or late stricture formation (**Figs. 193.4E, 193.4F**)
  - Major complication; occurs in up to 50% of patients; mortality rate 3–90%
    - 50% of leaks subclinical, usually heal without treatment; others require NGT placement and antibiotics
    - Larger leaks require drainage of peri-anastomotic fluid collections with pigtail catheter or chest tube
    - Uncontained leak (i.e., large leak with contrast media flowing freely into pleural space) may require surgical intervention (**Figs. 193.5, 193.6**)
  - Early postoperative period (two or three days): technical failure
  - Later postoperative period (three to seven days): from ischemic changes in stomach
- Mediastinal abscess/mediastinitis

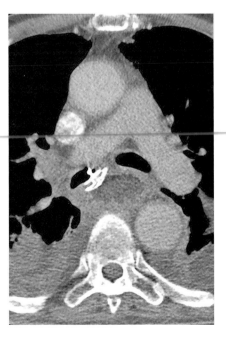

Fig. 193.5 Chest CT (mediastinal window) of a 70-year-old man several months out from an Ivor Lewis procedure with complicating fistula formation between the gastric tube in the prevertebral mediastinal space and the bronchus intermedius. The patient suffered repeated bouts of aspiration and sepsis and was too unstable for surgical repair. As a last resort, an Amplatzer ASD occluder device was placed to seal off the fistulous communication, as seen above.

- Chylothorax
  - Results from thoracic duct injury
  - Prevalence highest following trans-hiatal esophagectomy
  - Clinical clue: Chest tube drainage >200–400 mL per 8 hours
- Delayed emptying
  - Causes include failure to perform a pyloric drainage procedure; obstruction at the hiatus; redundant neoesophagus with resultant kinking or twisting
  - Radiologic clue: presence of a large air-fluid level in mediastinum (**Figs. 193.4A, 193.4B, 193.4C, 193.4D, 193.4E, 193.4F**)

Prognosis

- Esophageal resection is a high-risk procedure; high morbidity and mortality (3%)
- Overall five-year survival rates vary from 5% to 35%; recurrence rates after curative surgery range between 34% and 79%
- Postoperative radiation therapy may improve local control; chemotherapy may prevent or delay systemic metastasis
- *Locoregional recurrence* (21–68%)
  - *Local*—disease reoccurring at site of anastomosis, esophageal resection, and lymph node dissection
  - *Regional*—disease reoccurring within organs or lymph nodes adjacent to the esophagus; or in cervical or upper abdominal lymph nodes where no lymph node dissection had been performed
- *Distant recurrence*
  - *Hematogenous*—disease within a *solid organ* (e.g., liver, lung, bone, adrenal gland, kidney, brain, in descending order of frequency) or within the *pleura* (e.g., pleura-based nodules, masses, effusion, irregular pleural thickening)
  - *Transcelomic*—metastatic lesions develop within peritoneal cavity

■ Postoperative Imaging Surveillance

Esophagography

- Assess tumor recurrence at anastomotic site (3–9% of cases); nodular narrowing
- Limited due to inability to detect mural disease and lymphadenopathy

MDCT

- May detect recurrent disease before symptoms develop
- Soft-tissue mass(es) or as intramural nodular wall thickening of stomach or esophagus at anastomosis site
- Overall accuracy in determining recurrence: 87%

Whole-Body FDG PET/Integrated PET-CT

- Useful adjunct to conventional imaging studies
- May demonstrate metabolic activity indicative of recurrent tumor before anatomic changes become evident on conventional imaging
- Superior to conventional imaging in detection of distant metastases
- Limited by lack of sensitivity/inability to detect small (<1.0 cm) or necrotic metastases

Endoscopic Ultrasound

- More sensitive than upper endoscopy and CT for assessing anastomotic recurrence and locoregional nodal metastases

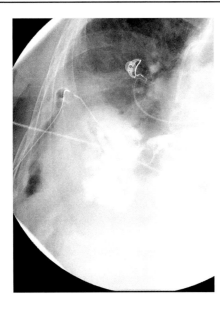

Fig. 193.6 Fluoroscopic spot view over the right thorax during esophagography in a 62-year-old man with mid-thoracic esophageal cancer and complicating postoperative esophagopleural fistula and empyema shows an uncontained large leak with free spillage of contrast into the pleural space. The patient had undergone an Ivor Lewis procedure nine days earlier

PEARLS

- Complex surgical procedures used in esophagectomy can grossly distort normal anatomic structures and landmarks, confounding image interpretation.
- Accurate diagnostic interpretation requires that radiologists be familiar with these procedures and the expected postoperative changes seen in these otherwise complex cases to recognize perioperative and postoperative complications.
- Distant recurrence occurs more frequently than locoregional recurrence with lower-third tumors; locoregional recurrence occurs more frequently for upper- or middle-third lesions.
- Most frequent location of lymph node metastases preoperatively include: right recurrent laryngeal nerve nodal chain, right paracardiac nodes, periesophageal nodes, and lesser curvature nodes.
- Most frequent location of lymph node recurrence postoperatively include left upper recurrent laryngeal nerve nodal chain, right supraclavicular, celiac, and abdominal paraaortic nodes.

Suggested Reading

1. Becker CD, Barbier PA, Terrier F, Porcellini B. Patterns of recurrence of esophageal carcinoma after transhiatal esophagectomy and gastric interposition. AJR Am J Roentgenol 1987;148(2):273–277

2. Carlisle JG, Quint LE, Francis IR, Orringer MB, Smick JF, Gross BH. Recurrent esophageal carcinoma: CT evaluation after esophagectomy. Radiology 1993;189(1):271–275

3. Kim TJ, Lee KH, Kim YH, et al. Postoperative imaging of esophageal cancer: what chest radiologists need to know. Radiographics 2007;27(2):409–429

4. Linden PA, Sugarbaker DJ. Section V: techniques of esophageal resection. Semin Thorac Cardiovasc Surg 2003;15(2):197–209

5. Stewart BW, Kleihues P. World Cancer Report. Lyon: IARC; 2003

INDEX

Note: Page numbers in **boldface** indicate primary diagnosis or main discussion. Page numbers followed by *f* and *t* indicate figures and tables, respectively.